FETAL AND NEONATAL BRAIN INJURY

Mechanisms,
Management,
and the Risks
of Practice

DAVID K. STEVENSON, M.D.
Associate Professor
Director, Newborn Nurseries

PHILIP SUNSHINE, M.D.
Harold K. Faber Professor

Department of Pediatrics
Stanford University School of Medicine
Stanford, California

1989
B.C. Decker Inc • Toronto • Philadelphia

Publisher   **B.C. Decker Inc**
3228 South Service Road
Burlington, Ontario   L7N 3H8

B.C. Decker Inc
320 Walnut Street
Suite 400
Philadelphia, Pennsylvania   19106

Sales and Distribution

United States and Puerto Rico
The C.V. Mosby Company
11830 Westline Industrial Drive
Saint Louis, Missouri   63146

Canada
McAinsh & Co. Ltd.
2760 Old Leslie Street
Willowdale, Ontario   M2K 2X5

Australia
McGraw-Hill Book Company Australia Pty. Ltd.
4 Barcoo Street
Roseville East 2069
New South Wales, Australia

Brazil
Editora McGraw-Hill do Brasil, Ltda.
rua Tabapua, 1.105, Itaim-Bibi
Sao Paulo, S.P. Brasil

Colombia
Interamericana/McGraw-Hill de Colombia, S.A.
Apartado Aereo 81078
Bogota, D.E. Colombia

Europe
McGraw-Hill Book Company GmbH
Lademannbogen 136
D-2000 Hamburg 63
West Germany

France
MEDSI/McGraw-Hill
6, avenue Daniel Lesueur
75007 Paris, France

Hong Kong and China
McGraw-Hill Book Company
Suite 618, Ocean Centre
5 Canton Road
Tsimshatsui, Kowloon
Hong Kong

India
Tata McGraw-Hill Publishing Company, Ltd.
12/4 Asaf Ali Road, 3rd Floor
New Delhi 110002, India

Indonesia
P.O. Box 122/JAT
Jakarta, 1300 Indonesia

Italy
McGraw-Hill Libri Italia, s.r.l.
Piazza Emilia, 5
I-20129 Milano MI
Italy

Japan
Igaku-Shoin Ltd.
Tokyo International P.O. Box 5063
1-28-36 Hongo, Bunkyo-ku,
Tokyo 113, Japan

Korea
C.P.O. Box 10583
Seoul, Korea

Malaysia
No. 8 Jalan SS 7/6B
Kelana Jaya
47301 Petaling Jaya
Selangor, Malaysia

Mexico
Interamericana/McGraw-Hill de Mexico, S.A. de C.V.
Cedro 512, Colonia Atlampa
(Apartado Postal 26370)
06450 Mexico, D.F., Mexico

New Zealand
McGraw-Hill Book Co. New Zealand Ltd.
5 Joval Place, Wiri
Manukau City, New Zealand

Panama
Editorial McGraw-Hill Latinoamericana, S.A.
Apartado Postal 2036
Zona Libre de Colon
Colon, Republica de Panama

Portugal
Editora McGraw-Hill de Portugal, Ltda.
Rua Rosa Damasceno 11A–B
1900 Lisboa, Portugal

South Africa
Libriger Book Distributors
Warehouse Number 8
''Die Ou Looiery''
Tannery Road
Hamilton, Bloemfontein 9300

Southeast Asia
McGraw-Hill Book Co.
348 Jalan Boon Lay
Jurong, Singapore 2261

Spain
McGraw-Hill/Interamericana de Espana, S.A.
Manuel Ferrero, 13
28020 Madrid, Spain

Taiwan
P.O. Box 87–601
Taipei, Taiwan

Thailand
632/5 Phaholyothin Road
Sapan Kwai
Bangkok 10400
Thailand

United Kingdom, Middle East and Africa
McGraw-Hill Book Company (U.K.) Ltd.
Shoppenhangers Road
Maidenhead, Berkshire
SL6 2QL England

Venezuela
McGraw-Hill/Interamericana, C.A.
2da. calle Bello Monte
(entre avenida Casanova y Sabana Grande)
Apartado Aereo 50785
Caracas 1050, Venezuela

NOTICE

The authors and publisher have made every effort to ensure that the patient care recommended herein, including choice of drugs and drug dosages, is in accord with the accepted standards and practice at the time of publication. However, since research and regulation constantly change clinical standards, the reader is urged to check the product information sheet included in the package of each drug, which includes recommended doses, warnings, and contraindications. This is particularly important with new or infrequently used drugs.

Fetal and Neonatal Brain Injury: Mechanisms, Management, and the Risks of Practice   ISBN 1–55664–117–6

Library of Congress catalog card number: 88–51778   10 9 8 7 6 5 4 3 2 1

CONTRIBUTORS

GEORGE A. ALBRIGHT, M.D.

Clinical Professor of Anesthesia and Obstetrics, Northwestern University Medical School and Northwestern Memorial Hospital; Director of Anesthesia, Prentice Women's Hospital, Chicago, Illinois
Effects of Anesthesia on the Fetus and Neonate

GEOFFREY ALTSHULER, M.B., B.S., M.D.

Professor of Pathology and Clinical Professor of Pediatrics, University of Oklahoma Health Sciences Center, Oklahoma City, Oklahoma
The Medicolegal Imperative: Placental Pathology and Epidemiology

ANN M. ARVIN, M.D.

Associate Professor of Pediatrics, Stanford University School of Medicine; Co-Director, Division of Pediatric Infectious Diseases, Stanford University Medical Center, Stanford, California
Congenital Infections as Causes of Neurologic Sequelae: Prevention, Diagnosis, and Treatment

WILLIAM E. BENITZ, M.D.

Assistant Professor of Pediatrics, Stanford University School of Medicine; Associate Director of Nurseries, Stanford University Hospital, Stanford, California
Fetal Injury from Drug Abuse in Pregnancy: Alcohol, Narcotic, Cocaine, and Phencyclidine
Immediate Management
Extended Management

FORREST C. BENNETT, M.D.

Associate Professor of Pediatrics; Director, High Risk Infant Follow-up Program, Child Development and Mental Retardation Center, University of Washington School of Medicine, Seattle, Washington
Foreword

RICHARD E. BESINGER, M.D.

Instructor, Department of Obstetrics and Gynecology, Loyola University of Chicago Stritch School of Medicine; Attending Perinatologist, Loyola University Medical Center, Maywood, Illinois
Preterm Labor and Intrauterine Growth Retardation: Complex Obstetrical Problems with Low Birth Weight Infants

ROBERT R. CLANCY, M.D.

Associate Professor of Neurology and Pediatrics, University of Pennsylvania School of Medicine; Associate Neurologist, Children's Hospital of Philadelphia and Hospital of the University of Pennsylvania, Philadelphia, Pennsylvania
Neonatal Seizures

RONALD S. COHEN, M.D., F.A.A.P.

Clinical Assistant Professor of Pediatrics, Stanford University School of Medicine, Stanford; Director, Newborn Intensive Care, Santa Clara Valley Medical Center, San Jose, California
Fetal Injury from Drug Abuse in Pregnancy: Alcohol, Narcotic, Cocaine, and Phencyclidine
Hypoglycemia and Brain Injury

DIETER R. ENZMANN, M.D.

Associate Professor of Radiology, Stanford University School of Medicine, Director of Neuroradiology, Director of Magnetic Resonance Imaging, Stanford University Medical Center, Stanford, California
Imaging of Hypoxic-Ischemic Cerebral Damage

JAMES E. FERGUSON II, M.D.

Assistant Professor of Obstetrics and Gynecology, University of Virginia School of Medicine, Charlottesville, Virginia
Preterm Labor and Intrauterine Growth Retardation: Complex Obstetrical Problems with Low Birth Weight Infants
Complications of Labor and Delivery: Selected Medical and Surgical Considerations

LORRY R. FRANKEL, M.D.

Assistant Professor of Pediatrics, Stanford University School of Medicine; Director, Pediatric Intensive Care, Stanford University Hospital, Stanford, California
Immediate Management
Extended Management

RONALD N. GIBSON, B.S.

Research Associate, Department of Gynecology and Obstetrics, Stanford University School of Medicine, Stanford, California
Fetal Responses to Asphyxia

AMNON GOLDWORTH, Ph.D.

Professor of Philosophy, San Jose State University,
San Jose, California
The Appropriateness of Intensive Care Applications

RICARDO R. GONZÁLEZ-MÉNDEZ, Ph.D.

Research Associate, Division of Neonatology, Department
of Pediatrics, Stanford University Medical Center,
Stanford, California
New Noninvasive Technologies to Evaluate Brain Function

ALLEN A. HERMAN, M.B., Ch.B., Ph.D.

Visiting Scientist, Epidemiology Branch, Prevention
Research Program, National Institute of Child Health and
Human Development, National Institutes of Health,
Bethesda, Maryland
*The Medicolegal Imperative: Placental Pathology and
Epidemiology*

R. HAROLD HOLBROOK Jr., M.D.

Assistant Professor and Chief, Maternal–Fetal Medicine,
Stanford University School of Medicine,
Stanford, California
Fetal Responses to Asphyxia

JOHN A. KERNER Jr., M.D.

Associate Professor of Pediatrics, Stanford University
School of Medicine; Co-Director, Pediatric
Gastroenterology and Coordinator, Nutritional Support
Services, Stanford University Hospital and Children's
Hospital, Stanford, California
Nutritional Management

ANNELIESE F. KORNER, Ph.D.

Professor (Research), Psychiatry and the Behavioral
Sciences Division of Child Psychiatry and Child
Development, Stanford University School of Medicine,
Stanford, California
*The Scope and Limitations of Neurologic and Behavioral
Assessments of the Newborn*

ANJALI MALKANI, M.D.

Fellow in Pediatric Gastroenterology, Stanford University
School of Medicine, Stanford, California
Nutritional Management

EDWARD J. NOVOTNY Jr., M.D.

Associate Research Scientist and Lecturer, Department of
Neurology, Yale University School of Medicine;
Attending Neurologist, Yale–New Haven Hospital,
New Haven, Connecticut
Hypoxic-Ischemic Encephalopathy

CHARLES G. PROBER, M.D.

Associate Professor of Pediatrics, Stanford University
School of Medicine; Co-Director, Division of Pediatric
Infectious Diseases, Stanford University Medical Center,
Stanford, California
*Congenital Infections as Causes of Neurologic Sequelae:
Prevention, Diagnosis, and Treatment*

JOHN T. REPKE, M.D.

Assistant Professor of Gynecology and Obstetrics and
Pediatrics, The Johns Hopkins University School of
Medicine; Attending Physician and Director of Obstetrics
Clinics, The Johns Hopkins Hospital,
Baltimore, Maryland
*Preterm Labor and Intrauterine Growth Retardation:
Complex Obstetrical Problems with Low Birth Weight
Infants*
*Complications of Labor and Delivery: Selected Medical and
Surgical Considerations*

WILLIAM D. RHINE, M.D.

Fellow, Division of Neonatology, Department of
Pediatrics, Stanford University Medical Center,
Stanford, California
New Noninvasive Technologies to Evaluate Brain Function

HERBERT C. SCHWARTZ, M.D.

Professor of Pediatrics, Division of Hematology–
Oncology, Stanford University School of Medicine,
Stanford, California
*Hematologic Disorders: Anemia, Polycythemia, and
Hyperbilirubinemia*

DAVID K. STEVENSON, M.D.

Associate Professor of Pediatrics, Stanford University
School of Medicine; Director, Newborn Nurseries,
Stanford University Medical Center, Stanford, California
*Fetal Injury from Drug Abuse in Pregnancy: Alcohol,
Narcotic, Cocaine, and Phencyclidine*
Immediate Management
Extended Management
Hypoglycemia and Brain Injury
*Hematologic Disorders: Anemia, Polycythemia, and
Hyperbilirubinemia*
New Noninvasive Technologies to Evaluate Brain Function
The Appropriateness of Intensive Care Applications

PHILIP SUNSHINE, M.D.

Harold K. Faber Professor of Pediatrics, Stanford
University School of Medicine; Stanford, California
Epidemiology of Perinatal Asphyxia

BARRY R. THARP, M.D.

> Professor of Neurology and Pediatrics, Stanford University School of Medicine; Head, Division of Pediatric Neurology and Director, EEG Laboratory, Stanford University Medical Center, Stanford, California

> *Electroencephalography in the Assessment of the Premature and Full-Term Infant*
> *Etiology and Timing of Static Encephalopathies of Childhood (Cerebral Palsy)*

RONALD L. THOMAS, M.D.

> Clinical Instructor, Department of Obstetrics and Gynecology, Uniformed Services University of the Health Sciences, Bethesda and Instructor, Department of Obstetrics and Gynecology, The Johns Hopkins University School of Medicine, Baltimore; Director, Division of Maternal–Fetal Medicine, Department of Obstetrics and Gynecology, Naval Hospital, Bethesda, Maryland

> *Complications of Labor and Delivery: Selected Medical and Surgical Considerations*

STEVEN L. WEINSTEIN, M.D.

> Clinical Instructor, Department of Neurology, Stanford University School of Medicine; Physician Specialist, Department of Pediatric Neurology, Stanford University Medical Center, Stanford, California

> *Etiology and Timing of Static Encephalopathies of Childhood (Cerebral Palsy)*

''Supported in part by Grant RR-81 from the General Clinical Research Centers Program, Division of Research Resources, National Institutes of Health, and the Christopher Taylor Harrison Research Fund.''

Foreword

Forrest C. Bennett, M.D.

The title of this book speaks for itself and for the realities of contemporary perinatology, neonatology, and neuroscience. Historic, unresolved scientific debates concerning the mechanisms and timing of brain injury and the specific etiologies of brain dysfunction have suddenly become central to and partially responsible for the medical malpractice litigation epidemic of the 1980s. The courtroom, rather than the laboratory, is the arena where these complex neurologic questions are regularly publicly debated. Opposing neuroscientists are in great demand as expert witnesses. Issues of probable causation versus probable preventability are frequently overlapped and confused. Profound decisions regarding the mechanisms and appropriate management of fetal and neonatal brain injury are being rendered daily by judges and lay juries rather than by scientific investigations. Our honest uncertainties and disagreements and incomplete knowledge about human central nervous system function, including varying susceptibility and response to potential insults, provides a fertile field for current litigants. If this scenario strikes some as unappealing or even dangerous, it nevertheless constitutes and reflects present societal attitudes and practices. As such, it demands the serious attention and continuing education of all biomedical and behavioral professionals who deal with issues relating to early brain damage and its short- and long-term consequences. That is the rationale for this timely, comprehensive book.

The human brain is susceptible to a wide variety of genetic, developmental, and acquired abnormalities and insults. These brain injuries can occur prenatally, perinatally and/or neonatally, or postnatally. The permanent neurosensory residua of these abnormalities and insults vary in type and severity but basically involve dysfunctions in one or more areas of development (i.e., motor, cognitive, language and/or learning, socioemotional) and/or in aspects of behavior (i.e., temperament, conduct, activity level, selective attention). A particular developmental or behavioral dysfunction (e.g., cerebral palsy) is generally not unique to or indicative of a specific causative agent; conversely, a potential causative agent (e.g., asphyxia) may be followed by a wide range of outcomes from apparently normal development through the full spectrum of major and minor neurosensory impairments. For example, while asphyxia is certainly capable of causing cerebral palsy, most cases of cerebral palsy are not related to asphyxia, and most newborns who have suffered an asphyxial episode do not develop cerebral palsy. There is frequently a substantial gap in time between the onset of the brain abnormality and the appearance and identification of the resultant developmental and behavioral dysfunctions, particularly in the case of more minor, subtle sequelae which may escape detection throughout infancy and early childhood.

Because of these incredible brain complexities and variabilities, precise causal relationships between prior events and eventual outcomes frequently cannot be reliably constructed. Nevertheless, in light of current medicolegal realities, it is incumbent upon perinatologists, neonatologists, child neurologists, developmental pediatricians, and other physicians active in the diagnosis and management of potential brain injuries to participate with scientific rigor in a careful, cautious attempt to establish probable cause or broad category of disorder on a "more likely than not" basis for individual cases. Even in the absence of absolute precision and certainty, which rarely exists when considering mechanisms of fetal and neonatal brain injury, accumulated interdisciplinary knowledge allows one to make informed, probable etiologic linkages in most cases.

How can one adequately prepare oneself for this important differential diagnostic task? What additional knowledge or synthesis is presently required to improve this individual case review process? I believe it is virtually impossible to render competent opinions in this area without a thorough understanding of the types of permanent neurosensory impairments that may follow brain injury or maldevelopment. In order to facilitate our understanding of the epidemiology of these chronic neurodevelopmental disabilities, we critically need standard definitions and categorization systems. For example, in both patient care and clinical research, we must strive for simplified, uniform ways to talk about cerebral palsy and its main subtypes (i.e., clinical syndromes); we must distinguish specific levels of mental retardation; we must begin to classify and recognize central communication disorders (i.e., specific language disorders, central processing disorders, language and/or learning disorders) as potential long-term sequelae of a variety of brain insults.

In addition, we critically need to become more specific and precise in our thinking and writing about the types and severities of neurodevelopmental disabilities associated with certain congenital or acquired brain abnormalities or injurious agents. While these association patterns do not guarantee etiologic certainty, they are extremely useful adjuncts to overall case consideration. For example, we must carefully distinguish motor disability from mental disability in each case and specify which one, or both, apply. Asphyxia, a common cause of cerebral palsy and associated mental retardation and seizure disorders, rarely results in mental retardation alone without accompanying motor disability.[1-3] Mental retardation alone or in association with a chronic seizure disorder, but without cerebral palsy, predominantly results from a variety of prenatal defects in brain development, probably in most cases on a genetic or developmental basis.[4] Thus, the relatively simple function of differentiating between mental retardation with or without cerebral palsy has enormous implications in terms of causation, developmental needs, and prognosis. Subsuming both mental and motor disabilities under the indiscriminate label "static encephalopathy" could obscure these epidemiologic distinctions.

Accordingly, in our careful attempts to better delineate etiologic pathways, we must not fall into the trap of casually labeling as "cerebral palsy" the almost universal hypotonia and motor delays seen in infants and young children with mental retardation. The primary brain impairment associated with Down syndrome and many other genetic disorders is mental retardation, not cerebral palsy. Confusing these two developmental concepts will only lead to erroneous causation suppositions.

As another example of our need for increased specificity when describing neurodevelopmental disabilities, differentiating between the two major types of cerebral palsy, i.e., spastic (pyramidal) and athetoid (extrapyramidal), enhances etiologic considerations.[5,6] While mixtures and overlaps of these two basic forms of motor disability may follow a variety of brain insults or developmental abnormalities, the association of severe extrapyramidal cerebral palsy with average or near-average mental abilities is uniquely encountered as a consequence of acute, total intrapartum asphyxia or, less commonly today, bilirubin encephalopathy (kernicterus). In summary, if the primary neurodevelopmental disability is mental retardation, one's thinking should be oriented first and foremost to the early prenatal period, while, if the primary disability is cerebral palsy, strong etiologic consideration must be given to acquired perinatal or neonatal events. When the two disabilities occur relatively equally together (sometimes referred to as psychomotor

retardation), potential causes span all time periods from early prenatal to late postnatal and include the full spectrum of specific etiologies.

It is also useful and important to distinguish the patterns of neurodevelopmental disability associated with term infants who have experienced perinatal and/or neonatal complications from those disability patterns seen in surviving low birth weight, preterm infants. The classic "disease of immaturity," i.e., spastic diplegia type of cerebral palsy, is often seen in preterm infants with preserved mental capabilities and remains highly correlated with gestational age, particularly between 28 and 34 weeks gestation.[7,8] It has been increasingly recognized that spastic diplegia of prematurity is not exclusively related to complications in the neonatal intensive care unit, but often reflects compromised prenatal status, i.e., lack of fetal well-being, which, in some cases, may have contributed to the onset of premature labor.[9] It is not uncommon to encounter preterm infants with spastic diplegia who suffered virtually no respiratory distress and did not sustain an intracranial hemorrhage, but who may have been slightly growth retarded at birth.[10] Thus, all preterm survivors, regardless of the length or severity of neonatal course, are at some increased risk for the development of spastic diplegia and merit close neuromotor monitoring during the first two years of life. In contrast, term infants who develop the spastic diplegia type of cerebral palsy frequently do so following a documented asphyxial, traumatic, or infectious brain insult and, typically, are left with both permanent motor and mental disabilities.

We need an expanded realization of the complete spectrum of neurodevelopmental and neurobehavioral disabilities associated with brain injuries. While most clinical investigations focus on major handicapping conditions identified in the early years of life (i.e., cerebral palsy, mental retardation, vision and/or hearing impairment), an increasing body of evidence is revealing a vast array of "new morbidities" which become increasingly apparent after three years of age and which occur with increased prevalence following acquired brain insults. These more subtle developmental and behavioral sequelae may be seen in addition to previously established major disabilities or may develop independently over time in children who escaped major impairments. These "minor" central nervous system handicapping conditions include reduced or borderline intelligence, a variety of specific speech and language problems, coordination and balance deficits, perceptual disorders, socioemotional immaturities, and school underachievement secondary to learning disabilities and/or attention deficits. Considered together they constitute a numerically substantial, yet often overlooked and underreported, group of permanent dysfunctions which impact children's family, academic, and social lives.

These "new morbidities" are not unique to acquired brain injuries since they frequently share strong familial patterns of occurrence which presumably reflect mixed genetic and environmental influences. They are not specific to any particular time period of development, i.e., prenatal versus perinatal versus postnatal. They are not specific to any one cause of brain damage. Nevertheless, they frequently represent the eventual common pathway of brain dysfunction that may follow a variety of brain insults. For example, long-term follow-up investigations of low birth weight, preterm infants are consistently identifying such later childhood morbidities as language delays, visual-motor perceptual problems, attention deficits, conduct disorders, and specific learning disabilities in such areas as reading and mathematics.[11] While the exact etiologic mechanisms of these later morbidities are often difficult to differentiate precisely, it is clear that, as a group, they occur with increasing prevalence as birth weight and gestational age decrease and also with increasing prevalence as the severity and duration of perinatal and/or neonatal complications (e.g., asphyxia, intracranial hemorrhage, periventricular leukomalacia, infection, chronic lung disease) increase. That is, these more subtle brain dysfunctions are seen particularly in the smallest and sickest survivors of neonatal intensive care. While low socioeconomic status and adverse environmental experiences certainly add to the overall developmental and behavioral risk, permanent morbidities are regularly encountered in this population in the presence of optimal psychosocial status as well.

Recent investigations have described these same types of neurodevelopmental morbidities following other brain injuries. Potential fetal toxins such as tobacco, alcohol, narcotics, and a variety of anticonvulsant agents have been repeatedly demonstrated often to produce varying "minor" brain dysfunctions even in the absence of the classic syndromes which may accompany chronic fetal exposure.[12,13] Intrauterine infections, particularly cytomegalovirus, may result in a variety of neurosensory impairments even in children who manifest relatively few neonatal signs and symptoms.[14] Postnatal central nervous system infection (e.g., bacterial meningitis, viral meningoencephalitis) has been associated with language, learning, and behavioral problems and also with reduced intelligence when compared to sibling controls.[15–17] Severe head injury with prolonged loss of consciousness is frequently followed by developmental and behavioral deficits, particularly problems with attention and memory.[18] Chronic lead toxicity appears to cause permanent brain dysfunctions independent of the socioeconomic disadvantage that usually accompanies exposed populations.[19] The possible long-term neurodevelopmental effects of neonatal hyperbilirubinemia currently are debated even more vigorously in light of recent evidence demonstrating transient auditory electrophysiologic abnormalities in conjunction with moderately elevated neonatal bilirubin levels.[20] While investigations of infants experiencing fetal and/or neonatal asphyxial insults with resultant hypoxic-ischemic encephalopathy have focused almost exclusively on the major triad of cerebral palsy,

mental retardation, and epilepsy, accumulating reports and clinical experiences strongly suggest that more subtle neurodevelopmental morbidities frequently follow this type of insult and are presently underreported and insufficiently examined.[21,22] In summary, nearly identical brain dysfunctions may be the residua of very temporally and mechanistically different specific causes.

I further believe it is virtually impossible to render competent medicolegal opinions in this area without a thorough understanding of the difference between risk and disability and the neurologic markers which must connect the two if causal inferences are to be reliably drawn. Risk, as a descriptive concept in the context of neurodevelopmental disabilities, indicates an association between some personal characteristic, event, exposure, or behavior and the subsequent identification of a disability. The term is not used to denote a necessary or definitive outcome. Instead, at-risk identifies an increased potential or possibility that an individual with a specific intrinsic characteristic or exposed to a specific extrinsic agent or event will eventually develop a disability compared to an individual not at-risk. The analytic concept of risk differs from the descriptive aspect by assigning a numerical value to an individual's risk potential. Therefore, if a specific characteristic or event associated with the development of a particular disability has a risk ratio of greater than 1.00, then an elevated possibility exists for the disability to occur when the target characteristic or event is present.

There are several important "risks" to consider when applying the concept of risk to medicolegal reviews. Most individual neurodevelopmental risk factors will not be followed by the disability for which the child is at increased risk, i.e., the prevalence of most disabilities following established risk factors is considerably less than 50 percent, and most at-risk children, for a variety of brain compensatory and resiliency reasons, do not develop permanent disabilities. Second, because of the relative infrequency of most individual neurodevelopmental risk factors (e.g., low birth weight, asphyxia, toxins) in the general population, the majority of children overall who develop a particular disability will usually come from the much larger, presumed low-risk group who did not demonstrate the initial risk factor. This is particularly true for major, severe neurodevelopmental disabilities such as cerebral palsy and mental retardation which typically present in the absence of any identifiable risk factors. Clustering risk factors and combining both biologic and environmental risks (so-called "doubly vulnerable" population) certainly increases the likelihood of eventual disability, especially those more subtle, later neurodevelopmental morbidities.

Thus, while individual risk factors will *possibly* be followed by one or more neurodevelopmental disabilities, by themselves they will not *probably* be directly responsible in most cases. That is to say, additional intervening evidence must exist to reliably link risk to disability and to scientifically and medicolegally convert a possible risk-disability association into a probable cause and effect relationship. In the case of potential acquired brain injuries, it must be demonstrated that the risk agent or event was temporally closely followed by evidence of acute neurologic depression and/or deterioration (e.g., reduction in state of consciousness, alterations of muscle tone, autonomic nervous system instability, apnea, seizure activity) which, despite often apparently resolving, eventually evolved, over varying periods of time, into a permanent disability. The presence of relatively immediate neurologic abnormalities and signs of acute brain dysfunction following a potential risk, e.g., intrapartum asphyxia, provides confirmatory evidence of the gravity of the event and renders causal linkages with a subsequent disability as plausible; conversely, the virtual absence of signs or symptoms of acute neurologic compromise makes risk-disability causal linkages unlikely.

Taking as an example a common perinatal scenario, intrapartum fetal heart rate abnormalities as detected electronically or by auscultation constitute a risk factor for the development of certain disabilities, particularly cerebral palsy. By themselves, these heart rate abnormalities (e.g., loss of variability, decelerations, accelerations) neither identify nor predict disabilities, only risks. If, however, they are followed by many of the classic signs and symptoms of perinatal asphyxia (e.g., low Apgar scores, need for positive pressure resuscitation following delivery, metabolic acidosis, hypotonia-hypertonia, apnea, neonatal seizures, delayed feeding, systemic organ dysfunctions), the likelihood increases that a definite brain injury occurred which, depending upon the severity of irreversible damage sustained, may or may not result in permanent cerebral palsy. In this case the sequence of events makes it both scientifically sound and medicolegally reasonable to causally link the intrapartum asphyxia and cerebral palsy providing that no other competing etiologic mechanisms are evident. If, on the other hand, fetal heart rate abnormalities are not followed after delivery by signs of acute neurologic disturbance but, instead, by an essentially uncomplicated neonatal course, it then becomes both scientifically illogical and medicolegally irresponsible to automatically causally link a future disability with this risk factor.

The current medicolegal climate surrounding "birth injuries" has produced a somewhat concerning type of scientific response. The original description of infantile cerebral palsy in the mid-19th century is usually credited to Dr. William John Little, one of the founders of orthopedic surgery in England. In his classic treatise, "On the Influence of Abnormal Parturition, Difficult Labours, Premature Birth, and Asphyxia Neonatorum on the Mental and Physical Condition of the Child, Especially in Relation to Deformities,"[23] Little clearly articulated his opinions that asphyxia during the labor and delivery process and prematurity were the primary causes of the various cerebral palsy clinical syndromes. This article was not well accepted by the London Obstetrical Society. For many years this point of view was so popularized that,

typically, physicians and the general public alike would automatically associate cerebral palsy with birth-related asphyxia or trauma without careful scrutiny of the circumstances of each individual case. It was only following such individual investigation that the large number of completely unexplained cases of cerebral palsy became recognized, and the cerebral palsy causation pendulum slowly moved away from a strictly perinatal explanation to a broader, more complex interpretation which acknowledged the presence of intrinsic and extrinsic prenatal disorders of brain development.

Unfortunately, partially motivated and fueled by the 1980s medical malpractice crisis involving so-called "bad baby" cases, an increasing volume of reports utilizing the National Institutes of Health Collaborative Perinatal Project data from 25 years ago,[24] consensus conference publications,[25] and editorials[26] seems, at times, to be attempting to move this etiologic pendulum too far in the opposite direction. This contemporary scientific response to a serious medicolegal dilemma, which threatens access to pregnancy care and turns every disabled child into a potential litigant, often appears to be forcing prenatal (or idiopathic) explanations from inadequate data and minimizing the role of intrapartum asphyxia except in the most extreme cases. This approach strikes me as unfounded and hazardous as the narrow perinatal viewpoint and threatens to underestimate in physicians' minds the diverse neurodevelopmental consequences of asphyxia. A more rational posture would seem to be a compromise which acknowledges the importance of considering each case individually, thoroughly examining each major time period (i.e., prenatal, perinatal, postnatal) for etiologic clues, and recognizing that many permanent neurodevelopmental disabilities result from a *combination* of factors which may cumulatively injure the brain during fetal, intrapartum, and neonatal life.

As I stated at the outset, our knowledge of the mechanisms and pathophysiology of brain injury is still incomplete with many mysteries yet to be revealed. Despite new and improved brain imaging capabilities, many children with severe mental and/or motor neurodevelopmental disabilities probably secondary to prenatal defects in brain development will be found to have normal cranial studies.[27] Unfortunately, this absence of a specific etiology or syndrome often appears weak medicolegally, is interpreted by some to be nothing more than diagnosis by exclusion of other possibilities, and allows for substantially less valid etiologic hypotheses to be seriously entertained. Sophisticated neuropathologic techniques are increasingly revealing the neuronal pathologies (e.g., reduced dendritic arborization and synaptic organization, failure of neurotransmitter or neuroreceptor production, cellular heterotopias) which, in future years, are likely to be demonstrated to be the ultrastructural and functional bases for many severe brain disorders currently classified as idiopathic. "In vivo" we must continue to struggle with incomplete information for now.

This is also the present status with regard to the critical scientific and medicolegal task of timing probable brain injuries, particularly those caused by asphyxia. Currently available laboratory tests and brain imaging methodologies do not, in most cases, differentiate between chronic intrauterine and acute intrapartum asphyxia. It remains extremely difficult and often impossible to quantitatively apportion percentages of asphyxial brain injury and resultant neurodevelopmental disabilities in an infant who has experienced both chronic uteroplacental insufficiency and acute intrapartum deterioration. Neuropathologic documentation of prenatal brain damage is increasingly possible at autopsy, but specific correlations in survivors are lacking.[28] We need more precise timing markers, such as improved fetal function tests, both to answer these types of questions and also to plan more effectively obstetric interventions.

Our knowledge of the capabilities, mechanisms, and limits of brain "plasticity" and recovery from injury is still in its infancy. It is clear that seemingly similar insults may have dramatically different outcomes. Some of this disparity certainly relates to our continued imprecision in clinically determining the extent of actual brain injury as opposed to potential brain injury. For example, our clinical definitions of asphyxia remain general and imprecise without being able to readily measure the severity or duration of cerebral hypoxia-ischemia. However, it is also possible that a portion of the observed disparity in neurodevelopmental outcome results from differences in brain resiliency. A number of studies show that considerable plasticity, modifiable by environmental influences, occurs in the formation of certain connections within the nervous system.[29] In all likelihood, plasticity is a continuous remodeling of some aspects of the synaptic organization that occurs throughout life. Evidence exists suggesting that more optimal child-rearing environments may reduce the ultimate impact of less severe brain injuries. Gender differences also appear to exist with boys demonstrating greater brain vulnerability than girls in terms of permanent neurodevelopmental sequelae.[30] What mechanisms might underlie these observed differences? Are there types of early experiential interventions capable of supporting and facilitating brain recovery in some modest fashion? Even though there is no evidence of "growing new neurons" following brain injury, can subsequent synaptogenesis and the formation of new neural pathways be enhanced and in which cases and under which set of circumstances? We need answers to these questions to guide our rehabilitative efforts.

Never before has an improved awareness and understanding of fetal and neonatal brain injury been more imperative for physicians and other child development professionals. The risk of malpractice, interpreted reasonably or unreasonably, is all too real. This book comprehensively updates the epidemiologic, etiologic, diagnostic, and prognostic information available today in this controversial area. It highlights state-of-the-art technologies and recent advances with potential clinical utility. It deals with the key issue of which brain injuries are likely to be prevented by optimal prenatal, perinatal, and neonatal management and where the limits of preventability currently exist. The book does not answer all of our questions about the complexities of the immature, developing brain, but it is "must" reading for the primary care practitioner, the tertiary neuroscientist, and the expert witness alike.

REFERENCES

1. Freeman JM, Nelson KB. Intrapartum asphyxia and cerebral palsy. Pediatrics 1988; 82:240–249.
2. Volpe JJ. Perinatal hypoxic-ischemic brain injury. Pediatr Clin North Am 1976; 23(3):383–397.
3. Brown JK, Purvis RJ, Forfar JO, Cockburn F. Neurological aspects of perinatal asphyxia. Dev Med Child Neurol 1974; 16:567–580.
4. Opitz JM. Mental retardation: biologic aspects of concern to pediatricians. Pediatr Rev 1980; 2(2):41–50.
5. Stanley F, Alberman E, eds. The epidemiology of the cerebral palsies. Clin Dev Med 1984; 87.
6. Vining EPG, Accardo PJ, Rubenstein JE, Farrell SE, Roizen NJ. Cerebral palsy: a pediatric developmentalist's overview. Am J Dis Child 1976; 130:643–649.
7. Bennett FC. Neurodevelopmental outcome of low birthweight infants. In: Kelley VC, ed. Practice of pediatrics. Philadelphia: Harper & Row, 1984:1.
8. Atkinson S, Stanley FJ. Spastic diplegia among children of low and normal birthweight. Dev Med Child Neurol 1983; 25:693–708.
9. Hagberg G, Hagberg B, Olow I. The changing panorama of cerebral palsy in Sweden 1954–1970. III. The importance of fetal deprivation of supply. Acta Pediatr Scand 1976; 65:403–408.
10. Bennett FC, Chandler LS, Robinson NM, Sells CJ. Spastic diplegia in premature infants: etiologic and diagnostic considerations. Am J Dis Child 1981; 135:732–737.
11. Bennett FC. Neurodevelopmental outcome in low birthweight infants: the role of developmental intervention. In: Guthrie RD, ed. Clincis in critical care medicine. Neonatal intensive care. New York: Churchill Livingstone, 1988.
12. Iosub S, Fuchs M, Bingol N, Gromisch DS. Fetal alcohol syndrome revisited. Pediatrics 1981; 68:475–479.
13. Wilson GS, Desmond MM, Verniaud WM. Early development of infants of heroin-addicted mothers. Am J Dis Child 1973; 126:457–462.
14. Saigal S, Lunyk O, Larke RPB, Chernesky MA. The outcome in children with congenital cytomegalovirus infection: a longitudinal follow-up study. Am J Dis Child 1982; 136:896–901.
15. Feldman HM, Michaels RH. Academic achievement in children 10 to 12 years after *Haemophilus influenzae* meningitis. Pediatrics 1988; 81:339–344.
16. Sells CJ, Carpenter RL, Ray CG. Sequelae of central nervous system enterovirus infections. N Engl J Med 1975; 293:1–4.
17. Sell SHW, Webb WW, Pate JE, Doyne EO. Psychological sequelae to bacterial meningitis: two controlled studies. Pediatrics 1972; 49:212–217.
18. Mahoney WJ, D'Souza BJ, Haller JA, Rogers MC, Epstein MH, Freeman JM. Long-term outcome of children with severe head trauma and prolonged coma. Pediatrics 1983; 71:756–762.
19. McMichael AJ, Baghurst PA, Wigg NR, Vimpani GV, Robertson EF, Roberts RJ. Port Pirie cohort study: environmental exposure to lead and children's abilities at the age of four years. N Engl J Med 1988; 319:468–475.
20. Nakamura H, Takada S, Shimabuku R, Matsuo M, Matsuo T, Negishi H. Auditory nerve and brainstem responses in newborn infants with hyperbilirubinemia. Pediatrics 1985; 75:703–708.
21. Skov H, Lou H, Pederson H. Perinatal brain ischemia: impact at four years of age. Dev Med Child Neurol 1984; 26:353–357.
22. Towbin A. Organic causes of minimal brain dysfunction: perinatal origin of minimal cerebral lesions. JAMA 1971; 217:1207–1214.

23. Little WJ. On the influence of abnormal parturition, difficult labours, premature birth, and asphyxia neonatorum on the mental and physical condition of the child, especially in relation to deformities. Trans Obstet Soc Lond 1862; 3:293–344.

24. Nelson KB, Ellenberg JH. Antecedents of cerebral palsy: multivariate analysis of risk. N Engl J Med 1986; 315:81–86.

25. Freeman JM, ed. Prenatal and perinatal factors associated with brain disorders. NIH publication No. 85–1149, 1985.

26. Paneth N. Birth and the origins of cerebral palsy. N Engl J Med 1986; 315:124–126.

27. Moeschler JB, Bennett FC, Cromwell LD. Use of the CT scan in the medical evaluation of the mentally retarded child. J Pediatr 1981; 98:63–65.

28. Ellis WG, Goetzman BW, Lindenberg JA. Neuropathologic documentation of prenatal brain damage. Am J Dis Child 1988; 142:858–866.

29. Moore RY. Normal development of the nervous system. In: Freeman JM, ed. Prenatal and perinatal factors associated with brain disorders. NIH publication No. 85–1149, 1985.

30. Brothwood M, Wolke D, Gamsu H, Benson J, Cooper D. Prognosis of the very low birthweight baby in relation to gender. Arch Dis Child 1986, 61:559–564.

CONTENTS

POSSIBLE CAUSES OF ACQUIRED FETAL AND NEONATAL BRAIN INJURY

1 Epidemiology of Perinatal Asphyxia 2
   Philip Sunshine

2 Preterm Labor and Intrauterine Growth Retardation: Complex Obstetrical Problems with Low Birth Weight Infants 11
   Richard E. Besinger
   John T. Repke
   James E. Ferguson II

3 Complications of Labor and Delivery: Selected Medical and Surgical Considerations 34
   Ronald L. Thomas
   James E. Ferguson II
   John T. Repke

4 Effects of Anesthesia on the Fetus and Neonate 46
   George A. Albright

5 Fetal Injury from Drug Abuse in Pregnancy: Alcohol, Narcotic, Cocaine, and Phencyclidine 57
   Ronald S. Cohen
   William E. Benitz
   David K. Stevenson

6 Fetal Responses to Asphyxia 65
   R. Harold Holbrook Jr.
   Ronald N. Gibson

7 Congenital Infections as Causes of Neurologic Sequelae: Prevention, Diagnosis, and Treatment 79
   Charles G. Prober
   Ann M. Arvin

MANAGEMENT OF THE DEPRESSED OR NEUROLOGICALLY DYSFUNCTIONAL INFANT

8 Immediate Management 94
   William E. Benitz
   Lorry R. Frankel
   David K. Stevenson

9 Extended Management 104
   William R. Benitz
   Lorry R. Frankel
   David K. Stevenson

10 Hypoxic-Ischemic Encephalopathy 113
   Edward J. Novotny Jr.

11 Neonatal Seizures 123
   Robert R. Clancy

12 Hypoglycemia and Brain Injury 141
   Ronald S. Cohen
   David K. Stevenson

13 Hematologic Disorders: Anemia, Polycythemia, and Hyperbilirubinemia 147
   David K. Stevenson
   Herbert C. Schwartz

14 Nutritional Management 159
   Anjali Malkani
   John A. Kerner Jr.

ASSESSING THE CAUSES OF PERMANENT NEUROLOGIC DISABILITY AND THE RISKS OF PRACTICE

15 Electroencephalography in the Assessment of the Premature and Full-Term Infant 175
   Barry R. Tharp

16 New Noninvasive Technologies to
    Evaluate Brain Function 185
        William D. Rhine
        Ricardo R. González-Méndez
        David K. Stevenson

17 Imaging of Hypoxic-Ischemic
    Cerebral Damage 196
        Dieter R. Enzmann

18 Etiology and Timing of Static
    Encephalopathies of Childhood
    (Cerebral Palsy) 221
        Steven L. Weinstein
        Barry R. Tharp

19 The Scope and Limitations of Neurologic
    and Behavioral Assessments of the
    Newborn 239
        Anneliese F. Korner

20 The Medicolegal Imperative:
    Placental Pathology and
    Epidemiology 250
        Geoffrey Altshuler
        Allen A. Herman

21 The Appropriateness of Intensive
    Care Applications 264
        David K. Stevenson
        Amnon Goldworth

POSSIBLE CAUSES OF ACQUIRED FETAL AND NEONATAL BRAIN INJURY

1 Epidemiology of Perinatal Asphyxia

Philip Sunshine, M.D.

Asphyxia
   Correlative Signs of Asphyxia
      Meconium
      Fetal Blood Gas Levels
      Neonatal Neurologic Syndrome
Seizures
Cerebral Palsy
Epidemiology of Mental Retardation
Conclusion

In 1985 Dr. John M. Freeman[1] noted that in the United States alone 750,000 young people were afflicted with cerebral palsy and 850,000 children had mental retardation. He also noted that 10 percent of all school-age children were handicapped, and that neurologic and communicative disorders in the United States cost society approximately $114 billion dollars per year.

Perinatal asphyxia and birth injuries have been the major factors leading to neurologic and intellectual impairment in the pediatric population.[2-4] Although this potential causal relationship has been recognized since Little's description of infants and children with "neurological deformities" in 1862,[5] the strength of this claim can be challenged. This is due to dilemmas regarding the association of perinatal injuries with subsequent development of neurologic disabilities, the main one being the difficulty in assessing the duration and severity of the asphyxial period.[6,7] Even with the advent of electronic fetal heart monitoring and the measurement of scalp and cord pH and base deficits, not all the factors contributing to asphyxia may be evident or recognized.

Often a thorough investigation attempting to identify the cause of the asphyxia either is not carried out or is incomplete and the diagnosis of perinatal asphyxia is made by default. Furthermore, long-term follow-up in the asphyxiated infant is often lacking, and except for a few studies, little is known of the subsequent development of these patients. Although severely affected infants are most likely to be enrolled in intervention and follow-up programs, those with a history of mild to moderate asphyxia often do not participate in long-term evaluation. Finally, an infant or child may be identified as having neurologic or intellectual impairment, and then a retrospective analysis is instituted to identify the etiology of the abnormality. In many instances a definitive causative factor is not found, but there are suggestions that some "irregularities" of practice occurred during the perinatal period. Thereupon these findings provide the basis for the assumption that perinatal asphyxia was responsible for the child's impairment, and that if alternative approaches had been undertaken in the intrapartum period, little if any damage would have resulted. Unfortunately such reasoning has prevailed over the years despite the lack of substantive supporting data, and numerous litigations have been instituted in the belief that retrospective associations represent cause and effect relationships.

We readily recognize infants who have been subjected to severe intrauterine stress, who are depressed at the time of birth, and who remained obtunded in the neonatal period. These infants often have seizures with aberrant electroencephalographic patterns and have a significant incidence of subsequent neurologic handicaps. These infants fit the classic clinical scenario of the neonate with hypoxic-ischemic encephalopathy.[2]

But what about the neonate who is depressed at birth but who responds readily to resuscitation and has a relatively uneventful neonatal course? If such an infant is later found to have neurologic disabilities, can one implicate abnormalities in the perinatal period as being the "proximal cause" of the sequelae? The data provided in Chapter 10 suggest that episodes of mild and moderate asphyxia are not associated with handicaps, and that even following severe asphyxia, most infants, if they survive, have normal neurologic function.

It is critical that we devise criteria in order to better understand the factors that contribute to the development of the "brain damaged child" and not be unduly influenced by circumstantial evidence. It is also critical to recognize that the events leading to difficulties in the prematurely born infant may be different from those in the infant born at term. Depending on the gestational age, the preterm infant is three to 30 times more likely to develop cerebral palsy than the infant born at term,[8-10] and often the problems in the small infant arise in the immediate postpartum period rather than in the intrapartum period. Thus, in attempts to evaluate etiology, pathogenesis, intervention, and management, one must consider that similar events may have different consequences depending on the patient's capacity to respond and which are frequently determined by gestational age. However, infants with evidence of intrauterine growth retardation also form a significant portion of the patients with cerebral palsy, suggesting that the underlying cause or causes of their difficulties may be very different from those in infants who are appropriately grown.

ASPHYXIA

As noted by Paneth and Stark,[6,7] the fundamental problem in assessing the relationship between asphyxia and subsequent neurologic outcome has been the difficulty in assessing the degree of asphyxia. Various techniques have been used to identify the asphyxiated infant, including the time to initiate spontaneous ventilation, the time that positive pressure ventilation was required to sustain the infant, and the use of the neonatal scoring system developed by Apgar.[11,12] Scott,[13] defining severe asphyxia in infants who were apparently stillborn or who required more than 20 minutes to establish spontaneous respirations, included both preterm and term infants in the evaluation. Scott also noted that, although half the infants died, three-quarters of the survivors were apparently normal, a surprising finding considering the dire condition of the infants at birth (Table 1-1).

The newborn scoring system developed by Virginia Apgar was used to identify infants who were depressed and who required resuscitative efforts. Although Apgar did not design the scoring system to be used as a tool to evaluate outcome and subsequent neurologic damage, the system has been utilized by many for correlation with ultimate outcome. It was so utilized in the National Collaborative Perinatal Project of the National Institutes for Neurological Diseases and Stroke (NCPP).[14] Although the Apgar scoring system is not perfect, because it can be influenced by factors that are not necessarily related to asphyxia, it remains the standard by which neonates are evaluated immediately after birth as well as their response to appropriate therapy. The long-term neurologic outcome, especially in term infants, has not correlated well with low scores at one, five, and even 10 minutes, but the correlation improves significantly for infants who have persistently low scores

(0 to 3) 15 and 20 minutes after birth.[8] If one uses an Apgar score of 7 or less at five minutes to indicate asphyxia, the incidence of asphyxia in the NCPP study is found to be almost 5 percent (see Table 1-1).

In 1980 MacDonald and co-workers[15,16] evaluated 38,405 consecutive deliveries and defined neonatal asphyxia in infants who required more than one minute of positive pressure ventilation before sustained respiration occurred. They found 447 infants with asphyxia, an overall incidence of 1.16 percent. The more immature the infant, the greater the incidence, severity, and mortality associated with asphyxial episodes (see Table 1-1).

Peters and co-workers[17,18] evaluated 17,196 infants born during the week of April 5, 1970 through April 11, 1970 in the United Kingdom. These investigators used the time required for the onset of regular respirations to evaluate asphyxia. The times were less than one minute, one to three minutes (mild to moderate asphyxia), and more than three minutes (severe asphyxia). The mortality rates were very low in infants who required either less than one minute or one to three minutes to breathe; however, there was an increase in mortality in infants who required more than three minutes to institute normal respiration. The incidence of mild to moderate asphyxia was 18 percent and of severe asphyxia, 4 percent. The overall mortality was most pronounced in very low birth weight infants. The subsequent follow-up demonstrated an increased incidence of cerebral palsy not only in infants of low birth weight but also in larger infants as well especially in those requiring more than three minutes to institute spontaneous respiration (see Table 1-1).

Correlative Signs of Asphyxia

Several signs or findings have been correlated to some extent with the severity of asphyxia in the intrapartum period. These have included the presence of meconium in the amniotic fluid, evidence of acidosis as measured in cord blood, the presence of the neonatal neurologic syndrome, and the occurrence of seizures in the first three days of life. Each is discussed separately.

Meconium

The presence of meconium in the amniotic fluid has long been thought to indicate fetal stress. Meconium is found in 8 to 20 percent of all deliveries, being uncommonly encountered in preterm gestations and more frequently encountered in the postdate baby. If meconium is found at birth of infants at 34 weeks' gestation or younger, significant intrauterine stress or intrauterine

TABLE 1-1 Incidence of Perinatal Asphyxia, Mortality, and Handicaps in Survivors[57]

Authors	Years of Study	Definition of Asphyxia	No. of Patients	Incidence of Asphyxia	Deaths (%)	Outcome in Survivors (%)		
						Normal	Mild to Moderate Damage	Severe Damage
Neligan et al, 1974 comm.[58]	1960–1962	Delay greater than 5 min to establish respiration	13,203	27/1,000 (includes prematures)	21	95.4	0.5	4
Neligan et al, 1974 hospital study[59]	1961–1970	Cardiac arrest or delay greater than 20 min to establish respiration	20,793	1.8/1,000	52	77		23
Scott, 1976[13]	1966–1971	Apparent stillborn or delay greater than 20 min to establish respiration	12,389	3.8/1,000	52	74		26
Nelson and Ellenberg, 1981[8]	1959–1966	Apgar scores 6 or less at 5 min (all weights)	49,498	47/1,000	24	96.4		3.6
		Apgar score 0 – 3 at 5 min (all weights)	49,498	15.7/1,000	44	94.7		5.3
		Apgar score 0 – 3 at 10 min or later (all weights)	49,498	15.4/1,000	76	76	10	14
Peters et al, 1984[17]	4/4/70– 4/11/70	More than 3 min to establish respiration (all weights)	16,333	45/1,000	6.0	86		14
Mulligan et al[15] and McDonald et al 1980[16]	1970–1975	More than 1 min positive pressure ventilation	38,405	11.6/1,000	46.1*	81.5		18.5
MacDonald et al, 1985[43]	1981–1983	Neonatal seizures	13,084	3/1,000	23	80		20

*89% <30 weeks. 18% >36 weeks.
Modified from Dennis J. The long-term effects of intrapartum cerebral damage. In: Crawford JW, ed. Risks of labour. Chichester: John Wiley, 1985:157.

infection must be suspected. In term and post-term infants meconium staining is usually light and the fetus and newborn are essentially symptom free. However, heavy, thick meconium passed early in labor tends to be associated with increased fetal and neonatal morbidity and death.[19]

The presence of meconium per se in term infants is not predictive of neurologic sequelae; if fact, Nelson and Ellenberg[20] noted that less than 0.5 percent of the infants weighing more than 2,500 gm and having meconium staining had neurologic sequelae. In studies in the Netherlands, the presence of meconium-stained amniotic fluid had no predictive value in regard to outcome, the development of neurologic symptoms in the newborn period, or acidosis as measured by the pH of cord blood.[21,22] Even when the presence of meconium was ascertained and used in conjunction with either Apgar scores or cord pH values or both, the finding did not alter the incidence of subsequent neurologic abnormalities.

Fetal Blood Gas Levels

Stewart Clifford[23] was one of the first clinicians to suggest that neurologic abnormalities in the neonate are not necessarily due to birth trauma but rather to the accumulation of lactic and carbonic acids secondary to the hypoxic-anoxic episode. He also noted that, in addition to damage occurring in the central nervous system, every organ and tissue in the body could be affected to some degree. Since his observations, which subsequently have been supported by studies in laboratory animals,[24-27] it has been postulated that the accumulation of lactic acid is correlative with the abnormalities seen in hypoxic-ischemic encephalopathy.

Studies by Sykes and co-workers[28] and Silverman and co-workers[29] questioned whether Apgar scores truly reflected neonatal asphyxia. In both studies, each evaluating over 1,000 neonates, a correlation between the Apgar score at one minute and the presence of significant acidosis was lacking. In the study by Sykes and co-workers[28] only 20 percent of the neonates with Apgar scores of 6 or less had cord pH values of 7.10 or less. Of infants whose cord pH value was 7.10 or less, 22 percent had Apgar scores of 6 or less. Similar results were obtained by Silverman and co-workers,[29] who noted that the metabolic state of the fetus as measured by the umbilical artery pH level was not closely related to the Apgar score unless a severe degree of biochemical abnormality was encountered, i.e., a pH value less than 7.05.

In studies carried out in Groningen, Dijxhoorn and co-workers[21] found similar results in appropriately grown neonates. They found that measurements of the arterial or venous pH or the maternal-fetal difference in pH alone could not be used as predictors of neonatal neurologic depression. However, in infants who were small for gestational age, the incidence of fetal acidosis was greater than in appropriate-for-gestational-age infants but was not necessarily correlated with severe neonatal depression.[22]

It appears from the major studies that have attempted to correlate cord pH, Apgar scores, and neurologic outcomes that only when there is evidence of extreme abnormality is there any correlation with short-term outcome. Unfortunately the long-term outcome in patients in whom these correlates have been measured has not yet been ascertained.[10] In addition, data to document that the persistence of acidosis leads to tissue damage are also lacking.

Neonatal Neurologic Syndrome

If significant intrapartum asphyxia has occurred, the infant should demonstrate neurologic abnormalities in the neonatal period. It is often difficult to ascertain such abnormalities in preterm infants, especially those who have cardiopulmonary abnormalities and who are receiving assisted ventilation. Often these infants cannot be distinguished from other prematurely born infants with similar cardiopulmonary abnormalities. However, in the term or near-term infant signs of encephalopathy are readily discerned. Sarnat and Sarnat[30] developed an infant scoring system that categorizes the patients into three states of "postasphyxial encephalopathy"—mild, moderate, and severe. Although they correlated many of the findings with electroencephalographic changes, one can use their classification even if the electroencephalograms are not evaluated.

Patients with mild encephalopathy often are hyperirritable and have hyperactive reflexes, tachycardia, poor sucking, but no evidence of seizures. Patients with severe encephalopathy are stuporous, flaccid, and hypotonic; there are no Moro, oculovestibular, or tonic neck reflexes. The infants do not suck and often show decerebrate posturing. These patients are often in need of assisted ventilation and cardiotonic support and remain in this state for days to weeks. The electroencephalographic pattern usually demonstrates burst suppression or is isopotential. Patients with moderate encephalopathy tend to be in the middle of these two extremes, have mild hypotonia and weak or incomplete reflexes, and often have focal or multifocal seizures.

The neurologic outcome in these infants is related to the severity of the neonatal symptoms. Robertson and Finer[31] reported that infants with mild symptoms had no handicaps at follow-up; 80 percent of those with moderate encephalopathy were without handicap; and those with severe encephalopathy either died or had moderate to severe neurologic sequelae.

Levene and co-workers,[32] using slightly different criteria to grade severity, also defined three separate classes of postasphyxial encephalopathy. They noted that the overall incidence of postasphyxial encephalopathy was six per 1,000 live births. Severe encephalopathy was found in 2.1 births per 1,000, but only two of the 11 babies who died in this study were in the severe postasphyxial encephalopathy group. In this study 23 percent of the infants with postasphyxial encephalopathy had "unremarkable" Apgar scores at one and five minutes. In Levene's study 25 percent of the patients had evidence of intrauterine growth retardation, whereas 29 percent of Robertson and Finer's patients were similarly affected.[31]

Thus, if a neonate shows evidence of asphyxia as demonstrated by aberrant fetal heart rate patterns, low Apgar scores, or delayed onset of respirations, but has little if any evidence of neurologic depression or abnormalities in the immediate neonatal period, it is highly unlikely that the patient will demonstrate significant neurologic sequelae.[2,31,33] Analyzing the data from the NCPP study, Nelson and Ellenberg[33] substantiated previous observations and stated that infants who are depressed at birth but who do not demonstrate evidence of neonatal encephalopathy do not have an increased risk of cerebral palsy as they develop.

SEIZURES

The onset of seizures within the first two to three days of life has been thought to indicate the quality of perinatal care.[34,35] More likely, however, seizures have more correlation with long-term neurologic handicaps, since these infants are 15 to 17 times more likely to have neurologic sequelae than newborns without seizures.[36] The incidence of neonatal seizures has been reported to vary between 1.3 per 1,000 and 14 per 1,000 live births, but more recent data suggest that the incidence does not exceed 9 per 1,000.[37] Over 60 percent of neonatal seizures occur within the first 48 hours of life and, except for those occurring secondary to bacterial meningitis, have a more ominous outcome, in terms of mortality and neurologic sequelae, than those occurring later in the neonatal period.[38,39] The overall mortality varies from 9 to 35 percent (Table 1–2).

The etiology of neonatal seizures varies as well. Even though many investigators suggest that the early onset of seizures is due primarily to intrapartum events, other etiologic factors have been incriminated as well. In a study in Leicester, England, Levine and Trounce[40] found that, although intrapartum or postnatal asphyxia accounted for 53 percent of the patients, hemorrhage (15 percent), infection (8 percent), metabolic aberrations (5 percent), hypoglycemia (3 percent), and stroke (5 percent) also contributed to the problem. Only 8 percent of these patients had seizures of unexplained origin, a finding at variance with the incidences reported in Stockholm[41] (29 percent) and Australia[37] (64 percent). Typically infants who suffer from severe hypoxic-ischemic encephalopathy have seizures beginning in the first 48 hours after birth. These seizures are recurrent and extremely difficult to control. These patients have excessive mortality, and the survivors often have significant incidences of neurologic impairment. Conversely, patients who have a single seizure of a fleeting nature should have an excellent outcome, especially if the seizures do not recur.

As noted by Niswander and co-workers,[42] even when mothers were managed appropriately during the intrapartum period, early onset seizures occurred in their offspring. In the Dublin randomized study described by MacDonald et al,[43] the incidence of early-onset seizures was twice as great in the intermittently monitored population as in those whom electronic fetal heart rate monitoring was employed. However, the mortality and the incidence of severe disability in the survivors of neonatal seizures at one year of age were identical in the two groups studied.

Keegan and co-workers[44] identified 66 infants with neonatal seizures, 34 of whom were term births, and retrospectively evaluated the perinatal events that occurred in the infants. The term infants had lower one and five minute Apgar scores than control infants and had increased incidences of placenta previa, abruptio placentae, and postdatism. Abnormal fetal heart rate patterns were noted in 85 percent of these patients, with an absence of variability in 59 percent or an abnormal pattern with absence of variability in 53 percent. In the patients with aberrant fetal heart rate patterns there was appropriate intervention in over 80 percent of the cases. Despite intervention, all infants had seizures and almost half (42 percent) the survivors had significant neurologic handicaps. Even more disconcerting was the number of infants with seizures who did not demonstrate fetal heart rate patterns suggestive of fetal distress and thus no intervention was indicated. These observations suggest that either the event leading to the seizures occurred prior to the onset of labor or the event (or events)

occurred in infants with lesser degrees of fetal heart rate abnormality than are currently recognized.

CEREBRAL PALSY

The incidence of cerebral palsy varies to some degree depending on the severity of the disorder. In the NCPP study the incidence of moderate to severe cerebral palsy in infants who survived the neonatal period was 3.2 per 1,000 live births.[8-10] The incidence reported in Liverpool by Pharoah and co-workers[45] varied from 1.18 to 1.97 per 1,000 live births. In Sweden, Hagberg and co-workers[46] described the incidence over a 20-year period and noted that it initially fell from 1.9 to 1.4 per 1,000 but over the last 10 years of the study increased to 2 per 1,000. Stanley and Watson[47] in Western Australia demonstrated that the incidence of cerebral palsy in their population remained stable at approximately 2.5 per 1,000 live births even though the perinatal mortality had decreased by 65 percent, that fetal monitoring had been introduced, and that there had been a more liberal approach regarding the use of cesarean section. The incidence of cerebral palsy in infants weighing less than 1,500 gm was about 20 times that in infants born at term, and infants weighing 1,500 to 2,500 gm had an incidence three to four times that in term infants.

In attempting to correlate the development of cerebral palsy with Apgar scores in term infants, Nelson and Ellenberg[8] demonstrated that the incidence increased significantly when the low Apgar scores persisted for more than 10 minutes (Table 1–3). If the scores were 0 to 3 at five minutes but increased to 4 or more by 10 minutes, the incidence of cerebral palsy was less than 1 percent in the survivors. Only when the score remained low for 15 minutes or more did the incidence of cerebral palsy increase significantly. Conversely, 55 percent of the patients who developed cerebral palsy had one minute Apgar scores of 7 to 10; 73 percent of the patients had Apgar scores of 7 to 10 at five minutes.

In an attempt to identify risk factors that would predict cerebral palsy, Nelson and Ellenberg[10] in a review of the NCPP data found that 5 percent of the population at greatest risk contributed 37 percent of the patients with cerebral palsy. Over two-thirds of the patients with cerebral palsy did not emanate from this group; even more significant was the fact that over 97 percent of the patients identified in the high risk population group did not have cerebral palsy.

These investigators, in focusing in on this high risk cohort, could predict 13 percent of the patients with cerebral palsy on the basis of prepregnancy factors and 34 percent on the basis of both prepregnancy and pregnancy factors. The additional information derived from data regarding labor, delivery, and the neonatal period increased this predictability to 37 percent, a negligible increase.

TABLE 1–2   Incidence and Outcome in Infants with Neonatal Seizures

Author	Incidence	Mortality	Incidence of Handicaps in Survivors
Eriksson and Zetterson, 1979[41]	1.5/1,000 full-term deliveries; all infants < 4 weeks of age	14%	41%
Finer et al, 1981[60]	3.22/1,000 of inborn; total of 65 infants inborn and outborn 37 weeks or more	8%	50% (14% mild, 17% moderate, 19% severe)
Holden et al, 1982[36] (NCPP data)	5/1,000	34.8%; two-thirds died in neonatal period	13% cerebral palsy; 19% mental retardation; 33% epilepsy; 13% mental retardation, cerebral palsy, or epilepsy
Goldberg, 1983[37]			?
1971–1974	2/1,000	33.5%	
1975–1977	6/1,000	17.5%	
1978–1980	8.6/1,000	18.5% Mortality due to cerebral hypoxia: overall 50%	
Derham et al, 1985[35]	1.6/1,000 Infants > 37 weeks—seizures within 48 hours after birth	35%	36%
Minchom et al, 1987[38]	1.3/1,000 live births >37 weeks; seizures within 48 hours after birth	9.2%	22.4% (4% mild, 8% moderate, 10% severe)
Grant[39] and MacDonald et al, 1985[43]	Electronically monitored, 1.8/1,000 Auscultation, 4.1/1,000	25% 22%	25% 11%
Curtis et al[61] (101,829 term infants)	0.87/1,000	18%	25%

Thus, if most of the patients with cerebral palsy seem to come from a rather low risk population, what are the etiologic factors involved in cerebral palsy? Holm,[48] in reviewing 142 patients in the northwestern United States, found that in more than 50 percent of the cases disabilities were due to prenatal abnormalities, 10 percent to postnatal problems, and about 33 percent to perinatal abnormalities.

Using clinical criteria to identify the specific types of cerebral palsy and timing of etiology, Holm suggested that in about 50 percent of the patients with hemiplegia, 15 percent of those with spastic diplegia, 37 percent of those with spastic quadriplegia, 50 percent of those with athetosis, and 50 percent of those with mixed findings, the origin was "prenatal complications." In almost all the patients with ataxia and hypotonia the problems were the result of prenatal factors. Perinatal problems tended to manifest primarily as spastic diplegia (prematurely born) and quadriplegia.

Finally, Blair and Stanley[49] reviewed 183 patients in Western Australia and compared them with a control group of patients born during the same period (1975 to 1980). They estimated that in only 15 of the 183 patients (8 percent) was spastic cerebral palsy attributable to intrapartum asphyxia, a much lower incidence than had been postulated. Nelson[50,51] in a systematic review of the NCPP data found that the incidence of cerebral palsy associated with intrapartum asphyxia was in the range of 3 to 15 percent and that, if all factors were taken into

consideration, it did not exceed 20 percent. Thus, improvement in obstetrical care and intrapartum monitoring and appropriate neonatal resuscitation have a rather limited effect in decreasing the overall incidence of cerebral palsy. Nelson and Ellenberg[33] also noted that patients who had significant late pregnancy or birth complications, but who were asymptomatic or had transient symptoms in the neonatal period, did not have an increased incidence of cerebral palsy compared with patients without any risk factors (2.4 per 1,000 versus 2.3 per 1,000).

TABLE 1–3   Correlation of Apgar Scores of 0–3 and the Risk of Death and Cerebral Palsy in Survivors Among Infants Weighing More Than 2,501 Gm at Birth (NCPP Data)

Apgar Scores 0–3 Time Period (Minutes)	Live-born Infants	Death (%)	Known to 7 years	% Cerebral Palsy
1	1,729	3.1	1,330	0.7
5	286	7.7	217	0.9
10	66	18.2	43	4.7
15	23	47.8	11	9.1
20	39	59.0	14	57.1

Modified from Nelson KB, Ellenberg JH. Apgar scores as predictors of chronic neurologic disability. Pediatrics 1981; 68:38.

EPIDEMIOLOGY OF MENTAL RETARDATION

Using IQ measurements alone, epidemiologists have defined severe mental retardation as an IQ score below 50 and mild mental retardation as a score between 50 and 69. As proposed by Paneth and Stark,[6] the prevalence of severe mental retardation is remarkably consistent—between 3 and 4 per 1,000 school-age children. This type of retardation is often associated with motor handicaps, abnormal features or appearance, and seizures. These patients generally are found with equal frequency in all socioeconomic classes and most commonly are retarded as a result of "biologic insult to the brain."

Patients with mild mental retardation most commonly come from the most disadvantaged socioeconomic classes, have learning problems, and often require special classes or schooling in order to reach their ultimate levels of achievement. Associated neurologic handicaps may be found in as many as 30 percent of these patients, epilepsy being the most common finding.[52]

The incidence of mild mental retardation has been stated to be 23 to 30 per 1,000 in the school-age population and is closely related to socioeconomic class. In Sweden the incidence of this type of mental retardation was only 4 per 1,000.[52] It appears that alterations in the socioeconomic environment may have a significant effect in lowering the incidence of mild mental retardation.

Hagberg and Kyllerman[52] noted that patients with the fetal alcohol syndrome make up almost 10 percent of those with mild mental retardation and almost 1 percent of the patients with severe mental retardation. As more of these patients are being recognized in the United States, it is possible that an increased percentage will be found in both the mild mental retardation and severe mental retardation groups. Similarly, as the number of infants delivered of cocaine abusing mothers increases, it is possible that these patients may also contribute to the number of mentally retarded infants and children encountered.

Both Hagberg and Kyllerman[52] and Paneth and Stark[7] have studied the etiologic factors in mental retardation and noted that perinatal events could account for 10 percent of the cases of severe and mild mental retardation. Similarly, postnatal difficulties (after the first month of life) could account at most for 10 percent of the patients with both types of retardation. In most of the patients the origin of severe mental retardation lies in prenatal problems, including chromosomal abnormalities (40 percent), biochemical inborn errors of metabolism (3 to 5 percent), and intrauterine infections (5 percent). It is highly unlikely that severe mental retardation in infants who do not have cerebral palsy arises as a result of intrapartum asphyxia.

CONCLUSION

Although intrapartum asphyxia contributes in some ways to neurologic and intellectual impairment, the degree to which it contributes has been grossly overstated. By current standards it is estimated that intrapartum difficulties contribute in less than 15 percent of patients with cerebral palsy and severe mental retardation and that in most situations both abnormalities are present in the same individual.

Even though physicians, attorneys, and the lay public often have blamed inadequate obstetrical and pediatric care as the basis for cerebral palsy and severe mental retardation, current data do not support this belief. Often a diagnosis of cerebral palsy or severe mental retardation is made and a retrospective evaluation of the perinatal period is carried out. The neonate may be found to be depressed (low Apgar scores), aberrant fetal heart rate tracings may be found, and a retrospective evaluation of intrapartum events ensues. Unfortunately many cases have been brought to litigation on the basis of these findings, and "experts" in both perinatology and neonatal medicine have lent credence to casual interpretations, even when they are not justified by the data.

In addition, although electronic monitoring of fetal heart rates has been utilized to reduce the incidence of intrapartum asphyxia, neonatal mortality, and the subsequent development of neurologic handicaps in survivors, the data do not show that such intervention actually has been successful in the overall reduction of these events.[53-55] Electronic fetal heart rate monitoring undoubtedly has been useful in selected populations, especially in the prematurely born infant and possibly in the intrauterine growth-retarded infant in improving the outcome, and not as an adjunct in improving the outcome in low risk populations.

In a recent publication Freeman and Nelson[56] examined adverse intrapartum events and the subsequent development of neurologic disabilities. They listed criteria for implicating intrapartum events as leading to damage in the infant. These include documentation of marked and protracted intrapartum asphyxia; the presence of neonatal encephalopathy with evidence of the neonatal neurologic syndrome; evidence of asphyxial injury to other organ systems; evidence that the child's neurologic abnormalities are based on intrapartum asphyxia; and evidence that an evaluation to exclude other abnormalities has been carried out.

With the recent development of improved imaging techniques, I would add another stipulation: Structural abnormalities, if present, must be explained on the basis of intrapartum asphyxia and shown not to be due to developmental aberrations. Additionally, intrapartum asphyxia is almost never implicated as a causative factor in patients with severe mental retardation who do not have concurrent evidence of cerebral palsy. Lastly, patients who are small for gestational age contribute significantly to the number of patients with neonatal asphyxia, the neonatal neurologic syndrome, cerebral palsy, and neonatal seizures. Attempts to improve early recognition and possible intervention in pregnancies complicated by intrauterine growth retardation would potentially enhance the outcome in these patients.

REFERENCES

1. Freeman JM. Preface. In: Freeman JM, ed. Prenatal and perinatal factors associated with brain disorders. PHS, NIH Publication 85-1149. Washington, DC: Department of Health and Human Services, 1985.

2. Volpe JJ. Neurology of the newborn. 2nd ed. Philadelphia: WB Saunders, 1987.

3. Brann AW. Factors during neonatal life that influence brain disorders. In: Freeman JH, ed. Prenatal and perinatal factors associated with brain disorders. PHS, NIH Publication 85-1149. Washington, DC: Department of Health and Human Services, 1985:263.

4. Brann AW Jr. Hypoxic ischemic encephalopathy (asphyxia). Pediatr Clin North Am 1986; 33:451.

5. Little WJ. On the influence of abnormal parturition, difficult labours, premature birth, and asphyxia neonatorum on the mental and physical condition of the child especially in relation to deformities. Trans Obstet Soc London 1861–1862; 3:293.

6. Paneth N, Stark R. Mental retardation, cerebral palsy, and intrapartum asphyxia. In: Cohen WR, Friedman EA, eds. Management of labor. Baltimore: University Park Press, 1983:143.

7. Paneth N, Stark RI. Cerebral palsy and mental retardation in relation to indicators of perinatal asphyxia. An epidemiologic overview. Am J Obstet Gynecol 1983; 147:960.

8. Nelson KB, Ellenberg JH. Apgar scores as predictors of chronic neurologic disability. Pediatrics 1981; 68:38.

9. Nelson KB, Ellenberg JH. Antecedents of cerebral palsy. Multivariate analysis of risk. N Engl J Med 1986; 315:81.

10. Nelson KB, Ellenberg JH. Intrapartum events and cerebral palsy. In: Kubli F, Patel N, Schmidt W, Linderkamp O, eds. Perinatal events and brain damage in surviving children. Berlin: Springer-Verlag, 1988:139.

11. Apgar V. A proposal for a new method of evaluation of the newborn infant. Curr Res Anaesth Analg 1953; 32:260.

12. Apgar V, James LS. Further observations on the newborn scoring system. Am J Dis Child 1962; 104:419.

13. Scott H. Outcome of very severe birth asphyxia. Arch Dis Child 1976; 51:712.

14. Niswander KR, Gordon M. Collaborative perinatal study of the National Institute for Neurological Disease and Stroke. The women and their pregnancies. Vol I. Philadelphia: WB Saunders, 1972.

15. MacDonald HM, Mulligan JC, Allen AC, et al. Neonatal asphyxia. I. Relationship of obstetric and neonatal complications to neonatal mortality in 38,405 consecutive deliveries. J Pediatr 1980; 96:898.

16. Mulligan JC, Painter MJ, O'Donoghue PA, et al. Neonatal asphyxia. II. Neonatal mortality and long-term sequelae. J Pediatr 1980; 96:903.

17. Peters TJ, Golding J, Lawrence CJ, et al. Factors associated with delayed onset of regular respiration. Early Hum Dev 1984; 9:209.

18. Peters TJ, Golding J, Lawrence CJ, et al. Delayed onset of regular respiration and subsequent development. Early Hum Dev 1984; 9:225.

19. Meis PJ, Hall M III, Marshall JR, et al. Meconium passage: a new classification for risk assessment during labor. Am J Obstet Gynecol 1978; 131:509.

20. Nelson KB, Ellenberg JH. Obstetric complications as risk factors for cerebral palsy or seizure disorders. JAMA 1984; 251:1843.

21. Dijxhoorn MJ, Visser GHA, Huisjes HJ, et al. The relationship between pH values and neonatal neurological morbidity in full-term appropriate-for-dates infants. Early Hum Dev 1985; 11:33.

22. Dijxhoorn MJ, Visser GHA, Touwen BCL, et al. Apgar score, meconium and acidaemia at birth in small-for-gestational age infants born at term, and their relation to neonatal neurological morbidity. Br J Obstet Gynaecol 1987; 94:873.

23. Clifford SH. The effects of asphyxia on the newborn infant. J Pediatr 1941; 18:567.

24. Dawes GS. Foetal and neonatal physiology. Chicago: Year Book, 1968:141.

25. Myers RE. Two patterns of perinatal brain damage and their conditions of occurrence. Am J Obstet Gynecol 1972; 112:246.

26. Myers RE. Experimental models of perinatal brain damage: relevance to human pathology. In: Gluck L, ed. Intrauterine asphyxia and the developing fetal brain. Chicago: Year Book, 1977:37.

27. Brann AW Jr, Myers RE. Central nervous system findings in the newborn monkey following severe in-utero partial asphyxia. Neurology 1975; 25:327.

28. Sykes GS, Molloy PM, Johnson P, et al. Do Apgar scores indicate asphyxia? Lancet 1982; 1:494.

29. Silverman F, Surdan J, Wasserman J, et al. The Apgar score: is it enough? Obstet Gynecol 1985; 66:331.

30. Sarnat HB, Sarnat MS. Neonatal encephalopathy following fetal distress. A clinical and electroencephalographic study. Arch Neurol 1976; 33:696.

31. Robertson C, Finer N. Term infants with hypoxic-ischemic encephalopathy: outcome at 3-5 years. Dev Med Child Neurol 1985; 27:473.

32. Levene HL, Kornberg J, Williams THC. The incidence and severity of post-asphyxial encephalopathy in full-term infants. Early Hum Dev 1985; 11:21.

33. Nelson KB, Ellenberg JH. The asymptomatic newborn and risk of cerebral palsy. Am J Dis Child 1987; 141:1333.

34. Dennis J, Chalmers I. Very early neonatal seizure rate: a possible epidemiological indicator of the quality of perinatal care. Br J Obstet Gynaecol 1982; 89:418.

35. Derham RJ, Matthews TG, Clarke TA. Early seizures indicate quality of perinatal care. Arch Dis Child 1985; 60:809.

36. Holden KR, Mellits ED, Freeman JM. Neonatal seizures. 1. Correlation of prenatal and perinatal events with outcomes. Pediatrics 1982; 70:165.

37. Goldberg HJ. Neonatal convulsions—a 10 year review. Arch Dis Child 1983; 58:967.

38. Minchom P, Niswander K, Chalmers I, et al. Antecedents and outcome of very early neonatal seizures in infants born at or after term. Br J Obstet Gynaecol 1987; 94:431.

39. Grant A. The relationship between obstetrically preventable intrapartum asphyxia, abnormal neonatal neurological signs and subsequent motor impairment in babies born at or near term. In: Kubli F, Patel N, Schmidt W, Linderkamp O, eds. Perinatal events and brain damage in surviving children. Berlin: Springer-Verlag, 1988:149.

40. Levine MI, Trounce JQ. Cause of neonatal convulsions. Towards more precise diagnosis. Arch Dis Child 1986; 61:78.

41. Eriksson M, Zetterstrom R. Neonatal convulsions. Incidence and causes in the Stockholm area. Acta Paediatr Scand 1979; 68:807.

42. Niswander K, Elbourne D, Redman C, et al. Adverse outcome of pregnancy and the quality of obstetric care. Lancet 1984; 2:827.

43. MacDonald D, Grant A, Sheridan-Pereira M, et al. Dublin randomized controlled trial of intrapartum fetal heart rate monitoring. Am J Obstet Gynecol 1985; 152:524.

44. Keegan KA, Waffarn F, Quilligan EJ. Obstetric characteristics and fetal heart rate patterns of infants who convulse during the newborn period. Am J Obstet Gynecol 1985; 153:732.

45. Pharoah POD, Cooke T, Rosenbloom I, et al. Trends in birth prevalence of cerebral palsy. Arch Dis Child 1987; 62:379.

46. Hagberg B, Hagberg G, Olow I. The changing panorama of cerebral palsy in Sweden. IV. Epidemiological trends 1959–1978. Acta Paediatr Scand 1984; 73:433.

47. Stanley FJ, Watson LD. Cerebral palsy in Western Australia: trends, 1968–1981. Am J Obstet Gynecol 1988; 158:89.

48. Holm V. The causes of cerebral palsy—a contemporary perspective. JAMA 1982; 247:1473.

49. Blair E, Stanley FJ. Intrapartum asphyxia: a rare cause of cerebral palsy. J Pediatr 1988; 112:515.
50. Nelson KB. Cerebral palsy: what is known regarding cause? Ann NY Acad Sci 1986; 477:22.
51. Nelson KB. What proportion of cerebral palsy is related to birth asphyxia? J Pediatr 1988; 112:572 (editorial).
52. Hagberg B, Kyllerman M. Epidemiology and mental retardation—a Swedish survey. Brain Dev 1983; 5:441.
53. Quilligan E. Fetal monitoring: is it worth it? Obstet Gynecol 1976; 45:96.
54. Leveno KJ, Cunningham EG, Nelson S, et al. A prospective comparison of selective and universal electronic fetal monitoring in 34,995 pregnancies. N Engl J Med 1986; 315:615.
55. Prentice A, Lind T. Fetal heart rate monitoring during labour—too frequent intervention, too little benefit. Lancet 1987; 2:1375.
56. Freeman JM, Nelson KB. Intrapartum asphyxia and cerebral palsy. Pediatrics 1988; 82:240.
57. Dennis J. The long-term effects of intrapartum cerebral damage. In: Crawford JW, ed. Risks of labour. Chichester: John Wiley, 1985:157.
58. Neligan G, Prudham D, Steiner H. The formative years: birth, family and development in Newcastle-upon-Tyne. London: Oxford University Press, 1974.
59. Steiner N, Neligan G. Perinatal cardiac arrest. Quality of the survivors. Arch Dis Child 1975; 50:696.
60. Finer WN, Robertson CM, Richards RT, et al. Hypoxic-ischemic encephalopathy in term neonates: perinatal factors and outcome. J Pediatr 1981; 98:112.
61. Curtis PD, Matthews TG, Clarke TA, et al. Neonatal seizures: the Dublin collaborative study. Arch Dis Child 1988; 63:1065.

2

Preterm Labor and Intrauterine Growth Retardation: Complex Obstetrical Problems with Low Birth Weight Infants

Richard E. Besinger, M.D., John T. Repke, M.D., and James E. Ferguson II, M.D.

Obstetrical Aspects of Prematurity
Neonatal Aspects of Prematurity
Premature Rupture of Membranes
Preterm Labor
    Bed Rest, Hydration, and Sedation
    Beta-Mimetic Drugs
        Ritodrine
        Terbutaline
        Other Beta-Agonist Drugs
    Magnesium Sulfate
    Prostaglandin Synthetase Inhibitors
    Calcium Channel Blocking Drugs
    Combination Therapy
Intrauterine Growth Retardation

Low birth weight is a major contributor to perinatal morbidity and mortality in modern obstetrics. Approximately 80 percent of the perinatal deaths that occur in nonanomalous infants are directly related to prematurity. In the near-term infant, low birth weight as a sequela of intrauterine growth retardation (IUGR) is also a major contributor to perinatal morbidity and mortality. Although the classic definition of prematurity refers to birth weights less than 2,500 gm in births occurring prior to the 37th week of gestation, we use the term low birth weight in this chapter to describe infants who weigh less than 2,500 gm at birth regardless of gestational age. Very low birth weight infants typically are those weighing less than 1,500 gm at birth. This chapter focuses on the perinatal management of the "small baby" as a consequence of prematurity and IUGR.

Birth weight is influenced by a number of important factors in addition to gestational age, including race, parity, fetal sex, and other intrauterine environmental factors. Because of difficulties in accurately assigning gestational age, it is often difficult to determine the origins of a "small baby" whose mother presents in labor. In the absence of accurate gestational dating, the query of the practicing obstetrician is whether this small baby is actually preterm and appropriate for its gestational age or a near-term fetus who happens to be small-for-gestational-age secondary to IUGR. Since ultrasonography in later pregnancy is notoriously inaccurate in determining gestational age, early clinical and ultrasonic dating is mandatory if this clinical dilemma is to be resolved correctly.

The incidence of low birth weight and very low birth weight infants has remained fairly constant since 1950.[1] Approximately 75 in 1,000 live-born infants can be categorized as low birth weight, with an additional 11 in 1,000 live-borns weighing less than 1,500 gm. A slight decline in the incidence of low birth weight infants was noted in the 1970s, with the major improvement occurring in near-term, low birth weight infants.[2] Despite the relatively constant incidence of low birth weight infants over the past three decades, a significant improvement in neonatal mortality has been realized. In 1950 the neonatal mortality associated with low birth weight for this group of neonates approximated 20 in 1,000 live births, with corresponding figures in 1980 approaching 8 in 1,000 live births. This dramatic improvement in mortality figures is most likely attributable to the advent of intensive care for the compromised neonate.[1] However, this apparent clinical success is not without significant cost—more than $2 billion being spent in the United States for neonatal care in 1982.[3] Most of this expenditure has been earmarked for the treatment of low birth weight infants.

The most feared complications associated with the delivery of low birth weight infants are developmental disabilities. Such major handicaps as cerebral palsy and mental retardation, evidence of sensory impairment, or the more subtle findings of minimal cerebral dysfunction are the result of damage to the developing brain. Before the advent of neonatal intensive care, more than half the survivors with birth weights less than 1,500 gm were handicapped.[4] Consequently there has been concern that improving neonatal survival incidences for premature or low birth weight infants will result in the survival of more handicapped children. However, several reviews of the outcome in extremely premature infants born in recent decades do not confirm these concerns.[4-9] It appears that of the surviving extremely small neonates who received neonatal intensive care, fewer than 15 percent will have severe neurologic handicaps. Since the etiologies of these developmental disabilities are attributable to a complex array of antepartum, intrapartum, and neonatal factors, the major goal for the practicing obstetrician in the prevention of these maladies is to insure optimal conditions for the neonate at birth.

OBSTETRICAL ASPECTS OF PREMATURITY

Premature labor and preterm rupture of membranes (PROM) are major etiologic factors in preterm delivery. Although a variety of maternal diseases and complications occasionally necessitate obstetrical intervention at an early gestational age, noniatrogenic causes of preterm delivery make up the majority of the cases.[10] Reproducible maternal risk factors associated with preterm delivery include low socioeconomic status, nonwhite race, maternal age less than 18 years or greater than 40 years, low prepregnancy maternal weight, and smoking.[11]

The incidence of preterm birth correlates strongly with prior obstetrical outcome. A history of one preterm birth is associated with a risk of recurrence approximating 20 to 40 percent.[12] Several risk scoring systems based on historical and epidemiologic variables have been proposed to identify patients at risk for preterm delivery.[11,13] However, none of these systems has reached the level of discrimination necessary to be recommended for routine clinical use, and none is yet applicable for universal use in varying populations. Pregnancy complications such as placenta previa, placental abruption, polyhydramnios, multiple gestations, cervical incompetence, uterine malformation, and an anomalous fetus are associated with preterm delivery. A relationship between preterm delivery and coitus has been suggested in some studies.[14,15]

Approaches to the prevention of preterm birth have been widely varied in their focus. Since preterm labor and PROM are not mutually exclusive entities, prevention strategies generally have applied to both etiologic factors. Cervical cerclage has been advocated in the treatment of recurrent preterm losses, but its use for the prevention of preterm births should be restricted to patients with classic cervical incompetence. Two recent prospective randomized trials of cerclage for patients at high risk for preterm delivery failed to show any benefit from cervical cerclage.[16,17] Actually the theoretic risks of increased infection and increased uterine irritability could lead to an increased incidence of preterm delivery. The weekly use of 17-hydroxyprogesterone caproate (Delalutin) has been advocated as a prophylactic treatment for prematurity. Although several prospective studies suggest that the use of synthetic progesterones may prevent preterm delivery, the data remain controversial.[18-20] Similarly, the prophylactic use of standard tocolytic drugs in patients at high risk of preterm delivery has not been extensively evaluated. Preliminary studies with low doses of beta-mimetic drugs have failed to demonstrate any significant effect on prematurity incidences in singleton gestations,[21] whereas the prophylactic use of such tocolytic drugs in twin gestations may be more effective.[22]

Uterine activity prior to overt preterm labor may be an important predictor of preterm delivery. It has been demonstrated that women who progress into preterm labor have an increased frequency of uterine contractions beginning in the second trimester of pregnancy. With the advent of sophisticated ambulatory tocodynamometers, it may now be possible to identify prelabor uterine activity in patients at high risk for preterm delivery.[23,24] Such a system may be advantageous, since tocolytic therapy is more successful when preterm labor is recognized and treated early. However, several recent randomized trials comparing home monitoring systems and close nursing contact have failed to demonstrate an advantage in the use of such a home monitoring system.[25,26] Once uterine activity has been recognized, real-time evaluation of fetal breathing may identify individuals at risk for progressive preterm delivery.[27,28] In the absence of fetal breathing, preterm patients with uterine contractions are likely to progress into active labor and deliver within a short time. By contrast, when fetal breathing is recognized, the prospects for continuing the pregnancy are good.

Once preterm labor or PROM becomes manifest, treatment strategies revolve around the premise that a delay in delivery will allow for continued fetal maturation. Since an inverse relationship exists between survival incidence and gestational age, this decision seems prudent.[29] However, the risks of maternal sepsis, maternal reactions to tocolytic drugs, fetal sepsis, and intrauterine demise of the compromised fetus must be factored in any decision to delay delivery. Still, the potential benefits to be gained in terms of neonatal morbidity and mortality by delaying delivery are great, particularly between the gestational ages of 24 and 28 weeks.[30,31]

Once preterm delivery appears imminent, the obstetrician should consider glucocorticoids for the enhancement of fetal pulmonary maturity. Both animal studies and controlled prospective trials in humans have shown that antenatal steroid administration in selected populations reduces the incidence of respiratory distress syndrome (RDS) and the mortality incidence in infants delivered before 32 weeks.[32,33] To obtain maximal benefit from glucocorticoids, the infant must be delivered at least 24 hours after the first dose administered, must be of nonwhite race, and must be female. The beneficial effects appear to wear off seven days following treatment.[33] Dexamethasone and betamethasone are the usual medications of choice.

The major short-term side effects include the risk of pulmonary edema in mothers who are receiving tocolytic drugs and intravenous fluid therapy concurrently, as well as an increased incidence of maternal and neonatal infection. Another potential complication of maternal glucocorticoid administration is short-term impairment of glucose tolerance. Long-term follow-up of infants receiving intrauterine steroid therapy for enhancement of pulmonary maturity has failed to show impairment in physical, cognitive, and psychosocial development.[34] Recently, combined maternal administration of corticosteroids and thyroid releasing hormone has been advocated for the acceleration of fetal lung maturation.[35] Despite the apparent benefit in the use of corticosteroids, their universal clinical use remains controversial; improvement in the perinatal outcome following the administration of steroids may be highly dependent on the population in which it is utilized.

Once it appears that preterm delivery is imminent, the issue of intrapartum fetal heart rate monitoring must be considered. In general, the same criteria utilized during fetal heart rate monitoring to diagnose fetal distress in the term fetus are applicable to the preterm fetus.[36,37] Periodic fetal heart rate patterns and baseline variability can be used to predict umbilical artery pH's, but are in no way predictive of central nervous system hemorrhage, RDS, or neonatal death.[37] Any interpretation of fetal heart rate patterns must be tempered by considering the gestational age, the presence of chorioamnionitis, or the use of beta-mimetic tocolytic drugs.[36] An increased incidence of fetal distress is evident in patients with PROM and may represent the loss of the protection that amniotic fluid normally provides for the umbilical cord.[38] The clinical evidence suggests that the preterm infant can tolerate stress associated with normal labor and that a normal fetal heart rate pattern predicts a good fetal outcome in the absence of unrelated perinatal complications. In the presence of ominous fetal heart rate patterns, further intrapartum evaluation or prompt delivery is mandated. Despite these concerns over intrapartum fetal compromise as evidenced by fetal heart rate monitoring, a recent randomized intrapartum trial of electronic fetal heart rate monitoring during preterm labor showed no difference in outcome when compared with intermittent auscultation.[39]

The delivery route for the very low birth weight infant remains controversial. The lack of randomized prospective clinical trials addressing this issue makes any clinical recommendation concerning delivery route precarious. It is generally accepted that when preterm labor has begun and the fetus is in a cephalic presentation, cesarean section is not superior in terms of neonatal morbidity and mortality when compared with vaginal delivery.[40-44] It does not appear that survival or morbidity is influenced by the mode of delivery when the very low birth weight fetus is in a vertex presentation. The eventual neonatal outcome in this group of patients is more likely a consequence of gestational age rather than route of delivery. When the fetus is in a breech presentation, there may be an advantage to performing cesarean delivery if fetal viability is not an overwhelming issue.[41,44] Most studies suggest that vaginal breech delivery in this group of fetuses may be associated with increased perinatal morbidity. However, the conflicting information in the literature allows for significant individualized interpretation regarding the delivery route in the very low birth weight infant.

NEONATAL ASPECTS OF PREMATURITY

Once the preterm infant has been delivered, it is faced with the task of adapting to an extrauterine environment with organ systems that are physiologically immature. The main treatment goal of the practicing neonatologist is to provide supportive care so as to allow maturation of these organ systems. We have just begun to appreciate the developmental consequences of supporting immature organ systems, as well as the consequences of our therapeutic interventions.

RDS continues to be the most common clinical problem encountered in the preterm neonate. Its incidence varies inversely with gestational age, and there is a slight male preponderance.[45] The syndrome is characterized by progressive respiratory insufficiency with increasing oxygen demands, which appear within the first six hours of life.[45,46] It is the result of an inadequate amount or inadequate production of mature pulmonary surfactant.[47] Pulmonary surfactant decreases the surface tension within the alveolus and allows for the expansion of lung tissue. Lack of surfactant predisposes to atelectasis, hypoventilation, and a mismatch of ventilation and perfusion, which in turn leads to hypercarbia, hypoxia, and acidosis. Capillary endothelial damage with leakage of fibrin and formation of hyaline membranes as seen under microscopic examination represents the hallmark of the disease. The major surfactants in the fetal lung include phosphatidylcholine, phosphatidylinositol, and phosphatidylglycerol.[48] Phosphatidylcholine and sphingomyelin form the basis of the lecithin-sphingomyelin ratio, which, in addition to phosphatidylglycerol, can be measured in amniotic fluid.

The diagnosis of classic RDS can be difficult and at times is confirmed retrospectively. Roentgenographic evidence is confirmed by the presence of air bronchograms, a reduced lung volume, a ground glass appearance, and perhaps a total white-out of the neonatal chest x-ray features.[45]

The mainstay of management in neonates with RDS is aggressive respiratory support. Mild forms of the disease may require only oxygen administration by a head hood. However, ventilatory assistance with intermittent mechanical ventilation and continuous positive airway pressure may be required.[49] Careful fluid management, correction of acid-base abnormalities, and maintenance of adequate oxygenation must be attended to carefully. The use of diuretics has been shown to ameliorate the course of RDS.[50] Mechanical ventilation should be continued until maturation of surfactant occurs, usually within 72 hours after delivery. Oxygen administration should be monitored closely to prevent pulmonary oxygen toxicity, and the infant should be weaned from mechanical ventilation as rapidly as possible to prevent complications such as pneumothorax, pulmonary interstitial emphysema, or the development of chronic lung disease. In the very low birth weight infant, significant structural immaturity of the pulmonary tree and surfactant deficiency commonly coexist.[51] Recently human surfactant replacement in the preterm neonate has provided encouraging results and may further decrease the morbidity and mortality in this common neonatal condition.[52,53]

Patent ductus arteriosus is also a common entity in the premature infant. Its incidence is closely related to coexisting RDS. Patency of this vessel can be considered physiologically normal for this group of neonates, since the mechanisms of closure of the ductus arteriosus are immature.[54] A patent ductus arteriosus allows for a left to right shunt of cardiac output that leads to hyperperfusion of the lungs, pulmonary edema, decreased lung compliance, and subsequent alterations in pulmonary gas exchange. The clinical signs include bounding pulses, a systolic murmur, hyperdynamic cardiac function, and systemic hypoperfusion. The presence of a patent ductus arteriosus is commonly confirmed by Doppler echocardiography. Prostaglandin synthetase inhibitors are currently used to close a patent ductus arteriosus, but the very low birth weight infant may be refractile to such therapy.[55] Surgical ligation can be performed in infants when medical therapy has failed and when this is warranted by the current clinical status.[56]

Unfortunately intraventricular hemorrhage (IVH) is a frequent event in the preterm infant. The overall incidence is inversely related to gestational age and has been reported to occur in 40 to 60 percent of infants with gestational ages less than 34 weeks.[57] Risk factors for the development of IVH include asphyxia, hypoxia, acidosis, anemia, and severe RDS.[58,59] Current hypotheses in regard to the pathogenesis revolve around the reported lack of connective tissue supporting the germinal matrix blood vessels, impaired autoregulation of cerebral blood flow, and hypoxia-induced capillary damage to the periventricular capillaries.[59]

Clinically, IVH should be suspected in a preterm neonate with the acute onset of acidosis, hypotension, and hypoventilation and a drop in the hematocrit reading. The presence of IVH can be confirmed easily by ultrasonic studies of the neonatal cranium through the fontanelles. IVH has been described in isolated cases prior to birth but commonly becomes manifest within the first 48 hours of life. A grading system has been proposed. Grade I signifies subependymal hemorrhage only; grade II, IVH without ventricular dilatation; grade III, IVH with ventricular dilatation; and grade IV, IVH with parenchymal hemorrhage.[60] Posthemorrhagic hydrocephalus is found in approximately 20 percent of the patients with severe IVH.[57] The poorest neurologic outcome is observed in infants with grade III and IV disease.[61-63]

The treatment is directed at preventing further compression of blood flow in the periventricular brain matter. Serial lumbar punctures, diuretics, and osmotic drugs have been advocated in the presence of IVH with ventricular dilatation.[59] In cases of persistent or severe ventriculomegaly, a ventricular peritoneal shunt may be required.

The etiology of IVH is probably multifactorial but is clearly related to prematurity. The role of hypoxia in utero and the mode of delivery as contributing factors is still undefined. The primary goal for obstetricians should be to prevent IVH in patients at risk. Recently the antenatal administration of phenobarbital has been shown to decrease the incidence of IVH in infants at risk.[64]

Thermal regulation is also a considerable problem for the extremely premature neonate. The preterm infant is poorly equipped to generate heat because of its lack of glycogen and brown fat reserves. The relative lack of subcutaneous fat and the increased surface area in these neonates are also contributing factors. Hypothermia can produce hypoglycemia, metabolic acidosis, and an increased requirement for oxygen. Therefore, it is mandatory that close monitoring of the infant's response to its thermal environment be included in all treatment of the preterm neonate.

The development of hyperbilirubinemia in the preterm infant is extremely common because of hepatic immaturity, increased enterohepatic circulation of bilirubin, and a decreased red blood cell survival incidence. Treatment is critical in preterm infants because of the greater tendency to develop kernicterus than term infants. Kernicterus may develop in the presence of low levels of free and total bilirubin, suggesting the relative immaturity of the blood-brain barrier. Risk factors associated with hyperbilirubinemia include hypoalbuminemia, hypothermia, hypoxia, and sepsis. Treatment is directed toward prevention with the early use of phototherapy. In addition, exchange transfusion may be required.

Apnea, defined as the lack of spontaneous respiration for longer than 15 seconds, occurs frequently in the preterm infant.[65] The idiopathic apnea of prematurity is probably due to the relative immaturity of the brainstem. Although it is commonly present after birth, the onset of apnea in a previously stable infant may reflect the onset of sepsis, acidosis, or pulmonary dysfunction. Therapy includes tactile stimulation, assisted ventilation, and the administration of methylxanthines to improve the sensitivity of the neonatal respiratory center to carbon dioxide.[65]

Necrotizing enterocolitis is an acute inflammatory disease of the gastrointestinal tract observed in the extremely unstable preterm infant. Infants at risk include those experiencing acidosis, hypoxia, or hypotension, the presence of an umbilical catheter, and the early onset of oral or tube feedings.[66] Typically the infant develops emesis, feeding residuals, abdominal distention, and frank or occult blood in the stool.[67] Signs of sepsis, apnea, and bradycardia are also present. Shock and disseminated intravascular coagulation may occur.[67] Abdominal x-ray findings can be pathognomonic when a pattern of ileus, pneumatosis intestinalis, or evidence of perforation is present.

Once a diagnosis has been made, intravenous fluid support, antibiotics, and close monitoring should be initiated. Feedings should be discontinued whenever necrotizing enterocolitis is being considered as a potential problem. Otherwise, supportive measures with parenteral nutrition, serum and blood replacement, and the use of pressor drugs may be required. Surgical intervention is indicated in cases of intestinal perforation.

The pathogenesis of necrotizing enterocolitis is probably related to hypoperfusion of the bowel and the presence of pathogenic organisms in the neonatal intestine.[66] Low blood flow to the mesenteric vessels occurs in the presence of compromised cardiac output, hypoxia, or acidemia. This allows for mucosal injury and predisposes to bacterial proliferation within the bowel wall. Eventually a cascade of endotoxemia, perforation, and disseminated intravascular coagulation occurs.[68] Once again, prevention is the best approach to necrotizing enterocolitis. Prevention of acidosis and hypoxia and withholding of feedings in the compromised preterm infant significantly decrease the incidence of this disease.[67] With the advent of total parenteral nutrition, withholding of oral feedings in the compromised infant is prudent.

Chronic complications as a consequence of prematurity have been described as more premature neonates overcome their acute problems. Bronchopulmonary dysplasia can be present in infants who have received prolonged mechanical ventilation and oxygen supplementation.[69] Clinically bronchopulmonary dysplasia is characterized by tachypnea and hypoventilation. It is the result of increased airway resistance, decreased pulmonary compliance, intrapulmonary shunting, and a persistent oxygen requirement. Chest x-ray films commonly demonstrate emphysematous and atelectatic changes. The incidence of this complication is estimated to be 3 to 8 percent in infants with severe RDS.[70] Its pathophysiology probably lies in continuous exposure to oxygen and mechanical ventilation, which prove toxic to the respiratory epithelium.

Impaired phagocytosis of the hyaline membranes present in the RDS produces squamous metaplasia of the respiratory epithelium and peribronchial muscle hypertrophy. This leads to local fibrosis and eventual obliterative disease of the bronchial tree. If continuous lung damage occurs, interstitial fibrosis, bullous emphysema, and pulmonary hypertension may become persistent problems. It is reasonable to consider this chronic lung disease as a multifactorial disease caused by pulmonary immaturity, primary parenchymal disease, oxygen toxicity, barotrauma, and possibly infectious etiologies. Prevention remains the best treatment, by reducing oxygen supplementation and ventilator pressures when clinically possible.[71] Once chronic lung disease has developed, treatment is symptomatic and includes oxygen support, positive pressure ventilation as necessary, and diuretics in cases of pulmonary hypertension.

Retinopathy of prematurity is still a chronic problem despite recent restrictions on oxygen supplementation in the premature infant.[72] The pathogenesis of this disease is probably related to immature vascular development of the retina, since retinopathy of prematurity persists despite careful monitoring of oxygen levels.[73] The amount of cicatricial retinopathy subsequently determines the degree of visual handicap.[74] Minimal disease is usually correctable by lenses to correct myopia. However, significant retinopathy can result in the severe vision disturbances. If retinal detachment is extensive, the visual handicap can be profound. Ophthalmologic examination of all premature infants exposed to oxygen is recommended.

Although mortality data relating to the care of the premature neonate are easily obtained, the changing incidence of morbidity with improved neonatal care is less readily determined at this time. Severe medical complications, including cerebral palsy, mental retardation, chronic lung disease, and retinopathy of prematurity, occur in a small proportion of survivors, but the proportion of infants with lesser morbidity, such as minimal cerebral dysfunction, learning disabilities, and other postneonatal deficiencies, is less clearly defined. Once again, it needs to be emphasized that the obstetrician's goal in the treatment of preterm labor is to delay delivery if indicated, or if delivery is unavoidable to provide the neonatologist with an infant in optimal condition so as to minimize these complications.

PRETERM RUPTURE OF MEMBRANES

PROM is commonly defined as the leakage of amniotic fluid through the cervix beginning prior to the onset of labor in gestations prior to 37 weeks.[75,76] Once a patient presents with a history of uncontrolled leakage of fluid through the vagina, a sterile speculum examination for confirmation of PROM is mandatory. The presence of gross amniotic fluid in the vagina, an alkaline pH in the normally acidotic vagina, and microscopic ferning when this vaginal fluid is air dried are all confirmatory findings.[77] The presence of bleeding, meconium, or seminal fluid can negate the usefulness of these clinical tests.[78] Digital examination should not be performed because of the increased risk of infection unless delivery is anticipated in the immediate future.[79] Ultrasonic evaluation of the amniotic fluid may be useful when findings on clinical examination of the vagina are equivocal. Intra-amniotic injection of Evan's blue dye or indigo carmine dye during amniocentesis can be utilized to confirm or rule out the diagnosis of PROM.

The etiology of PROM is unknown at this time. It has been suggested that alterations in collagen content in the amniotic membranes may predispose to this entity.[80] Women who experience PROM have also been shown to have lower serum copper and zinc levels, which may be important in regulating and maintaining collagen.[81] A more important etiologic factor is probably the presence of subclinical infection and an abnormal proteolytic response.[82] That a large number of patients with PROM and preterm labor experience chorioamnionitis,[83] that repeated vaginal examinations may predispose to PROM,[84] and that significant numbers of pathogens are commonly isolated in patients with PROM support this view.[85,86] Group B *Streptococcus, Ureaplasma, Mycoplasma, Chlamydia*, and a variety of anaerobic species have been implicated. The prophylactic use of erythromycin in patients with documented *Ureaplasma-Mycoplasma* colonization appears to reduce prematurity incidences. Still, the association between PROM and infection remains poorly delineated. However, an approximate 20 percent recurrence incidence in cases of PROM suggests that recurring infection may be responsible.[87]

The clinical dilemma for the practicing obstetrician in PROM is balancing maternal risks of infection against fetal risks of immaturity and sepsis. Clinical chorioamnionitis usually can be diagnosed by the presence of maternal fever, a purulent vaginal discharge, uterine tenderness, leukocytosis, and positive bacterial cultures.

Although bacteremia, sepsis, and septic shock can occur, most cases of maternal chorioamnionitis respond well to delivery of the infected fetus and membranes, along with the intravenous administration of antibiotics.[88] However, the diagnosis of subclinical chorioamnionitis can be difficult, and several clinicians recently have recommended amniocentesis for culture and fetal lung maturity studies in these troublesome cases.[89,90] However, since reaccumulation of amniotic fluid is absent in a majority of these patients, the practicality of this technique may be limited.[91]

The main risk to the preterm fetus in the presence of PROM remains prematurity. In fetuses with suspected pulmonary immaturity, it is prudent to delay delivery as long as possible.[92-94] In PROM prior to 36 weeks, labor ensues in approximately 80 percent of the patients within 48 hours after rupture of membranes. The latency period exceeds two weeks in only 10 to 15 percent of pregnancies. However, if PROM occurs prior to 28 weeks, the average latency period can be as long as three weeks.[92] Latency periods tend to be longer and the risk of infection less in pregnancies characterized by the reaccumulation of amniotic fluid.[95] It has been demonstrated in multiple studies that delaying delivery in the presence of PROM for only 24 to 48 hours produces a lower incidence of RDS, suggesting that surfactant production is stimulated in these fetuses.[96,97] For this reason a short-term course of tocolytic therapy for 24 to 48 hours in patients without overt chorioamnionitis may be appropriate in order to maximize fetal lung function.

Other fetal complications include developmental abnormalities when PROM occurs in gestations prior to 26 weeks. Specifically, pulmonary hypoplasia can be a significant risk when extreme oligohydramnios is present prior to 26 weeks.[98] Skeletal deformities related to compression of the fetus are also common during prolonged PROM.[99] When PROM occurs prior to 25 weeks' gestation, the likelihood of neonatal survival is low.[98] Approximately 25 percent of these fetuses may survive the neonatal period with significant morbidity. Other risks to the fetus associated with PROM include occult or frank cord prolapse and a higher incidence of fetal distress in the presence of labor as a result of cord compression.

Congenital infections and sepsis can develop in fetuses when chorioamnionitis is present. Fetuses can respond to intrauterine infection with tachycardia and exhibit nonreassuring fetal heart rate patterns and decreased biophysical activity.[100,101] Despite concern about the effects of chorioamnionitis on neonates, long-term follow-up in exposed preterm infants has failed to demonstrate significant developmental abnormalities attributable to chorioamnionitis alone.[102] Recently several studies have shown that nonstress fetal heart rate testing and biophysical profile testing can be used to predict early chorioamnionitis and allow for timely intervention.[100,101] Early intervention in these cases theoretically will allow for an improved outcome and earlier treatment of the septic fetus.

Management of PROM remains one of the most controversial areas in obstetrics.[103] Any management decision must involve weighing the risks of PROM to the mother and undelivered fetus against the risk of prematurity to an immature neonate. The presence or absence of PROM must be established with certainty by the practitioner. Once a confirmatory sterile vaginal examination has been performed and cervical cultures have been obtained, a real-time ultrasound examination to confirm dates and relative oligohydramnios should be performed. If a free flowing vaginal sample of amniotic fluid can be obtained, this should be sent for lecithin-sphingomyelin ratio and phosphatidylglycerol determinations. If a gestational age prior to 35 weeks is suspected and fetal pulmonary function either by vaginal sampling or subsequent amniocentesis remains immature, conservative management should be considered. If the gestational age is greater than 35 weeks or mature fetal lung parameters exist, plans for delivery should be considered. The undelivered patient should be monitored carefully for impending chorioamnionitis with serial maternal temperature readings, examinations for uterine tenderness, and serial white blood cell counts. Amniocentesis for culture or serial use of C-reactive protein analysis should be considered to evaluate patients suspected of having asymptomatic chorioamnionitis. Serial fetal heart rate strips and biophysical profiles may be helpful in identifying impending chorioamnionitis. Delivery should be contemplated whenever progressive labor, overt chorioamnionitis, or fetal compromise becomes evident.

The use of maternally administered corticosteroids in the presence of PROM has been suggested by some clinicians. However, prospective randomized studies comparing steroid therapy and timed delivery after 48 hours with expectant management demonstrate no apparent clinical benefit from steroid administration.[104,105] These studies also suggest an increased risk of neonatal sepsis and postpartum endometritis in pregnant patients receiving steroids ante partum. There is no evidence to suggest abnormal cognitive development in school children exposed to antenatal steroid therapy.[106]

Another area of controversy is the use of tocolytic drugs in the presence of PROM. Classically obstetricians have been reluctant to utilize tocolytic drugs in these patients because they may mask clinical evidence of chorioamnionitis. However, there are data suggesting that pregnancies in which short-term tocolytic therapy is used may exhibit a decreased incidence and severity of neonatal RDS. However, recent long-term studies using oral tocolytic therapy in a randomized fashion failed to demonstrate significant improvement in the neonatal outcome or extension of the latency period following PROM.[107-109]

The use of antibiotics in the presence of PROM is also controversial. There is a paucity of data in this area, and the effectiveness of in utero treatment or prophylaxis of chorioamnionitis remains unknown. It is generally recommended that women with chorioamnionitis who are in labor be treated with antibiotics. However, recent studies utilizing either intravenous therapy or intra-amniotic instillation of antibiotics suggest that this approach to PROM may be reasonable.[110,111]

PRETERM LABOR

The identification and treatment of preterm labor illustrate one of the central dilemmas in obstetrics today. For the practicing obstetrician it is often difficult to justify the use of heroic intervention to prevent a preterm birth when a controlled preterm delivery with subsequent care of the neonate might be better. Such heroic intervention with powerful tocolytic medications appears to have an insignificant effect on the incidence of general low birth weight in a variety of populations,[112,113] but may benefit the appropriately selected patient. Even if an ideal inhibitor of preterm labor were available, the maximal reduction of preterm delivery would only be 10 to 20 percent because most patients are not candidates for tocolysis. Medical and obstetrical contraindications to tocolytic therapy preclude the use of these drugs in many patients. However, the use of beta-adrenergic drugs to prolong gestation appears to be effective in lowering the combined maternal and neonatal medical costs of treating preterm labor prior to 34 weeks' gestation.[114]

Multiple factors are thought to be involved in the initiation of human preterm labor. Prostaglandins, catecholamines, increased formation of gap junctions, premature cervical maturation, alterations in estrogen-progesterone ratios, and changes in uterine blood flow have all been implicated in the initiation of preterm labor.[115] Preterm labor is also associated with identifiable maternal conditions, such as abruptio placentae, uterine anomaly, polyhydramnios, multiple gestations, and subclinical chorioamnionitis.[116-119] Since the triggering event of preterm labor is usually unknown, the therapy is therefore empiric in nature.

The most widely used definition for preterm labor is the presence of six to eight uterine contractions per hour associated with documented cervical change. There is inherent difficulty in diagnosing true preterm labor, since a placebo response approximating 20 to 50 percent is observed in cases of threatened preterm labor.[120] Various parameters are used for measuring the success of tocolytic therapy, including birth weight, short-term and long-term delays in delivery, and perinatal survival incidences. However, evaluation of the efficacy of tocolytic drugs is difficult because cervical dilatation and gestational age at the start of treatment differ from patient to patient. It appears that tocolysis success incidences are inversely related to the degree of cervical dilatation. Therefore, only randomized, controlled clinical trials can be used to prove the efficacy of drugs given to inhibit preterm labor.

In 1980 the United States Food and Drug Administration approved ritodrine hydrochloride for the inhibition of preterm labor. Of all the tocolytic drugs discussed in this chapter, this is the only one approved so far, and the other drugs should be considered experimental. However, the use of approved drugs for nonlabelled indications is entirely appropriate when effectiveness has been reported extensively in the medical literature. The apparent lack of an ideal tocolytic drug has led to widespread use of a variety of medications in the treatment of preterm labor.

Certain criteria must be fulfilled before a patient is considered a candidate for attempted pharmacologic arrest of preterm labor. Reported gestational ages through which preterm labor should be stopped vary from 20 to 36 weeks, with corresponding estimated fetal weights of 500 to 2,500 gm. At each institution the survival incidences in the neonatal nursery at each specific gestational age should be known and compared with the risk of attempted tocolysis. Ultrasonography is indicated if the gestational age is uncertain and particularly if IUGR is suspected. If fetal lung maturity is in question, amniocentesis to document pulmonary maturity should be considered. The presence of a live fetus without life-threatening anomalies should also be assured. Obstetrical contraindications to tocolysis include preeclampsia, suspected IUGR, placental abruption, fetal distress, and chorioamnionitis. It is important to realize that initiation of tocolysis may be hazardous rather than protective to the fetus in an unfavorable uterine environment. The initial measures recommended when tocolysis is indicated are noted in Table 2–1.

Let us look at the pharmacologic measures in clinical use today for the inhibition of preterm labor.

TABLE 2–1   Initial Measures Recommended When Tocolysis Is Initiated

Bed rest
Admission weight
Baseline vital signs
Sterile speculum examination to exclude
    rupture of membranes
Intravenous access line
Continuous fetal monitoring for fetal heart
    rate and contractions
Aerobic cervical culture
Electrocardiogram
Ultrasonography
Laboratory studies
    Complete blood count
    Electrolyte levels
    Glucose level
    Urinalysis

Bed Rest, Hydration, and Sedation

In a significant percentage of patients with suspected preterm labor, uterine contractions subside with bed rest, hydration, and sedation. In a recent nonrandomized study of this phenomenon, 55 percent of the patients responded to this pretherapy, while 45 percent required tocolytic therapy.[120] Medications such as narcotics and barbiturates do not relax the myometrium and may actually cause an oxytocic effect.[121] Since these drugs can cause central nervous system depression and respiratory difficulties in the preterm infant if given prior to delivery, they should be used judiciously. A one-hour observation period prior to initiating tocolytic therapy should be used if the criteria for the diagnosis of preterm labor have not been met. Intravenous hydration during this period should not exceed 500 cc, since its only purposes are to prevent ketosis, ensure adequate maternal intravascular volume, and improve uteroplacental blood flow in anticipation of tocolytic therapy. Further hydration may predispose to the development of pulmonary edema and ultimately may delay the administration of tocolytic drugs.

Beta-Mimetic Drugs

A variety of beta-adrenergic drugs are used for preterm labor. Irrespective of the drug used, the obstetrician must have a thorough knowledge of beta-adrenergic effects in order to use these powerful drugs safely. Beta-adrenergic agonists act on intermembranous beta receptors in a variety of cells, which activate the enzyme adenylcyclase and cause an increase in intracellular cyclic AMP levels.[122] The increased level of cyclic AMP initiates a series of cellular reactions that reduce intracellular calcium levels, thereby decreasing the sensitivity of the myosin-actin contractile unit in the uterus. These receptors are also found in the heart, small intestine, adipose tissue, uterus, blood vessels, bronchioles, and diaphragm. Therefore, intravenous administration of the beta-mimetic drug can stimulate beta receptors in multiple organ systems and is ultimately responsible for the clinically significant side effects associated with these medications.[122] Most common are maternal cardiovascular side effects such as hypotension, tachycardia, and arrhythmia.[123,124] The activation of vascular beta-adrenergic receptors leads to vasodilatation, resulting in diastolic hypotension. This produces a reflex compensatory increase in the heart rate, stroke volume, and cardiac output and increases the systolic blood pressure.[125] Because of concern about cardiac stimulation, such therapy is contraindicated in patients with cardiac disease.

Cardiac arrhythmias have also been reported with these drugs.[124] Arrhythmias commonly reported include supraventricular tachycardia, atrial fibrillation, atrial premature contractions, and ventricular ectopy. Therefore, a careful cardiac history should be taken and screening electrocardiography performed to rule out underlying cardiac irregularities prior to initiation of this therapy.

Beta-mimetic drugs also may increase the risk of myocardial ischemia because they increase myocardial muscle oxygen consumption by increasing the heart rate and myocardial contractility.[126] Although chest pain is a relatively common symptom associated with these drugs, only a few investigators have reported electrocardiographic changes indicative of myocardial ischemia. Transient ST segment depression is the most common observation and appears to be dose related with resolution occurring after discontinuation of therapy.[125,126] Clinical evidence suggests that inadequate coronary blood flow may be responsible. Despite these concerns and clinical observations, there has never been evidence of myocardial damage as shown by elevated cardiac enzyme levels or cardiac-specific myoglobin.[127]

As the clinical use of these drugs has become more widespread, it has become evident that pulmonary edema during tocolytic therapy is a major life-threatening complication.[125,128] This complication has been observed in up to 5 percent of the patients receiving intravenous beta-mimetic therapy.[125] It occurs with and without concurrent maternal glucocorticoid therapy for fetal lung maturation. Multiple gestations, anemia, hypertension, and the need for blood transfusions are risk factors for the development of pulmonary edema. The pathophysiology of this serious complication is not well understood but does not appear to be related to cardiac failure. Several investigators suggest that increased pulmonary capillary permeability and fluid overload may be responsible. Significant salt and water retention secondary to the effects of beta-mimetic therapy on kidney function has been described.[129] Infection is a leading cause of lung injury in adults and may be another reason for the increase in pulmonary capillary permeability observed in patients with preterm labor. If pulmonary edema becomes evident, the tocolytic medication should be discontinued, oxygen should be administered, and attempts to effect a diuresis should be undertaken. Ventilatory support and invasive arterial blood gas monitoring may be required. Careful input and output monitoring, minimal pretherapy hydration, and frequent chest examinations may lessen the risk of developing this life-threatening complication.

The other major category of complications associated with these beta-mimetic medications is metabolic in nature. Alterations in maternal glucose, insulin, potassium, and lactic acid metabolism have been described.[125,130–132] Parenteral administration of these medications results in an acute rise in the plasma glucose concentration and is probably mediated by pancreatic stimulation to secrete glucagon.[130,131] Concurrent insulin release also occurs and parallels the level of induced hyperglycemia.[132] With these alterations hypokalemia develops as a direct result of hyperglycemia and hyperinsulinemia. These medications do not appear to increase urinary potassium excretion or alter aldosterone-mediated potassium urinary loss.[131]

In addition to intracellular migration of potassium due to alterations in glucose-insulin metabolism, these drugs may have a direct effect on the membranous sodium-potassium ion pump. Since the total body potassium is not decreased with beta-mimetic therapy, potassium replacement therapy is rarely necessary. However, it should be considered when serum levels are low prior to initiation of therapy, when a cardiac arrhythmia is present, or when a potassium wasting diuretic has been administered. These medications also lead to glycogenolysis and lipolysis, which result in increased lactate production without significant changes in the maternal pH.[132]

Because of these metabolic alterations induced with beta-adrenergic drugs, their use in known insulin-dependent diabetics is controversial.[133] The significant metabolic alterations seem to parallel the severity of insulin deficiency in these patients, and it may be prudent to avoid these medications in this population. However, careful control of glucose can be obtained with concurrent intravenous insulin administration and careful monitoring of metabolic parameters.

Other maternal effects described with these drugs include increased maternal transaminase elevations, paralytic ileus, cerebral vasospasm in patients with a history of migraine syndrome, and respiratory arrest in those with myasthenia gravis.

Placental transfer of these beta-mimetic drugs is rapid and induces a similar beta-adrenergic response in the fetus.[134] Heart rate elevation is common and is presumed to be secondary to direct beta-receptor stimulation in the fetal heart. Metabolic alterations are also a concern, and reactive hypoglycemia after birth may not be an uncommon occurrence. However, there is no evidence of induced hypokalemia or alterations in the fetal acid-base status attributable to these medications.[135] Tocolytic therapy should be discontinued once cervical dilatation of 4 to 5 cm has been obtained. It is prudent to discontinue medications at that time, since this minimizes the risk of significant neonatal drug levels.

Alterations in uteroplacental blood flow have been described with these drugs, with varying results. Although some investigators report an increase in uteroplacental blood flow,[136] others report a decrease.[137] These conflicting results are probably due to differences in the drugs used, the duration of infusion of medication, the concurrent use of sedation or anesthesia, and the method of blood flow determination. For the most part, changes in uteroplacental blood flow secondary to beta-mimetic drugs are not associated with clinically significant alterations in fetal hemodynamics.

Depression of the fetal central nervous system as manifested by Apgar scores has not been reported with any of these medications.[138] Likewise, no significant alteration of the umbilical pH at the time of delivery has been described with beta-mimetic therapy.[135] Long-term developmental evaluation of infants exposed to these drugs in utero has been reported.[139-142] The developmental progress assessed after one to nine years does not significantly differ from the progress observed in preterm control subjects. No significant alterations in growth, head circumference, neurologic development, or psychomotor or social development have been associated with these medications. An interesting benefit in utilizing these tocolytic drugs is that their administration has been associated with a decreased incidence of RDS.[143,144] This phenomenon appears to be the result of increased release of surfactant, as opposed to increased production prior to birth.

The development of tolerance to the metabolic and cardiovascular side effects of beta-adrenergic drugs has been well documented. Because of this biologic phenomenon of receptor desensitization, some investigators suggest that the capacity of these tocolytic drugs to arrest premature labor may be only transitory.[145] Let us look more specifically at the efficacy and potential side effects with each beta-mimetic drug used in clinical practice today.

Ritodrine

In 1980 the United States FDA approved ritodrine hydrochloride for the inhibition of preterm labor. That decision culminated more than 10 years of clinical research with ritodrine in the United States by various investigators employing different clinical protocols at a variety of medical centers.

The first prospective double-blind, placebo-controlled study of ritodrine was performed in Europe as a multicenter trial in 1971.[146] Preterm delivery was delayed for at least seven days in 80 percent of the ritodrine group and in 48 percent of the placebo group. In 1972 a series of prospective randomized, double-blind studies compared ritodrine with ethanol or placebo at a variety of medical centers throughout the United States.[147,148] A total of 313 singleton patients were studied, and this constituted the phase III clinical trials for the FDA approval process. Statistically significant prolongation of preterm pregnancy was shown with ritodrine when compared with alcohol and placebo controls. This study also showed that the offspring of ritodrine-treated mothers demonstrated a significantly reduced incidence of neonatal death and RDS. There also was a significantly higher incidence in those reaching 36 weeks of gestation or exhibiting birth weights greater than 2,500 gm.

Subsequent randomized clinical trials examining the efficacy of ritodrine have produced contradictory results. In one study involving 29 patients receiving parenteral doses of ritodrine or placebo, there was no significant extension of pregnancy or increased birth weight.[149] In another comparison 129 patients in preterm labor received three different regimens of ritodrine administration; 44 patients receiving placebo and bed rest failed to demonstrate any difference in delay of delivery, birth weight, or neonatal mortality.[150] Several other recent studies have raised similar questions regarding the efficacy of ritodrine in the treatment of preterm labor.[151,152]

In comparative studies involving terbutaline and ritodrine for the arrest of preterm labor, it appeared that the intravenous administration of these drugs produced comparable results.[153,154] Similarly, several short-term comparison studies of ritodrine and intravenous doses of magnesium sulfate also showed no statistical difference in the incidence of success with tocolytic therapy.[153,155,156]

Oral maintenance therapy with ritodrine appears to be successful in preventing recurrent preterm labor and allows for ambulatory management of these patients. In one study involving 60 patients who received either oral doses of ritodrine for maintenance or placebo, there was a significant difference in the mean interval from initiation of therapy to the first relapse or delivery; in patients receiving maintenance ritodrine therapy this first relapse occurred at 25.9 days as compared with 5.8 days in the placebo group.[157] A comparison study of oral doses of terbutaline and oral doses of ritodrine in maintenance therapy suggested that oral maintenance with terbutaline may be more effective.[154]

Ritodrine is usually given intravenously at a rate of 50 μg per minute, and the dose is increased every 20 minutes until uterine contractions have ceased, unacceptable side effects have developed, or a maximal dose of 350 μg per minute has been achieved. After uterine contractions have stopped, the intravenous dosage is reduced to the lowest infusion rate that will allow for continued uterine quiescence and that rate is maintained for 12 to 24 hours. Maternal intravenous infusion of ritodrine reaches therapeutic levels quickly with an initial phase half-life of six to nine minutes followed by a biphasic elimination phase with a half-life of two to three hours.[147,154] Ritodrine is excreted in a free conjugated form primarily in the urine. There is a rapid and appreciable transplacental transfer of the intravenous ritodrine dose, with a mean fetal-to-maternal concentration ratio of 1.17.[158] Once maternal administration of ritodrine has been discontinued, ritodrine levels in the umbilical cord at delivery remain significant for up to five hours.[159] Therefore, once tocolysis has failed and delivery is imminent, intravenous ritodrine therapy should be discontinued to minimize neonatal drug levels.

Oral maintenance with ritodrine is initiated with either 10 mg every two hours or 20 mg every four hours.

Most clinicians find that monitoring of the maternal pulse can be used to titrate the oral dose required for adequate tocolysis, as evidenced by a maternal pulse rate of more than 100 beats per minute or 20 percent above baseline. Although metabolic alterations with oral doses appear to be minimal, maternal and fetal cardiovascular responses to oral administration remain significant.[160]

Despite the lack of clinical evidence that ritodrine is more effective than any other tocolytic drug or that it is associated with a lower incidence of maternal and fetal side effects, ritodrine remains the only FDA-approved drug for tocolytic therapy in the United States today.

Terbutaline

Terbutaline also can inhibit uterine contractions and has been shown to be effective in treating preterm labor. In the first double-blind placebo-controlled study, reported in 1976, 30 patients received intravenous therapy for at least eight hours, maintenance subcutaneous therapy being continued until 36 weeks.[161] Eighty percent of the terbutaline-treated patients achieved 36 weeks' gestation, whereas only 20 percent of the placebo-treated patients achieved a similar gestational age. A similar double-blind, placebo-controlled study failed to show any efficacy with terbutaline.[162] In comparison studies with ethanol, intravenous terbutaline therapy yielded a mean prolongation of pregnancy of 15 days as compared with 10 days in the ethanol group.[163] Comparison studies of terbutaline and magnesium have demonstrated similar tocolytic efficacy.[153,164,165]

Terbutaline is given intravenously at a rate of 10 μg per minute, and the dose is increased every 20 minutes until contractions have ceased, unacceptable side effects develop, or a maximal dose of 25 μg per minute has been achieved. Maternal infusion of terbutaline reaches therapeutic levels rapidly, with a mean terminal half-life of 3.7 hours.[166] Both free and conjugated forms of terbutaline are excreted in the urine, and significant variations in serum concentrations have been noted. In view of this finding, terbutaline infusion should be titrated on an individual basis to maximize uterine inhibition and minimize maternal side effects. There is rapid transplacental transfer of terbutaline, with maternal-fetal equilibration after one hour.[166] Therefore, once preterm delivery seems inevitable, intravenous terbutaline therapy should be discontinued to minimize neonatal levels of the drug.

Subcutaneous administration of terbutaline has been advocated as an alternative to intravenous infusion.[167] Terbutaline is rapidly absorbed after subcutaneous administration, with an absorptive half-life of seven minutes. A commonly used regimen is 0.25 mg given subcutaneously every 20 to 60 minutes until contractions subside. A randomized comparison of intravenous and subcutaneous administration of terbutaline has revealed similar efficacies and side effects.[168] The ease of administration and avoidance of intravenous hydration make subcutaneous administration a reasonable alternative to intravenous therapy.

Parenteral administration of terbutaline can be continued for 12 to 24 hours after uterine activity has ceased. Thereafter, oral maintenance therapy should be begun with 2.5 to 5 mg given every four to six hours. Once again, this dose can be titrated by monitoring the maternal pulse rate.

Maternal side effects are similar with either terbutaline or ritodrine. Most randomized comparison studies show no difference in the incidence of tachycardia, hypotension, chest pain, arrhythmia, hypokalemia, or jitteriness.[154,157] Recent studies report significant alterations in maternal glucose tolerance with long-term oral terbutaline therapy, which has not been observed with oral ritodrine therapy.[169] However, the large cost differential and the minimal difference in side effects between these two medications may warrant the substitution of terbutaline for ritodrine during maintenance therapy.

Other Beta-Agonist Drugs

Pharmacologic alterations of beta-adrenergic medications have produced a variety of selective tocolytic drugs. These include isoxsuprine, fenoterol, salbutamol, hexaprenaline, and orciprenaline. Although all produce significant tocolytic effects, controlled clinical trials have not been performed. Of all these drugs, hexaprenaline appears to have the least effect on the maternal cardiovascular system.

Magnesium Sulfate

Physiologists have known for some time that magnesium has the potential to decrease muscle contractility.[170] In vitro studies have shown that magnesium decreases the frequency of depolarization of myometrial smooth muscle cells and uncouples the ATP-linked activation of the actin-myosin contractile units. Calcium influx across-cell membranes appears to be of low magnitude in the uterus, and it is hypothesized that most of the calcium required to initiate cellular contractility comes from intracellular stores in the sarcoplasmic reticulum.[171] Magnesium ions compete with low-affinity calcium binding sites on the outside of the sarcoplasmic reticulum membrane and block the transport of calcium within this specialized organelle. This alteration of calcium storage within the myometrial cell seems a likely explanation for the tocolytic effect observed with magnesium sulfate.

Placebo-controlled clinical trials to demonstrate the efficacy of magnesium sulfate as a tocolytic drug have been limited. In one study involving 31 patients who received intravenous doses of magnesium sulfate and nine patients receiving a placebo infusion, delivery was delayed for more than 24 hours in 77 percent of the magnesium-treated group and in 44 percent of the placebo-treated group.[172] In this study the incidence of success was inversely related to the degree of cervical dilation. Another placebo-controlled clinical trial involving 35 patients failed to show any significant difference in delivery outcome.[164] Several comparison studies have shown that magnesium sulfate is an efficacious tocolytic drug. In a comparison study with intravenous alcohol administration there was a significant improvement in the outcome with magnesium sulfate.[172] Several other comparison studies with terbutaline or ritodrine failed to show a significant difference in outcome with either intravenous magnesium or intravenous beta-mimetic therapy.[153,155,156] These studies have consistently demonstrated that tocolytic success incidences with intravenous magnesium sulfate therapy are comparable to those obtained with beta-mimetic therapy.

More recent studies with magnesium sulfate infusion rates as high as 5 gm per hour have not demonstrated an improvement in tocolytic efficacy when compared with earlier studies using infusion rates of 2 gm per hour. Most of these studies showed that maternal side effects associated with magnesium therapy were minimal, and a distinct clinical advantage, when compared with beta-mimetic therapy, was clearly evident.[153,155]

The incidence of maternal side effects is low when intravenous magnesium sulfate therapy is maintained in a nontoxic range. In one study only 2 percent of the patients receiving magnesium sulfate had side effects significant enough to necessitate discontinuation of intravenous therapy, as compared with 38 percent of those receiving ritodrine and 60 percent receiving terbutaline.[153]

Transient hypotension associated with a feeling of heat and flushing is the most common side effect and is usually associated with a loading bolus of magnesium sulfate.[173] There are no significant cardiac side effects, and cardiac output remains unchanged with magnesium therapy.[173] Maternal hypothermia has been described following the infusion of magnesium sulfate, as well as maternal paralytic ileus with prolonged administration. Pulmonary edema has been described with magnesium sulfate therapy and steroid administration but is considered a rare occurrence. Maternal serum concentrations of ionized and nonionized calcium appear to fall dramatically with the infusion of magnesium sulfate.[173] This is probably the result of increased renal excretion of calcium and alterations in serum parathyroid hormone levels. Despite these apparent physical alterations, several large uncontrolled clinical studies with magnesium sulfate therapy have shown that this tocolytic drug is safe and well tolerated.[174,175]

Magnesium sulfate appears to increase uteroplacental blood flow in animal models.[173] This is probably related to the vasodilator properties of magnesium sulfate on smooth muscle in the blood vessels. This makes it a potentially useful tocolytic drug in cases of maternal bleeding or suspected uteroplacental insufficiency. Significant transplacental transfer of magnesium to the fetus occurs, and a decrease in fetal heart rate variability as a dose-related phenomenon has been described.[173] Otherwise, fetal side effects associated with magnesium sulfate appear to be minimal.

Although magnesium levels associated with maternal magnesium sulfate infusions are rarely toxic to the newborn, significant neonatal hypotonia and drowsiness may be related to neonatal hypermagnesemia.[176,177] This is usually associated with maternal magnesium infusion lasting longer than 24 hours, intramuscular injections, and premature infants. There is not a reproducible correlation between maternal magnesium levels and umbilical cord levels at birth. Maternal magnesium infusion does not appear to cause neonatal hypocalcemia, nor is there evidence of hypotension or reactive hypoglycemia in the exposed neonate. There are no known long-term follow-up studies of infants who have received magnesium sulfate infusion.

Magnesium sulfate is administered intravenously as an initial 4 gm loading dose over a 15 to 20 minute period, with a subsequent continuous infusion rate of 2 to 6 gm per hour. An average serum magnesium level of 4.8 mg per deciliter is obtained with an infusion rate of 3 gm per hour.[155] Therefore, higher infusion rates may be necessary to obtain therapeutic serum magnesium levels. Magnesium is eliminated almost entirely by renal excretion of the drug; 75 percent of the administered magnesium sulfate dose is excreted during the time of bolus infusion, and 90 percent is excreted within 24 hours after treatment.[178] All patients receiving these higher doses of magnesium sulfate should be monitored closely for loss of deep tendon reflexes and respiratory depression. With impaired renal function or higher infusion rates, it is necessary to check the serum magnesium levels frequently in order to prevent maternal toxicity. The loss of deep tendon reflexes occurs in the 8 to 10 mg per deciliter range, and respiratory depression is seen with doses in the range of 10 to 15 mg per deciliter. At doses above this level, cardiac conduction defects and cardiac arrest can occur.

The main disadvantage in the clinical use of magnesium sulfate as a tocolytic drug is the lack of an oral preparation for use once initial uterine contractions have subsided. Most clinicians utilize oral doses of a beta-mimetic drug for maintenance therapy following the arrest of preterm labor with intravenous magnesium sulfate therapy. Others advocate continuous long-term magnesium sulfate infusions, and several patients have received such therapy for up to 13 weeks.[179]

Sequential therapy with magnesium sulfate in patients who fail to respond to beta-mimetic therapy has been advocated by some clinicians. Although significant progression in cervical dilatation can occur before magnesium sulfate therapy can be instituted, it appears that sequential use of these drugs does not decrease the chance for successful therapy.

In conclusion, there is substantial evidence that magnesium sulfate is a reasonable and safe tocolytic drug for the inhibition of preterm labor. Although magnesium sulfate generally has been regarded as an alternative therapy to treat individuals who fail to benefit from beta-mimetic therapy, it offers several distinct advantages as a first-line tocolytic drug. These include minimal side effects in the mother and neonate, lack of deleterious alterations in uteroplacental blood flow, and the widespread clinical experience with magnesium among obstetricians for seizure prophylaxis in pre-eclampsia. With further clinical experience, magnesium sulfate may someday be used routinely as a primary tocolytic drug.

Prostaglandin Synthetase Inhibitors

Prostaglandin synthetase inhibitors have also been shown to be effective in inhibiting preterm labor. However, concern about the effect of prostaglandin synthetase inhibitors on the fetus has limited their clinical use. Indomethacin is the most widely used prostaglandin synthetase inhibitor in clinical use today. Prostaglandins appear to be important modulators of uterine contractility. Elevated prostaglandin metabolite levels have been measured in patients with preterm labor.[180] The production of prostaglandins is associated with uterine contractility and appears to be linked to calcium entry across smooth muscle membranes.[171] Indomethacin, Naprosyn, and fenoprofen exert a marked depressant effect on uterine contractility in excised uterine muscle strips. Administration of indomethacin or ritodrine during labor in humans results in a significant reduction in serum prostaglandin levels.[181,182]

The most extensive clinical experience with indomethacin as a first-line tocolytic drug was reported in 1984 and involved 252 patients with intact membranes in preterm labor.[183] Of these, 88 percent obtained prolongation of pregnancy for longer than one week. The majority of patients who successfully responded to indomethacin in this study had an initial cervical dilatation of less than 3 cm.

Controlled clinical studies have demonstrated the efficacy of indomethacin in the inhibition of preterm labor. In a prospective randomized, double-blind study of 30 patients, indomethacin was found to be significantly more effective than placebo in inhibiting preterm labor during a 24-hour course of therapy.[184] Another controlled, double-blind study of 36 patients confirmed these results.[185] A comparison study with alcohol, salbutamol, and indomethacin involving 62 patients revealed that a combination of ethanol and indomethacin inhibited labor for more than 48 hours in 70 percent of the cases, as compared with 60 percent with salbutamol and 32 percent with ethanol alone.[186]

Indomethacin usually is administered initially as a 50 mg oral loading dose, followed by 25 mg every four to six hours.[187] It is rapidly absorbed after oral administration, peak plasma concentrations occurring within 90 minutes to two hours. The half-life excretion of indomethacin in nonpregnant adults is approximately 2.2 hours.[188] It is readily transferred across the placental unit to the fetus and appears in the fetal blood within 15 minutes. Fetal concentrations of indomethacin equilibrate with maternal levels within five hours.[187]

Maternal side effects from indomethacin are minimal.[187] This medication does not alter the maternal heart rate or blood pressure. The most common maternal complaints with oral therapy are nausea and heartburn. Indomethacin has a reversible effect on maternal platelet function but does not appear to lead to increased maternal perinatal hemorrhage.[187] Indomethacin should be avoided in patients with a history of peptic ulcer disease or bleeding disorders.

Indomethacin does not appear to alter uteroplacental blood flow significantly.[187] The major fetal and neonatal complications theoretically associated with prostaglandin synthetase inhibitors are premature closure of the ductus arteriosus and neonatal primary pulmonary hypertension. Although the literature regarding ductus arteriosus physiology is contradictory, the preponderance of studies point to a relative resistance to closure of the ductus arteriosus at an early gestational age.[189,190] Recent uncontrolled reports of in utero Doppler flow studies in the fetus suggest some degree of ductus constriction when maternal indomethacin therapy is administered.[191] However, intrauterine fetal demise or fetal hydrops associated with maternal indomethacin therapy has not been described. Indomethacin also can induce a persistent fetal circulation in the neonate by causing persistent constriction of the pulmonary vasculature. Several anecdotal cases have been reported; however, the majority of clinical experience with this tocolytic drug has failed to substantiate this potential complication. In two large clinical studies of indomethacin utilized prior to 34 weeks of gestation in 464 patients, no cases of premature ductus closure or persistent fetal circulation were reported.[185,190]

Other potential perinatal complications include impaired renal function in the fetus with resultant oligohydramnios, enhanced bleeding in the neonate, and hyperbilirubinemia. Although a variety of case reports have addressed these issues, there does not appear to be an increased incidence of oligohydramnios, neonatal bleeding, or significant hyperbilirubinemia with maternal indomethacin therapy for tocolysis.

In summary, prostaglandin synthetase inhibitors appear to be effective and easily administered as tocolytic drugs in the treatment of preterm labor. Indomethacin is extremely well tolerated by the mother, and most severe adverse side effects reported with the fetus and neonate are anecdotal. It is recommended that this tocolytic drug be discontinued after the 34th week of gestation, which appears to minimize fetal-neonatal side effects. Further evaluation of prostaglandin synthetase inhibitors could show that the risk-benefit ratio for these tocolytic drugs justifies their routine clinical use.

Calcium Channel Blocking Drugs

Calcium channel blocking drugs such as nifedipine, nicardipine, and verapamil are capable of inhibiting uterine contractions. Nifedipine has been shown to suppress both prostaglandin- and oxytocin-induced uterine activity in isolated human and animal myometrial preparations.[192]

Clinical experience in the treatment of preterm labor with these drugs has been limited. To date, no controlled randomized clinical trials have been reported to confirm their efficacy. The first clinical experience with nifedipine was reported in Europe in 1980.[193] Ten patients with suspected preterm labor were administered this drug until uterine activity subsided. In all 10 patients preterm labor was arrested in the 72-hour study period. Similar results have been observed in patients given nifedipine for the simultaneous treatment of preterm labor and hypertension.[194] A clinical study in the United States involving 13 patients who failed to benefit from other tocolytic therapies reported that delivery was delayed for more than 48 hours in 69 percent of the patients given oral doses of nifedipine.[195]

This diverse group of drugs appears to prevent entry of extracellular calcium into the smooth muscle cells. These drugs apparently block the passage of calcium through voltage-dependent channels and may suppress calcium release from the intracellular sarcoplasmic reticulum, in addition to increasing calcium extrusion from the smooth muscle cell.[171] These medications may cause smooth muscle relaxation, which is nonspecific and can result in peripheral vasodilatation. Additionally, some of these drugs cause slowing of atrioventricular conduction in the heart.

The physiologic alterations associated with nifedipine are mainly systemic hypotension and reflex tachycardia, as well as headache and cutaneous flushing. These hemodynamic alterations appear to be similar to and perhaps less than those induced with ritodrine. Recently a small randomized clinical trial comparing nifedipine and ritodrine showed that cardiac stimulation and vasodilation were less pronounced with calcium blocking drugs and that calcium blocking drugs were not associated with hypokalemia.[196] The volume expansion status appeared to be similar with the two medications.

The major concern restricting the clinical use of calcium channel blocking drugs is the effect on uteroplacental blood flow. Animal studies using nifedipine, however, have demonstrated minimal alterations in placental perfusion.[197] In patients who have received nifedipine during pregnancy, no adverse fetal or neonatal side effects have been described.

Nifedipine is active orally and can be administered parenterally. The usual oral dosage is 10 to 20 mg every four to six hours. The maternal mean half-life of nifedipine appears to be 76 minutes.[198] Both oral and sublingual doses of nifedipine result in significant maternal serum concentrations, and transplacental transfer of these drugs has been confirmed. There appears to be substantial interpatient and intrapatient variability in serum levels, which probably relates to differences in maternal and neonatal metabolism.[198] Sublingual administration may be preferable, because it allows some control of administration when maternal hypotension becomes manifest.

In summary, calcium blocking drugs represent an apparently powerful class of tocolytic drugs. However, concern over their effect on the fetus and newborn, as well as their unproven clinical efficacy, mandates that they be considered experimental at this time.

Combination Therapy

The simultaneous use of several tocolytic drugs has been studied in a limited fashion. The reasoning behind such use lies in the potential for additive tocolytic effects, the ability to decrease individual tocolytic drug dosages, and the hope of decreasing potential side effects. Although combination therapy has been utilized in routine clinical practice, the number of controlled studies in the literature has been limited.

The adjunctive use of magnesium sulfate with ritodrine therapy for the inhibition of preterm labor has been evaluated with conflicting results.[199-202] The simultaneous use of these two drugs after failure of single agent tocolytic therapy has been advocated by some investigators. In one randomized comparison study involving 64 patients, delivery was delayed longer than one week in 31 percent of the ritodrine group compared with 59 percent with combination therapy.[199] These authors reported that the maternal and fetal side effects did not differ in the two groups, and the dose requirement with ritodrine, as well as the total duration of therapy, was less in the combination therapy group.

In a similar blind study involving 50 patients, adjunctive therapy with magnesium sulfate did not appear to alter the metabolic changes associated with ritodrine.[200] However, other investigators have failed to show improved efficacy in delaying delivery when simultaneous therapy had been utilized.[200-202] The most disturbing aspect of the concurrent use of ritodrine and magnesium is the significant cardiac side effects in patients receiving combination therapy.[202] Because of the potential for serious maternal side effects and conflicting results in terms of efficacy, the concurrent use of magnesium and ritodrine is not currently recommended.

Preterm Labor and Intrauterine Growth Retardation

The additive effects of calcium channel blockers and ritodrine have also been investigated. Since verapamil has the capacity to alter cardiac conduction in the human heart, it has been used to inhibit the cardiovascular side effects of ritodrine during the treatment of preterm labor. In a double-blind, randomized trial involving 83 patients receiving ritodrine and verapamil and 99 patients receiving ritodrine and placebo, there was no apparent difference in prolongation of pregnancy.[203] However, there was a significant decrease in the incidences of maternal side effects attributable to intravenous ritodrine therapy. In 60 percent of the patients who received ritodrine alone, there was significant patient intolerance, whereas patients who received combination therapy showed no appreciable intolerance. No untoward fetal effects from verapamil therapy were reported in this study.

Concurrent ritodrine and indomethacin use has been advocated by other investigators. In a double-blind, randomized trial of ritodrine and a regimen of ritodrine and indomethacin involving 44 patients, there appeared to be a significant increase in the mean number of days gained from initiation of therapy.[204] In addition, the number of pregnancies achieving 37 weeks and the number of recurrences were significantly different in the two groups. A similar randomized trial involving 120 patients showed a significant increase in the number of days gained.[205]

Although this represents a small number of studies involving combination tocolytic therapy, further investigation and clinical experience ultimately may prove that combination therapy is beneficial in improving efficacy and decreasing maternal and fetal side effects. Until that time, combination tocolytic therapy should be used with caution in the clinical setting.

INTRAUTERINE GROWTH RETARDATION

As mentioned, it is often exceedingly difficult to distinguish between a baby who is "small" on the basis of being preterm and appropriate for gestational age and a baby who is term and small for gestational age. It is estimated that one-third of all infants born in the United States each year weighing less than 2,500 gm are actually at term but growth retarded.[206] IUGR was a poorly understood process until approximately 25 years ago when Lubchenco et al[207] first established normative data for the comparison of gestational age with birth weight. These fetal growth curves allowed Battaglia and Lubchenco[208] to define small-for-gestational-age infants, i.e., those with birth weights below the 10th percentile for gestational age.

Growth retardation is considered to be present when a fetus has a restriction or limitation of growth despite greater developmental potential. Although the term "growth retardation" has often been used syn-

onymously with "small for gestational age," clearly not all small-for-gestational-age fetuses suffer from growth retardation (Table 2–2). Some fetuses that are small for gestational age are constitutionally small. That is, these fetuses suffer from no pathologic process but are small because of the limited growth potential inherited from their parents.

A variety of criteria have been used to define IUGR. A birth weight less than the 10th percentile for gestational age should be uniformly adopted and utilized.[209] It should be further noted that in the antepartum period, IUGR is only suspected; definitive diagnosis requires the evaluation of birth weight at delivery and the exclusion of constitutionally small-for-gestational-age infants. Because all conclusions concerning (suboptimal) fetal-neonatal growth relate to gestational age, the importance of establishing an accurate gestational age cannot be overstated. A closely related issue is the selection of appropriate birth weight standards. Whenever possible, population-specific data should be utilized to evaluate fetal-neonatal growth.[210]

IUGR can be divided into two clinical subtypes: symmetrical and asymmetrical. Symmetrical growth retardation generally results when there is an early fetal insult, such as a congenital infection. This type of growth retardation is therefore "intrinsic" to the fetus. Asymmetrical growth retardation occurs later in pregnancy and is largely due to pathologic processes, such as maternal vascular disease, that are "extrinsic" to the fetus. In symmetrical growth retardation all biometric aspects of fetal growth are symmetrically and uniformly reduced. In symmetrical growth retardation, there is frequently "sparing" of fetal brain and head growth. Although the head growth may be unaffected, these fetuses demonstrate a diminution in the cross-sectional area of the abdomen reflecting impaired liver glycogen

TABLE 2–2 Gestational Age, Size,* and Functional Growth†

Gestational Age: Preterm, Term, Post-term
  AGA
    Growth retardation
    Macrosomia
  SGA
    Constitutional
    Growth retardation
      Symmetrical
      Asymmetrical
  LGA
    Constitutional
    Macrosomia

*Size: AGA—appropriate for gestational age; SGA—small for gestational age; LGA—large for gestational age.
†Functional growth: Constitutional—normal course of growth for an infant destined to be small or large; growth retarded—small owing to a pathologic process; macrosomic—large owing to a pathologic process.
From Gant NF. Inappropriate fetal growth: diagnosis and management of fetal growth retardation. In: Pritchard JA, MacDonald PC, Gant NF. Williams Obstetrics. 17th ed. Norwalk, Connecticut: Appleton & Lange, 1984:2.

storage secondary to a reduction in the blood supply to the liver and other visceral organs. This adaptation to uteroplacental insufficiency is caused by the chronic redistribution of fetal cardiac output favoring brain growth, and heart and adrenal perfusion.[211]

When IUGR is suspected, a careful search must be conducted in an attempt to elucidate the underlying etiology. Maternal, fetal, or placental factors, or any combination thereof, may contribute to IUGR. Common maternal factors associated with IUGR include pregnancy-induced hypertension, anemia, poor weight gain, low prepregnancy weight, a history of IUGR, cyanotic heart disease, chronic hypertension, and renal disease.[212] Any factor that interferes with the physiologic exchange in intervillous perfusion may cause IUGR.[213] Maternal factors such as vascular disease, especially when complicated by hypertension, frequently lead to late-onset asymmetrical IUGR with associated oligohydramnios.[214] Smoking, hypertension, and preeclampsia together account for more than half of all cases of IUGR in some reported studies.[215]

Fetal factors account for approximately 20 percent of all cases of growth retardation and usually result in symmetrical growth retardation. In general, these are intrinsic causes; however, an extrinsic cause such as severe maternal vascular disease resulting in uteroplacental insufficiency, if active early enough, can also cause symmetrical growth retardation. Fetal infection with cytomegalovirus or rubella virus early in pregnancy can have devastating consequences on both fetal growth and development. Additional fetal factors include radiation exposure in the embryonic period and chromosomal abnormalities such as trisomy 13 and 18. Placental factors that may cause IUGR include multiple gestation, abruptio placentae, chronic placental infarction, and placenta previa. Any absolute or relative decrease in the placental mass may affect the quality of substrate available to fetus. In cases of multiple gestation there is a decrease in the placental mass relative to the fetal mass, and IUGR occurs in as many as 30 percent of twin pregnancies.[216]

Because of the markedly increased perinatal morbidity and mortality associated with IUGR, it would be ideal if, in all cases, the diagnosis could be suspected ante partum so that appropriate care might improve the outcome.[210] It is disappointing to learn that despite the general awareness of IUGR and associated etiologic factors, only 30 to 40 percent of the cases are diagnosed ante partum.[217]

A careful history is of obvious importance to the clinician in attempting to identify underlying maternal factors that could suggest a risk for IUGR. A history of maternal risk factors, such as hypertension, smoking, drug or alcohol abuse, or diabetes with vascular disease, should be sought. Furthermore, it has been reported that the previous birth of a growth-retarded infant is associated with a 25 to 30 percent chance of recurrence of IUGR, even when no other maternal risk factors exist.[218] Lag in the fundal height measurement is a physical finding that is helpful in the recognition of possible IUGR. Belizan et al[219] constructed normal curvilinear fundal height parameters for their population and noted that the 10th percentile birth weight was associated with a fundal height approximately 4 cm below that expected for gestational age. Utilizing the fundal height measurements in a patient population at increased risk for IUGR, they were able to predict IUGR at delivery with an 86 percent sensitivity. Other investigators, however, have been unable to reproduce these laudatory results.[206,217]

Ultrasonography has become an invaluable tool in the antepartum evaluation of possible IUGR. Early studies used the biparietal diameter alone in an attempt to recognize IUGR.[220] Symmetrical growth retardation was described as "low profile" and asymmetrical retardation as "late flattening." Although use of the biparietal diameter alone to diagnose IUGR was an improvement over purely historical and physical findings, it is clear that biparietal diameter growth alone cannot be used as the sole criterion in the diagnosis because it may be inaccurate more than half the time (Table 2–3).

TABLE 2–3   Value of Sonographic Criteria in Detecting Intrauterine Growth Retardation

Criterion	Sensitivity* (%)	Specificity* (%)	Predictive Value Positive (%)	Negative (%)
Advanced placental grade	62	64	16	94
Elevated FL/AC	34–49	78–83	18–20	92–93
Low TIUV	57–80	72–76	21–24	92–97
Small BPD	24–88	62–94	21–44	92–98
Small BPD and advanced placental grade	59	86	32	95
Slow rate of BPD growth†	75	84	35	97
Low EFW	89	88	45	99
Decreased AFV	24	98	55	92
Elevated HC/AC	82	94	62	98

FL/AC—fetal length/abdominal circumference ratio; BPD—biparietal diameter; AFV—amniotic fluid volume; TIUV—total intrauterine volume; EFW—estimated fetal weight; HC/AC—head circumference/abdominal circumference ratio.
*A range of values is given for a criterion when different studies apply that criterion in two or more ways.
†One study (Crane et al) found 100% sensitivity and specificity. This study has been omitted since it included only four growth-retarded fetuses.
From Benson CB, Doubilet PM, Saltzman DH. Intrauterine growth retardation: predictive value of US criteria for antenatal diagnosis. Radiology 1986; 160:415–417.

Because clinical experience and animal studies have shown growth-retarded fetuses to have reduced hepatic glycogen stores and liver mass with a consequent reduction in the abdominal diameter,[221] several investigators have used abdominal diameter-circumference alone or in combination with head circumference or abdominal circumference ratios to identify growth-retarded fetuses (see Table 2–3). Warsof et al[222] believe that abdominal circumference measurements alone are most predictive of IUGR, and that determination of the biparietal diameter in conjunction with the abdominal circumference does not improve the accuracy.

The total intrauterine volume has also been recommended in an attempt to detect intrauterine growth retardation. The total intrauterine volume is calculated by measuring the greatest length, width, and height of the uterus and multiplying it by the constant 0.5233.[223] The rationale for its use follows from the fact that in pregnancies complicated by growth retardation, in addition to the fetus being small, frequently the placenta is small and the amniotic fluid volume is reduced. Consequently one might expect the total intrauterine volume to be a sensitive predictor. Although there was initial enthusiasm, more recent investigators have found a sensitivity of only 70 percent and a predictive value of an abnormal test of only 41 percent.[224] Additionally this technique is somewhat burdensome to use because it requires a static contact ultrasound unit.

Ultrasonic placental grading has also been used in an attempt to diagnose IUGR in utero. Utilizing the initial grading scheme of Grannum,[225] Kazzi et al[226] used placental grade, clinical risk factors, and the biparietal diameter in an attempt to identify fetuses with IUGR. In their overall study population they found a sensitivity of 59 percent; the predicted value of an abnormal test was 52 percent. Fetuses with IUGR frequently have been found to have reduced quantities of, or no, amniotic fluid. This is thought to be caused by chronic hypoxia in utero, resulting in a redistribution of fetal blood flow from the fetal kidneys with resultant oliguria and consequent reduced amniotic fluid volume.

Because of this clinical finding Manning et al[227] evaluated the significance of oligohydramnios (defined as the broadest pocket of amniotic fluid of less than 1 cm) to predict IUGR. In a group of patients at risk for IUGR they noted a sensitivity of 83 percent and a positive predictive value of 90 percent. Philipson et al,[228] however, in attempting to utilize this criterion to screen for IUGR in their population, noted a maximal projected sensitivity of only 16 percent. Estimated fetal weights below the 10th percentile for gestational age are frequently helpful in identifying suspected growth-retarded fetuses in utero. Using the biparietal diameter and abdominal circumference to estimate fetal weight, Ott and Doyle[229] noted a sensitivity of 89.9 percent in the diagnosis of growth-retarded infants and an overall specificity of 79.8 percent.

Umbilical artery velocimetry studies have been introduced recently and may be helpful in the diagnosis of growth retardation in utero. These studies analyze the ratio of peak systolic and least diastolic blood flow velocities. The umbilical placental circulation is a high flow–low resistance vascular bed in which the increasing volume flow of advancing gestation is caused by a fall in the distal resistance.[230] In uncomplicated pregnancies the placental vascular resistance generally decreases as term approaches, and because of the inverse relationship between resistance and flow velocity, the systolic-diastolic ratio decreases.

Several investigators have noted that growth-retarded fetuses can be detected accurately by utilizing umbilical artery Doppler studies.[230,231] Fleischer et al[231] noted a sensitivity of 78 percent and a specificity of 83 percent using umbilical artery velocimetry studies to diagnose IUGR. Giles et al[232] identified a specific microvascular lesion in the placenta in pregnancies complicated by growth retardation, characterized by obliteration of small muscular arteries in tertiary stem villi. They also found an associated reduction in diastolic flow velocities, reflected by an increase in the systolic-to-diastolic ratio, indicative of the increased placental resistance.

The management of the fetus suspected of being growth retarded in utero is complicated and difficult. If the fetus is term or near term, and the obstetrician can be assured of pulmonary maturity, there is little to be gained from continued in utero existence, and delivery should be strongly considered. If the fetus is preterm, the goal is to allow continued in utero growth and development as long as there is no evidence of acute fetal or maternal compromise. To do so, the obstetrician must evaluate and treat problems contributing to IUGR, institute monitoring of fetal well-being, evaluate fetal growth serially, and determine the optimal timing and route of delivery.

In order to evaluate and treat problems contributing to IUGR, a careful anatomic fetal ultrasound examination should be performed to rule out structural abnormalities. Careful evaluation of the biometric parameters and amniotic fluid volume is critical. If the fetus is symmetrically growth retarded or has structural abnormalities, because of the increased likelihood of a chromosomal abnormality, consideration should be given to karyotyping the fetus, obtaining cells by either amniocentesis or cordocentesis, depending on the gestational age.[233] Moreover, cordocentesis also allows for the evaluation of possible congenital infection and determination of fetal oxygenation and acid-base balance.[234]

A recent study indicated that there are distinct in utero differences detected by cordocentesis in amino acid concentrations between appropriate and small-for-gestational-age fetuses.[235] These differences may have future diagnostic and therapeutic implications. If the maternal history indicates a correctable cause of IUGR, such as malnutrition or drug ingestion, steps should be taken to alleviate the insult, for instance, discontinuing the offending drug(s) and supplementing the diet. Maternal bed rest should be used routinely but is most likely to benefit fetuses with growth retardation on an "extrinsic" basis.

In discussions with the mother about suspected suboptimal growth, we strongly caution against the use of the term "growth retardation." The negative connotation associated with the word "retardation" could easily alarm the patient and cause a chronic state of increased anxiety, catechol secretion, and resultant diminution in uterine perfusion.

Monitoring of fetal well-being on a weekly or, if indicated, more frequent basis can be accomplished utilizing a variety of different testing shemata.[236] The obstetrician should use the method with which he or she is most familiar. Fetal movement counts, nonstress testing, contraction stress testing, biophysical profile scoring, and Doppler umbilical artery velocimetry studies offer reliable alternatives. Fetal growth should be evaluated serially at two- to three-week intervals, depending on the stage of gestation in which suboptimal fetal growth is suspected. The critical issue is to demonstrate continued growth in the biparietal diameter and abdominal diameter and a progressive increase in the estimated fetal weight. Fetal growth parameters should be plotted in relation to gestational age. An arrest in biparietal diameter growth over three weeks or the finding of oligohydramnios should lead to the strong consideration of delivery.[237]

Finally the obstetrician needs to determine the optimal timing and route of delivery. Consideration of the ideal timing of delivery presupposes that the obstetrician is certain of the gestational age. Gestational age can be determined most accurately in the first trimester of pregnancy. However, frequently this critical information is unknown, and the obstetrician is faced with a "small" baby who may be growth retarded, constitutionally small, or appropriately grown with a less advanced gestational age than originally suspected. Recent preliminary findings suggest that determination of the transverse fetal cerebellar width may serve as an independent indicator of gestational age. Unlike other fetal biometric parameters, cerebellar width is unaffected by IUGR and may be used as a standard against which other fetal growth parameters may be compared.[238] Although determining the ideal time for delivery is probably the most difficult issue in managing fetuses with suspected IUGR, if fetal surveillance is reassuring, the maternal condition is stable, and the fetus is growing in utero, the fetus may remain undelivered. However, if signs of fetal compromise develop, the risks of continued in utero existence must be weighed against the risks of immaturity and serious consideration given to preterm delivery. Ideally several antenatal surveillance tests should indicate fetal compromise before delivery is planned in a preterm immature fetus.

The route of delivery depends on the condition of the cervix and the ability to monitor the fetus closely during labor. Because growth-retarded fetuses seem to have a diminished tolerance for hypoxia, we recommend continuous intrapartum electronic monitoring during labor.[239] It is critically important to have neonatal facilities and personnel available to care for a potentially compromised fetus or neonate. Neonatal complications may include hypothermia, polycythemia, hypoglycemia, and hypocalcemia.[240] It should be noted that despite optimal antepartum and intrapartum care, fetuses who are growth-retarded, as a group, have an increased incidence of major and minor handicaps and reduced potential for somatic growth. The long-term prognosis obviously depends on the underlying insult, the gestational age at delivery, the condition at birth, and the severity of growth retardation.[240] Early recognition and careful management, as outlined, should allow for further improvement in the perinatal outcome for these fetuses.

REFERENCES

1. Lee KS, Panet HN, Gartner L, et al. Neonatal morbidity: an analysis of recent improvements in the United States. Am J Public Health 1980; 70:15.
2. Kessel S, Villar J, Berendes H, Nugent R. The changing pattern of low birth weight in the United States. JAMA 1984; 251:1978.
3. Walker D, Feldman A, Vohr B, Oh W. Cost-benefit analysis of neonatal intensive care for infants weighing less than 1,000 grams at birth. Pediatrics 1984; 74:20.
4. Hack M, Famaroff AA, Merkatz IR. The low birth weight infant—evolution of a changing outlook. N Engl J Med 1979; 301:1162.
5. Davies PA, Stewart AL. Low birth weight infants: neurologic sequelae and later intelligence. Br Med Bull 1975; 31:85.
6. Stewart AL, Reynolds EOR. Improved prognosis for infants of very low birth weight. Pediatrics 1974; 54:724.
7. Stewart AL, Reynolds EOR, Lipschomb AA. Outcome for infants of very low birth weight: survey of world literature. Lancet 1981; 1:1038.
8. Kitchens WH, Ryan MM, Rickerts A, et al. A longitudinal study of very low birth weight infants. Section IV. An overview of performance at eight years of age. Dev Med Child Neurol 1980; 22:172.
9. Luthy DA, Shy KK, Strikland D, et al. Status of infants at birth and risk for adverse neonatal outcomes and long-term sequelae: a study in low birth weight infants. Am J Obstet Gynecol 1987; 157:676.
10. Arias F, Tomich P. The etiology and outcome of low birth weight of preterm infants. Obstet Gynecol 1982; 60:277.
11. Papiernak E, Kaminski M. Multifactorial study of the risk of prematurity at 32 weeks of gestation. J Perinat Med 1974; 2:30.
12. Keirse M, Rush R, Anderson A, Turnbull A. Risk of preterm delivery in patients with previous preterm delivery and/or abortion. Br J Obstet Gynaecol 1978; 85:81.
13. Creasy RC, Gummer BA, Liggins GC. A system for predicting spontaneous preterm birth. Obstet Gynecol 1980; 55:692.
14. Naeye R. Coitus and associated amniotic fluid infections. N Engl J Med 1974; 301:1198.
15. Kiebanwoff M, Nugent R, Rhoads G. Coitus during pregnancy: is it safe? Lancet 1984; 2:914.
16. Rush RW, Issacs S, McPherson K, et al. A randomized trial of cervical cerclage in women at high risk of spontaneous preterm delivery. Br J Obstet Gynaecol 1984; 91:724.
17. Lazar P, Gueguen S, Dretfus J, et al. Multicentered controlled trial of cervical cerclage in women at moderate risk of preterm delivery. Br J Obstet Gynaecol 1984; 91:731.

18. Hauth J, Gilstrap L, Brekken A. Effects of 17-alpha-hydroxy-progesterone caproate on pregnancy outcome in an active duty military population. Am J Obstet Gynecol 1983; 146:187.

19. Johnson J, Lee P, Zachary A, et al. High risk prematurity—Progestin treatment and steroid studies. Obstet Gynecol 1979; 54:412.

20. Yemini M, Borenstein R, Dreazen E, et al. Prevention of premature labor by 17-alpha-hydroxy-progesterone caproin. Am J Obstet Gynecol 1985; 151:574.

21. Walters AW, Wood C. A trial of oral ritodrine for the prevention of premature labor. Br J Obstet Gynaecol 1977; 84:26.

22. O'Leary JA. Propyhlactic tocolysis of twins. Am J Obstet Gynecol 1986; 154:904.

23. Katz M, Neuman R, Gill P. Assessment of uterine activity in ambulatory patients at high risk for preterm labor and delivery. Am J Obstet Gynecol 1986; 154:44.

24. Katz M, Gill PJ, Neuman RB. Detection of preterm labor by ambulatory monitoring of uterine activity for the management of oral tocolysis. Am J Obstet Gynecol 1986; 154:1253.

25. Morrison JC, Martin JN Jr, Martin RW, et al. Prevention of preterm birth by ambulatory assessment of uterine activity: a randomized study. Am J Obstet Gynecol 1987; 156:536.

26. Iams JD, Johnson FF, O'Shaughnessy RW, West LC. A prospective random trial of home uterine activity monitoring in pregnancies at increased risk of preterm labor. Am J Obstet Gynecol 1987; 157:638.

27. Castle BM, Turnbull AC. The presence or absence of fetal breathing movements predicts the outcome of preterm labor. Lancet 1983; 2:471.

28. Besinger RE, Compton AA, Hayashi RH. The presence or absence of fetal breathing movements as a predictor of outcome in preterm labor. Am J Obstet Gynecol 1987; 157:753.

29. Goldenberg RL, Nelson KG, Davis RO, Koski J. Delay and delivery: influence of gestational age and the duration of delay on perinatal outcome. Obstet Gynecol 1984; 64:480.

30. Milligan J, Shennan A, Hoskins E. Perinatal intensive care: where and how to draw the line. Am J Obstet Gynecol 1984; 148:499.

31. Worthington D, Davis LE, Grausz JP, et al. Factors influencing survival and morbidity with very low birth weight delivery. Obstet Gynecol 1983; 62:550.

32. Liggins GC, Howie RN. A control trial of antepartum glucocorticoid treatment for the prevention of respiratory distress syndrome in premature infants. Pediatrics 1972; 50:515.

33. Collaborative Group on Antenatal Steroid Therapy. Effects of antenatal dexamethasone administration and prevention of respiratory distress syndrome. Am J Obstet Gynecol 1981; 141:276.

34. Collaborative Group on Antenatal Steroid Therapy. Effects of antenatal dexamethasone administration in the infant: long-term follow-up. J Pediatr 1984; 104:259.

35. Ballard P. Combined hormonal treatment and lung maturation. Semin Perinatol 1984; 8:283.

36. Westgren M, Holmquist P, Svenningsen NW, Ingemarsson I. Intrapartum fetal monitoring in preterm deliveries: prospective study. Obstet Gynecol 1982; 60:99.

37. Braithwaite NDJ, Milligan GE, Shennan AT. Fetal heart rate monitoring and neonatal mortality in the very preterm infant. Am J Obstet Gynecol 1986; 154:250.

38. Moberg LJ, Garite TJ, Freeman RK. Fetal heart rate patterns and fetal distress of patients with preterm premature rupture of membranes. Obstet Gynecol 1984; 64:60.

39. Luthy DA, Shy KK, vanBelle G, et al. A randomized trial of electronic fetal monitoring in preterm labor. Obstet Gynecol 1987; 69:687.

40. Barrett JM, Boehm FH, Vaughn MK. The effective type of delivery on neonatal outcome in singleton infants of birth weights of one thousand grams or less. JAMA 1983; 250:625.

41. Yu VYH, Bajuk B, Cutting D, et al. Effect of mode of delivery on outcome of very-low-birth weight infants. Br J Obstet Gynaecol 1984; 91:633.

42. Kitchens W, Ford GW, Doyle LW, et al. Cesarean section or vaginal delivery at 24-25 weeks' gestation: comparison of survival in neonatal and two year morbidity. Obstet Gynecol 1985; 66:149.

43. Newton ER, Haering WA, Kennedy JL, et al. Effect of mode of delivery on morbidity and mortality in infants at an early gestational age. Obstet Gynecol 1986; 67:507.

44. Effer S, Saigal S, Rand C, et al. Effective delivery method on outcome in very low birth weight breech infants: is improved survival related to cesarean section or other perinatal care maneuvers? Am J Obstet Gynecol 1983; 145:123.

45. Farrell PM, Avery ME. Hyaline membrane disease. Am Rev Respir Dis 1975; 3:657.

46. Mannino FL, Gluck L. The management of respiratory distress syndrome. In: Thibault DW, Gregory GA, eds. Neonatal pulmonary care. Menlo Park, California: Addison-Wesley, 1979:56.

47. Stark AR, Frantz ID III. Respiratory distress syndrome. Pediatr Clin North Am 1986; 33:533.

48. Kulovich MV, Hallman MV, Gluck L. The lung profile. I. Normal pregnancy. Am J Obstet Gynecol 1979; 135:57.

49. Gregory GA, Kitterman JA, Phibbs RH, et al. Treatment of the idiopathic respiratory-distress syndrome with continuous positive airway pressure. N Engl J Med 1971; 284:1333.

50. Yeh TF, Shibli A, Lev ST, et al. Early furosemide therapy in preterm infants with respiratory distress syndrome: a randomized trial. J Pediatr 1984; 105:603.

51. Edwards DK, Jacob J, Gluck L. The immature lung: radiographic appearance, course and complication. Am J Roentgenol 1980; 135:659.

52. Hallman M, Merritt TA, Schneider H, et al. Isolation of human surfactant from amniotic fluid and a pilot study of its efficacy and respiratory distress syndrome. Pediatrics 1983; 71:473.

53. Merritt TA, Hallman M, Bloom BT, et al. Prophylactic treatment of very premature infants with human surfactant. N Engl J Med 1986; 315:785.

54. Cunningham MD, Ellison RC, Zierler S, et al. Perinatal risk assessment for patent ductus arteriosus in premature infants. Obstet Gynecol 1986; 68:41.

55. Friedman WF, Hirschklau MJ, Printz MP, et al. Pharmacologic closure of patent ductus arteriosus in the premature infant. N Engl J Med 1976; 295:526.

56. Salomon NW, Anderson RM, Copeland JG, et al. A rational approach to ligation of patent ductus arteriosus in the neonate. Chest 1979; 75:671.

57. Ahmann PA, Lazzara A, Dykes F, et al. Intraventricular hemorrhage: incidence and an outline. Ann Neurol 1980; 7:118.

58. Tejani N, Rebold B, Tuck S, et al. Obstetrical factors in the causation of periventricular-intraventricular hemorrhage. Obstet Gynecol 1984; 64:510.

59. Volpe JJ. Neonatal intraventricular hemorrhage. N Engl J Med 1981; 304:886.

60. Shankaran S, Slovis T, Benoard MP, et al. Sonographic classification of intracranial hemorrhage. A prognostic indicator of mortality, morbidity and short-term neurologic outcome. J Pediatr 1982; 100:469.

61. Bejar R, Curbelo V, Coen RW, et al. Diagnosis and follow-up of intraventricular and intracerebral hemorrhages by ultrasound studies of infant brains through the fontanelles and sutures. Pediatrics 1980; 66:661

62. Papile LA, Munsick-Bruno G, Schaefer A. Relationship of cerebral intraventricular hemorrhage and early childhood handicaps. J Pediatr 1983; 103:272.

63. Lowe JA, Galbraith RS, Sauerbrei EE, et al. Motor and cognitive development of infants with intraventricular hemorrhage, ventriculomegaly and periventricular parenchymal lesions. Am J Obstet Gynecol 1986; 155:750.

64. Morales WJ, Coerten J. Prevention of intraventricular hemorrhage and very low birth weight infants by maternally administered phenobarbital. Obstet Gynecol 1986; 68:295.

65. Kattwinkel J. Apnea in the neonatal period. Pediatr Rev 1980; 2:115.

66. Brown EG, Sweet AY. Neonatal necrotizing enterocolitis. Pediatr Clin North Am 1982; 29:1149.

67. Walsh MC, Kliegman RM, Fanaroff AA. Necrotizing enterocolitis: a practitioner's perspective. Pediatr Rev 1988; 9:219.

68. Seigel JD, McCracken GH. Sepsis neonatorum. N Engl J Med 1981; 304:642.

69. Phillips AGS. Oxygen plus pressure plus time: the etiology of bronchial pulmonary dysplasia. Pediatrics 1975; 55:44.

70. Tooley WH. Epidemiology of bronchopulmonary dysplasia. J Pediatr 1979; 95:851.

71. Rhodes PG, Graves GR, Patel DM, et al. Minimizing pneumothorax and bronchial pulmonary dysplasia in ventilated infants with hyaline membrane disease. J Pediatr 1983; 103:634.

72. Lucey JF, Damgman D. A re-examination of the role of oxygen in retrolental fibroplasia. Pediatrics 1984; 73:82.

73. Shohat M, Reisner SH, Crinkler R, et al. Retinopathy of prematurity: incidence and risk factors. Pediatrics 1983; 72:159.

74. Kalina RE. Treatment of retrolental fibroplasia. Surv Ophthalmol 1980; 24:229.

75. Rudd EG. Premature rupture of the membranes. A review. J Reprod Med 1985; 30:841.

76. Gibbs RS, Blanco JD. Premature rupture of membranes. Obstet Gynecol 1982; 60:671.

77. Smith R. Techniques for detection of ruptured membranes: a review and preliminary report. Obstet Gynecol 1976; 48:172.

78. Reese EA, Chervenak F, Moya F, et al. Amniotic fluid arborization: effect of blood meconium and pH alterations. Obstet Gynecol 1984; 64:248.

79. Schutti M, Treffers P, Kloostman G, Soepatmi S. Management of premature rupture of membranes: the risk of vaginal examination to the infant. Am J Obstet Gynecol 1983; 146:395.

80. Skinner S, Campo SG, Liggins G. Collagen content of human amniotic membranes: effective gestation length and premature rupture. Obstet Gynecol 1981; 57:487.

81. Kiilholma P, Gronroos M, Erkkola R, et al. The role of calcium, copper, iron and zinc in preterm delivery and premature rupture of fetal membranes. Gynecol Obstet Invest 1984; 17:194.

82. Lonky NM, Hayashi RH. A proposed mechanism for premature rupture of membranes. Obstet Gynecol Surv 1988; 43:22.

83. Minkoff H. Prematurity: infection is an etiologic factor. Obstet Gynecol 1983; 62:137.

84. Lenihan JP Jr. Relationship of antepartum pelvic examinations to premature rupture of membranes. Obstet Gynecol 1984; 63:33.

85. Minkoff H, Grunebaum AN, Schwarz RH, Feldman J, et al. Risk factors for prematurity and premature rupture of membranes: a prospective study of the vaginal flora in pregnancy. Am J Obstet Gynecol 1984; 150:965.

86. Regan J, Chao S, James LS. Premature rupture of membranes, preterm delivery, and group B streptococcus colonization of mothers. Am J Obstet Gynecol 1981; 141:184.

87. Naeye R. Factors predispose to premature rupture of membranes of fetal membranes. Obstet Gynecol 1982; 60:93.

88. Koh KS, Chan FH, Monfared AH, et al. The changing perinatal and maternal outcome in chorioamnionitis. Obstet Gynecol 1979; 53:730.

89. Broekhuizen FF, Gilman M, Hamilton PR. Amniocentesis for Gram stain and culture in preterm premature rupture of the membranes. Obstet Gynecol 1985; 66:316.

90. Feinstein SJ, Vintzileos AM, Lodeiro JG, et al. Amniocentesis with premature rupture of membranes. Obstet Gynecol 1986; 68:147.

91. Yeast JD, Garite T, Dorchester W. The risks of amniocentesis in the management of preterm rupture of membranes. Am J Obstet Gynecol 1984; 149:505.

92. Johnson JWC, Daikoku NH, Niebyl JR, et al. Premature rupture of the membranes and prolonged latency. Obstet Gynecol 1981; 57:547.

93. Graham RL, Gilstrap LC III, Hauth JC, et al. Conservative management of patients with premature rupture of fetal membranes. Obstet Gynecol 1982; 59:607.

94. Andreyko JL, Chen CP, Shennan AT, Milligan JE. Results of conservative management of premature rupture of the membranes. Am J Obstet Gynecol 1984; 148:600.

95. Vintzileos AM, Campbell WA, Nochimson DJ, Weinbaum PJ. Degree of oligohydramnios and pregnancy outcome in patients with premature rupture of the membranes. Obstet Gynecol 1985; 66:162.

96. Curet L, Rao B, Zachman R, et al. Association between ruptured membranes, tocolytic therapy and respiratory distress syndrome. Am J Obstet Gynecol 1984; 148:263.

97. Nelson L, Meis P, Hatjis C, et al. Premature rupture of membranes: a prospective randomized evaluation of steroids, latent phase, and expectant management. Obstet Gynecol 1985; 66:55.

98. Taylor J, Garite TJ. Premature rupture of membranes before fetal viability. Obstet Gynecol 1984; 64:615.

99. Nimrod C, Varela-Gittings F, Machin G, et al. The effect of very prolonged membrane rupture on fetal development. Am J Obstet Gynecol 1984; 148:540.

100. Vintzileos AM, Campbell WA, Nochimson DJ, Weinbaum PJ. The use of the nonstress test in patients with premature rupture of the membranes. Obstet Gynecol 1986; 149:53.

101. Vintzileos AM, Campbell WA, Nochimson DJ, et al. Fetal biophysical profile versus amniocentesis in predicting infection in preterm premature rupture of the membranes. Obstet Gynecol 1986; 68:488.

102. Morales WJ. The effect of chorioamnionitis on the developmental outcome of preterm infants at one year. Obstet Gynecol 1987; 70:183.

103. Capeless EL, Mead PB. Management of preterm premature rupture of membranes: lack of a national consensus. Am J Obstet Gynecol 1987; 157:11.

104. Garite TJ, Freeman R, Linzey E, et al. Prospective randomized study of corticosteroids in the management of premature rupture of membranes and the premature gestation. Am J Obstet Gynecol 1981; 141:408.

105. Iams J, Talbert M, Barrows H, Sachs L. Management of preterm prematurely ruptured membranes: a prospective randomized comparison of observation versus steroids and timed delivery. Am J Obstet Gynecol 1985; 151:32.

106. MacArthur G, Howie R, Dezoete J, Elkins J. School progress and cognate development of six year old children whose mothers were treated antenatally with betamethasone. Pediatrics 1982; 70:99.

107. Christensen KV, Ingmarson I, Leideman T, et al. Effects of ritodrine on labor after premature rupture of membranes. Obstet Gynecol 1980; 55:187.

108. Garite TJ, Keegan KA, Freeman RK, Nageotte MP. Randomized trial of ritodrine tocolysis versus expectant management of patients with premature rupture of membranes at 25–30 weeks gestation. Am J Obstet Gynecol 1987; 157:388.

109. Levy DL, Warsaw SL. Oral ritodrine and preterm premature rupture of membranes. Obstet Gynecol 1985; 66:621.

110. Romero R, Scioscia AL, Edberg SC, Hobbins JC. Use of parenteral antibiotic therapy to eradicate bacterial colonization of amniotic fluid in premature rupture of membranes. Obstet Gynecol 1986; 67:15S.

111. Ogita S, Imanaka M, Sugawa T. Clinical effectiveness of newly devised cervical indwelling catheter in managing premature rupture of the membranes—a Japanese collaborative work. Abstract 31 presented at the Eighth Annual Meeting, Society of Perinatal Obstetricians, Las Vegas, Nevada, February 1988.

112. Boylan T, Odriscoll K. Improvement in perinatal mortality rate attributed to spontaneous preterm labor without use of tocolytic agents. Am J Obstet Gynecol 1983; 145:781.

113. Tejani NA, Verma UL. Effects of tocolysis on incidents of low birth weight. Obstet Gynecol 1983; 61:556.

114. Korenbrot CC, Aalto LH, Laros RK Jr. The cost effectiveness of stopping preterm labor with beta adrenergic treatment. N Engl J Med 1984; 310:691.

115. Garfield RH. Control of myometrial function in preterm versus term labor. Clin Obstet Gynecol 1984; 27:572.

116. Harris BA, Gore H, Flowers CE Jr. Peripheral placental separation: a possible relationship to preterm labor. Obstet Gynecol 1985; 66:774.

117. Hameed C, Tejani N, Verma UL, et al. Silent chorioamnionitis as a cause of preterm labor refractile tocolytic therapy. Am J Obstet Gynecol 1984; 149:726.

118. McGregor JA. Prevention of preterm birth: new initiatives based on microbial-host interactions. Obstet Gynecol Surv 1988; 43:1.

119. Gravett MG, Hummell D, Eschenbach DA, et al. Preterm labor associated with sub-clinical amniotic fluid infection and with bacterial vaginitis. Obstet Gynecol 1986; 67:229.

120. Valenzuela G, Kline S, Hayashi RH. Follow-up of hydration and sedation in the pre-therapy of premature labor. Am J Obstet Gynecol 1983; 147:396.

121. Sica-Blanco Y, Rozada H, Remedio MR. Effects of meperidine on uterine contractility of pregnancy and pre-labor. Am J Obstet Gynecol 1967; 97:1096.

122. Roberts JM. Current understanding in pharmacologic mechanisms in the prevention of preterm birth. Clin Obstet Gynecol 1984; 27:592.

123. Katz M, Robertson MA, Creasy RK. Cardiovascular complications associated with terbutaline treatment for preterm labor. Am J Obstet Gynecol 1981; 139:605.

124. Benedetti TJ. Maternal complications of parenteral beta-sympathomimetic therapy for premature labor. Am J Obstet Gynecol 1983; 145:1.

125. Hosenpud JD, Morton MJ, O'Grady JP. Cardiac stimulation during ritodrine hydrochloride tocolytic therapy. Obstet Gynecol 1983; 62:52.

126. Michalak D, Kline V, Marquette GP. Myocardial ischemia: a complication of ritodrine tocolysis. Am J Obstet Gynecol 1983; 146:861.

127. Meinen K. Radioimmunoassay procedure of serum myoglobin in cases of long-term tocolysis with beta-sympathomimetics. Gynecol Obstet Invest 1981; 12:37.

128. Benedetti TJ, Hargrove JC, Rosene KA. Maternal pulmonary edema during premature labor inhibition. Obstet Gynecol 1982; 59:33S.

129. Hankins GD, Hauth JC, Keuhl T. Ritodrine hydrochloride infusion in pregnant baboons to sodium and water compartment alterations. Am J Obstet Gynecol 1983; 147:254.

130. Hancock PJ, Setzer ES, Beutoum SN. Physiologic and biochemical effects of ritodrine therapy on the mother and neonate. Am J Perinatol 1985; 2:1.

131. Kirkpatrick C, Quenon M, Desir D. Blood anions and electrolytes during ritodrine infusion in preterm labor. Am J Obstet Gynecol 1980; 138:523.

132. Spellacy WN, Cruz AC, Buhi WC, et al. The effects of ritodrine infusion on maternal metabolism: measurements of levels of glucose, insulin, glucagon, triglycerides, cholesterol, placental lactogen and chorionic gonadotropin. Am J Obstet Gynecol 1978; 131:637.

133. Miodovnik M, Peros N, Holroyde JC, Siddiqi TA. Treatment of preterm labor in insulin-dependent women. Obstet Gynecol 1985; 65:621.

134. Unbehaun V. Effects of betamimetic tocolytic agents on the fetus. J Perinat Med 1974; 2:17.

135. Humphrey M, Chang A, Gilbert M, et al. The effects of intravenous ritodrine on acid-base status of the fetus during the second stage of labor. Br J Obstet Gynaecol 1975; 82:234.

136. Brettes JP, Renaud R, Gandar R. A double-blind investigation into the effects of ritodrine and uterine blood flow during the third trimester of pregnancy. Am J Obstet Gynecol 1976; 124:164.

137. Thiagarajah S, Harbert GM, Bourgeois FJ. Magnesium sulfate ritodrine hydrochloride: systemic and uterine hemodynamic effects. Am J Obstet Gynecol 1985; 153:666.

138. Huisjes HJ, Touwen BCL. Neonatal outcome after treatment with ritodrine: a controlled study. Am J Obstet Gynecol 1983; 147:250.

139. Karlsson K, Krantz M, Hamberger L. Comparison of various betamimetics on preterm labor, survival and development of the child. J Perinat Med 1980; 8:19.

140. Karlsson K. Beta receptor agonist in pregnancy. Long-term effects in preterm children. Acta Obstet Gynecol Scand (Suppl) 1982; 108:71.

141. Polwczyk D, Tejani N, Lauersen N, et al. Evaluation of seven to nine year old children exposed to ritodrine in utero. Obstet Gynecol 1984; 64:485.

142. Svenningsen NW. Follow-up studies of preterm infants after maternal beta receptor agonist treatment. Acta Obstet Gynecol Scand (Suppl) 1982; 108:67.

143. Boog G, Gandar R. Betamimetic drugs and possible prevention of respiratory distress syndrome. Br J Obstet Gynaecol 1975; 82:285.

144. Cabero L, Giralt E, Navarro E, et al. A betamimetic drug and human fetal lung maturation. Eur J Obstet Gynecol Reprod Biol 1979; 9:261.

145. Berg G, Andersson RGG, Ryden G. Beta-adrenergic receptors in human myometrium during pregnancy; changes in the number of receptors after beta-mimetic treatment. Am J Obstet Gynecol 1985; 151:392.

146. Wesselius-deCasparis A, Thiery M, Sian A, et al. Results of double-blind, multicenter study of ritodrine in premature labor. Br Med J 1971; 3:144.

147. Bardens TP, Peter JB, Merkatz IR. Ritodrine hydrochloride: a betamimetic agent for use in preterm labor. I. Pharmacology, clinical history, administration, side effects and safety. Obstet Gynecol 1980; 56:1.

148. Merkatz IR, Peter JB, Barden TP. Ritodrine hydrochloride: a betamimetic agent for use of preterm labor. II. Evidence of efficacy. Obstet Gynecol 1980; 56:7.

149. Spellacy WN, Cruz AC, Birke SA, et al. Treatment of preterm premature labor with ritodrine: a randomized controlled study. Obstet Gynecol 1979; 54:220.

150. Larsen JF, Hansen MK, Hesseldahl H, et al. Ritodrine and the treatment of premature labor. A clinical trial compared with a standard treatment with three regimens involving the use of ritodrine. Br J Obstet Gynaecol 1980; 87:949.

151. Levino KJ, Guzick DS, Hankins GD, et al. Single center randomized trial of ritodrine hydrochloride for preterm labor. Lancet 1986; 1:1293.

152. Larsen JF, Eldon K, Lange AP, et al. Ritodrine in the treatment of preterm labor: second Danish multiple center study. Obstet Gynecol 1986; 67:607.

153. Beall MH, Edgar BW, Paul RH, et al. Comparison of ritodrine, terbutaline and magnesium sulfate for suppression of premature labor. Am J Obstet Gynecol 1985; 153:854.

154. Caritis SN, Toig G, Heddinger LA, et al. A double-blind study comparing ritodrine and terbutaline in the treatment of premature labor. Am J Obstet Gynecol 1984; 154:7.

155. Hollander DI, Nagey DA, Pupkin MJ. Magnesium sulfate and ritodrine hydrochloride: a randomized comparison. Am J Obstet Gynecol 1987; 156:631.

156. Tchilinguirian NG, Najem R, Sullivan GB, et al. The use of ritodrine and magnesium sulfate in the arrest of premature labor. Int J Gynaecol Obstet 1984; 22:117.

157. Creasy RK, Goldbus MS, Larros RK Jr. Oral ritodrine maintenance in the treatment of preterm labor. Am J Obstet Gynecol 1980; 137:212.

158. Gross TL, Kuhnert BR, Kuhnert PM, et al. Maternal and fetal plasma concentrations of ritodrine. Obstet Gynecol 1985; 65:793.

159. Caritis SN, Linn SL, Toig G, et al. Pharmacodynamics of ritodrine in pregnant women during premature labor. Am J Obstet Gynecol 1983; 147:752.

160. Schreter P, Caspte E, Snir E, et al. Metabolic effects of intramuscular and oral administration of ritodrine. Obstet Gynecol 1981; 57:730.

161. Ingemarsson I. Effects of terbutaline on premature labor. A double-blinded placebo-controlled study. Am J Obstet Gynecol 1975; 125:520.

162. Howard TE Jr, Killam AP, Penny LL, et al. A double-blind randomized study of terbutaline in premature labor. Milit Med 1982; 147:305.

163. Caritis SN, Carson D, Greebon D, et al. Comparison of terbutaline and ethanol in the treatment of preterm labor. Am J Obstet Gynecol 1982; 142:183.

164. Cotton DB, Strassner HT, Hill LM, et al. Comparison of magnesium sulfate, terbutaline and placebo for the inhibition of

preterm labor: randomized study. J Reprod Med 1984; 29:92.

165. Miller JM Jr, Keane MWD, Horger EO III. A comparison of magnesium sulfate and terbutaline for the arrest of premature labor. J Reprod Med 1982; 27:348.

166. Lyrenas S, Grahnen A, Lindberg B, et al. Pharmacokinetics of terbutaline during pregnancy. Eur J Clin Pharmacol 1986; 29:619.

167. Stubblefield PG, Heyl PS. Treatment of preterm labor with subcutaneous terbutaline. Obstet Gynecol 1982; 59:457.

168. Moise KJ Jr, Dorman K, Giebel R, et al. A randomized study of intravenous versus subcutaneous/oral terbutaline in the treatment of preterm labor. Abstract 276 presented at the seventh annual meeting, Society of Perinatal Obstetricians, Orlando, Florida, February, 1987.

169. Main EK, Main DM, Gabbe SG. Chronic oral terbutaline tocolytic therapy is associated with maternal glucose intolerance. Am J Obstet Gynecol 1987; 157:644.

170. Hall DG, McGaughery HS Jr, Corey EL, et al. Effects of magnesium therapy and the duration of labor. Am J Obstet Gynecol 1959; 78:27.

171. Carsten ME, Miller JD. A new look at uterine muscle contractions. Am J Obstet Gynecol 1987; 157:1303.

172. Steer CM, Petrie RH. A comparison of magnesium sulfate and alcohol prevention of preterm labor. Am J Obstet Gynecol 1977; 129:1.

173. Petrie RH. Tocolysis using magnesium sulfate. Semin Perinatol 1981; 5:266.

174. Elliott JP. Magnesium sulfate as a tocolytic agent. Am J Obstet Gynecol 1983; 147:277.

175. Spisso KR, Harbert GM, Thiagarajah S. The use of magnesium sulfate as a primary tocolytic agent to prevent premature delivery. Am J Obstet Gynecol 1982; 142:840.

176. Stone SR, Pritchard JA. Effects of maternally administered magnesium sulfate on the neonate. Obstet Gynecol 1970; 35:574.

177. Rasch DK, Hooper PA, Richardson CJ, et al. Neurobehavioral effects of neonatal hypermagnesemia. J Pediatr 1982; 100:272.

178. Cruikshank DP, Pitkin RM, Dowell NE, et al. Urinary magnesium, calcium and phosphate excretion during magnesium sulfate infusion. Obstet Gynecol 1981; 58:430.

179. Wilkins IA, Goldenberg JD, Phillips RM, et al. Long term use of magnesium sulfate as a tocolytic agent. Obstet Gynecol 1986; 67:38S.

180. White CM, Ghodgaonkar RB, Dubin NH, et al. Prostaglandin F metabolite concentrations as a prognostic factor of preterm labor. Obstet Gynecol 1986; 67:496.

181. Fuchs AR, Husslein P, Somolough L, et al. Plasma levels of oxytocin and 13, 14-dihydro-15-ketoprostaglandin $F2_a$ in preterm labor and the effect of ethanol and ritodrine. Am J Obstet Gynecol 1987; 144:753.

182. Zuckerman H, Reiss U, Atad J, et al. Effect of indomethacin on plasma levels of prostaglandin F_2 alpha in women in labor. Br J Obstet Gynaecol 1977; 84:339.

183. Zuckerman H, Shalev E, Gilliet G, et al. Further studies of inhibition of preterm labor with indomethacin I. J Perinat Med 1984; 12:19.

184. Niebyl JR, Blake DA, White RD, et al. The inhibition of preterm labor with indomethacin. Am J Obstet Gynecol 1980; 136:1014.

185. Zuckerman H, Shalev E, Gilliet G, et al. Further studies of inhibition of preterm labor with indomethacin. II. Double-blind study. J Perinat Med 1984; 12:25.

186. Spearing G. Alcohol, indomethacin and salbutamol. Obstet Gynecol 1979; 53:171.

187. Repke, JR, Niebyl JR. Role of prostaglandin synthetase inhibitors in the treatment of preterm labor. Semin Reprod Endocrinol 1985; 3:259.

188. Alvan G, Orme M, Bertilsson L, et al. Pharmacokinetics of indomethacin. Clin Pharmacol Ther 1975; 18:364.

189. Goode BM, Dossetor JFB. Effects on the fetus of indomethacin given to suppressed labor. Lancet 1979; 2:1187.

190. Dudley DKL, Hardie MJ. Fetal and neonatal effects of indomethacin use as a tocolytic agent. Am J Obstet Gynecol 1985; 151:181.

191. Moise KJ Jr, Hohta JC, Dawod S, et al. Indomethacin in the treatment of preterm labor: effects on the human ductus arteriosus. Abstract 14 presented at the seventh annual meeting, Society of Perinatal Obstetricians, Orlando, Florida, February 1987.

192. Ulmsten U, Andersson KE, Foreman A. Relaxing effects of nifedipine on non-pregnant human uterus in vitro and in vivo. Obstet Gynecol 1978; 52:436.

193. Ulmsten U, Andersson KE, Wingerup L. Treatment of premature labor with calcium antagonist nifedipine. Arch Gynecol 1980; 229:1.

194. Ulmsten U. Treatment of normotensive and hypertensive patients with preterm labor using oral nifedipine, a calcium antagonist. Arch Gynecol 1984; 236:69.

195. D'Alton ME, Jillson AE, Hou S, et al. Treatment of preterm labor with the calcium antagonist nifedipine. Abstract 61 presented at the Fifth Annual Meeting, Society of Perinatal Obstetricians, Las Vegas, Nevada, February 1985.

196. Ferguson JE II, Holbrook RH Jr. Prospective randomized comparison of cardiovascular and metabolic effects associated with nifedipine and ritodrine tocolysis. Presented at annual meeting, Society for Gynecologic Investigation, Toronto, Canada, 1986.

197. Veille JC, Bissonnett JM, Hohimer AR. The effects of the calcium channel blocker nifedipine on uterine blood flow in the pregnant goat. Am J Obstet Gynecol 1986; 154:160.

198. Ferguson J, Schutz T, Pershe R, et al. Nifedipine pharmacokinetics during preterm labor tocolysis. Presented at annual meeting, Society of Gynecologic Investigation, Baltimore, Maryland, 1988.

199. Hatjis CG, Nelson LH, Meis PJ, et al. Addition of magnesium sulfate improves effectiveness of ritodrine in preventing preterm delivery. Am J Obstet Gynecol 1984; 150:142.

200. Ferguson JE II, Holbrook H Jr, Stevenson DK, et al. Adjunctive magnesium sulfate infusion does not alter metabolic changes associated with ritodrine tocolysis. Am J Obstet Gynecol 1987; 156:103.

201. Ogburne PL Jr, Hansen CA, Williams PP, et al. Magnesium sulfate and betamimetic dual agent tocolysis in preterm labor after single agent failure. J Reprod Med 1985; 30:583.

202. Ferguson JE II, Hensleigh PA, Kredenster D. Adjunctive use of magnesium sulfate with ritodrine for preterm labor tocolysis. Am J Obstet Gynecol 1984; 148:166.

203. Rodriquez-Escudero FS, Arawguren C, Benito JA. Verapamil to inhibit the cardiovascular side effects of ritodrine. Int J Gynecol Obstet 1981; 19:333.

204. Gamissans O, Canas E, Cararach V, et al. A study of indomethacin combined with ritodrine in threatened preterm labor. Eur J Obstet Gynecol Reprod Biol 1978; 8:123.

205. Katz Z, Lancet M, Yemini M, et al. Treatment of premature labor contractions with combined ritodrine indomethacin. Int J Gynaecol Obstet 1983; 21:337.

206. Daikoku NH, Johnson JWC, Graf C, et al. Patterns of intrauterine growth retardation. Obstet Gynecol 1979; 54:211.

207. Lubchenco LO, Hansman C, Dressler M, Boyd E. Intrauterine growth as estimated from liveborn birth-weight data at 24 to 42 weeks of gestation. Pediatrics 1963; 32:793.

208. Battaglia FC, Lubchenco LO. A practical classification of newborn infants by weight and gestational age. J Pediatr 1967; 71:159.

209. Seeds JW. Impaired fetal growth: definition and clinical diagnosis. Obstet Gynecol 1984; 64:303.

210. Williams RL, Creasy RK, Cunningham GL, et al. Fetal growth and perinatal viability in California. Obstet Gynecol 1982; 59:624.

211. Meschia G. Supply of oxygen to the fetus. J Reprod Med 1979; 23:160.

212. Galbraith RS, Karchmar EJ, Piercy WN, et al. The clinical prediction of intrauterine growth retardation. Am J Obstet Gynecol 1979; 133:281.

213. Resnik R. Maternal diseases associated with abnormal fetal growth. J Reprod Med 1978; 21:315.

214. Belton SR, Ferguson JE II, Catanzarite VA. Neurofibromatosis and pregnancy: report of a case complicated by intrauterine

growth retardation and oligohydramnios. Am j Obstet Gynecol 1984; 149:468.

215. Scott A, Moar V, Ounsted M. The relative contributions of different maternal factors in small-for-gestational-age pregnancies. Eur J Obstet Gynecol Reprod Biol 1981; 12:157.

216. Houlton MCC, Marivate M, Philpott RH. The prediction of fetal growth retardation in twin pregnancy. Br J Obstet Gynaecol 1981; 88:264.

217. Tejani N, Mann LI. Diagnosis and management of the small-for-gestational-age fetus. Clin Obstet Gynecol 1977; 20:943.

218. Tejani N. Recurrence of intrauterine growth retardation. Obstet Gynecol 1982; 59:329.

219. Belizan JM, Villar J, Nardin JC, et al. Diagnosis of intrauterine growth retardation by a simple clinical method: measurement of fundal height. Am J Obstet Gynecol 1978; 131:643.

220. Campbell S, Dewhurst CJ. Diagnosis of the small-for-dates fetus by serial ultrasonic cephalometry. Lancet 1971; 2:1002.

221. Evans MI, Mukherjee AB, Schulman JD. Animal models of intrauterine growth retardation. Obstet Gynecol Surv 1983; 38:183.

222. Warsof SL, Cooper DJ, Little D, Campbell S. Routine ultrasound screening for antenatal detection of intrauterine growth retardation. Obstet Gynacol 1986; 67:33.

223. Gohari P, Berkowitz RL, Hobbins JC. Prediction of intrauterine growth retardation by determination of total intrauterine volume. Am J Obstet Gynecol 1977; 127:255.

224. Chinn DH, Filly RA, Callen PW. Prediction of intrauterine growth retardation by sonographic estimation of total intrauterine volume. J Clin Ultrasound 1981; 9:175.

225. Grannum PA, Berkowitz RL, Hobbins JC. The ultrasonic changes in the maturing placenta and their relation to fetal pulmonary maturity. Am J Obstet Gynecol 1979; 133:915.

226. Kazzi GM, Gross TL, Sokol RJ. Fetal biparietal diameter and placental grade: predictors of intrauterine growth retardation. Obstet Gynecol 1983; 62:755.

227. Manning FA, Hill M, Platt LD. Qualitative amniotic fluid volume determination by ultrasound: antepartum detection of intrauterine growth retardation. Am J Obstet Gynecol 1981; 139:254.

228. Philipson EH, Sokol RJ, Williams T. Oligohydramnios: clinical associations and predictive value for intrauterine growth retardation. Am J Obstet Gynecol 1983; 146:271.

229. Ott WJ, Doyle S. Ultrasound diagnosis of altered fetal growth by the use of normal ultrasonic fetal weight curves. Obstet Gynecol 1984; 63:201.

230. Trudinger BJ, Giles WB, Cook CM. Flow velocity waveforms in the maternal uteroplacental and fetal umbilical placental circulations. Am J Obstet Gynecol 1985; 152:155.

231. Fleischer A, Schulman H, Farmakides G, et al. Umbilical artery velocity waveforms and intrauterine growth retardation. Am J Obstet Gynecol 1985; 151:502.

232. Giles WB, Trudinger BJ, Baird PJ. Fetal umbilical artery flow velocity waveforms and placental resistance: pathological correlation. Br J Obstet Gynaecol 1985; 92:31.

233. Hogge WA, Thiagarajah S, Brenbridge AN, Harbert GM. Fetal evaluation by percutaneous blood sampling. Am J Obstet Gynecol 1988; 158:132.

234. Pardi G, Buscaglia M, Ferrazzi E, et al. Cord sampling for the evaluation of oxygenation and acid-base balance in growth-retarded human fetuses. Am J Obstet Gynecol 1987; 157:1221.

235. Cetin I, Marconi AM, Bozzetti P, et al. Umbilical amino acid concentrations in appropriate and small for gestational age infants: a biochemical difference present in utero. Am J Obstet Gynecol 1988; 158:120.

236. Repke JT. Ferguson JE II. Fetal monitoring and fetal distress. In: Albright GA, Ferguson JE II, Joyce TH III, Stevenson DK, eds. Anesthesia in obstetrics: maternal, fetal, and neonatal aspects. Boston, Massachusetts: Butterworths, 1986:551.

237. Bastide A, Manning F, Harman C, et al. Ultrasound evaluation of amniotic fluid: outcome of pregnancies with severe oligohydramnios. Am J Obstet Gynecol 1986; 154:895.

238. Reece EA, Goldstein I, Pilu G, Hobbins JC. Fetal cerebellar growth unaffected by intrauterine growth retardation: a new parameter for prenatal diagnosis. Am J Obstet Gynecol 1987; 157:632.

239. Lin C-C, Moawad AH, Rosenow PJ, River P. Acid-base characteristics of fetuses with intrauterine growth retardation during labor and delivery. Am J Obstet Gynecol 1980; 137:553.

240. Chiswick ML. Intrauterine growth retardation. Br Med J 1985; 291:845.

3

Complications of Labor and Delivery: Selected Medical and Surgical Considerations

Ronald L. Thomas, M.D., James E. Ferguson II, M.D., and John T. Repke, M.D.

Antepartum and Intrapartum Considerations
Presentation
    External Version of a Breech Presentation
Normal Labor
Abnormal Labor
Maternal Infectious Diseases
    Group B Streptococcal Infection
    Herpes
Maternal Immune Thrombocytopenia
Acid-Base Considerations in Labor
Delivery Considerations
    Episiotomy
    Forceps and Vacuum Use
Management of Meconium
Macrosomia
Shoulder Dystocia and Brachial Plexus Injury
Management Decisions: A Perspective

Potential complications of labor and delivery can be recognized through information from the history, laboratory, and physical examination, but many times complications are recognized only after they occur, retrospectively. One conceptual approach to the recognition of potential complications is a temporal one, which divides the "at risk interval" into antepartum, intrapartum, and delivery. This chapter attempts to place topics that are not frequently covered in reviews of risk assessment into the categories of major clinical emphasis.

ANTEPARTUM AND INTRAPARTUM CONSIDERATIONS

Medical and surgical disorders of the mother and fetus can have implications for the obstetrician and the intrapartum management plan. Certain conditions, such as fetal anomalies and specific high risk maternal conditions (e.g., severe cardiac disease), usually result in the entire management's being shifted to a tertiary care institution. Other high risk conditions, however, frequently present as emergencies to the practicing obstetrician or are common, albeit high risk, conditions that may be managed outside a referral center; these can result in management dilemmas. Other more detailed reference articles address the management of fetal malformations such as omphalocele, gastroschisis, hydrocephalus, neural tube defects, and other anomalies. Other reviews cover a variety of maternal conditions that may be associated with an adverse perinatal outcome. However, there are conditions that specifically result in intrapartum management dilemmas; some of these are discussed here.

PRESENTATION

Fetal malpresentations are a significant source of both fetal and maternal morbidity. Certain clinical circumstances should increase one's suspicion of malpresentation. Some of the more common associations are summarized in Tables 3–1 and 3–2.

The incidence of malpresentation (unstable, oblique, transverse lie) at term is approximately 0.33 percent.[1] This contrasts sharply with the incidence of 2 percent at 32 weeks.[2] Early diagnosis is imperative and has a major impact on fetal mortality; a reduction from 27.5 to 9.2 percent was reported in one study comparing late with early diagnosis of fetal malpresentation.[3] Delayed diagnosis may allow cord prolapse, which is 20 times more prevalent with an abnormal lie than with a

TABLE 3-1   Fetal Etiologies of Malpresentation

Uterine volume–fetal size disproportions
  Hydramnios
  Macrosomia
  Hydrocephalus
  Multiple gestations
  Placenta previa
  Anencephaly
Inherent fetal activity deficits
  Chromosomal abnormalities, trisomies
  Myotonic dystrophy

Adapted from Seeds JW. Malpresentations. In: Gabbe SG, Niebyl JR, Simpson JL, eds. Obstetrics: normal and problem pregnancies. New York: Churchill Livingstone, 1986:453.

vertex presentation.[2] The route of delivery may have a significant impact on perinatal mortality. Cesarean delivery has been compared with the past practice of internal podalic version and extraction, and abdominal delivery is associated with significant reductions in perinatal mortality. The question of version in these instances is addressed subsequently.

Malpresentation is generally thought of as it applies to the presenting part, but attitudinal abnormalities of vertex presentations can be just as significant. Deflection abnormalities can be of any degree, but face and brow presentations are the two major categories. Face presentations occur with an average incidence of 0.2 percent.[1] Perinatal mortality is reported to be as high as 5 percent.[4] An extremely high rate of fetal malformation is found in this circumstance, with incidences ranging as high as 60 percent.[5] Although vaginal delivery is possible, cesarean section incidences of up to 60 percent are reported.[6] As with other malpresentations, early recognition probably leads to a lower perinatal mortality.[7] The persistent mentum posterior presentation, at least at term, is of special note, since in this case vaginal delivery is not safe or warranted.[8]

Brow presentations are even more unusual, with an incidence of 1 in 1,500.[9] This presentation may convert to a face or occiput presentation during the course of

TABLE 3-2   Maternal Etiologies of Malpresentation

Historical
  Grand multiparity; presumably decreased ability to maintain tone allows increased fetal mobility and, as such, greater risk of nonvertex presentation
  Previous malpresentation: this suggests abnormal pelvic abdominal anatomy not directing to a normal vertex lie

Anatomic
  As above, with suggestion of pelvic contracture not allowing descent of the vertex
  Leiomyomas or other pelvic tumor distorting either the uterine cavity or the pelvic abdominal cavity
  Uterine malformation, congenital

Adapted from Seeds JW. Malpresentations. In: Gabbe SJ, Niebyl JR, Simpson JL, eds. Obstetrics: normal and problem pregnancies. New York: Churchill Livingstone, 1986:453.

labor. Less than half these patients ultimately deliver vaginally.[10,11]

Prolongation, protraction, and arrest disorders are most common with deflection malpresentations, perhaps in part because of the increased occurrence of cephalopelvic disproportion. A general rule is to avoid oxytocin augmentation and proceed to cesarean delivery in patients with dysfunctional labor and a deflection abnormality.

Brief mention will be made of compound presentation, although this is rarely seen in term labor. The repercussions of this malpresentation in the premature fetus can be devastating. The overall incidence ranges from 1 in 377 to 1 in 1,213.[10,12-14] By definition, a limb precedes the presenting part. An arm prolapsing with the vertex fortunately is most common and carries the best prognosis. The perinatal mortality in this category averages 93 in 1,000,[10] with the foot and breech combination higher (17 to 19 percent).[13] The most common morbid complication in these patients is cord prolapse.[12] Although retraction of the prolapsing limb may spontaneously occur and allow safe vaginal delivery, cesarean section is still required in many cases for either cord prolapse or an arrest of labor.[10]

The breech presentation demonstrates several of the etiologic factors already mentioned in Tables 3–1 and 3–2. Clearly prematurity predisposes to a breech presentation, with an incidence declining from 25 percent before 28 weeks[15] to 7 percent at 32 weeks.[8] Certain types of breech presentations are even more commonly associated with prematurity; given a premature breech, 50 percent are footling or incomplete forms.[15] Twenty percent of the patients have a history of a previous breech presentation.[8] As with all persistent malpresentations, consideration should be given to the possible presence of a fetal congenital malformation or chromosomal abnormality.

The basic mechanisms of labor are not inherently different with a breech presentation if vaginal delivery is being considered. With incomplete and complete breech presentations, cord prolapse and cord compression with resultant fetal distress are always of concern. Many obstetricians advocate elective cesarean delivery for all nonfrank breech presentations.[1] Recently Bingham and Lilford[16] reviewed the risks and benefits of selected breech deliveries and concluded that a well-supported argument could be made for primary cesarean delivery of all breeches. Clearly the morbidity and mortality following vaginal delivery for the unselected breech fetus favor the abdominal route. Just as clearly, vaginal delivery favors a maternal outcome with reduced morbidity and mortality. As social trends and family size change, and patient expectations continue to increase, obstetricians may begin to alter historical practice. Thorough assessment and counseling must be part of any planned vaginal breech delivery at term. The special additional concerns for premature vaginal breeches are beyond the scope of this chapter.

External Version of a Breech Presentation

Breech presentations, which account for approximately 3.5 percent of presentations at the onset of labor,[17] continue to be a common indication for cesarean delivery. The purpose of external cephalic version is to reduce the number of breech presentations and thus reduce the frequency of cesarean delivery. The practice of external cephalic version is one that has existed since Aristotle's time and is a topic of renewed interest in the 1980s. The incidence of success with external version is reported to range between 30 and 98 percent.[17] This wide variation undoubtedly exists because of differences in candidate selection and technique. There are clear contraindications to external cephalic version; Table 3-3 lists some of the more common ones.

Specific influences on the incidence of success can include parity, placental location, volume of amniotic fluid, and type of breech.[22] Knowledge of these factors may be helpful when one is counseling a patient prior to version. Whether tocolysis at the time of external cephalic version is required is questionable. Robertson et al[23] have obtained successful results without tocolysis, with no significant difference between two groups in a randomized study. Whenever external cephalic version is considered, one is in effect balancing the fetal morbidity and mortality of vaginal breech delivery against the risks of cesarean breech delivery and the risks with external cephalic version with or without success. Obviously considerations of maternal morbidity and mortality are extremely important, and there is no question that vaginal delivery is safer than cesarean delivery. The morbidity and mortality associated with external cephalic version are extremely low. This technique is reviled by a few; however, it clearly is an acceptable option when there are no fetal or maternal contraindications and when it is performed by obstetricians experienced with the techniques of external cephalic version.

NORMAL LABOR

As with most observations in medicine, our understanding of "abnormal" is based to a large extent on the definition of "normal." Friedman's classic work remains the standard by which normal labor is judged.[24] A representation of the Friedman labor curve is shown in Figure 3-1.

Labor can be defined most simply as a series of organized uterine contractions that cause a change in cervical dilatation and effacement. This change in cervical findings marks the beginning of the latent phase or preparatory division of labor. This is followed by the active phase or dilatational division of labor in which rapid cervical dilatation occurs. The active phase of labor ends at full cervical dilatation. Stage II of labor encompasses the period between full dilatation and retraction of the cervix and delivery. Stage III involves delivery of the placenta. This ideal labor curve provides only a framework in which to discuss abnormalities. Normal labor curves may fall to either side of the "ideal" labor curve. Also, there may be differences between the labor expected in nulliparous and multiparous patients (Fig. 3-2).

ABNORMAL LABOR

Diagnosing abnormal labor allows specific therapeutic measures to be applied under some circumstances and in other cases simply identifies cases of high risk labor that merit closer observation. Abnormalities of labor fall into three basic categories: prolongation disorders, protraction disorders, and arrest disorders. As labor patterns for nulliparous patients and multiparous patients vary, so do the diagnostic criteria for labor disorders. The most common patterns of abnormal labor are summarized in Table 3-4. Certain observations and generalizations can be made regarding progress or lack of progress in labor. Abnormalities of the latent

TABLE 3-3   Contraindications to External Cephalic Version

Maternal	Fetal
Diabetes or abnormal glucose tolerance test result[18]	Well-engaged breech[18]
Cardiac disease[18]	Abnormal antepartum testing, non–stress test[18]
Hypertensive disease[17]	Intrauterine growth retardation[18]
Hyperthyroidism[19]	
Obesity[17,20,21]	Oligohydramnios[18]
Multiple pregnancy[17]	Rh isoimmunization[17]
Patient refusal[18]	
Rupture of membranes[18]	
Previous uterine scar[19]	
Third trimester bleeding[19]	
Placenta previa[18]	

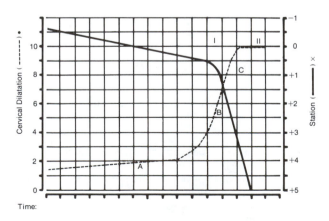

Figure 3-1   Divisions and stages of labor. *A*, Preparatory division. *B*, Dilatational division. *C*, Pelvic division. I, Stage I. II, Stage II.

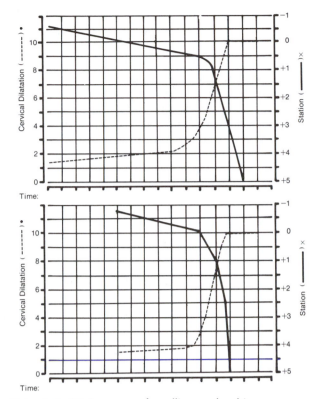

Figure 3-2 Friedman curves for nullipara and multipara.

phase are important for two reasons: First, prolongation of this phase is unique as a labor abnormality in that it does not have a negative prognosis for further dysfunctional labor patterns. Second, the latent phase of labor is the most sensitive to exogenous influences, such as sedation and analgesia; thus, this prolongation disorder is commonly iatrogenic.

Protraction disorders are much less frequent than latent phase prolongation. These disorders—protraction of dilation and protraction of descent—are prognostically much more significant, since cesarean delivery is most commonly the final outcome. The actual etiology of these dysfunctional patterns is unknown, but certain observations have been made. Relative malpres-

entations appear more commonly with protraction disorders, and once they are noted, attempts to correct apparently ineffectual contraction patterns through oxytocin augmentation are particularly unsuccessful.[25] Some investigators suggest that unwarranted midforceps assistance in this group may contribute to unfavorable fetal outcomes. [24-27]

Arrest disorders are perhaps most obvious. Clinical evaluation of these patients, however, may require the greatest obstetrical skill. Approximately half these patients require cesarean delivery.[25] Those with the best prognosis for vaginal delivery are those with disorders that are iatrogenic secondary to excessive sedation or analgesia. These patients respond well to the use of oxytocin for labor augmentation. Unfortunately, even in cases of absolute cephalopelvic disproportion, oxytocin augmentation may also result in continued cervical dilatation. It is important in these cases not to proceed to a traumatic and difficult forceps delivery.

Certain observations can provide important clinical clues to relative fetal-maternal proportions. The Müller-Hillis maneuver has been espoused as a technique to assess cephalopelvic disproportion in the active phase of labor.[28] It is performed at contraction peak with fundal pressure to determine whether there is additional room for pelvic descent. In cases of vertex impaction without descent, a diagnosis of cephalopelvic disproportion must be entertained. As always, cephalopelvic disproportion is a retrospective diagnosis, and often only the findings at cesarean section reveal the actual etiology to be macrosomia or malpresentation. Another clinical situation suggestive of cephalopelvic disproportion is the nulliparous patient in active labor with an unengaged vertex; this atypical finding warrants close observation.

Table 3-5 summarizes management decisions that can be used in addressing various patterns of dysfunctional labor.

MATERNAL INFECTIOUS DISEASES

Several maternal infectious diseases may have an impact on intrapartum decision making by the obstetrician. The two that we shall discuss are the two that most

TABLE 3-4   Patterns of Abnormal Labor

	Nullipara	Multipara
Prolongation, latent phase	>20 hr	>14 hr
Protraction, dilatational division; active phase	Dilatation slope ≤1.2 cm/hr	Dilatation slope ≤1.5 cm/hr
Protraction, descent phase	Descent ≤2 cm/hr	Descent ≤2 cm/hr
Prolongation, deceleratory portion of active phase	≤3 hr	≤1 hr
Arrest, dilatational division; active phase	No change in examination for longer than 2 hr	
Arrest, descent phase	No descent for longer than 1 hr	
Failure of descent	No descent in deceleratory phase or in stage II of labor	

Adapted from Friedman EA. Dysfunctional labor. In: Cohen WR, Friedman EA, eds. Management of labor. Baltimore: University Park Press, 1983;11.

TABLE 3-5   Management of Dysfunctional Labor

Prolongation of latent phase	Therapeutic rest or oxytocin augmentation if medically indicated
Protraction disorder	Expectancy with cesarean section with diagnosis of cephalopelvic disproportion
Arrest disorder	Oxytocin augmentation if no evidence of cephalopelvic disproportion; cesarean delivery with cephalopelvic disproportion

Adapted from Friedman EA. Dysfunctional labor. In: Cohen WR, Friedman EA, eds. Management of labor. Baltimore: University Park Press, 1983;11.

commonly generate discussion in labor and delivery units and are most frequently a cause of concern to patients—maternal group B streptococcal infection and maternal herpes simplex viral infection.

Group B Streptococcal Infection

Group B streptococci are currently the most frequent cause of life-threatening neonatal infection in the United States. Maternal colonization incidences have ranged from 8 to 31 percent, vertical transmission from mother to infant being most likely in cases of heavy colonization.[29] Although it has been suggested that group B streptococcal colonization in the mother may increase the incidence of prematurity, the preponderance of evidence does not support this contention. However, early-onset group B streptococcal infection is the most important factor contributing to neonatal mortality in the United States today.[30,31] It is also a significant cause of neonatal morbidity, which may include respiratory distress, pneumonia, necrotizing enterocolitis, and intraventricular hemorrhage. In an effort to try to minimize early-onset neonatal group B streptococcal infection, it has been recommended that mothers in high risk groups receive intrapartum antibiotic treatment. These high risk groups have included patients with premature labor or prolonged rupture of the membranes and patients with intrapartum fever.[32] This type of intrapartum chemoprophylaxis has been demonstrated to interrupt the vertical transmission of group B streptococci from mother to infant.

Herpes

Herpes, perhaps more than any other infectious disease, has generated considerable anxiety and concern for obstetricians and patients alike. In part this may be because of the uncertainty of the prevalence of herpes within a population, making it impossible to ascertain with accuracy the risk for the development of herpes in a newborn who might be exposed to the virus. Women who experience a primary herpes simplex virus type II infection during pregnancy place their infants at considerable risk because of an increased likelihood of premature labor as well as the possibility of delivery through an infected cervix.[1] These possibilities have led to the recommendation that women experiencing a primary genital herpes infection during pregnancy be treated with antiviral drugs.[33]

Alternatively it appears that women who experience recurrences of genital herpes have a very low risk of transmitting the virus to their neonates. This in turn has led to the recommendation that antiviral therapy not be given to pregnant women experiencing recurrences of genital herpes, and that antiviral therapy may not be indicated in neonates born to mothers with recurrent genital herpes infections.[34] Because of its very high associated morbidity and mortality, the major concern has always been the development of disseminated neonatal herpes. Newer information has led to a modification of our approach to the management of patients with a history of genital herpes in the antepartum and intrapartum periods. These revised recommendations have been published in the American College of Obstetricians and Gynecologists' statement from the committee on obstetrics and maternal and fetal medicine.[35] Adherence to these guidelines may significantly reduce physician and patient anxiety as well as medicolegal exposure.

MATERNAL IMMUNE THROMBOCYTOPENIA

Since the early 1970s it has been recommended that, in order to prevent neonatal intraventricular hemorrhage and subsequent brain injury, infants of mothers with immune thrombocytopenic purpura be delivered by cesarean section.[36,37] Since that time, advances in obstetrical technology have allowed for an alternative approach to this problem. Since the maternal platelet count and the presence or absence of antiplatelet antibodies, either direct or indirect, have not been consistently associated with the neonatal platelet count or function, it became necessary to have alternative methods of assessing neonatal platelet status. Two approaches are available for doing this. One approach involves intrapartum blood sampling of a fetal scalp vein for determination of a platelet count. Another method involves percutaneous umbilical blood sampling and subsequent analysis of the fetal platelet count.

A report by Laros and Kagan[38] suggests that cesarean section should not be utilized routinely for the delivery of infants of mothers with immune thrombocytopenic purpura because of uncertainty whether, in fact, cesarean section protects these infants from subsequent intraventricular hemorrhage. This further raises the issue of whether vaginal delivery is acceptable for these patients even with a normal fetal platelet count and, if so, whether that includes the use of vacuum extraction and midpelvic forceps operations. The answers to these questions are not currently known. To recognize the dual need of taking proper care of the patient (both patients) and minimizing medicolegal exposure, we advocate the following policy:

1. Women who have immune thrombocytopenic purpura are offered percutaneous umbilical blood sampling, prior to the onset of labor, fetal scalp blood sampling in early labor, or elective cesarean section after the risks and benefits of each of these approaches have been fully discussed.

2. Maternal platelet counts, the presence or absence of antiplatelet antibodies, and current steroid use are not involved in the decision concerning the route of delivery.

3. If fetal platelet counts have not been determined prior to delivery, our pediatric staff is notified at the earliest possible time of impending delivery in these patients so that they can be prepared to deal with the potential bleeding problems that can result if a neonate is born with profound thrombocytopenia.

ACID-BASE CONSIDERATIONS IN LABOR

One of the goals in the management of labor and delivery is to avoid fetal asphyxia. Clearly certain fetuses engender suspicion and warrant close monitoring throughout labor. These fetuses include those with suspected anomalies, postdatism, pregnancies complicated by uteroplacental insufficiency or significant maternal disease, and those in which there is a clear suspicion of intrauterine growth retardation.

Today the dominant assessment technique is continuous electronic fetal monitoring during labor and delivery. Three major factors are evaluated during this monitoring—the baseline fetal heart rate, variability, and periodic changes. Whenever there are baseline changes involving tachycardia or bradycardia, further evaluation is necessary. The same is true when there is a decrease in variability. Short-term variability can be evaluated with the new third generation fetal monitors. Variability in general remains the most sensitive indicator of fetal status.[39]

When normal long-term variability is documented, one can be assured in more than 99 percent of the cases that the fetus is not asphyxiated.[40-42] Periodic changes of the early, variable, and late type also can be evaluated for evidence of fetal asphyxia. Early decelerations are most unusual and generally are a result of head compression. Late decelerations routinely suggest fetal hypoxemia. In all cases the potential exists for asphyxia.[43] In every case when late decelerations are noted, further evaluation is mandatory, and plans for delivery must be entertained. In utero resuscitation employing maternal oxygen administration, intravenous hydration, exaggeration of the left lateral position, and discontinuation of oxytocin, if it is being employed, frequently abolishes late deceleration in which variability has been maintained. In repetitive late decelerations with loss of variability unresponsive to in utero resuscitation when vaginal delivery cannot be effected in a very short period of time, consideration must be given to urgent cesarean delivery. Variable decelerations are less worrisome; they generally suggest cord vulnerability, and if they are brief in duration and the variability remains normal, careful surveillance of the fetus can continue without the need for immediate delivery.

When there is a suspicion of fetal asphyxia and delivery is not imminent, scalp pH determination may be warranted. The scalp capillary blood pH has a good correlation with the cord pH, and a normal scalp pH of 7.25 to 7.35 correlates well with a normal fetal arterial pH of 7.27 to 7.28 and is generally slightly lower than the normal fetal venous value of 7.38.[44,45] Of major concern is that, with significant fetal asphyxia, i.e., a pH of 6.9 or lower, there is irreversible cell damage.[46] Obviously intervention before this endpoint is desirable. Fortunately there are many false positive results in evaluating fetal heart rate deceleration patterns. Forty percent of the fetuses with late decelerations have normal cord pH's,[40,47] although the evaluation of variability may refine interpretation somewhat. When a normal fetal scalp sample is obtained (pH 7.25 or more), 92 percent of the neonates have normal Apgar scores. Conversely, when the fetal scalp pH is less than 7.20, 80 percent of the Apgar scores are abnormal (6 or less). A scalp pH between 7.20 and 7.25 lies in a gray zone and warrants repeating the determination in 30 minutes.[43]

Another technique for evaluation is scalp stimulation.[48] When variability is absent and the tracing suggests fetal hypoxemia, as Clark et al[48] noted, fetal heart rate acceleration in response to scalp stimulation is suggestive of a normal pH, and fetal scalp sampling may not be warranted. A more recent application involves vibroacoustic stimulation, and the data currently available suggest that, when fetal heart rate acceleration occurs in response to acoustic stimulation, the fetal acid-base status is normal and fetal scalp sampling again may not be indicated.[49] In both these situations a lack of response has a false positive value of 50 percent or greater.

Current sensitivities and specificities of the techniques available for monitoring the fetal acid-base status in labor are not ideal but when used in combination generally allow for delivery of an uncompromised infant.

DELIVERY CONSIDERATIONS

Episiotomy

Episiotomy has been noted to be the most common operation performed in obstetrics outside of clamping the cord.[50] Although it was originally described in 1742 as a procedure performed only in cases of extreme resistance,[51] it came into uniform use after 1918 when Pomeroy [52] suggested that it be incorporated into routine obstetrical practice. Two years later DeLee[53] continued to recommend episiotomy coupled with the universal prophylactic use of outlet forceps. In the majority of women delivering infants in the United States, episiotomies are performed routinely.

In the current atmosphere of the informed patient, an introspective look is being taken at all procedures, including episiotomy. Thacker and Banta[54] have extensively reviewed more than a century of the English literature dealing with the performance of episiotomy and have found no evidence to support routine use of the procedure. These findings do not imply that episiotomies have no indications; there is agreement that episiotomy reduces traction required for forceps delivery and clearly reduces the length of the second stage of labor.[55] Episiotomies cannot be considered entirely benign, since 20 percent or more of nulliparous patients and more than 10 percent of multiparous patients experience extensions of the episiotomy with resultant third or fourth degree lacerations.[56] This incidence of episiotomy extension is similar to that reported by Beynon[57] three decades ago. The same study indicates that third and fourth degree lacerations are extremely rare when midline episiotomies are not performed.[56] A recent review of fourth degree laceration breakdown and its repair demonstrates that this relatively common trauma is not an insignificant concern.[58]

There are proponents of routine episiotomy and prophylactic episiotomy. The 18th edition of *Williams Obstetrics* supports the use of midline episiotomy to avoid a perineal tear. A historical observation equates the increase in the use of episiotomy with a decrease in the incidence of subsequent symptomatic pelvic relaxation. However, this observation fails to take into account the decreasing family size and lower parity of today's patient. Although a causal relationship between episiotomy use and a lower incidence of pelvic relaxation has been suggested, it has never been proved.[59]

Perhaps one of the more interesting views about episiotomy is provided by Bottoms and Sokol:[60] "episiotomy may be considered a plastic surgical procedure designed to preserve the appearance and function of the introitus as a sexual organ." If an incision were truly to decrease the incidence of pelvic musculature distention, it would be more appropriate to perform a procto-episiotomy in every case, with division of the levators, thus opening the fascial ring of the pelvic floor. By the time the fetal vertex actually reaches the perineum, little of the major pelvic supporting tissue is left unstretched and untraumatized.

The applicability of episiotomy or outlet forceps in premature deliveries is perhaps less controversial. Clearly, if fetal distress occurs (and it may be more likely in these premature infants) or if forceps are to be used to protect the fetal calvarium and assist delivery, an episiotomy should be performed routinely. Bishop et al,[61] in one of the early reports from the collaborative study of cerebral palsy, suggested that "early and generous episiotomy at the appropriate time, followed by the gentle use of outlet forceps, not only offers the premature infant the best chance for survival but also provides protection from traumatic experiences that may result in decreased motor and mental ability as well as in an increased incidence of abnormal neurologic symptoms." This summary was applied to a group of fetuses weighing less than 2,500 gm, and though applicable in 1965 when the article appeared, it may not be quite so applicable today. In fact in a recent study, Barrett et al[62] were unable

to find a difference in morbidity or mortality in infants weighing 751 to 1,000 gm regardless of whether they were delivered with or without forceps or episiotomy. Another report by Huff et al[63] suggests that outlet forceps did, in fact, provide significant protection from intracranial hemorrhage in their study group of 41 patients delivering between 26 and 33 weeks. One hypothesis suggests that forceps use and episiotomy performance enforce more delicate handling and delivery of the fetus and therefore have an indirect effect in improving the fetal outcome.

The use of episiotomy at term is clearly a decision that involves informed consent and that must be made with involvement by the patient. Esthetically and sexually it may have advantages, but medically there are probably few indications. The procedure itself cannot be considered completely benign, and practitioners should not lose sight of this fact. In the case of the premature infant, control and gentleness of delivery are probably more important than episiotomy and forceps application in improving the outcome. Routine use of episiotomy will continue to be indicated in cases of forceps application and in situations, such as fetal distress or maternal disease, requiring a shortening of the second stage of labor. Physician experience will dictate the cases in which episiotomy can be used to avoid significant or serious perineal tears.

Forceps and Vacuum Use

The topic of operative vaginal delivery is as highly charged as any in modern obstetrics. In no other decade would patients readily accept and even request cesarean delivery over forceps application. Emotions among obstetricians are equally strong in regard to midforceps applications. Current trends and philosophies in obstetrics are reflected by journal publications and reference textbook attention to this subject. It has been more than a decade since any major standard reference text has been published dealing solely with forceps application. In contrast, new texts glorifying "high tech" obstetrics, i.e., vaginal ultrasound and Doppler studies of the fetus, fill publishers' displays. A review of journals over the past five years regarding midforceps delivery ranges from the more positive "Midforceps Delivery: A Critical Review,"[64] calling for well-controlled, prospective studies, to a clearly negative view, "Midforceps Delivery: No?"[27]

A brief description is warranted before continuing. "Low forceps" indicates an application made when the fetal sagittal suture is directly in the anterior-posterior plane and the vertex is visible between contractions or maternal expulsion efforts without parting the maternal labia. "High forceps" implies that the fetal biparietal diameter has not passed through the pelvic inlet. Unfortunately all other applications are combined into the category of "midforceps." This clearly creates difficulty in addressing or comparing collected data and outcomes. Although some studies make an effort to separate "difficult" from "easy" midforceps delivery, there is no uniform classification that addresses station of the vertex, position, or degree of asynclitism.

The conclusion we have drawn after review of the literature relating to midforceps deliveries is that the procedure does have certain clear indications, such as fetal distress, but, in contrast, its use cannot be justified to shorten the second stage of labor merely as a patient or physician convenience. Friedman's recent extensive review found uniform evidence of risk with midforceps delivery (although not statistically significant in some series),[27] and various authors interpretations have ranged from condemnation to the conclusion that "there is virtually no inherent danger in the operative procedure itself."[65] Although the use of midforceps in affecting deliveries will continue, indications will probably become more limited, and only the passage of time will determine whether midforceps delivery goes the way of high forceps applications.

The misgivings that obviously exist about midforceps applications do not exist at present for low or "outlet" forceps delivery. This procedure, once applied widely for "prophylaxis," began with DeLee's published recommendation in 1920[53] and remains primarily an elective procedure. The most common "indications" today for outlet forceps application include maternal exhaustion and what is unfortunately described as "terminal fetal bradycardia."

Currently there is increasing interest in comparing vacuum extraction with forceps applications, and most preliminary data support the use of the newer Silastic cups for indications similar to those for forceps. Historically vacuum cup extraction, with its first use credited to Simpson in 1849[66,67] gained little momentum as a useful procedure until the mid-1950s. This was due in large part to modifications reported by Malmstrom[68] and early favorable publicity.[69] Slow American acceptance followed these early reports.[69-71] In the 1980s favorable reports began to appear again in both the British and American literature.[72,73]

Following these reports, additional modifications have occurred, specifically, the introduction of the Silastic vacuum apparatus. This apparatus appears to eliminate some of the scalp trauma previously reported.[74] There may be circumstances in which the vacuum extractor has clear advantages. These are suggested by observations supporting the less traumatic autorotation from occiput posterior and occiput transverse presentations that occur with vacuum extraction, advantages in correcting flexion abnormalities, advantages in the correction of asynclitism, and also the significant advantage of less need for analgesia or anesthesia. One clear contradiction to vacuum use is the presence of a premature fetus. The use of vacuum in this circumstance clearly increases the danger of neonatal jaundice and may have other unacceptable effects as well.[75]

Practice trends, such as those reviewed by Broekhuizen et al[76] indicate an increase in the use of vacuum, with a concomitant decline in forceps applications. Their review also suggests that, although failure incidences are similar, there is a clear tendency for vacuum extractors to be used at higher stations and in situations in which the preapplication position is not occiput anterior. As expected, the incidence of maternal trauma is less in the vacuum group.

Several observations made during the initial reports of vacuum extraction were worrisome. Shoulder dystocia was more common in the vacuum group, probably reflecting the higher station of application and perhaps a more significant relative cephalopelvic disproportion. Also, "cosmetic injuries" ("chignon") were more common with vacuum use. Many of these early reports used the Malmstrom metal vacuum extractor rather than the currently used Silastic cup, which may effectively eliminate many of these concerns. Vacuum extraction has replaced midforceps usage in at least some institutions.

MANAGEMENT OF MECONIUM

The presence of meconium stained amniotic fluid at the time of delivery remains a delivery room emergency. When recognized during the intrapartum period, meconium staining should promote action on the part of the obstetrician to better assess the intrapartum fetal status. This should include continuous intrapartum electric fetal heart rate monitoring, which usually dictates placement of a fetal scalp electrode to allow for better assessment of fetal heart rate variability. In the setting of thick meconium with an uninterpretable or nonreassuring fetal heart rate tracing, further efforts to evaluate the fetal acid-base status should be undertaken and, if not possible, delivery by cesarean section performed. It should be recognized, however, that although fetal heart rate abnormalities may worsen the prognosis in the fetus with meconium stained amniotic fluid, meconium staining in and of itself does not worsen the prognosis associated with a specific fetal heart rate pattern.[77]

Identifying meconium as a potential risk factor assists the obstetrician in more careful management for labor and delivery of that fetus. In post-term pregnancies or even in the non–high risk pregnancy, the obstetrician should always be prepared at the time of delivery for the possible finding of meconium staining. The use of DeLee suction on the perineum has been demonstrated to be preferable to the use of a suction bulb,[78] and oral or oronasal suctioning has been demonstrated to be more efficacious than nasal suctioning alone.[79]

The obstetrician also must be aware that the timing of meconium passage frequently has implications in regard to neonatal prognosis. Meconium staining beginning subsequent to the time of initial rupture of membranes tends to be associated far less frequently with fetal acidosis or depressed Apgar scores. However, the presence of meconium staining in conjunction with abnormal fetal heart rate patterns, including repeated variable decelerations, absence of periodic accelerations, and reduced baseline variability, suggests inadequate fetal compensation for the stresses of labor and has been associated with low Apgar scores.[80] When meconium staining is noted or in situations in which meconium staining is very likely (for example, in postdated pregnancies), a pediatrician qualified to perform neonatal resuscitation should be notified and should be physically present at the time of the infant's delivery. An anesthesiologist may substitute in this role when a pediatrician cannot be present.

In the event of meconium aspiration, there is potential for a pediatric emergency requiring intensive resuscitative efforts in an effort to minimize asphyxia and minimize the risk of subsequent pulmonary hypertension in the neonate. Carson et al[81] have recommended that all infants born in the presence of meconium undergo laryngoscopy, including visualization of the vocal cords and direct tracheal suctioning. The general policy at our institutions has included the following: Vigorous crying infants born with a history of thin meconium do not necessarily require special resuscitative measures, and infants who seem to be depressed at birth and have a history of meconium staining should undergo suctioning of the oropharynx with visualization of the vocal cords and tracheal suctioning when appropriate. Gregory et al[82] have reported a 10 percent incidence of meconium obtained from below the cords even after no meconium was identified at the level of the vocal cords. This finding suggests that perhaps all infants with a history of thick meconium should undergo suctioning below the level of the vocal cords.

The presence of thick meconium and aggressive neonatal resuscitation frequently result in a low one-minute Apgar score. This has frequently resulted in disagreement between the obstetrician and the pediatrician with regard to the implications of the Apgar score. The obstetrician must keep in mind that a low one-minute Apgar score in the presence of vigorous resuscitative efforts and neonatal intubation does not necessarily imply improper obstetrical management. In fact, a depressed one-minute Apgar score may work in favor of the baby so that respiratory efforts are not made at the time of crucial suctioning. The practice of determining umbilical cord blood gas levels at all high risk deliveries, including deliveries associated with meconium staining, allows for the more accurate assessment of the neonatal condition. The measurement of pH, P_{O_2}, and P_{CO_2} values in specimens from the umbilical artery and umbilical vein gives more reliable information with regard to the immediate predelivery acid-base status of the infant than does a one-minute Apgar score.

In summary, when a potentially asphyxiated infant is expected, a resuscitation team should be present in the delivery room. Meconium staining represents a high risk situation, whereas meconium aspiration represents a pediatric emergency. When meconium has been identified, DeLee suctioning at the perineum is recommended, the baby being handed to the resuscitation team immediately after completion of the delivery, avoiding stimulation. Once meconium aspiration has occurred, mortality rates as high as 28 percent have been reported, most of these secondary to neonatal pulmonary hypertension and complications associated with this hemodynamic disorder.[83]

In evaluating the Apgar score, one must remember that a low Apgar score may suggest asphyxia, but it may not necessarily reflect the duration of asphyxia. Umbilical cord gas levels and delivery room observations may assist in establishing the duration of asphyxia. Full-term infants at risk for developing neurologic sequelae show some evidence of neurologic abnormality within the first week of life, most presenting within the first 12 hours. This occurs regardless of the Apgar score. In full-term infants the incidence of cerebral palsy is approximately 1 percent with an Apgar score of 0 to 3 at five minutes; the longer the score remains low, the greater the significance.[84]

MACROSOMIA

Macrosomia is routinely defined as a birth weight greater than 4,500 gm.[85-88] Although occasionally macrosomia is defined as a weight greater than 4,000 gm,[89] the more classic definition is the former. The incidence of macrosomia has remained relatively constant over the past several decades and continues to be 1.3 to 1.7 percent.[85-87]

The triad of clinical observations associated with fetal macrosomia includes maternal obesity, diabetes mellitus, and postdatism.[86] Other clinical findings that should also raise suspicion include a maternal registration weight greater than 200 pounds, previous macrosomia, white race, multiparity, and (when known) a male fetus.[85] Even without historical factors, fetal macrosomia should be considered whenever the fundal height at term measures more than 40 cm.[90]

There is no argument that significant fetal morbidity and mortality can be associated with macrosomia. This significant difference in outcome between macrosomic infants and control infants seems to be isolated to the route of delivery, i.e., vaginal birth.[90] In a report by Modanlou et al[87] 45 percent of the macrosomic infants that were admitted to the neonatal intensive care unit were admitted specifically because of delivery complications, including Erb's palsy, meconium aspiration, and asphyxia.

One of the more common complications associated with macrosomia is shoulder dystocia, with an incidence ranging from 6 to 18.3 percent.[90] In cases in which shoulder dystocia has led to Erb's palsy, permanent damage has been observed in as few as 6 percent[91] and in as many as 20 percent.[92] The two major maternal complications continue to be postpartum hemorrhage (as frequent as up to a 15.5 percent incidence) and cesarean delivery (as frequent as 22.5 percent).[86]

The absolute difference in increasing cesarean deliveries may not significantly alter the outcome. Boyd et al[89] studied two groups of infants weighing more than 4,000 gm separated by 15 years. There appeared to be no reduction in trauma or asphyxia in comparing complications in the more recent group with those observed in the older group. This leads to two hypothetical solutions: First, it may be worthwhile to scan patients routinely at 26 to 38 weeks' gestation when macrosomia is observed to be developing and to induce labor at that time, before excessive fetal weight gain,[89] or, second, to perform cesarean delivery before labor leads to dystocia, fetal distress, and associated morbidity.[87]

Probably the most important consideration in reducing the significant fetal morbidity in fetal macrosomia is recognition. Several techniques have been introduced, including ultrasound prediction of fetal weight using abdominal circumference and other biometric paramaters,[93] determination of femur length–abdominal circumference ratios in cases in which fetal dates are not known,[94] and simultaneous follow-up of the biparietal diameter and abdominal circumference in known risk groups.[95] In all cases the key to avoiding maternal and fetal morbidity and mortality appears to be predelivery diagnosis of fetal macrosomia.

In the past the accuracy of prenatal diagnosis has been as poor as 20 percent.[85] It is hoped that, with new ultrasound techniques and obstetrician awareness, a significant improvement can be made in this historical record. As always, patients need to be effectively counseled and informed decisions have to be made, balancing the risk of cesarean delivery with its associated maternal morbidity against vaginal delivery of a macrosomic infant with its potential short-term neonatal morbidity, including meconium aspiration, asphyxia, and nerve palsies, and long-term morbidity, including permanent nerve palsies.

SHOULDER DYSTOCIA AND BRACHIAL PLEXUS INJURY

As with many issues in obstetrics, one approach to reducing the incidence of shoulder dystocia and brachial plexus injury has been to attempt to better identify the patients at risk. One such group of patients, those with infants in the breech presentation, have been discussed elsewhere. The challenge is to identify the patient at risk for shoulder dystocia who presents with a singleton fetus in a vertex presentation. Better identification of the macrosomic infant and avoidance of midpelvic opera-

tions in pregnancies complicated by macrosomia will reduce the incidence of shoulder dystocia.

At least one study has demonstrated that, when shoulder dystocia accompanied the midpelvic delivery of an infant in excess of 4,000 gm, 47 percent of such deliveries were complicated by birth injury.[96] A review of brachial plexus injury at The Johns Hopkins Hospital suggested that the incidence of Erb's palsy is not decreasing despite an increase in the incidence of cesarean section, a decreased incidence of vaginal breech deliveries, and a decreased number of forceps deliveries. It was also noted that midforceps operations accounted for 50 percent of the forceps associated cases of Erb's palsy. Nulliparous patients have seemed to be at particular risk for Erb's palsy, although in this series neither dysfunctional labor nor a prolonged second stage of labor seemed to identify a patient at risk for Erb's palsy. Additionally it was noted that cesarean section is not always protective against the development of Erb's palsy.[97]

One may speculate that no reliable predictive factors exist to aid the clinician in preventing Erb's palsy. However, recognition that the nulliparous patient with a large baby is at particular risk and that abandonment of midforceps operations may further reduce the risk may help to diminish the incidence of this injury. This approach will result in a slightly increased incidence of cesarean section. The clinician, however, must recognize that Erb's palsy and shoulder dystocia cannot be predicted 100 percent of the time. The most important medicolegal consideration may be to attempt to recognize the patient who may have risk factors for shoulder dystocia, and therefore brachial plexus injury, and be familiar with the manuevers that are employed in an effort to deal with unexpected shoulder dystocia.[98]

To conclude, there are many intrapartum decisions that can affect maternal, fetal, and subsequent neonatal welfare. Many of these decisions have not only medical implications but medicolegal implications. Although physicians frequently find themselves in the position of having to be an advocate for both mother and fetus, it is necessary to recognize that forced obstetrical procedures may have serious consequences for the physician. Court orders for cesarean section rest on questionable legal grounds, and in some cases the decision for cesarean section may rest on questionable medical grounds.[99]

MANAGEMENT DECISIONS: A PERSPECTIVE

The use and misuse of the Apgar score has also created a new medical practice environment. This has been addressed by a committee statement from The American College of Obstetricians and Gynecologists.[100] Consumer groups, both locally and at the national level, question the need for high incidences of cesarean section. Additionally there is even published information suggesting that obstetrical decisions may have profound behavioral implications on the infants who are the products of such decisions. In short, the medicolegal environment is changing, and obstetricians must be ready to face that change. Our best protection to meet the challenge is to practice quality medicine based on scientific fact, when available, or to establish standards of care when scientific evidence is lacking. Ultimately our goal is to improve the health care of women and to improve the general health of the entire next generation.

To put this into some perspective, we quote from an article by Jacobson et al[101] that summarizes findings the authors found both "astounding and alarming." They conclude that "irrespective of what mechanism may transfer the trauma from birth to adulthood, we conclude that obstetric procedures should be carefully evaluated and possibly modified so as to prevent eventual self-destructive behavior." Clearly our challenges for the next decade and the next century are formidable.

REFERENCES

1. Seeds JW. Malpresentations. In: Gabbe SG, Niebyl JR, Simpson JL, eds. Obstetrics: normal and problem pregnancies. New York: Churchill Livingstone, 1986:453.
2. Johnson CE. Transverse presentation of fetus. JAMA 1964; 187:642.
3. Cockburn KG, Drake RF. Transverse and oblique lie of the fetus. Aust NZ J Obstet Gynaecol 1968; 8:211.
4. Dede JA, Friedman EA. Face presentation. Am J Obstet Gynecol 1963; 87:515.
5. Browne ADH, Carney D. Management of malpresentations in obstetrics. Br Med J 1964; 393:1295.
6. Cucco UP. Face presentation. Am J Obstet Gynecol 1966; 94:1085.
7. Copeland GN, Nicks FI, Christakos AC. Face and brow presentations. NC Med J 1968; 29:507.
8. Pritchard JA, MacDonald PC, eds. Williams obstetrics. 16th ed. New York: Appleton-Century-Crofts, 1980.
9. Abell DA. Brow presentations. Afr Med J 1973; 47:1315.
10. Cruikshank DP, White CA. Obstetric malpresentations — 20 years' experience. Am J Obstet Gynecol 1973; 116:1097.
11. Levy DL. Persistent brow presentation — a new approach to management. South Med J 1976; 69:191.
12. Breen JL, Wiesmeien E. Compound presentation — a survey of 131 patients. Obstet Gynecol 1968; 32:419.
13. Goplerud J, Eastman NJ. Compound presentation. Obstet Gynecol 1953; 1:59.
14. Weissberg SM, O'Leary JA. Compound presentation of the fetus. Obstet Gynecol 1973; 41:60.
15. Collea JV. Current management of breech presentation. Clin Obstet Gynecol 1980; 23:525.
16. Bingham P, Lilford RJ. Management of the selected term breech presentation: assessment of the risk of selected vaginal delivery versus cesarean section for all cases. Obstet Gynecol 1987; 69:965.
17. Savona-Ventura C. The role of external cephalic version in modern obstetrics. Obstet Gynecol Surv 1986; 41:393.
18. Stine LE, Phelan JP, Wallace R, et al. Update on external cephalic version performed at term. Obstet Gynecol 1985; 65:642.
19. Dyson DC, Ferguson JE II, Hensleigh P. Antepartum external cephalic version under tocolysis. Obstet Gynecol 1986; 67:63.
20. Hofmeyer GJ. Effect of external cephalic version in late pregnancy on breech presentation and cesarean section rate: a controlled trial. Br J Obstet Gynaecol 1983; 90:392.
21. Van Dorsten JP, Schifrin BS, Wallace RL. Randomized controlled trial of external cephalic version with tocolysis in late pregnancy. Am J Obstet Gynecol 1981; 141:417.
22. Ferguson JE II, Armstrong MA, Dyson DC. Maternal and fetal factors affecting success of antepartum external cephalic version. Obstet Gynecol 1987; 70:722.
23. Robertson AW, Kopelman JN, Read JA, et al. External cephalic version at term: is a tocolytic necessary? Obstet Gynecol 1987; 70:896.
24. Friedman EA. The functional divisions of labor. Am J Obstet Gynecol 1971; 109:274.
25. Friedman EA. Dysfunctional labor. In: Cohen WR, Friedman EA, eds. Management of labor. Baltimore: University Park Press, 1983:11.
26. Friedman EA, Sachtleben-Murray MR, Dahrouge D, Neff RK. Long-term effects of labor and delivery on offspring: a matched-pair analysis. Am J Obstet Gynecol 1984; 150:941.
27. Friedman EA. Midforceps delivery: no? Clin Obstet Gynecol 1987; 30:93.
28. Hillis DS. Diagnosis of contracted pelvis. IMJ 1938; 74:131.
29. Boyer KM, Gadzala CA, Burd LI, et al. Selective intrapartum chemo-prophylaxis in neonatal group B streptococcal early onset disease. I. Epidemiologic rationale. J Infect Dis 1983; 148:795.
30. Lee KS, Paneth N, Gartner LM, et al. Neonatal mortality: an analysis of the recent improvement in the United States. Am J Public Health 1980; 70:15.
31. Williams RL, Chen PM. Identifying sources of the recent decline in perinatal mortality rates in California. N Engl J Med 1982; 306:207.
32. Boyer KM, Gadzala CA, Kelly PD, Gotoff SP. Selective intrapartum chemoprophylaxis of neonatal group B streptococcal early onset disease. III. Interruption of mother to infant transmission. J Infect Dis 1983; 148:810.
33. Brown ZA, Vontver LA, Benedetti J, et al. Effects on infants of a first episode of genital herpes during pregnancy. N Engl J Med 1987; 317:1246.
34. Prober CG, Sullender WM, Yasukawa LL, et al. Low risk of herpes simplex virus infections in neonates exposed to the virus at the time of vaginal delivery to mothers with recurrent genital herpes simplex virus infections. N Engl J Med 1987; 316:240.
35. American College of Obstetricians and Gynecologists' statement. Perinatal herpes simplex virus infections, July 1987.
36. Territo M, Finklestein J, Oh W, et al. Management of autoimmune thrombocytopenia in pregnancy and in the neonate. Obstet Gynecol 1973; 41:579.
37. Murray JM, Harris RE. The management of the pregnant patient with idiopathic thrombocytopenic purpura. Am J Obstet Gynecol 1976; 126:449.
38. Laros RK, Kagan R. Route of delivery for patients with immune thrombocytopenic purpura. Am J Obstet Gynecol 1984; 148:901.
39. Martin CD Jr. Physiology of clinical use of fetal heart rate variability. Clin Perinatol 1982; 9:339.
40. Schimrin BS, Dane L. Fetal heart rate pattern: prediction of Apgar score. JAMA 1972; 219:1322.
41. Zanini B, Paul RH, Huey JH. Intrapartum fetal heart rate: correlation with scalp pH and the preterm fetus. Am J Obstet Gynecol 1980; 136:43.
42. Paul RH, Suidan AK, Yeh S, et al. Clinical fetal monitoring. VII. The evaluation of significance of intrapartum baseline fetal heart rate variability. Am J Obstet Gynecol 1975; 123:206.
43. Manning FA, Lange IR, Morrison I, et al. Determination of fetal health: methods for antepartum and intrapartum fetal assessment. Curr Probl Obstet Gynecol 1983; 7:1.
44. Cohen W, Schifrin B. Diagnosis and management of fetal distress during labor. Semin Perinatol 1978; 2:155.
45. Lofgren O, Jacobson L. TCPO₂ monitoring of the fetus and mother during normal labor. Birth Defects 1979; 15:193.
46. Beard RW, Morris ED, Clayton SP. pH and fetal capillary blood as an indicator of the condition of the fetus. J Obstet Gynaecol Br Commonwealth 1967; 74:812.

47. Wood C. Fetal scalp sampling: its place in management. Semin Perinatol 1978; 2:169.

48. Clark SL, Gimobsky ML, Miller FC. The scalp stimulation test: a clinical alternative to fetal scalp blood sampling. Am J Obstet Gynecol 1984; 148:274.

49. Smith CV, Nguyen HN, Phelan JP, et al. Intrapartum assessment of fetal wellbeing: a comparison of fetal acoustic stimulation with acid-based determinations. Am J Obstet Gynecol 1986; 155:726.

50. Pritchard JA, MacDonald PC, Gant NF, eds. Williams obstetrics. 17th ed. New York: Appleton-Lange, 1985.

51. Ould F. A treatise of midwifery. Dublin: Milton & Head, 1742. Cited in Laufe LE, Leslie DC. The timing of episiotomy. Am J Obstet Gynecol 1972; 114:773.

52. Pomeroy RH. Shall we cut and reconstruct the perineum for every primipara? Am J Obstet Dis Women Child 1918; 78:211.

53. DeLee JB. The prophylactic forceps operation. Am J Obstet Gynecol 1920; 1:34.

54. Thacker SB, Banta HD. Benefits and risks of episiotomy: an interpretive review of the English literature, 1860–1980. Obstet Gynecol Surv 1983; 36:322.

55. Laufe LE, Leslie DC. The timing of episiotomy. Am J Obstet Gynecol 1972; 114:773.

56. Thorp JM, Bowes WA, Brame RG, et al. Selected use of midline episiotomy: effect on perineal trauma. Obstet Gynecol 1987; 70:260.

57. Beynon CL. The normal second stage of labour. J Obstet Gynaecol Br Emp 1957; 64:815.

58. Hauth JC, Gilstrap LC, Ward SC, et al. Early repair of an external sphincter ani muscle and rectal mucosal dehiscence. Obstet Gynecol 1986; 67:806.

59. Goodlin RC. On protection of the maternal perineum during birth. Obstet Gynecol 1983; 62:393.

60. Bottoms SF, Sokol RJ. Mechanisms and conduct of labor. In: Iffy L, Kaminetzky HA, eds. Principles and practice of obstetrics and perinatology. Vol. 2. New York: John Wiley, 1981:825.

61. Bishop EH, Israel SL, Briscoe CC. Obstetric influences on the premature infant's first year of development; a report from the collaborative study of cerebral palsy. Obstet Gynecol 1965; 26:628.

62. Barrett JM, Boehm FH, Vaughn WK. The effect of type of delivery on neonatal outcome in singleton infants of birth weight of 1,000 g or less. JAMA 1983; 250:625.

63. Huff DL, Thurnau GR, Sheldon R. The outcome of protective forceps deliveries of 26–33 week infants. Abstract 45, Society of Perinatal Obstetricians, Orlando, Florida, February 5–7, 1987.

64. Richardson DA, Evans MI, Cibils LA. Midforceps delivery: a critical review. Am J Obstet Gynecol 1983; 145:621.

65. Dudley AG, Markham SM, McNie TM. Elective versus indicated midforceps delivery. Obstet Gynecol 1971; 37:19.

66. Ott WJ. Vacuum extractor. Obstet Gynecol Surv 1975; 30:643.

67. Kappy KA. Vacuum extractor. Clin Perinatol 1981; 8:79.

68. Malmstrom T. Vacuum extractor: an obstetrical instrument. Acta Obstet Gynecol Scand 1954; 33:1.

69. Lang P. The vacuum extractor: value in relation to forceps and range of indications. Acta Obstet Gynecol Scand 1961; 43 (Suppl):57.

70. Kelly JV, Mishell DR. Experience with the vacuum extractor. Surg Gynecol Obstet 1964; 114:609.

71. Matheson GW, Davajan V, Mishell DR. The use of the VE: a reappraisal. Acta Obstet Gynecol Scand 1965; 47:155.

72. Chamberlain G. Forceps and vacuum extraction. Clin Obstet Gynecol 1980; 7:511.

73. Vacca A, Grant A, Wyatt G. Portsmouth operative delivery trail: a comparison of vacuum extraction and forceps delivery. Br J Obstet Gynaecol 1983; 90:1107.

74. Maryniak GM, Frank JB. Clinical assessment of the Kobayashi vacuum extractor. Obstet Gynecol 1984; 64:431.

75. Rosemann G. Vacuum extraction of premature infants. S Afr J Obstet Gynecol 1969; 7:10.

76. Broekhuizen FF, Washington JM, Johnson F, et al. Vacuum extraction versus forceps delivery: indications and complications, 1979 to 1984. Obstet Gynecol 1987; 69:338.

77. Krebs HB, Petres RE, Dunn LJ, et al. Intrapartum fetal heart rate monitoring. III. Association of meconium with abnormal fetal heart rate patterns. Am J Obstet Gynecol 1980; 137:936.

78. Gage JE, Taeusch HW, Treves S, Caldicott W. Suctioning of upper airway meconium in newborn infants. JAMA 1981; 246:2590.

79. Pfenninger E, Dick W, Brecht-Krauss D, et al. Investigation of intrapartum clearance of the upper airway in the presence of meconium contaminated amniotic fluid using an animal model. J Perinat Med 1991; 12:57.

80. Meis PJ, Hobel CJ, Ureda JR. Late meconium passage in labor —a sign of fetal distress? Obstet Gynecol 1982; 59:332.

81. Carson BS, Losey RW, Bowes WA, Simmons MA. Combined obstetric and pediatric approach to prevent meconium aspiration syndrome. Am J Obstet Gynecol 1976; 126:712.

82. Gregory GA, Gooding CA, Phibbs RH, Tooley WH. Meconium aspiration in infants—a prospective study. J Pediatr 1974; 85:848.

83. Vidyasagar D, Yeh TF, Harris V, Pildes RS. Assisted ventilation in infants with meconium aspiration syndrome. Pediatrics 1975; 56:208.

84. Nelson KB, Ellenberg JH. Apgar scores as predictors of cerebral palsy. Pediatrics 1981; 68:36.

85. Parks DG, Ziel HK. Macrosomia: a proposed indication for primary cesarean section. Obstet Gynecol 1978; 52:407.

86. Spellacy WN, Miller S, Winegar A, Peterson PQ. Macrosomia —maternal characteristics and infant complications. Obstet Gynecol 1985; 66:158.

87. Modanlou HD, Dorchester WL, Thorosian A, Freeman RK. Macrosomia—maternal, fetal, and neonatal implications. Obstet Gynecol 1980; 55:420.

88. Nathanson JN. The excessively large fetus as an obstetric problem. Am J Obstet Gynecol 1950; 60:54.

89. Boyd ME, Usher RH, McLean FH. Fetal macrosomia: prediction, risk, proposed management. Obstet Gynecol 1983; 61:715.

90. Posner AC, Friedman S, Posner LB. The large fetus: a study of 547 cases. Obstet Gynecol 1955; 5:268.

91. Gordon M, Rich H, Deutschberger J, Green M. The immediate and long-term outcome of obstetric birth trauma. I. Brachial plexus paralysis. Am J Obstet Gynecol 1973; 117:51.

92. Sack RA. The large infant: a study of maternal, obstetric, fetal, and newborn characteristics; including a long-term pediatric follow-up. Am J Obstet Gynecol 1969; 104:195.

93. Deter RL, Hadlock FP. Use of ultrasound in the detection of macrosomia: a review. J Clin Ultrasound 1985; 13:519.

94. Hadlock FP, Harrist RB, Fearneyhough TC, et al. Use of femur length/abdominal circumference ratio in detecting the macrosomic fetus. Radiology 1985; 154:503.

95. Tamura RK, Sabbagha RE, Depp R, et al. Diabetic macrosomia: accuracy of third trimester ultrasound. Obstet Gynecol 1986; 67:828.

96. Benedetti TJ, Gabbe SG. Shoulder dystocia—a complication of fetal macrosomia and prolonged second stage of labor with mid-pelvic delivery. Obstet Gynecol 1978; 52:526.

97. Repke JT, Niebyl JR, King TM. Brachial plexus injury: a review of the Johns Hopkins Hospital experience, 1972–1982. Abstract 146, Society of Perinatal Obstetricians, San Antonio, Texas, February 1984.

98. Gonik B, Stringer CA, Held B. An alternate manuever for the management of shoulder dystocia. Am J Obstet Gynecol 1983; 145:882.

99. Kolder VEB, Gallagher J, Parsons NT. Court ordered obstetrical interventions. N Engl J Med 1987; 316:1192.

100. American College of Obstetricians and Gynecologists Committee. Use and misuse of the Apgar score, November 1986.

101. Jacobson B, Eklund G, Hamberger L, et al. Perinatal origin of adult self-destructive behavior. Acta Psychiatr Scand 1987; 76:364.

4

Effects of Anesthesia on the Fetus and Neonate

George A. Albright, M.D.

Maternal Anesthetic Catastrophes
    General Anesthesia
        Preoxygenation
        Failed Endotracheal Intubation
        Pulmonary Aspiration
        Circulatory Failure
    Regional Anesthesia
        Total Spinal, Subdural, and Massive
            Epidural Blocks
        Local Anesthetic Reactions
        Test Dose
Indirect Drug Effects
    Labor and Delivery
    Placental Perfusion
        Hypotension
        Uterine Hypertonus–Uterine Artery Spasm
Direct Drug Effects
    Systemic Medication
    Local Anesthetics
        Fetal Scalp Injection
    Neurobehavioral Effects

The selection of analgesic and anesthetic techniques for the management of labor pain should be based on need, effectiveness, and contribution to maternal and perinatal mortality and morbidity. The risks of obstetrical anesthesia depend in large measure on the availability and training of anesthesia personnel in the delivery unit. When psychoanalgesia and systemic medication are inadequate, obstetricians may be forced to administer paracervical blocks (risking fetal bradycardia), to permit relatively untrained personnel to administer inhalation anesthetics, or to provide their own regional anesthesia.

Perinatal mortality and morbidity may result from maternal anesthetic catastrophes, or they may be due to the direct or indirect effects of analgesic and anesthetic drugs. Acute failure of the maternal cardiopulmonary system markedly interferes with the placental exchange of oxygen and carbon dioxide, necessitating prompt delivery of the fetus. Unfortunately efforts to oxygenate the mother, secure the airway, and stabilize the cardiovascular system may be difficult and protracted and delay unduly the operative delivery of the infant.

Even though obstetrical patients are generally young and in good health, they represent an at-risk population for anesthesia. Obstetrical anesthetic procedures may have to be carried out in relatively uncooperative patients or in response to acute fetal distress or obstetrical shock. This sense of urgency may result in maternal anesthetic catastrophes owing to inadequate preanesthetic evaluation or checking of anesthesia equipment and supplies; inadequate preparation, monitoring, and testing of the patient; and less than cautious administration of anesthesia. Anesthetic accidents resulting from unintentional injection of the wrong drug (e.g., epinephrine instead of ephedrine) and administration of general anesthesia with hypoxic gas mixtures (turning off oxygen instead of nitrous oxide) do occur and are difficult if not impossible to defend in litigation. A properly prepared and properly notified anesthesiologist can safely anesthetize a healthy parturient without delaying emergency delivery if an assistant is available to apply cricoid pressure. Otherwise, delay is preferable to risking preventable maternal anesthetic catastrophes.

Regional techniques should not be instituted unless there are trained personnel and equipment immediately available for full cardiopulmonary resuscitation. Oxygen, suction, and blood pressure apparatus should be physically present in any room in which a patient is to receive a regional anesthetic for labor pain relief. An Ambu bag, preferably, should be in the room or immediately available along with a "crash cart" in the delivery suite. An anesthesia cart containing the necessary supplies to institute regional anesthesia and emergency drugs and equipment is a convenient method to permit the safe administration of analgesic dosages of local anesthetics in the labor room. The surgical dosage of local anesthetics should be administered only in the delivery room (except for 3 percent chloroprocaine in cases of acute fetal distress) where equipment and facilities are optimal for the recognition and treatment of local anesthetic–induced seizures or cardiovascular collapse and, if necessary, for emergency cesarean section.

The fetus and neonate may be affected as a result of anesthetic effects on the course of labor, placental perfusion, and placental transfer of the anesthetic drug.

Placental perfusion is decreased because of hypotension secondary to peripheral vasodilatation (systemic medication, autonomic blockade) and uterine hypertonus or uterine artery spasm secondary to paracervical block, vasopressor drugs, reflex release of endogenous catecholamines, or unintentional intravascular injection of local anesthetics. Placentally transferred local anesthetics are not associated with significant perinatal depression unless the perinate is severely hypoxic and acidotic. However, unintentional fetal scalp injection (paracervical or pudendal blocks, caudal epidural anesthesia) has been associated with perinatal mortality.

MATERNAL ANESTHETIC CATASTROPHES

The adverse effect of maternal anesthetic catastrophes on the neonatal outcome was clearly demonstrated by case histories of bupivacaine-induced maternal seizure and cardiac arrest that occurred in the United States during the 1970s and early 1980s. Clinical data relating to 44 cases of maternal cardiac arrest documented the difficulty in cardiopulmonary resuscitation of the term pregnant woman and the poor neonatal outcome if delivery was delayed. Marx[1] stressed the importance of left uterine displacement (manual displacement is preferable to a left pelvic tilt) and elevation of the legs during cardiopulmonary resuscitation of the term female and recommended early delivery of the infant to facilitate maternal resuscitation by release of caval compression.

Maternal cardiopulmonary collapse may occur during the induction of general anesthesia owing to severe hypoxia (inadequate inspired oxygen, failed endotracheal or unrecognized esophageal intubation, pulmonary aspiration, pulmonary edema with light anesthesia, and hypertension) and circulatory failure (drug overdose with hypovolemia or catecholamine depletion [drug abuse] and severe cardiac disease). It may also occur following the administration of regional anesthesia (total spinal [acute or late onset], subdural, or massive epidural block, local anesthetic drug reaction).

Regional anesthesia generally is considered safer for the mother than general anesthesia because of the risks of failed endotracheal intubation and pulmonary aspiration. However, anesthesiologists generally have administered general anesthesia for emergency delivery (secondary to acute maternal or fetal distress). Spinal anesthesia in the absence of contraindications (severe maternal hemorrhage and hypovolemia) has been demonstrated to be almost as quick as and to result in a better neonatal status than that with general anesthesia.[2] Thus, spinal anesthesia or the rapid injection of 3 percent chloroprocaine through a previously inserted epidural catheter is preferable to general anesthesia in patients who are at particular risk for pulmonary aspiration or who appear to have a poor airway. Furthermore, parturients whose anatomic features suggest difficulty with endotracheal intubation, who have a multiple gestation (emergency cesarean section for the second twin), or who already have demonstrated placental insufficiency during early labor benefit from placement of a "prophylactic" epidural catheter to avoid the need for general anesthesia if acute fetal distress develops.

General Anesthesia

Hypoxia may occur during the administration of general anesthesia owing to failure of the oxygen supply, hypoventilation, airway obstruction, or cardiovascular collapse. Women at term have an increased oxygen consumption (+20 percent) and a decreased functional reserve capacity, and the arterial oxygen tension may vary from 65 to 105 torr. Arterial oxygen tension decreases more rapidly with apnea in pregnant women than in nonpregnant women.[3] When the anesthetic mask is removed (for endotracheal intubation), room air is drawn into the lungs, with arterial desaturation occurring within several minutes. Maternal cyanosis may develop when preoxygenation is inadequate and the anesthetic mask is removed before the jaw is sufficiently relaxed, resulting in a time-consuming and often difficult endotracheal intubation, with increased likelihood of vomiting and pulmonary aspiration.

Preoxygenation

Preoxygenation provides an increase in the volume of oxygen stored in the functional reserve of the lung in order to delay the onset of arterial desaturation during apnea. It has been suggested that four deep (vital capacity) breaths of pure oxygen within 30 seconds would be as effective as the traditional three to five minutes of tidal oxygen breathing for maintaining oxygenation during routine endotracheal intubation.[4,5] However, recent studies have indicated that, when apnea is prolonged (difficult intubation, obstructed airway), arterial desaturation occurs more rapidly in both pregnant and nonpregnant patients preoxygenated with four breaths than in those preoxygenated for three minutes.[6,7] These studies also demonstrated a variable time to arterial oxygen desaturation (especially with the four breath technique), indicating the desirability of a minimum of three minutes of preoxygenation and the use of a pulse oxygen saturation monitor (pulse oximeter) for the induction of general anesthesia, particularly when a difficult endotracheal intubation is anticipated.

Failed Endotracheal Intubation

Failed endotracheal intubation and unrecognized esophageal intubation are the leading causes of anesthetic-related maternal mortality, surpassing pulmonary aspiration, which often accompanies a difficult or failed endotracheal intubation. Endotracheal intubation can be facilitated by proper positioning of the head and neck in a sniff position, allowing for both hyperextension (facilitating entry of the laryngoscope) and flexion of the head (facilitating visualization of the larynx). A variety of endotracheal handles and blades (laryngoscope lights can and do fail) should be available, as well as various sizes of endotracheal tubes with stylets (laryngeal edema from toxemia, infection, strenuous labor, or overhydration may admit only a 5 to 5.5 mm endotracheal tube) and a small laryngoscope handle or polio type of blade (enlarged breasts and increased diameter of the chest may obstruct entry of the laryngoscope). Endotracheal intubation is also facilitated by awaiting adequate jaw relaxation before removing the anesthetic mask. Generally a different approach (e.g., change in head position, different laryngoscope) should be tried for a repeat intubation attempt, since the first look in a given position is usually the best.

When the endotracheal tube is not seen to pass between the vocal cords, posterior displacement of the tube toward the palate (while the laryngoscope is still in the mouth) usually brings the tube and vocal cords into direct view.[8] Proper positioning of the endotracheal tube traditionally has been verified by observation of bilateral chest expansion, confirmed by bilateral and equal breath sounds in both axillas and on the anterior chest and the absence of breath sounds over the epigastrium. Since the epigastrium cannot be auscultated because of the abdominal "prep," final verification of proper placement of the endotracheal tube should be detection of a typical carbon dioxide exhalation curve and maintenance of normal arterial oxygen saturation (endotracheal tube not positioned in a main stem bronchus).

If endotracheal intubation cannot be accomplished in a reasonable length of time, the parturient must be oxygenated by mask with minimal positive pressure (to prevent inflation of the stomach) before hypoxia creates the risk of cardiac arrest. Rarely, total upper airway obstruction may ensue, necessitating placement of a large needle or catheter through the cricoid membrane or a cricothyrotomy to prevent cardiac arrest. Normally the patient should be awakened and nonemergency surgery performed under regional anesthesia or after an awake fiberoptic endotracheal intubation. When surgery cannot be postponed, general anesthesia given by mask (while cricoid pressure is maintained) is preferable to persisting with a difficult endotracheal intubation, which further delays delivery of the infant and risks pulmonary aspiration or hypoxic cardiac arrest.

Pulmonary Aspiration

The use of regional rather than general anesthesia for vaginal and abdominal delivery is the most constructive measure for the prevention of pulmonary aspiration, since all parturients should be considered "full stomach" patients. Anxiety, labor, analgesic drugs, and anatomic displacement of the stomach contribute to delayed gastric emptying or increased gastric secretions. Intragastric pressure is increased during pregnancy owing to the gravid uterus, and it is aggravated by the lithotomy or Trendelenburg position. The forceful application of fundal pressure at delivery may quickly stimulate vomiting. Progesterone relaxes and hiatal hernia interferes with the lower esophageal sphincter.

Since the need for general anesthesia never can be predicted, parturients should be given nothing by mouth and should be provided with an intravenous infusion of a dextrose-containing crystalloid solution during labor to provide for hydration and an energy source to minimize metabolic acidosis. Current practice recommends the administration of a nonparticulate antacid (sodium citrate) shortly before the induction of general anesthesia rather than the routine administration of colloidal antacids every two hours during labor and before surgery. Mortality and severe morbidity have been reported in patients who aspirate alkaline gastric contents containing colloid antacids.[9,10]

Since sodium citrate is not 100 percent effective in increasing gastric acidity to a safe level, other drugs have been recommended to reduce the risk of acid aspiration. Metoclopramide accelerates gastric emptying and increases the lower esophageal sphincter tone. H_2 receptor antagonists (cimetidine, ranitidine) reduce gastric acidity and gastric volume by blocking gastric histamine H_2 receptors. Because these drugs work by blocking production of newly formed gastric secretions (not those already in the stomach), there is a lag time of 45 to 90 minutes. Although these drugs have been administered to 10,000 to 12,000 patients without any significant side effects in either mothers or their offspring,[11] they generally are not administered routinely to all patients in labor but are reserved for patients who are scheduled for cesarean section under general anesthesia or who are at greater risk for emergency general anesthesia. The administration of sodium citrate, metoclopramide, and ranitidine before urgent general anesthesia provides maximal protection during endotracheal intubation and extubation.

Passage of a nasogastric tube and inducing vomiting with apomorphine before general anesthesia are unpleasant and do not guarantee that the stomach will be empty. An awake endotracheal intubation is time consuming, requires greater operator skill, and can be barbaric without premedication and local anesthesia, which may obtund laryngeal reflexes, permitting aspiration during the procedure. Fiberoptic laryngoscopy is not so traumatic, can be performed with local anesthesia, and yields a high incidence of success in experienced hands. It should be considered in any patient requiring general anesthesia in whom a difficult endotracheal intubation is anticipated.

The administration of anticholinergic drugs to reduce secretions (important if positive pressure ventilation is required after a failed endotracheal intubation) for a rapid sequence induction of anesthesia reduces lower esophageal sphincter tone, but this action can be neutralized by metoclopramide or ranitidine. The use of a small dose of a nondepolarizing muscle relaxant before administration of succinylcholine to prevent the increase in intra-abdominal pressure (rise in intragastric pressure) associated with abdominal fasciculations is controversial, since fasciculations increase both intragastric and lower esophageal sphincter pressure.[12]

When general anesthesia is required, a rapid-sequence induction, with cricoid pressure applied until a cuffed endotracheal tube is in place, should be used, followed by an awake extubation when the parturient can control her own airway. The application of cricoid pressure is considered the standard of care in the United States but is not uniformly practiced in other countries, since it may be ineffective if applied with inadequate pressure or it may interfere with endotracheal intubation if applied incorrectly or too vigorously.

The timing of application of cricoid pressure presents pitfalls with all approaches:

1. Application of a constant pressure tolerated by an awake patient at the start of induction may yield inadequate pressure.

2. Application of a gradually increasing pressure as tolerated may be inadequate or, if excessive, may stimulate vomiting before complete muscle paralysis occurs.

3. Application of pressure at the time of loss of the lid reflex, as originally recommended by Sellick,[13] will not prevent previous silent regurgitation. When active retching occurs, cricoid pressure should be maintained, not removed, since the theoretical possibility of esophageal rupture has not been reported.

I believe that smooth rapid induction of general anesthesia (adequate dosage of an induction drug and succinylcholine, and waiting until the jaw is relaxed before removing the mask) without positive pressure ventilation is the key to a successful induction of anesthesia. There is no quality control in the application of cricoid pressure, which is usually not administered by an anesthesiologist, may be grossly inadequate, or may interfere with endotracheal intubation. If the anatomic features appear to be distorted during a difficult intubation, cricoid pressure should be reduced, not increased, in response to more vigorous efforts with the laryngoscope to visualize the larynx.

Circulatory Failure

Cardiovascular collapse can occur during induction of general anesthesia owing to light anesthesia in the presence of hypertension. It may also result from a relative overdose of the induction drug in the presence of hypovolemia (severe bleeding, toxemia, or dehydration), catecholamine depletion as a result of chronic drug abuse,[14] and severe cardiac disease. Although thiopental (3 to 4 mg per kilogram is still the induction drug of choice for routine cesarean section, ketamine (1 mg per kilogram or less) is useful in the presence of hypovolemia or catecholamine depletion. Diazepam (15 to 20 mg) and etomidate (0.3 mg per kilogram are useful as induction drugs when ketamine is not appropriate (hypertension, coronary artery disease). The patient with a severe cardiac disorder may require slow induction of general anesthesia with a volatile drug (halothane, enflurane, isoflurane) or high dose fentanyl administration (valvular lesions, 20 to 30 μg per kilogram; myocardial ischemia, 50 to 75 μg per kilogram), accepting the increased risk of pulmonary aspiration and neonatal depression.

Light general anesthesia is provided for cesarean section to reduce fetal drug exposure, recognizing that the parturient will usually exhibit mild tachycardia and hypertension from the stress of endotracheal intubation and surgery. The hypertensive or toxemic patient who is not blood volume depleted may exhibit an exaggerated response, with severe hypertension risking a cerebrovascular accident or pulmonary edema from acute cardiac failure. These patients may require invasive monitoring; the hypertension should be controlled (diastolic pressure less than 110 torr), possibly with the intravenous administration of rapidly acting depressor drugs before induction of anesthesia. They require a larger than usual dosage of the induction drug (5 to 6 mg per kilogram of thiopental) and may benefit from the intravenous administration of lidocaine (1.0 to 1.5 mg per kilogram) and fentanyl before endotracheal intubation.[15]

Hemorrhage (placenta previa, abruptio placentae, or postpartum hemorrhage) is the most frequent cause of obstetrical shock. Other causes include cardiac failure, supine hypotensive syndrome, spinal shock, septic shock, amniotic fluid, air or blood clot embolism, and drug reactions.[16] Obstetrical blood loss is extremely difficult to estimate. A pulse rate increase may not occur until the blood loss reaches 2 liters, because parturients have a compensatory increase in blood volume (1,500 ml) during pregnancy. The fetus is at risk because compensatory hemodynamic changes preferentially maintain perfusion of the maternal vital organs at the expense of uterine perfusion.

Whenever a parturient with a viable fetus is bleeding, she should be maintained in the lateral position, provided with supplemental oxygen, and immediately cross matched for blood replacement, and a large caliber catheter(s) should be placed for rapid intravenous infusion of fluids. The urinary output, measured by an indwelling catheter, is an excellent clinical monitor of renal perfusion and can be used to follow the effectiveness of therapy to correct hypovolemia. The central venous pressure should be monitored as a guide to further fluid replacement when initial therapy is not successful in restoring an adequate urine output.

Parturients with lesser degrees of hemorrhage (not being actively transfused and vaginal delivery anticipated) may be managed with epidural anesthesia, preferably using a local anesthetic drug of short duration (chloroprocaine). When acute hemorrhage necessitates immediate delivery, a general endotracheal anesthetic should be administered using ketamine or etomidate as the induction drug, after initial rapid fluid and blood replacement.

The toxemic patient presents an unusual challenge for the anesthesiologist because she is unusually sensitive to catecholamines and may respond with acute hypertension to typical doses of vasopressor drugs (for the treatment of hypotension, unintentional intravascular injection of local anesthetic solutions containing epinephrine) or ergot compounds, or to endogenous release of catecholamines during endotracheal intubation under light general anesthesia. Conversely cardiovascular collapse may occur with routine induction doses of thiopental because of severe hypovolemia. When the blood volume status of a patient with severe preeclampsia is not known because of inadequate time for invasive monitoring, emergency general anesthesia can be provided by using a test dose of thiopental and titrating the subsequent dose to changes in sensorium or blood pressure while maintaining cricoid pressure, or by using 0.3 mg per kilogram of etomidate as the induction drug. If acute hypertension occurs during endotracheal intubation, an additional 50 to 75 mg of thiopental, 2.5 to 5.0 mg of chlorpromazine, or a 50 μg bolus of nitroprusside may be administered.

The use of epidural anesthesia in severe preeclampsia is controversial, although most obstetrical texts written since the late 1960s recommend its use when it is not contraindicated by other factors.[17] The safe administration of regional anesthesia in the toxemic patient for labor and cesarean section requires the absence of significant coagulopathy, a diastolic blood pressure less than 110 torr (controlled by vasodepressors), and an adequate circulating blood volume.[18] If the urinary output is inadequate, fluids should be administered to elevate a low central venous pressure before instituting regional anesthesia. Plasma expanders reduce the amount of crystalloid required as well as the risk of postpartum pulmonary edema.[19]

Regional Anesthesia

Anesthetic deaths caused by respiratory failure or spinal shock after regional anesthesia are considered to be preventable, since regional anesthesia should not impair the effectiveness of ventilation if the blood pressure is maintained and reasonable doses of local anesthetics are administered. Caplan et al[20] reported 14 patients who, within 30 minutes after injection of a spinal anesthetic, had rapidly progressive hypotension and bradycardia followed by severe brain damage or death, despite prompt institution of cardiopulmonary resuscitation. These investigators postulated that the hypoxia and hypercarbia associated with even modest respiratory insufficiency caused by additional intravenous doses of sedative drugs led to vasodilatation, failure of venous return, failure of compensatory tachycardia because of sympathetic block, the appearance of bradycardia and hypotension (unresponsive to atropine, ephedrine, and fluids), and rapid cardiac arrest. The poor outcome was attributed to a delay of almost eight minutes after the arrest in the administration of epinephrine (cardiopulmonary resuscitation is ineffective when the heart is empty).

Adverse effects of total spinal or massive epidural anesthetics can be prevented and complete recovery anticipated by the maintenance of adequate pulmonary exchange (artificial ventilation with oxygen) and blood pressure (fluids, pressor drugs). An exception may be sudden collapse with regurgitation and pulmonary aspiration before corrective measures can be instituted.

Local anesthetic-induced seizures are generally benign and respond to oxygenation, anticonvulsant drugs, and, if necessary, cardiovascular support. However, bupivacaine-induced seizures have resulted in 44 cases of maternal cardiac arrest with all concentrations of bupivacaine (0.25 percent, 1; 0.5 percent, 12; 0.75 percent, 31), with 30 deaths and seven patients who survived but sustained central nervous system damage.[21] Moreover, unpublished case histories suggest that bupivacaine-induced seizures without depression of the maternal cardiovascular system may result in fetal asphyxia and a poor outcome, presumably as a result of uterine hyperactivity or uterine artery spasm.[22] Abboud et al[23] reported a higher incidence of late decelerations (8 of 42) with epidural bupivacaine than with lidocaine (3 of 47) and chloroprocaine (none of 34) in the absence of maternal hypotension. Following the epidural administration of bupivacaine, two fetuses had prolonged heart rate decelerations lasting seven and 10 minutes, respectively, although the neonatal outcome was uniformly good in all groups.

Total Spinal, Subdural, and Massive Epidural Blocks

Severe hypotension after epidural administration of an anesthetic may be due to a total spinal block (unintentional placement of the drug in the spinal fluid), or a subdural injection (drug placed unintentionally in the potential space between the dura and the subarachnoid membranes), or a massive epidural block (excessive drug). A total spinal block results in apnea, dilatation of the pupils (blockade of the third nucleus), unconsciousness, and unobtainable blood pressure, usually within several minutes, if not promptly treated. However, subarachnoid injection of even 20 to 40 ml of lidocaine has been reported to produce a variable delay until maximal block occurs from 30 seconds to 45 minutes.[24] Furthermore, when a parturient is placed in the supine position, even with uterine displacement, following a gradually ascending high spinal block and in preparation for assisted mask ventilation or vaginal examination (looking for a prolapsed cord to explain sudden fetal distress), there may be a sudden further extension of the anesthetic level. Partial caval exclusion causes engorgement of epidural veins, which displaces cerebrospinal fluid (and local anesthetic) cranially, with sudden collapse.[25]

The clinical findings in subdural block are confusing, because some investigators have attributed any late-onset, long-duration high block resulting from relatively small amounts of local anesthetics intended for the epidural space to a subdural rather than an intrathecal block, even if there were signs of marked muscle paralysis and cardiovascular collapse.[26,27] However, radiographically confirmed subdural catheter (and local anesthetic) placement has resulted in subdural blocks that reached their highest level in 20 to 30 minutes and receded in 50 to 150 minutes. Motor block was minimal or absent, hypotension was easily treated or absent, and the block extended cranially (predominantly unilateral) rather than caudally.[28]

Massive epidural blocks are the result of excessive epidural doses, the speed of onset and the intensity of the block (which may mimic a spinal block) depending on the degree of overdosage. Although this usually occurs in older patients, the insulin-dependent juvenile diabetic scheduled for cesarean section is at risk for a massive epidural block because she may require only one-half to two-thirds of the regular dose.

When a patient receiving epidural anesthesia demonstrates respiratory distress or hypotension, or there is unexplained fetal distress, the cephalad extension of the sensory block and (if above T5) the motor strength of the hand grasp should be determined. These patients should be under continuous observation, kept in the lateral position, and provided with supplemental oxygen, fluids, and ephedrine (if necessary) to maintain the blood pressure while preparations are made to provide positive pressure mask or endotracheal ventilation with pure oxygen until the block has begun to wear off and the patient is stable.

Local Anesthetic Reactions

The initial signs and symptoms of central nervous system toxicity are usually excitation followed by depression (respiratory arrest). The patient should be asked if she is experiencing numbness of the tongue and circumoral tissues, lightheadedness and dizziness, visual and auditory disturbances, a metallic taste, drowsiness, or disorientation and should be observed for slurred speech, shivering, muscular twitching, tremors, or temporary unconsciousness. Early recognition of premonitory symptoms and signs and prompt treatment with hyperventilation and oxygenation may prevent a generalized convulsion.

Administered in large enough doses, local anesthetic drugs depress the heart directly by interfering with conduction and by decreasing myocardial contractility. When artificial respiration is maintained, the dose producing cardiac arrest may be several times larger than that which causes respiratory paralysis. However, small doses of bupivacaine (75 to 90 mg) have resulted in cardiac arrest in obstetrical patients. Immediate oxygenation and early abortion of the seizures are of critical importance to minimize the development of metabolic acidosis, which markedly aggravates the cardiotoxicity of bupivacaine. If cardiovascular collapse occurs, resuscitation may be difficult and prolonged. Specific drug therapy for local anesthetic–induced cardiotoxicity has not been established, although preliminary studies suggest that full doses of epinephrine reverse cardiac conduction block and that large doses of bretylium (20 to 30 mg per kilogram) are effective in the treatment of ventricular fibrillation.[29,30]

Test Dose

The use of a test dose for epidural anesthesia traditionally has been recommended to minimize the likelihood of total spinal anesthesia. Recently, unintentional intravascular injection has been regarded with greater concern because of the number of cases of maternal cardiac arrest from bupivacaine-induced seizures. The earliest sign of unintentional spinal anesthesia from high volume, low concentration drugs used for epidural anesthesia is not necessarily a high sensory block with muscle paralysis, but may be only patchy areas of hypesthesia and hypalgesia. Since the epidural catheter may migrate through the dura at any time, a repeated spinal test dose with a receding block is even less reliable and generally requires a larger amount of drug to be effective. Unfortunately there is no test dose of epidural local anesthetic solutions that will reliably and promptly indicate an intrathecal or intravascular injection in all patients without resulting in a high spinal block or a severe drug reaction in some patients.[31-33]

The use of 3 ml of hyperbaric 1.5 percent lidocaine with 15 μg of epinephrine is currently the best test dose for the detection of either an intrathecal or an intravascular injection.[34,35] However, the use of epinephrine as an intravascular test dose requires that the patient be continuously monitored with electrocardiography or a pulse monitor, and the cardiovascular effects of uterine contractions may be difficult to distinguish from changes in vital signs owing to the "epinephrine effect."[36,37] Furthermore, the safety of an intravascular injection of epinephrine in the obstetrical patient has been questioned. Hood et al[38] reported that intravenous doses of epinephrine (5, 10, and 20 μg per milliliter) resulted in a dose-related decrease in uterine blood flow of 30 percent to almost 60 percent, lasting longer than three minutes (although peak decreases lasted about one minute) in pregnant ewes.

The epinephrine test dose, like all other test doses, is not 100 percent reliable, and even if the results are negative, the needle or catheter may enter a blood vessel just before the therapeutic dose is given. Careful aspiration prior to, during, and after every drug administration, the use of an effective test dose, and, most important, the use of small (5 to 6 ml), slowly injected (over one to two minutes), closely spaced (two to three minutes apart) incremental doses (rather than large bolus administration of a local anesthetic dose merely because the test dose was negative) avoid or reduce the severity of toxic reactions and the incidence of unintentional intrathecal injections.

INDIRECT DRUG EFFECTS

The fetus and neonate may be affected owing to anesthetic effects on the course of labor and placental perfusion. Regional anesthesia for labor and delivery had been reported to prolong the course of labor (decreased uterine contractility), interfere with internal rotation of the fetal head (impaired sensory and motor block of the pelvic floor), and delay expulsion of the infant (absence of the "bearing down" reflex). The advantages of regional anesthesia in reducing or eliminating depressant drug effects on the fetus and neonate can be negated if placental perfusion is decreased by hypotension or uterine hyperactivity-uterine artery spasm.

Labor and Delivery

Regional anesthesia administered in early labor may completely inhibit uterine contractions. Local anesthetic solutions containing epinephrine (beta-adrenergic effect)

aggravate this effect and increase the propensity for regional anesthesia to interfere with uterine contractility during well-established labor. A number of studies have indicated that epidural anesthesia with or without epinephrine does not adversely affect the duration of labor, although uterine contractility may be diminished during the first 30 minutes after administration.[39-41] Furthermore, oxytocin augmentation overcomes any adverse effects of relief of labor pain on uterine contractility.

Epidural anesthesia in the absence of complications is associated with fewer alterations in the maternal acid-base status than in mothers who have undergone painful labor.[42-45] Several studies have reported a higher incidence of fetal bradycardia with epidural anesthesia than that in control groups.[46,47] However, these investigators did not administer a fluid load or maintain their patients in a lateral position until the onset of hypotension. Willcourt et al[48] reported that 9 percent of high risk parturients develop abnormal fetal heart rate patterns and low transcutaneous PO_2 levels associated with the onset of epidural anesthesia (bupivacaine, 0.5 percent) owing to a decrease in the maternal blood pressure or uterine hypertonus. However, these patients were placed in the supine position for 10 minutes before assuming a lateral position. Epidural anesthesia had no effect on fetal oxygenation when parturients were in the lateral position.

The marked increase in the use of forceps delivery with the introduction of epidural anesthesia may be attributable to their initial use in complicated labors, which commonly require forceps at delivery, inexperience in the need for delayed "bearing down" (the fetal head should be below the ischial spines or near the perineum), and not permitting a longer second stage, resulting in unnecessary forceps rotations and deliveries.[49-52] The basis for limiting the second stage of labor is found in studies in parturients without epidural anesthesia that demonstrated progressive fetal acidosis,[53] but this is not the case with epidural anesthesia. Phillips and Thomas[54] in a prospective study showed that patients in whom epidural anesthesia was discontinued had a decreased incidence of spontaneous vaginal delivery, a higher incidence of fetal distress, and a higher incidence of persistent malrotation than mothers who had epidural anesthesia for the second stage of labor.

Placental Perfusion

Placental perfusion is decreased as a result of hypotension secondary to peripheral vasodilatation (systemic medication, autonomic blockade) and uterine hypertonus-uterine arterial spasm secondary to paracervical block, vasopressor drugs, reflex release of endogenous catecholamines, or unintentional intravascular injection of local anesthetics.

Hypotension

The sympathetic blockade that invariably occurs with epidural anesthesia may cause visceral pooling of blood, a reduction in venous return, a lowering of the systemic blood pressure, and a decrease in uterine blood flow. A maternal systolic blood pressure less than 100 torr may be associated with fetal bradycardia. Fetal bradycardia develops invariably within five minutes after the maternal systolic blood pressure has fallen below 80 torr.[55]

In all patients receiving regional anesthesia an intravenous line should be in place, and they should be rapidly hydrated with non–dextrose-containing fluids (500 to 1,000 ml) and maintained in a lateral position or with left uterine displacement. Vital signs and patient responsiveness should be monitored frequently and regularly for 15 to 20 minutes or longer until the patient is stable (the block level has not increased over a five minute period) and then intermittently, since high blocks may have a rapid or slow onset, particularly with bupivaciane.[56] Fetal bradycardia that occurs with the onset of epidural anesthesia (10 to 20 minutes after the injection of a local anesthetic) in a hydrated parturient in the lateral position may be the result of a slight decrease in the uterine blood flow secondary to a small decrease in the mean arterial pressure (without compensatory placental vasodilation). These fetuses are at risk from a marginal uteroplacental blood supply and should be monitored carefully and delivered expeditiously.

Uterine Hypertonus–Uterine Artery Spasm

The etiology of paracervical block fetal bradycardia is controversial: Pharmacologic toxic bradycardia may result from an excessive fetal plasma concentration of local anesthetic, and hypoxic bradycardia may be the result of decreased placental perfusion secondary to uterine hypertonus or uterine arterial vasoconstriction. However, Morishima et al[57] have demonstrated in pregnant baboons that paracervical bradycardia occurs in association with a reduced uteroplacental blood flow and elevated uterine activity. Baxi et al[58] demonstrated, with a continuous transcutaneous oxygen electrode, that paracervical block bradycardia is accompanied by a decline in human fetal oxygen tension.

When the use of a paracervical block is restricted to parturients whose fetuses previously had normal heart rate patterns and acid-base status, and if the fetal bradycardia is not severe and persistent (so that delivery can be delayed until the heart rate fully recovers), the outcome for fetuses who develop bradycardia is not compromised. However, when the fetus is already compromised or the degree and duration of fetal bradycardia are excessive (heart rate less than 60 beats per minute for longer than four minutes), emergency delivery may be necessary to prevent intrauterine or neonatal death.

When the cardiac output is increased as a result of sympathetic stimulation or endogenous catecholamine release (anxiety, pain, or in response to aortocaval occlusion), uterine arterial vasoconstriction may result in a decrease in placental perfusion. When dehydration, metabolic acidosis, or hypovolemia is present, maternal compensatory mechanisms are often ineffective, with a marked decrease in placental perfusion. Acute moderate hemorrhage (500 to 750 ml within 15 minutes) causes minimal changes in maternal vital signs but inevitably decreases placental blood flow. Acute severe hemorrhage (1,500 ml within 15 minutes) usually decreases the maternal systemic pressure despite intense peripheral vasoconstriction, with a marked decrease in the placental flow.

Vasopressors are used most frequently in obstetrics as anesthetic adjuvants to prevent or treat hypotension secondary to spinal or epidural anesthesia. Vasopressors not only maintain or increase arterial blood pressure but may also increase uterine vascular and myometrial tone, thereby increasing uterine vascular resistance. These changes could reduce uterine blood flow. Hence, there is considerable controversy regarding the appropriate use of vasopressors in obstetrics.

In animals the treatment of hypotension (secondary to spinal anesthesia) with methoxamine, phenylephrine, angiotensin, or norepinephrine diminished uterine blood flow and led to fetal asphyxia.[59] Ephedrine, mephentermine, and metaraminol restored uterine blood flow toward normal. However, the return of uterine blood flow never exceeded 90 percent of prespinal levels in ewes and averaged only 80 percent of prespinal levels in primates.[60,61]

Skepticism should be the rule in extrapolating animal uterine blood flow data to human placental blood flow. Although it is controversial, human uterine vessels (unlike those of the ewe) do dilate with beta-adrenergic stimulation, making the interpretation of uterine blood flow data in sheep studies questionable. Marx et al[62] clearly demonstrated that ephedrine prophylaxis or treatment of spinal hypotension had no adverse effect on the clinical or biochemical neonatal status. Fetal acidosis and depression develop if significant and prolonged hypotension occurs, despite correction with or without ephedrine. Furthermore, 5 mg of ephedrine and 100 μg of phenylephrine to treat hypotension under epidural anesthesia for cesarean section have been shown to be equally effective in restoring blood pressure without differences between treatment groups in Apgar scores and umbilical cord blood acid-base status.[63]

The addition of epinephrine to local anesthetic solutions for epidural anesthesia in obstetrics remains controversial.[64-66] Wallis et al[67] demonstrated a transient 14 percent decrease in the uterine blood flow shortly after the onset of epidural anesthesia with chloroprocaine containing epinephrine, whereas uterine blood flow did not change in ewes receiving chloroprocaine (plain). Intervillous blood flow studies in humans have not demonstrated any significant reduction when epinephrine has been added to epidural anesthetics in the absence of concurrent hypotension.[68-70] No clinical studies have demonstrated any adverse effects on the neonates of mothers who epidurally received local anesthetics epidurally that contained epinephrine.

Fetal bradycardia, which occurs shortly after epidural injection of a local anesthetic in the absence of systemic hypotension, is probably the result of at least a partial unintentional intravascular injection. Greiss et al[71] have demonstrated a dose-related decrease in uterine blood flow following the intra-arterial injection of large doses of procaine, lidocaine, mepivacaine, and bupivacaine. The resultant blood concentrations were generally similar to those that might occur following the unintentional intravascular administration of local anesthetics as a complication of paracervical block or epidural anesthesia.

DIRECT DRUG EFFECTS

Perinatal mortality and morbidity may be increased because of the direct effects of analgesic or anesthetic drugs. Analgesic and anesthetic drugs administered to the parturient cross the placenta rapidly and produce time- and dose-related perinatal depression. Inhalation analgesia, in contrast to inhalation anesthesia, properly administered does not result in neonatal depression. Fetal hypoxia and acidosis potentiate the placental transfer and depressant effect of analgesic and anesthetic drugs.

Drug sensitivity is increased in the fetus and neonate, compared with that in adults, because of the greater permeability of the fetal blood-brain barrier, the absence or deficiency of microsomal enzymes, inefficient renal excretion, and asphyxia. Premature neonates are even more susceptible to these factors and also have higher blood concentrations, because they have smaller blood and tissue volumes in which the drugs can be distributed. The neonate who is depressed as a result of maternally administered drugs may hypoventilate or have respiratory apnea at birth, requiring assisted or controlled ventilation to produce normal exchange of respiratory gases and to eliminate anesthetics. When spontaneous or artificial ventilatory efforts are inadequate, hypoxia and acidosis develop, which potentiate the effects of depressant drugs and result in cardiovascular depression and eventual collapse.

Systemic Medication

Systemic medication, properly administered, is a valuable adjunct in the management of labor pain, although it may be associated with neonatal depression and interfere with early mother-infant interaction if they are too "sleepy" shortly after birth. Tranquilizers are administered in early labor to provide sedation. Opiates are administered during the active phase of labor to produce analgesia and mood modification. Medications should be administered by incremental rapid intravenous injections of small doses (12.5 mg of meperidine, 5.0 mg pentazocine, 0.25 mg of butorphanol) at the start of uterine contractions. Placental transfer of drugs is reduced when intravenous doses are injected at the beginning of a uterine contraction. By the time the bolus of drug goes through the maternal central circulation into the uterine arteries, placental perfusion is arrested (uterine contraction is at its peak). Maternal distribution rapidly lowers the maternal plasma concentration before placental circulation is reestablished and the placental drug diffusion gradient is lowered significantly.

The maximal safe dosage has not been established, although it is rare that more than six to eight intravenous doses are required. Meperidine probably should not be used in a large dose for protracted labor because of its progressive metabolism to normeperidine, with the potential for enhanced neonatal depression. Neonates of heavily medicated mothers who are not acidotic at birth may still require active resuscitation, including endotracheal intubation, if respiration is depressed. Naloxone rapidly crosses the placenta, so that when delivery is unexpectedly imminent, narcotic depression of both the mother and the fetus may be reversed by maternal intravenous administration.[72] However, because maternal analgesia may be dissipated, it usually is preferable to wait and administer naloxone (10 to 20 μg per kg) to the depressed neonate.

Local Anesthetics

Placentally transferred local anesthetics are not associated with significant perinatal depression unless the mature fetus is severely hypoxic and acidotic. Animal studies indicate that the fetus can tolerate extremely high concentrations of lidocaine or mepivacaine (20 to 27 μg per milliliter for over 60 minutes) provided that acidosis and hypoxia are not present.[73,74] However, lidocaine in a concentration of less than 6 to 8 μg per milliliter causes severe fetal bradycardia in asphyxiated fetuses (pH less than 7.2). Sinclair et al[75] reported the disappearance of all signs of toxicity in neonates at a mepivacaine plasma level of 8 μg per milliliter following exchange transfusion and gastric lavage after unintentional fetal scalp injection. However, the acidotic premature ewe fetus demonstrated further deterioration even with low plasma concentrations of lidocaine.[76] Therefore, chloroprocaine (rapid plasma enzymatic degradation) is the local anesthetic of choice when one is administering local anesthetics to the mother of a premature fetus or whenever there is concern about direct fetal local anesthetic toxicity.

Fetal Scalp Injection

Unintentional direct fetal scalp injection of local anesthetics from a misplaced needle while attempting caudal, paracervical, or pudendal block has resulted in a poor neonatal outcome and perinatal death. Early recognition of the problem (needle puncture marks) in neonates who have unexplained depression within the first hour or two after delivery and appropriate support of oxygenation, ventilation, and medication for the control of seizures will improve the outcome.

Neurobehavioral Effects

Neurobehavioral assessment of neonates has demonstrated effects not only from general anesthetics and systemically administered medications but also after epidural anesthesia. However, transient neurobehavioral changes in healthy neonates have not been associated with mother-infant bonding or feeding difficulties, or subsequent impairment of neurologic or psychologic development of the offspring of medicated or anesthetized mothers. Ounsted et al[77] reported that among vaginal deliveries, no significant differences were found in the developmental status of children at the age of four years relating to the method of pain relief used during childbirth.

Mothers are enduring unnecessarily painful labor with its psychic trauma and physiologic stress, which may result in progressive maternal and fetal acidosis. A drug-free but acidotic neonate is a poor substitute for a healthy but "slightly drugged" neonate with transient neurobehavioral changes of unproven significance. Patients should not be denied superior analgesic or anesthetic techniques or drugs because of concern for neurobehavioral effects. Small amounts of systemic medication or properly administered regional anesthesia should have no significant effect on the course of labor or infant well-being.

REFERENCES

1. Marx GF. Cardiopulmonary resuscitation of late-pregnant women. Anesthesiology 1982; 56:156.
2. Marx GF, Luykx WM, Cohen S. Fetal-neonatal status following caesarean section for fetal distress. Br J Anaesth 1984; 56:1009.
3. Archer GW, Marx GF. Arterial oxygen tension during apnoea in parturient women. Br J Anaesth 1974; 46:358.
4. Gold MI, Duarte I, Murarchick S. Arterial oxygenation in conscious patients after 5 minutes and after 30 seconds of oxygen breathing. Anesth Analg 1981; 60:313.
5. Norris MC, Dewan DM. Preoxygenation for cesarean section: comparison of two techniques. Anesthesiology 1985; 62:827.
6. Gambee AM, Hertzka RE, Fisher DM. Preoxygenation techniques: comparison of three minutes and four breaths. Anesth Analg 1987; 66:468.
7. Russell GN, Smith CL, Snowdow SL, Bryson THL. Preoxygenation techniques. Anesth Analg 1987; 66:1337.
8. Ford RWJ. Confirming tracheal intubation — a simple manoeuvre. Can Anaesth Soc J 1983; 30:191.
9. Bond VK, Stoelting RK, Gupta CD. Pulmonary aspiration syndrome after inhalation of gastric fluid containing antacids. Anesthesiology 1979; 51:452.
10. Heaney GAH, Jones HD. Aspiration syndromes in pregnancy (correspondence). Anaesthesia 1979; 51:1145.
11. Moore J, McAuley DM, Johnston JR, Howe JP. H$_2$-receptor blockade and gastric hyperacidity during labor. Abstract of scientific paper presented at annual meeting, Society for Obstetric Anesthesia and Perinatology, San Antonio, Texas, 1984.
12. Smith G. Pretreatment with nondepolarizing muscle relaxant does not decrease gastric regurgitation following succinylcholine. Anesthesiology 1982; 56:408.
13. Sellick BA. Cricoid pressure to control regurgitation of stomach contents during induction of anesthesia. Lancet 1961; 2:404.
14. Samuels SI, Maze A, Albright GA. Cardiac arrest during cesarean section in a chronic amphetamine abuser. Anesth Analg 1979; 59:528.
15. Kautto U-M. Effect of combinations of topical anesthesia, fentanyl, halothane on N20 on circulatory intubation response in normo and hypertensive patients. Acta Anaesthesiol Scand 1983; 27:245.
16. Marx GF. Shock in the obstetric patient. Anesthesiology 1965; 27:423.
17. The experts opine. Is epidural block for labor and delivery and for cesarean section a safe form of analgesia in severe preeclampsia or eclampsia? Surv Anesthesiol 1986; 30:304.
18. Hodgkinson R, Husain FJ, Hayashi RH. Systemic and pulmonary blood pressure during caesarean section in parturients with gestational hypertension. Can Anaesth Soc J 1980; 27:389.
19. Joyce TH III, Loon M. Preeclampsia: effect of albumin 25% infusion. Anesthesiology 1981; 55:A313.
20. Caplan RA, Ward RJ, Posner K, Cheney FW. Unexpected cardiac arrest during spinal anesthesia: a closed claims analysis of predisposing factors. Anesthesiology 1988; 68:5.
21. Albright GA, Ferguson JE, Joyce TH, Stevenson DK. Anesthesia in obstetrics: maternal, fetal, and neonatal aspects. Boston: Butterworth, 1986:137.
22. Albright GA. What is the place of bupivacaine in obstetric epidural analgesia? Can Anaesth Soc J 1985; 32:392.
23. Abboud TK, Khoo SS, Miller F, et al. Maternal, fetal, and neonatal responses after epidural anesthesia with bupivacaine, 2-chloroprocaine, or lidocaine. Anesth Analg 1982; 61:638.
24. Evans TI. Total spinal anaesthesia. Anaesth Intensive Care 1974; 2:158.
25. Russell IF. Spinal anaesthesia for caesarean section. Br J Anaesth 1983; 55:309.
26. Conklin KA, van der Wal C. Epidural anesthesia with chloroprocaine. Anaesthesia 1980; 35:202.
27. Soni N, Holland R. An extensive lumbar epidural block. Anaesth Intensive Care 1981; 9:150.
28. Lee A, Dood KW. Accidental subdural catheterisation. Anaesthesia 1986; 41:847.
29. Kasten GW, Martin ST. Successful resuscitation after massive intravenous bupivacaine overdose in anesthetized dogs. Anesthesiology 1985; 64:491.
30. Wojtczak JA, Griffin RM, Pratilas MS, Kaplan JA. Is it possible to resuscitate a bupivacaine-intoxicated heart? Anesthesiology 1984; 61:A207.
31. Albright GA. Clinical aspects of bupivacaine toxicity. Report to the Anesthetic and Life Support Drugs Advisory Committee. Washington, DC: Department of Health and Human Services, 1983.
32. Soni V, Peeters C, Covino B. Value and limitations of test dose prior to epidural anesthesia. Reg Anaesth 1981; 6:23.
33. Stonham J, Moss P. The optimal test dose for epidural anesthesia (correspondence). Anesthesiology 1983; 58:389.
34. Abraham RA, Harris AP, Maxwell LG, Kaplow S. The efficacy of 1.5% lidocaine with 7.5% dextrose and epinephrine as an epidural test dose for obstetrics. Anesthesiology 1986; 64:116.
35. Moore DC, Batra MS. The components of an effective test dose prior to epidural block. Anesthesiology 1981; 55:693.

36. Chestnut DH, Weiner CP, Herreg JE, Wong J. Effect of intravenous epinephrine upon uterine blood flow velocity in the pregnant guinea pig. Anesthesiology 1986; 65:633.
37. Leighton BL, Norris MC, Sosis M, et al. Limitations of epinephrine as a marker of intravascular injection in laboring women. Anesthesiology 1987; 66:688.
38. Hood D, Dewan DM, James FM III. Maternal and fetal effects of epinephrine in gravid ewes. Anesthesiology 1986; 64:601.
39. Raabe N, Belfrage P. Epidural analgesia in labour. IV. Influence on uterine activity and fetal heart rate. Acta Obstet Gynecol Scand 1976; 55:305.
40. Willdeck-Lund G, Lindmark G, Nilsson BA. Effect of segmental epidural analgesia upon the uterine activity with special reference to the use of different local anaesthetic agents. Acta Anaesthesiol Scand 1979; 23:519.
41. Tyack AJ, Millar DR, Nicholas ADG. Uterine activity and plasma bupivacaine levels after caudal epidural analgesia. Br J Obstet Gynaecol 1973; 80:896.
42. Pearson JF, Davies P. The effect of continuous lumbar epidural analgesia on the acid-base status of maternal arterial blood during the first stage of labour. J Obstet Gynaecol 1973; 80:218.
43. Pearson JF, Davies P. The effect of continuous lumbar epidural analgesia on maternal acid-base balance and arterial lactate concentration during the second stage of labour. J Obstet Gynaecol 1973; 80:225.
44. Zador G, Nilsson BA. Low dose intermittent epidural anaesthesia with lidocaine for vaginal delivery. Acta Obstet Gynecol Scand (Suppl) 1974; 34:17.
45. Thalme B, Belfrage P, Raabe N. Lumbar epidural analgesia in labour. Acta Obstet Gynecol Scand 1974; 53:27.
46. McDonald JS, Bjorkman LL, Reed EC. Epidural analgesia for obstetrics: a maternal, fetal, and neonatal study. Am J Obstet Gynecol 1974; 120:1055.
47. Wingate MB, Wingate L, Iffy L, et al. The effect of epidural analgesia upon fetal and neonatal status. Am J Obstet Gynecol 1974; 119:1101.
48. Willcourt RJ, Paust JC, Queenan JT. Changes in fetal TCPO$_2$ values occurring during labour in association with lumbar extradural analgesia. Br J Anaesth 1982; 54:635.
49. Bailey PW, Howard FA. Epidural analgesia and forceps delivery: laying a bogey. Anaesthesia 1983; 38:282.
50. Crawford JS. Correspondence. Br J Obstet Gynaecol 1981; 88:685.
51. Maresh M, Choong KH, Beard RW. Delayed pushing with lumbar epidural analgesia in labour. Br J Obstet Gynaecol 1983; 90:623.
52. Studd JWW, Crawford JS, Duignan NM, et al. The effect of lumbar epidural analgesia on the rate of cervical dilation and the outcome of labour of spontaneous onset. Br J Obstet Gynaecol 1981; 88:685.
53. Livnat EJ, Fejgin M, Scommegna A, et al. Neonatal acid-base balance in spontaneous and instrumental vaginal deliveries. Obstet Gynecol 1978; 52:549.
54. Phillips KC, Thomas TA. Second stage of labour with or without extradural analgesia. Anaesthesia 1983; 38: 972.
55. Hingson RA, Hellman LM. Anesthesia for obstetrics. Philadelphia:JB Lippincott, 1956.
56. Skowronski GA, Rigg RJA. Total spinal block complicating epidural analgesia in labour. Anaesth Intensive Care 1981; 9:274.
57. Morishima HO, Covino BG, Yeh MN, et al. Bradycardia in the fetal baboon following paracervical block anesthesia. Am J Obstet Gynecol 1981; 140:775.
58. Baxi LV, Petrie RH, James LS. Human fetal oxygenation following paracervical block. Am J Obstet Gynecol 1979; 135:1109.
59. Greiss FC, Van Wilkes D. Effects of sympathicomimetic drugs and angiotensin on the uterine vascular bed. Obstet Gynecol 1964; 23:925.
60. Eng M, Berges PV, Parer JT, et al. Spinal anesthesia and ephedrine in pregnant monkeys. Am J Obstet Gynecol 1973; 115:1095.
61. James FM III, Greiss FC Sr, Kemp RA. An evaluation of vasopressor therapy for maternal hypotension during spinal anesthesia. Anesthesiology 1970; 33:25.
62. Marx GF, Cosmi EV, Wollman SB. Biochemical status and clinical condition of mother and infant at cesarean section. Anesth Analg 1969; 48:986.
63. Grant GJ, Ramanathan S, Turndorf H. Maternal hemodynamic effects of ephedrine and phenylephrine. Anesth Analg 1987; 66:S73.
64. Albright GA. Epinephrine should be used with the therapeutic dose of bupivacaine in obstetrics. Anesthesiology 1984; 61:217.
65. Marx GF. Cardiotoxicity of local anesthetics — the plot thickens. Anesthesiology 1984; 60:3.
66. Marx GF. Correspondence. Anesthesiology 1984; 61:218.
67. Wallis KL, Shnider SM, Hicks JS, Spivey HT. Epidural anesthesia in the normotensive pregnant ewe: effects on uterine blood flow and fetal acid-base status. Anesthesiology 1976; 44:481.
68. Albright GA, Jouppila R, Holmen AI, et al. Epinephrine does not alter human intervillous blood flow during epidural anesthesia. Anesthesiology 1981; 54:131.
69. Jouppila R, Jouppila P, Hollmen A, Kuikka J. Effect of segmental extradural analgesia on placental blood flow during normal labour. Br J Anaesth 1978; 50:563.
70. Jouppila R, Jouppila P, Kuikka J, Hollmen A. Placental blood flow during caesarean section under lumbar extradural analgesia. Br J Anaesth 1978; 50:275.
71. Greiss FC, Still GS, Anderson SG. Effects of local anesthetic agents on the uterine vasculatures and myometrium. Am J Obstet Gynecol 1976; 124:889.
72. Clark RB. Transplacental reversal of meperidine depression in the fetus by naloxone. J Arkansas Med Soc 1971; 68:128.
73. Morishima HO, Adamson K. Placental clearance of mepivacaine following administration to the guinea pig fetus. Anesthesiology 1967; 28:343.
74. Morishima HO, Heymann MA, Rudolph AM, et al. Transfer of lidocaine across the sheep placenta to the fetus. Am J Obstet Gynecol 1972; 112:72.
75. Sinclair JC, Fox HJ, Lentz JF. Intoxication of the fetus by a local anesthetic: a newly recognized complication of maternal and caudal anesthesia. N Engl J Med 1965; 273:1173.
76. Morishima HO, Pedersen H, Santos A, et al. Pharmacodynamics of lidocaine in the asphyxiated preterm fetal lamb. Anesthesiology 1986; 65:A372.
77. Ounsted M, Scott A, Moor V. Pain relief during childbirth and development at 4 years (correspondence). J R Soc Med 1981; 74:629.

5 Fetal Injury from Drug Abuse in Pregnancy: Alcohol, Narcotic, Cocaine, and Phencyclidine

Ronald S. Cohen, M.D., William E. Benitz, M.D., and
David K. Stevenson, M.D.

Alcohol
Narcotic
Cocaine
Phencyclidine

Thalidomide, a sedative, is probably the most important teratogenic drug that achieved extensive clinical use. The mechanism by which this drug induces hypoplasia of the limbs remains uncertain. Relatively few other drugs have actually been shown to have teratogenic effects (Table 5–1). Since 1962, drug regulations in the United States have reflected a concern for the potential role of foreign compounds in injuring the fetus when the pregnant woman is exposed to them purposely or inadvertently. Unless the chemical is destroyed or altered during placental passage, any drug administered to the mother should be presumed to cross the placenta and potentially affect the fetus, especially from about the fifth week of fetal life. Low molecular weight chemicals (i.e., most compounds that we would categorize as drugs) can cross the placenta easily, the concentration gradient being the major determining factor. Unfortunately information obtained about specific drugs through animal experimentation generally cannot be extrapolated from species to species, or even from strain to strain within the same species. Further extrapolation from the results of animal experimentation to human circumstances is even more problematic. Moreover, specific cause and effect relationships rarely are defined clinically despite extensive human experience, which is typically anecdotal and associative.

With respect to teratogenesis, the fetus is at greatest risk during the first three months of gestation. However, injuries resulting in long-term behavioral consequences, which become apparent only later in life, probably also occur, and vulnerability throughout gestation is variable. The mechanisms of teratogenesis generally are obscure and may be confounded by other factors affecting particularly the performance of the placenta or generally the nutritional state of the fetus. Pregnant women are commonly exposed to prescription drugs and over-the-counter drugs throughout pregnancy. Despite the 1962 drug regulations, this exposure incidence has been unchanged, or more likely has increased. Superimposed on this "usual" drug exposure incidence during pregnancy has been the exposure incidence for totally elective or "recreational" drugs. The latter kind of drug exposure frequently confounds our ability to understand the condition of the neonate as well as the long-term neurodevelopmental outcome. The purpose of this chapter is not to present an exhaustive review of drugs and their potential fetal effects, but to discuss a few of the most common "recreational" exposures and their consequences, as they confound our understanding of transitional physiology and the perinatal and long-term outcome. Because of their potential for abuse and current social practices, the compounds that have been selected for review are alcohol, narcotic, cocaine, and phencyclidine.

TABLE 5-1 Teratogenicity of Drugs

Drug	Exposed Infants Studied		Type of Defect	General Comment
	Total	Deformed		
Cancer Chemotherapeutic Agents (Nicholson, 1968; Shepard, 1974):				
Aminopterin and methylaminopterin	41	8	Cranial ossifications defect (5), small mandible (5), palate defect (1), hydrocephalus (1)	
Busulfan	30	10	Spontaneous abortion and prematurity (10), cleft palate (1), eye defect (1)	
Chlorambucil	5	1	Absence of ureter and kidney (1)	All potentially teratogenic; first trimester treatment more commonly associated with defects; defects during second and third trimester unknown; often given in combinations and to acutely ill mother; one infant developed leukemia at nine months of age
Colchicine	16	0		
Cyclophosphamide	4	2	Absence of digits	
Mercaptopurine	26	1	Cleft palate (1), eye defect (1)	
Nitrogen mustard	8	0		
Procarbazine	3	1	Small pelvic kidneys	
Trimethylene melamine	3	0		
Urethan	8	0		
Vinblastine	4	0		
Sedatives:				
Thalidomide	?	10,000	Phocomelia	Rat and mouse fetuses not sensitive; human, monkey, and rabbit sensitive; single dose capable of producing defects in humans
Chlordiazepoxide and meprobamate	2500	See comments	No pattern	One large study found four-fold increase in defects from pregnancies when treatment carried out in first 42 days; another large study could not confirm this
Diazepam	137	See comments	Cleft lip and palate	Two studies found four-fold increase in expected incidence of facial clefts among mothers ingesting this drug during first trimester
Androgens:				
Testosterone, including its ethinyl derivatives	Unknown; ? many	50	Masculinization of female genitalia	10–20 mg daily of ethinyl testosterone produces masculinization in about 15% of female fetuses; neither progesterone nor 17-hydroxyprogesterone produced masculinization
Diethylstilbestrol	Over 500	7–73%	Precancerous adenosis of vagina	Precancerous changes found in 30–73% of offspring exposed before ninth week of gestation but only in 7% exposed after 17th week; cancer rate in exposed subjects less than 0.01%, at least by age 22 years
Corticosteroids	688	5	Cleft palate (5)	Little or no teratogenic effect in man
Coumarin anticoagulants	Unknown	9	Small nose, stippled secondary epiphyses, occasional mental retardation, optic atrophy	No case reports have appeared yet in women treated after first trimester
Diphenylhydantoin and trimethadione	Many	? Increased	Hypoplasia of terminal digits, nails, cleft palate	A number of large prospective studies have shown no increase in defects; other studies have found small increase in all types of defects; terminal digital hypoplasia may occur in up to 30% of exposed offspring
Radioiodine	Few	5	Athyrotic cretinism	Therapeutic amounts only; diagnostic doses have not caused cretinism; can cause airway obstruction at birth if administered during third trimester; some reports have suggested, but other studies do not confirm, human teratogenicity
Iodides and thioamides	Moderate number	Common	Goiter in newborn	
Oral contraceptives, trace anesthetics, aspirin, lithium, quinine	Many	No increase in pattern		

From Quilligan EJ, Kretchmer N, eds. Fetal and maternal medicine. New York: John Wiley, 1980:410.

ALCOHOL

Although references to the fetal effects of maternal alcohol consumption can be found as far back as the Bible (Judges 13:7), the modern investigation of alcohol teratogenicity began about 20 years ago.[1,2] Since that time a relatively well-defined fetal alcohol syndrome has been delineated,[3,4] although much debate continues about the more subtle effects of alcohol on the developing fetus. The fetal alcohol syndrome is defined by intrauterine growth retardation, facial abnormalities, and central nervous system dysfunction; frequently other anomalies involving the heart, kidneys, and skeletal system are found.[5] The teratogenic effects of alcohol are variable, with many more infants showing a pattern of less severe injury termed the "fetal alcohol effect."

The abnormality of growth is usually global,[5] despite the initial report suggesting that length was affected more than weight.[2] In fact, a permanent deficit in adipose tissue may be found in patients with the fetal alcohol syndrome, resulting in a chronic "skinny" appearance. The abnormality of growth is permanent, many of the patients never achieving "catch-up" growth.[5]

The facial characteristics are most helpful in making the diagnosis of fetal alcohol syndrome in the newborn period. In addition to microcephaly, these patients have short palpebral fissures and midfacial hypoplasia.[3] The short palpebral fissure reflects abnormal growth of the eye, which may result in frank microphthalmia.[6] Clarren and Smith[5] state that they and 12 other investigators found short palpebral fissures in 73 to 91 percent of their patients, making this relatively objective finding extremely helpful in establishing the diagnosis of fetal alcohol syndrome. The deficient growth of the midfacial region generally results in a thin upper lip with a small philtrum and a flattened nasal bridge. The maxillary hypoplasia may be pronounced enough to result in epicanthal folds, anteverted nares, a relatively exaggerated distance between the nose and the upper lip, and even an underbite profile, although actual micrognathia is more the rule.[5] Occasionally hirsutism, cleft lip and palate, and minor external ear abnormalities have been reported.

Abnormal neurologic findings in the neonatal period have been ascribed to infants of alcoholics. A "withdrawal syndrome," similar to that described in animals, has been reported, consisting of tremors, hypertonia, irritability, abdominal distention, and eventually seizures.[7] It can occur in alcohol-exposed infants without features of the fetal alcohol syndrome.[8] This syndrome is in many ways similar to that seen in infants withdrawing from narcotics, but may be differentiated by the lack of yawning and diaphoresis, by the presence of abdominal distention rather than the diarrhea commonly seen with opiates, and by the more frequent presence of opisthotonus.[8,9]

The long-term neurodevelopmental outcome in infants with overt fetal alcohol syndrome is of great concern. Follow-up of 20 such infants showed an average IQ of 65, 60 percent of the patients having scores more than two standard deviations below the mean.[10] These authors correlated the severity of the developmental impairment with the severity of the dysmorphic features and with the degree of growth deficiency in terms of height. However, even infants with mild manifestations had a mean IQ of 82. Others have demonstrated that infants with features of the fetal alcohol syndrome (especially eye and midfacial findings) identified in the newborn period could be differentiated from matched controls at about one year of age by the delay in growth, mental development, and motor development.[11] The milder changes of the fetal alcohol effect also have been reported to be permanent and identifiable after long-term follow-up in the majority of cases.[12] Indeed, these investigators found more cases at four years of age than at birth, the incidence being related to the amount of alcohol exposure both immediately before the recognition of pregnancy and during the pregnancy. For four-year-olds whose mothers consumed more than 60 ml of alcohol per day during early pregnancy, there was roughly a 40 percent incidence of the fetal alcohol effect at follow-up. Even among patients with "normal" intelligence and mild though identifiable dysmorphic features, learning difficulties at school may be common.[13] It also may be of interest to note that long-standing alterations in the electroencephalogram ("hypersynchrony") have been reported in infants of alcoholic women.[14]

Consumption of large amounts of alcohol throughout pregnancy results in a significant incidence of the fetal alcohol syndrome in the offspring. The question is, what constitutes a large amount of alcohol? Clearly it remains difficult to quantify fetal alcohol exposure. Maternal self-scoring remains the most common method and is fraught with potential inaccuracies. Usually maternal consumption is expressed in terms of ounces (or milliliters) of absolute alcohol per day. Most would agree that a daily consumption in the range of 3 ounces of absolute alcohol daily would pose a significant risk of the fetal alcohol effect.[5] However, lower levels of ethanol ingestion very likely cause some increased risk of the fetal alcohol effect.[15] Decreased head circumference and mild developmental delay have been associated with an average daily alcohol consumption of less than 1 ounce.[16,17] Furthermore, a history of alcoholism alone may adversely affect fetal growth, even if the mother has stopped drinking.[18] Indeed, owing to individual variations in metabolism and susceptibility, it may be fair to say that there is no absolutely safe level of alcohol consumption during pregnancy, although the risks associated with a daily consumption of 1 ounce or less must be very small in most people.[19,20] Although the amount of alcohol consumed in the earliest stages of pregnancy has been linked to fetal outcome,[15,21] women who reduce their alcohol consumption during pregnancy may also reduce the risks to their unborn child.[19] However, the impact of "binge" drinking during pregnancy remains unclear.

NARCOTIC

Although references to the effects of alcohol on the fetus may be found in the Bible, narcotic or opiate abuse is the "classic" model of the effect of maternal self-medication on the fetus. These drugs probably have received the most attention in past years, and the effects of other drugs frequently are compared to the well-described neonatal aftermath of maternal narcotic-opiate addiction. Although the list of narcotic-opiate drugs with a potential for abuse is almost endless, most of the literature focuses on two—heroin and methadone. Since the effects of these drugs are similar, this discussion also focuses on these.

Research dealing with the effects of maternal addiction by its very nature is complicated and fraught with difficulty. Drug addicts tend to be secretive and wary of authority figures, health professionals included. Even with well-motivated subjects, accurate monitoring may be difficult, if not impossible. Precise knowledge of the dosage and composition of drugs obtained on the street clearly is not practical, as "pushers" do not subscribe to "truth in advertising" regulations. "Street drugs" frequently are adulterated with other agents that may have significant effects on the mother and her fetus. Similarly, illegally obtained drugs generally are not administered according to a precise and uniform regimen. Furthermore, a large proportion of heroin addicts also abuse other drugs such as alcohol, marijuana, tobacco, caffeine, cocaine, and "speed." Sorting out the relative importance of these different drugs in the etiology of any finding clearly is difficult. Frequently there may be further complications such as poverty, malnutrition, and prostitution.

Before directing our attention to the obvious concern of neonatal withdrawal, it is worth remembering that any pregnancy complicated by maternal addiction is a high risk gestation *per se*. Ostrea and Chavez[22] have reported a significant increase in obstetrical complications, such as meconium staining, maternal anemia, premature rupture of membranes, hemorrhaging, and multiple births. Neonatal complications other than withdrawal, including intrauterine growth retardation and low Apgar scores, were also found to be increased.

The withdrawal syndrome seen in infants addicted *in utero* has been reviewed extensively.[23-25] The cardinal symptoms include wakefulness, irritability, jitteriness, persistent crying, hyperactivity, hyperreflexia, hyperthermia and diaphoresis, excessive sucking, diarrhea and vomiting, rhinorrhea, tachypnea, hiccups, poor weight gain, and seizures. An additional sign to note is excoriation of the elbows and knees secondary to hyperactivity. When listed in this fashion, these findings may sound nonspecific; however, the clinical appearance when seen is distinctive and easily recognizable.

All infants suspected of being at risk for neonatal narcotic withdrawal should be evaluated frequently with a withdrawal scoring system, several of which have been described.[26-28] This allows for less interobserver variability and thus a more controlled regimen of care. Frequent reassessment of the withdrawal score (i.e., every four hours) is recommended, because the severity of the withdrawal symptoms may change rapidly. The importance of experienced nurses in the management of these babies cannot be overemphasized. During this period of evaluation and observation these patients also must be handled with care. Many can be treated successfully nonpharmacologically, and all patients should be treated this way initially. This requires decreasing the sensory input, swaddling, frequent small feedings, and careful monitoring. Such treatment may be all that is needed in 30 to 50 percent of the cases.[23] The use of a withdrawal scoring system decreases the use of pharmacotherapy and shortens the hospital stay of opiate-exposed neonates.[26]

The decision to treat pharmacologically should be made on the basis of an elevated withdrawal score despite careful handling. Generally the therapeutic options include paregoric (or another orally administered opiate), phenobarbital, chlorpromazine, and diazepam. The pros and cons relating to these various drugs have been reviewed.[24] Paregoric or morphine elixir is our choice and is widely used. The starting dose is 0.1 to 0.2 mg orally every three to four hours, titrated to the patient's clinical behavior. Phenobarbital is probably the second most commonly used drug, given as a loading dose of about 20 mg per kilogram in divided doses during the first day, followed by maintenance dosages of 2 to 5 mg per kilogram per day to maintain a serum level of 20 to 30 μg per milliliter for at least one week, after which the drug dosage is tapered while the withdrawal score is followed. Diazepam (1.0 to 2.0 mg orally every eight hours) also has been used to treat neonatal withdrawal. However, the parenteral use of diazepam is attended by concerns about potential toxicity of the benzoate in the carrier vehicle.[29] Controlled comparisons of the efficacy of these drugs are few, although paregoric has been reported to be superior in terms of preserving nutritive sucking behavior.[26,30] Although the use of chlorpromazine (0.7 to 0.8 mg per kilogram intramuscularly or orally every six hours) has also been described, concerns remain about the prolonged half-life of its metabolites.[24] Other opiates have been used successfully, including methadone.[31]

Many questions remain about the long-term outcome in infants addicted *in utero* to opiates. The data here also are somewhat difficult to interpret, because the socioeconomic environment plays such an important role in infant development. Again, cooperation with authorities, such as health workers, frequently is difficult to maintain.

COCAINE

Cocaine abuse has spread rapidly to all segments of the American population, and it is very likely the most widely abused "drug" in the United States, depending on whether such drugs as alcohol, tobacco, and caffeine are included in the analysis. At least 5 million Americans are regular cocaine users.[32,33] Part of the popularity of this particular drug is that it is so "versatile," the drug for everyone. It is available both in expensive forms and very cheaply as "crack." It can be snorted, smoked, and injected, taken straight or mixed with other drugs, and initially was touted widely as being nonaddictive and "chic." Part of its élan may be the result of the widespread perception of its acceptance in Hollywood and among sports figures. Disturbingly, the recent tragic deaths of some of these media figures, directly attributed to cocaine, have not seemed to diminish the glamor associated with this terrible drug. Furthermore, cocaine has become the most profitable drug for dealers and smugglers, further increasing its popularity.

The effects of cocaine on the neonate cannot be fully appreciated without understanding its effects on the adult and the fetus. In addition to being a local anesthetic and a central nervous system stimulant, cocaine has profound vasoconstrictive activity owing to blockade of norepinephrine reuptake at nerve endings. When it is administered systemically, by either application to mucous membranes or intravenous injection, a marked increase in the blood pressure and heart rate may occur. Direct placental vasoconstriction has been demonstrated.[34] As might be assumed with a drug that is readily absorbed across mucosa and that rapidly crosses the blood-brain barrier, cocaine rapidly diffuses across the placenta. Furthermore, because of the lower fetal than maternal pH, cocaine levels in the fetus actually may exceed those in the mother.[35] Additionally, lower levels of plasma cholinesterase activity in the fetus result in slower metabolism and excretion of cocaine.[36] Therefore, fetal cocaine exposure due to maternal abuse would likely be considerable.

Data relating to the teratogenicity of cocaine are sparse and somewhat confusing. In part this may reflect interspecies differences; for example, the evidence for teratogenicity is stronger in mice than in rats.[37,38] The literature relating to humans is also somewhat confusing: One of the early reports dealing with effects of cocaine use during pregnancy stated that "no evidence of teratogenicity was observed" and that "no evident, potentially life-threatening symptomatology was noted."[39] Many who cite this reference ignore the authors' warnings that "This is, however, a very small number of infants, and we need in the future to be more discriminating and precise in our observations" and "We offer our observations as a point of departure for further studies."

More recent data are much more worrisome. In a larger study involving 50 cocaine-abusing mothers, a significant decrease in birth weight, length, and head circumference was observed, as well as a significant increase in the number of congenital malformations.[40] These growth defects may or may not be specific; there was no significant difference in growth parameters between the offspring of cocaine-abusing and multi-drug-abusing mothers. The authors postulated that the deformations may be due to vasoconstriction secondary to cocaine, resulting in disruption of the blood supply to developing tissues. Skull defects, especially, were noted among the infants of cocaine users, paralleling the abnormalities reported in mice exposed at about the ninth day of gestation.[38] Mice also showed an increased incidence of fetal resorption,[38] and there may be an increased incidence of spontaneous abortion in human cocaine addicts.[41] The reports of hydronephrosis in the mouse and the "prune-belly" syndrome in humans also may represent similar teratogenic effects of cocaine in these species.[38,41]

Cocaine has other nonteratogenic but no less deleterious effects on the fetus. Acute placental abruption has been associated with cocaine use.[40-42] Although the mechanism is not clear, we suspect that vasoconstriction is the "guilty party" once again. The abruption in these reports frequently resulted in premature labor and fetal loss. Premature labor without abruption also has been noted in conjunction with maternal cocaine use, suggesting that this drug may have a direct effect on uterine contractility.[43] Perinatal, and presumably intrauterine, cerebral infarcts have been reported in association with maternal cocaine use.[44]

It remains unclear whether cocaine produces "withdrawal" in the neonate. In part this confusion results because there is so much multidrug abuse that it is difficult to distinguish the effect of cocaine from the effects of opiates or alcohol. Abnormal state organization, detected by the Brazelton Neonatal Behavioral Assessment Scale, poor feeding, sleeplessness, tremors, and irritability have been associated with maternal cocaine abuse.[41,43] Cocaine usually is detectable in the urine of the intrauterinely exposed neonate for several days post partum because of the slow rate of metabolism and excretion.[44] Generally it is detected as benzoylecgonine, the metabolite of cocaine (benzoylmethylecgonine).

Two important issues pertain to the long-term care of the infants of cocaine addicts. Cocaine crosses readily into breast milk, remains there for days after ingestion, and may cause neurologic symptoms and even convulsions in the breast-fed infant.[45,46] Also preliminary data from one center indicate that cocaine exposure in utero may be a risk factor in the sudden infant death syndrome.[47]

Cocaine use is much more prevalent than practitioners would like to believe, especially in young people. It crosses all socioeconomic barriers. The data available unfortunately are preliminary, based on small numbers, and frequently confused by obfuscating factors. Nevertheless, given what we have, the data are worrisome. If indeed this drug is as dangerous to the fetus, newborn, and infant as the data now appearing suggest, its very widespread use indicates that we shall be dealing with a large number of infants with these problems. It would not be all surprising if this turns out to be a much greater problem for obstetricians, pediatricians, and society than opiates ever were.

PHENCYCLIDINE

PCP or "angel dust," the street names for phenylcyclohexylpiperidine or phencyclidine hydrochloride, is a relative newcomer on the drug abuse scene, whose widespread abuse has been almost ignored by the media, the government, and the medical establishment because of the great attention attracted by cocaine. Nevertheless its use in young urban populations has grown dramatically in the 1970s and 1980s.[48–51] PCP is cheap and readily available because it can be synthesized fairly easily. Like cocaine, it is a "multiple choice" drug—it can be ingested, injected, or inhaled, and it frequently is mixed with other drugs. Although the consumer often knowingly mixes PCP with drugs like alcohol and heroin, PCP also is often used by dealers to adulterate marijuana and cocaine without the knowledge of the potential buyer. Therefore, it is not surprising that PCP use is frequently underreported.[50] In a study in Washington, D.C., teenagers at an adolescent clinic who agreed to anonymous urine screening, 24 percent of those testing positive for tetrahydrocannabinol also were positive for PCP, whereas none were positive for PCP in the absence of tetrahydrocannabinol.[52] Furthermore, although 91 percent of those testing positive for tetrahydrocannabinol reported trying marijuana, only 11 percent of those testing positive for PCP reported its use. Although it is possible these teenagers were motivated to hide PCP use, the high correlation of PCP use with marijuana use suggests that some were smoking PCP unknowingly.

The amount of PCP abuse varies widely from community to community within the United States. It is encountered much more frequently in major metropolitan areas than in rural areas and is more commonly seen in the Northeast and West than elsewhere in the country.[50] Along with Los Angeles, New York, and Washington, D.C., Santa Clara County, California, where we practice, apparently is a major focus of PCP usage. PCP abuse is second only to opiate addiction among those seen at the Santa Clara County's Drug Abuse Program, making up 23 percent of those treated. Nevertheless nationwide estimates are that in 1985, 2.9 percent of high

school seniors had tried PCP, almost five times as many as reported trying heroin.[50] PCP is also the most common drug of abuse in patients brought to emergency rooms for drug-related emergencies in these major metropolitan areas.[51]

Although animal studies were unable to demonstrate any teratogenic effects,[53] they have shown significant and permanent alterations in brain neurotransmitter levels after antenatal exposure to this drug.[54,55] They also have documented clearly that PCP crosses the placenta readily, resulting in very high levels in fetal tissues.[56]

PCP was first brought to the attention of the neonatal-perinatal world in the early 1980s. Golden et al[57] reported one case of an infant exposed in utero to PCP who had possibly dysmorphic facies, abnormal behavior, and eventual spastic quadriparesis. Unfortunately, as is not uncommon, this case was complicated by exposure to marijuana in utero and intrauterine growth retardation. The investigators also were unable to test for PCP in the child. Subsequently two additional cases were reported; these infants also had significant abnormalities of behavior and tone, and one was microcephalic.[58] Significantly, PCP was detected in the urine of both infants for at least three days after birth.

Long-term follow-up studies in regard to intrauterine PCP exposure in humans just now are starting to be published. Howard, Kropenske, and Tyler[59] recently described five pre-term and five full-term infants seen at UCLA. In the first two days of life all showed "deviant neurobehavioral symptoms" such as irritability, tremors, and hypertonicity, with bizarre eye movements also common. These patients were all removed from their mothers for the period of follow-up (18 months). Persistent abnormalities of fine motor activity, eye movement, and social behavior were found. Unfortunately this report deals with only 12 patients, and there is a considerable confounding effect from the maternal use of other drugs; nevertheless it raises major concerns. Chasnoff et al[60] recently reported (in abstract) eight PCP-exposed infants who demonstrated a significant fall-off in head growth after 18 months of age. Given the known effects of this drug on animal fetal brain development,[54,55] these reports seem particularly ominous.

In summary, when the condition of the neonate is considered, the possibility of fetal drug exposure needs to be considered. Even when the transition from fetus to newborn is apparently not affected in any clinically important way, the long-term outcome in the exposed infant may be greatly altered independent of or confounded by complicating perinatal factors. Although these potential drug exposures have been discussed with special reference to the pregnant mother, the influence of drug exposure of the father on the perinatal and long-term outcome needs to be considered. A review of this intriguing area has been previously presented.[61] A discussion of the paternal mediating mechanisms is beyond the scope of this chapter. Even if the mechanisms by which paternal drug exposure might cause fetal injury remain obscure, the social and behavioral factors introduced by the drug-abusing father into the family may have an important impact on neurodevelopmental outcome in the child and may confound any attempt to define cause and effect relationships through retrospective reviews. Great caution is warranted when interpreting the long-term consequences of fetal drug exposure.

REFERENCES

1. Lemoine P, Harousseau H, Borteyru JP, et al. Les enfants de parents alcooliques: anomalies observées. Quest Med 1968; 476.
2. Jones KL, Smith DW, Ulleland CN, et al. Pattern of malformation in offspring of chronic alcoholic mothers. Lancet 1973; 1:1267.
3. Jones KL, Smith DW. Recognition of the fetal alcohol syndrome in early infancy. Lancet 1973; 2:999.
4. Jones KL, Smith DW. The fetal alcohol syndrome. Teratology 1975; 12:1.
5. Clarren SK, Smith DW. The fetal alcohol syndrome. N Engl J Med 1978; 298:1063.
6. Hanson JW, Jones KL, Smith DW. Fetal alcohol syndrome: experience with 41 patients. JAMA 1976; 235:1458.
7. Pierog S, Chandavasu O, Wexler I. Withdrawal symptoms in infants with the fetal alcohol syndrome. J Pediatr 1977; 90:630.
8. Coles CD, Smith IE, Fernhoff PM, Falek A. Neonatal ethanol withdrawal: characteristics in clinically normal, nondysmorphic neonates. J Pediatr 1984; 105:445.
9. Robe LB, Gromisch DS, Losub S. Symptoms of neonatal ethanol withdrawal. Curr Alcohol 1981; 8:485.
10. Streissguth AP, Herman CS, Smith DW. Intelligence, behavior, and dysmorphogenesis in the fetal alcohol syndrome: a report on 20 patients. J Pediatr 1978; 92:363.
11. Golden NL, Sokol RJ, Kuhnert BT, Bottoms S. Maternal alcohol use and infant development. Pediatrics 1982; 70:931.
12. Graham JM Jr, Hanson JW, Darby BL, et al. Independent dysmorphology evaluations at birth and 4 years of age for children exposed to varying amounts of alcohol in utero. Pediatrics 1988; 81:722.
13. Shaywitz SE, Cohen DJ, Shaywitz BA. Behavior and learning difficulties in children of normal intelligence born to alcoholic mothers. J Pediatr 1980; 96:978.
14. Ioffe S, Childiaeva R, Chernick V. Prolonged effects of maternal alcohol ingestion on the neonatal electroencephalogram. Pediatrics 1984; 74:330.
15. Hanson JW, Streissguth AP, Smith DW. The effects of moderate alcohol consumption during pregnancy on fetal growth and morphogenesis. J Pediatr 1978; 92:457.
16. Davis PJM, Partridge JW, Storrs CN. Alcohol consumption in pregnancy. How much is safe? Arch Dis Child 1982; 57:940.
17. Gusella JL, Fried PA. Effects of maternal social drinking and smoking on offspring at 13 months. Neurobehav Toxicol Teratol 1984; 6:13.
18. Little RE, Streissguth AP, Barr HM, Herman CS. Decreased birth weight in infants of alcoholic women who abstained during pregnancy. J Pediatr 1980; 96:974.
19. Rosett HL, Weiner L. Alcohol and pregnancy: a clinical perspective. Ann Rev Med 1985; 36:73.
20. Mills JL, Graubard BI. Is moderate drinking during pregnancy associated with an increased risk for malformations? Pediatrics 1987; 80:309.
21. Little RE, Asker RL, Sampson PD, Renwick JH. Fetal growth and moderate drinking in early pregnancy. Am J Epidemiol 1986; 123:270.
22. Ostrea EM Jr, Chavez CJ. Perinatal problems (excluding neonatal withdrawal) in maternal drug addition: a study of 830 cases. J Pediatr 1979; 94:292.
23. Sweet AY. Narcotic withdrawal syndrome in the newborn. Pediatr Rev 1982; 3:285.
24. Committee on Drugs. Neonatal drug withdrawal. Pediatrics 1983; 72:895.
25. Finnegan LP, Connaughton JF Jr, Kron RE, Emich JP. Neonatal abstinence syndrome: assessment and management. Addic Dis 1975; 2:141.
26. Finnegan LP, Kron RE, Connaughton JF, et al. Assessment and treatment of abstinence in the infant of the drug-dependent mother. Int J Clin Pharmacol 1975; 12:19.
27. Lipsitz PJ, Blatman S. Newborn infants of mothers on methadone maintenance. NY State J Med 1974; 74:994.
28. Lipsitz PJ. A proposed narcotic withdrawal score for use with newborn infants: a pragmatic evaluation of its efficacy. Clin Pediatr 1975; 14:592.
29. Schiff D, Chan G, Stern L. Fixed drug combinations and the displacement of bilirubin from albumin. Pediatrics 1971; 48:139.
30. Kron RE, Litt M, Phoenix MD, Finnegan LP. Neonatal narcotic abstinence: effects of pharmacotherapeutic agents and maternal drug usage on nutritive sucking behavior. J Pediatr 1976; 88:637.
31. Koffler H, Coen RW. Personal communication.
32. Fishburne PM. National survey on drug abuse: main findings 1979. Rockville, Maryland: National Institute on Drug Abuse, 1980 [DHHS publication (ADM) 80-976].
33. Miller J. National survey on drug abuse. Washington, D.C.: Department of Health and Human Services, 1983 [DHHS publication (ADM) 83-1263].
34. Sherman WT, Gautieri RF. Effect of certain drugs on perfused human placenta. X. Norepinephrine release by bradykinin. J Pharm Sci 1972; 61:878.
35. Brown WU, Bell GC, Alper M. Acidosis, local anesthetics and newborn. Obstet Gynecol 1976; 48:27.
36. Chasnoff IJ, Bussey ME, Savich R, Stack CM. Perinatal cerebral infarction and maternal cocaine use. J Pediatr 1986; 108:456.
37. Fantel AG, MacPhail BJ. The teratogenicity of cocaine. Teratology 1982; 26:17.
38. Mahalik JP, Gautieri RF, Mann DE. Teratogenic potential of cocaine hydrochloride in CF-1 mice. J Pharm Sci 1980; 69:703.
39. Madden JD, Payne TF, Miller S. Maternal cocaine abuse and effect on the newborn. Pediatrics 1986; 77:209.
40. Bingol N, Fuchs M, Diaz V, et al. Teratogenicity of cocaine in humans. J Pediatr 1987; 110:93.
41. Chasnoff IJ, Burns WJ, Schnoll SH, Burns KA. Cocaine use in pregnancy. N Engl J Med 1985; 313:666.
42. Acker D, Sachs BP, Tracey KJ, Wise WE. Abruptio placentae associated with cocaine use. Am J Obstet Gynecol 1983; 146:220.
43. Oro AS, Dixon SD. Perinatal cocaine and methamphetamine exposure: maternal and neonatal correlates. J Pediatr 1987; 111:571.
44. Chasnoff IF, Bussey ME, Savich R, Stack CM. Perinatal cerebral infarction and maternal cocaine use. J Pediatr 1986; 108:456.
45. Chasnoff IJ, Lewis DE, Squires L. Cocaine intoxication in a breast-fed infant. Pediatrics 1987; 80:836.
46. Chaney NE, Franke J, Wadlington WB. Cocaine convulsions in a breast-feeding baby. J Pediatr 1988; 112:134.
47. Chasnoff IJ, Hunt C, Kletter R, Kaplan D. Increased risk of SIDS and respiratory pattern abnormalities in cocaine-exposed infants. Pediatr Res 1986; 20:425A.
48. Husson BS. Trends and epidemiology of drug abuse, Los Angeles County, California, 1980–1983. In: Epidemiology of drug abuse: trends in selected cities, June 1984. Rockville, Maryland: National Institute on Drug Abuse, 1984; I:84.
49. Jain NC, Budd RD, Budd BS. Growing abuse of phencyclidine: California "angel dust." N Engl J Med 1977; 297:673.
50. Johnston LD, O'Malley PM, Bachman JG. Drug use among American high school students, college students, and other young adults: national trends through 1985. Rockville, Maryland: National Institute on Drug Abuse, 1986 [Publication (ADM) 86-1450].

51. Crider R. Phencyclidine: changing abuse patterns. In: Clouet DH, ed. Phencyclidine: an update. Monograph 64. Rockville, Maryland: National Institute on Drug Abuse, 1986:163 [Publication (ADM) 86-1443].

52. Silber TJ, Iosefsohn M, Hicks JM, et al. Prevalence of PCP use among adolescent marijuana users. J Pediatr 1988; 112:827.

53. Goodwin PJ, Perez VJ, Eatwell JC, et al. Phencyclidine: effects of chronic administration in the female mouse on gestation, maternal behavior and the neonate. Psychopharmacology 1980; 69:63.

54. Tenor SR. Permanent alterations in 5-hydroxytryptamine metabolism in discrete areas of rat brain following exposure to drugs during the period of development. Life Sci 1974; 15:245.

55. Tonge SR. Neurochemical teratology: 5-hydroxyindole concentrations in discrete areas of rat brain after the pre- and neonatal administration of phencyclidine and imipramine. Life Sci 1973; 12:481.

56. Nicholas JM, Lipshitz J, Schreiber EC. Phencyclidine: its transfer across the placenta as well as into breast milk. Am J Obstet Gynecol 1982; 143:143.

57. Golden NL, Sokol RJ, Rubin IL. Angel dust: possible effects on the fetus. Pediatrics 1980; 65:18.

58. Strauss AA, Modanlou HD, Bosu SK. Neonatal manifestations of maternal phencyclidine (PCP) abuse. Pediatrics 1981; 68:550.

59. Howard J, Kropenske V, Tyler R. The long-term effects on neurodevelopment in infants exposed prenatally to PCP. In: Clouet DH, ed. Phencyclidine: an update. Rockville, Maryland: National Institute on Drug Abuse, 1986:237 [Monograph 64, Publication (ADM) 86-1443].

60. Chasnoff I, Burns W, Burns K. Late onset head growth deficiency in PCP-exposed infants. Pediatr Res 1986; 20:202A.

61. Joffe JM. Influence of drug exposure of the father on perinatal outcome. Clin Perinatol 1979; 6:21.

6

Fetal Responses to Asphyxia

R. Harold Holbrook Jr., M.D. and Ronald N. Gibson, B.S.

The Fetal Cardiovascular System and Oxygen Delivery
     to Fetal Organs
Fetal Responses to Hypoxia and Asphyxia
     Experimental Models of the Consequences of Fetal
          Hypoxia and Asphyxia
     Cardiovascular Responses
          Maternal Hypoxia
          Reduced Uterine Blood Flow
          Umbilical Cord Compression
          Special Circulations
               Umbilical, Hepatic, and Ductus Venosus Blood
                    Flow
               Pulmonary and Ductus Arteriosus Blood Flow
               Coronary Blood Flow
               Adrenal Blood Flow
               Cerebral Blood Flow
          Mechanisms of Response
     Endocrine and Metabolic Responses
     Behavioral Responses
     Effects of Hypoxia and Asphyxia on the Fetal Brain
          Animal Models
          Effects in Humans
     Chronic Intrauterine Hypoxia and Asphyxia

Our understanding of the causes of perinatal brain damage and the role hypoxia and asphyxia might play is incomplete. Neurologic deficits possibly associated with fetal hypoxia and asphyxia must be interpreted in light of the degree of stress, the gestational age, and the known responses of the fetus to asphyxia. Although animal experimentation can provide valuable information, caution always must be used in extrapolating findings from animal work to humans. Although epidemiologic studies of the etiology of cerebral palsy and mental retardation may suggest that asphyxia plays a role, our ability to reliably determine the presence and degree of fetal hypoxia and asphyxia is limited. Furthermore, most infants with suspected intrapartum hypoxia or asphyxia do not develop cerebral palsy or mental retardation,[1] even if they experience early neonatal seizures.[2] Many confounding factors are probably involved. It is possible that, in cases in which intrapartum

hypoxia or asphyxia occurs and there is brain damage, the damage is congenital in origin. Chronic hypoxia during pregnancy with or without repeated acute hypoxic episodes also may be responsible.[3] In fact, evidence suggests that substandard prenatal care and complications of labor and delivery account for a minor proportion of the cases of cerebral palsy.

Understanding the fetal responses to hypoxia or asphyxia is an important step in the evaluation of clinical situations suggestive of fetal compromise and in determining the possible role of intrapartum asphyxia in neonatal brain damage. Of particular importance is the correlation of physical findings and pathologic abnormalities with specific types and degrees of asphyxia. Although these studies are difficult to perform retrospectively in the human, animal models may help to elucidate many of the possible mechanisms and sequelae of fetal asphyxia.

The outcome of hypoxia and asphyxia in the fetus is varied. The fetus appears to be more resilient than the adult; outcomes associated with suspected asphyxia can range from no noticeable abnormality to seizures, slightly diminished physical or mental achievement, or specific deficits, including cerebral palsy, mental retardation, seizures, and death.

Presumably hypoxia and asphyxia can cause injury to the brain during pregnancy as well as during labor and delivery. Evidence of prepartum or postpartum insults should be sought even when there is probable intrapartum hypoxia or asphyxia. Other causes of specific neurologic deficits should be considered, including developmental defects, environmental insults, trauma, and infection.

When the terms *hypoxia, anoxia,* and *asphyxia* are used clinically and in literature pertaining to experimental studies, definitions are often vague and overlap. For the sake of clarity here, some terms should be defined specifically. Hypoxia refers to diminished oxygen delivery to tissues despite adequate blood flow. Anoxia is defined as the absence of oxygen delivery to tissues despite adequate blood flow. Asphyxia, in the case of the fetus, implies diminished gas exchange between the maternal and fetal circulations. This results in increased P_{CO_2} and decreased P_{O_2} and pH values in fetal blood. With hypoxia, anoxia, and asphyxia, as anaerobic metabolism is increased, there is an increase in the fixed acid concentration and a decrease in the pH. The arterial pH value can decrease as a result of both an increased P_{CO_2} and an increased fixed acid concentration. Because of changes in the fetal circulation and metabolic variables associated with asphyxia, a given level of asphyxia may not produce the same effects on different organs. The cardiovascular and metabolic status of the fetus therefore must also be considered (Fig. 6–1).

Hypoxia and asphyxia in the fetus can be of maternal, placental, or fetal origin. Precipitating causes of maternal origin include a decreased maternal P_{O_2} and decreased uteroplacental blood flow. The causes of decreased uteroplacental blood flow include hypotension, hypertensive disorders with vasospasm, uterine anomalies, and uterine hyperactivity. Placental causes can be manifestations of maternal disorders, such as hypertension. Specific placental abnormalities include decreased placental exchange, placenta previa, vasa previa, and abruptio placentae. There are several abnormalities of the umbilical cord other than those of abnormal insertion that can cause hypoxia and asphyxia, including cord prolapse, cord compression, a single umbilical artery, cord entanglement, and true knots of the cord. The causes of hypoxia and asphyxia of fetal origin include decreased levels of fetal hemoglobin due to hemolysis or fetal-maternal hemorrhage and cardiovascular abnormalities. This chapter provides an overview of clinical and experimental knowledge concerning fetal responses to hypoxia and asphyxia.

THE FETAL CARDIOVASCULAR SYSTEM AND OXYGEN DELIVERY TO FETAL ORGANS

There is a substantial gradient between the P_{O_2} of maternal uterine arterial blood (about 90 mm Hg in sheep) perfusing the intervillous spaces within the placenta and that of fetal umbilical venous blood (about 35 mm Hg in sheep) leaving the placenta (Table 6–1). However, owing to the greater affinity of fetal hemoglobin for oxygen and the resulting leftward shift of the fetal oxygen-hemoglobin dissociation curve, fetal blood becomes more saturated than maternal blood at a given P_{O_2} (Fig. 6–2). Because of the greater concentration of hemoglobin in fetal blood, the transfer of oxygen from the maternal to the fetal circulation is facilitated. Since in the tissues the fetus normally operates on a steeper portion of the oxygen-hemoglobin dissociation curve than does the adult, oxygen release is facilitated from fetal hemoglobin when the P_{O_2} drops. The same phenom-

TABLE 6–1   Representative Normal P_{O_2} Values in the Uterine and Umbilical Circulations of Sheep Breathing Atmospheric Air at Sea Level

Location	P_{O_2} (mm Hg)
Uterine artery	90
Uterine vein	50
Umbilical vein	35
Umbilical artery	22

From Meschia G. Placental respiratory gas exchange and fetal oxygenation. In: Creasy RK, Resnik R, eds. Maternal-fetal medicine. Philadelphia: WB Saunders, 1974:276.

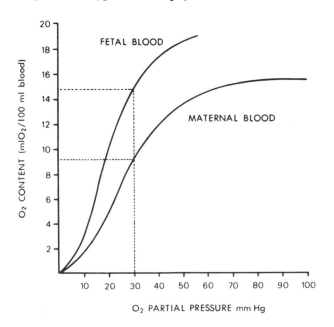

Figure 6–1   Maternal and fetal P_{O_2}-oxygen content curves. (From Parer JT. Uteroplacental and fetal physiology. In: Parer JT, Puttler OL, Freeman RK, eds. A clinical approach to fetal monitoring. Berkeley, California: Berkeley Bioengineering, 1974:17.)

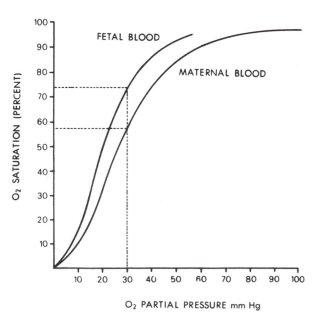

Figure 6–2   Maternal and fetal oxygen dissociation curves. (From Parer JT. Uteroplacental and fetal physiology. In: Parer JT, Puttler OL, Freeman RK, eds. A clinical approach to fetal monitoring. Berkeley, California: Berkeley Bioengineering, 1974:16.)

enon, however, may also cause a substantial decrease in the oxygen content of blood perfusing the fetus if the PO_2 value of blood in the maternal intervillous space falls. Despite these mechanisms for increased oxygen delivery and transport from mother to fetus, the oxygen content of fetal blood is reduced. Several mechanisms allow the fetus to maintain adequate oxygen delivery at low levels of oxygen content. Vital organs such as the heart and brain receive about double the adult levels of flow per unit of organ weight. Per unit of body weight, fetal cardiac output is normally more than double what it is in the adult, owing to both an elevated stroke volume (especially of the right ventricle) and a high heart rate. Oxygen delivery (oxygen delivery = oxygen content of blood × blood flow rate) is therefore maintained at sufficient levels. Normally the fetus receives an adequate oxygen supply, but it is quite vulnerable.

The oxygen saturation of blood from the placenta destined for fetal tissues decreases as it flows through the liver and combines with blood returning to the heart from the abdominal inferior vena cava, the superior vena cava, and the pulmonary and coronary circulations. This is compensated for in several ways in the fetal lamb. Although about half the umbilical venous blood flows through the liver (mainly through the left lobe), the rest bypasses the liver, flowing through the ductus venosus directly into the inferior vena cava.[4] It appears that streaming of ductus venosus blood occurs in the thoracic inferior vena cava. There is little mixing of the umbilical venous component (composing approximately one-third of the thoracic inferior vena cava flow[4,5] with the abdominal inferior vena cava component. Left hepatic venous blood, which is derived predominantly from umbilical venous blood, empties into the inferior vena cava at a point near the entrance of the ductus venosus and is distributed in a fashion similar to that of the ductus venosus flow.[6,7] The right lobe of the liver receives both portal and umbilical venous blood. Right hepatic venous blood is distributed in a manner similar to that of the abdominal inferior vena cava flow. In the right atrium, blood from the inferior vena cava, particularly the component derived from the umbilical vein, flows preferentially through the foramen ovale into the left atrium. The output from the left ventricle is distributed mainly to the heart, the upper limbs, and the head. The heart, brain, and upper carcass receive a significantly greater proportion of ductus venosus flow than of the abdominal inferior vena cava flow.[8] Therefore that component of the cardiac output with the greatest oxygen content is destined for the coronary and cerebral circulations. The superior vena cava return and the return from the coronary circulation flow almost entirely from the right atrium into the right ventricle. After passing into the pulmonary artery, some output from the right ventricle enters the pulmonary circulation, but most of it crosses the ductus arteriosus into the aorta where it is preferentially shunted to the placenta for reoxygenation. The

fetal pulmonary circulation receives only about 10 percent of the combined ventricular output. It is returned to the left atrium and reduces the oxygen content of blood destined for the cerebral and coronary circulations (Fig. 6–3).

The low oxygen content of fetal blood serves a purpose in that it maintains a high resistance in the pulmonary circulation and therefore a low pulmonary flow. It also maintains a high cerebral blood flow and keeps the ductus arteriosus and ductus venosus patent.

In the fetal circulation the left and right ventricles work in parallel and not in series as in the adult. Therefore the left and right ventricles do not require equivalent stroke volumes. In the fetus the combined total output of the two ventricles commonly is used to represent the fetal cardiac output.

In the fetal lamb, about 30 percent of the venous return to the heart is supplied by the return from the superior venae, lungs, and heart and 70 percent by the return from the inferior vena cava. About 40 percent of the inferior vena cava return crosses the foramen ovale, but less than 5 percent of the superior vena cava return does.[5] The output from the right ventricle is derived

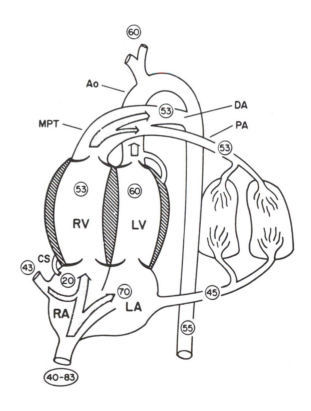

Figure 6–3 Oxygen saturation data relating to the fetal cardiac circulation. Ao, aorta. DA, ductus arteriosus. PA, pulmonary artery. MPT, main pulmonary trunk. RV, right ventricle. LV, left ventricle. CS, coronary sinus. RA, right atrium. LA, left atrium. (From Heymann MA. Biophysical evaluation of fetal status: fetal cardiovascular physiology. In: Creasy RK, Resnik R, eds. Maternal-fetal medicine. Philadelphia: WB Saunders, 1984:259.)

from 60 percent of the inferior vena cava flow, the coronary sinus return, and more than 95 percent of the superior vena cava flow. It composes about 65 percent of the combined total cardiac output. Only about 12 percent of the flow from the right ventricle into the pulmonary artery is distributed to the pulmonary circulation; the rest enters the descending thoracic aorta through the ductus arteriosus. A majority of the latter is distributed to the placenta; the rest is distributed to the lower fetal body. The output from the left ventricle is derived from the pulmonary venous return, about 40 percent of the inferior vena cava return, and less than 5 percent of the superior vena cava return. It composes about 35 percent of the total combined cardiac output. About 9 percent of the left ventricular output is distributed to the coronary circulation, about 62 percent to the brain and upper body, and the rest, about 29 percent to the lower body and placenta.

In the normoxemic, chronically instrumented fetal lamb late in gestation, the combined ventricular output is distributed approximately in the following manner: 40 percent, placenta; 8 percent, lungs; 3 percent, heart; 3 percent, brain; 0.1 percent, adrenals; 5 percent, gut; and 25 percent, carcass.[9]

The fetal heart is structurally and functionally different from the adult heart. The fetal coronary blood flow is high relative to that in the adult, and this maintains adequate oxygen delivery under normal conditions. However, the fetal heart is limited in its capacity to respond to stress.

Fetal cardiac muscle maintains a greater passive tension and develops a smaller active tension than adult cardiac muscle. Its velocity of shortening is also reduced. This is accounted for in part by a larger ratio of non-contractile to contractile components of the cardiac cells, a smaller diameter of cardiac cells, and less capacity to sequester intracellular calcium. The fetal heart therefore is working at or near its peak to meet normal needs.[10]

The extent and distribution of sympathetic fibers in near-term fetal sheep myocardium are significantly reduced compared with postnatal and adult myocardium[11,12,] and myocardial adrenergic receptor concentrations are at high levels.[13] No significant difference appears to exist in parasympathetic fibers.[11] Owing to the lack of complete sympathetic innervation of the fetal myocardium and the presence of a high concentration of adrenergic receptors, it is supersensitive to circulating catecholamines from the adrenals.

FETAL RESPONSES TO HYPOXIA AND ASPHYXIA

The response to hypoxia or asphyxia depends on the integration of neural, hormonal, and local control of the cardiovascular system. This in turn depends considerably on the gestational age of the fetus and its stage of development. The capacity of the fetus to withstand and compensate for hypoxia or asphyxia depends on the capacity of the cardiovascular system to maintain or increase organ perfusion and oxygen delivery, particularly to the heart and brain. Between a level of oxygen delivery that is insufficient to meet the needs of the heart and brain and that which is inadequate for aerobic metabolism of the rest of the body there will be an increase in the concentration of free acids. When hypoxia and asphyxia are severe enough to cause brain damage, they will also probably cause myocardial depression and damage. As the fetal arterial PO_2 decreases and cardiac output is redistributed, oxygen delivery becomes insufficient to meet the needs of less vital organs. Increased anaerobic metabolism causes an accumulation of metabolites and metabolic acidosis develops. This, in addition to any hypercapnia and respiratory acidosis, depresses cardiac function and in turn decreases organ perfusion and oxygen delivery. Cerebral blood flow autoregulation may become impaired, and eventually cerebral perfusion and oxygen delivery can become inadequate to meet metabolic needs.

Myers[14] has reported the effects of decreasing oxygen content in anesthetized term monkey fetuses. Decreases from a normal level of 10 to 12 volumes percent to 3 to 4 volumes percent for even extended periods cause no observable cardiovascular or neurologic alterations. Below 3 to 4 volumes percent, progressive cardiovascular changes occur. Between 0.8 and 1.5 volumes percent and at about 0.5 volumes percent brain damage is observed after periods longer than about 30 minutes. Below 0.5 volumes percent there is rapid decline and death. Therefore the degree of hypoxia required to produce brain damage is very close to the level that causes death. A combination of low arterial oxygen content and cerebral blood flow leads to a decline in oxygen delivery to the brain.

Experimental Models of the Consequences of Fetal Hypoxia and Asphyxia

There are considerable ethical and technical difficulties in studying responses to hypoxia and asphyxia in the human fetus and in predicting lesions that might result. Extrapolating data from animal models should always be done cautiously. Animal experimentation in this field has provided much useful information about the fetal responses and insight into the role hypoxia and asphyxia may play in perinatal brain damage. However, there are many questions left unanswered.

Our ability to study cardiovascular responses to hypoxia and asphyxia in experimental models owes much to the development of techniques for measuring cardiac output, distribution of cardiac output, and organ blood flow in fetal animals in utero using radionuclide-labeled microspheres.[15]

In sheep and other species in which uterine vessels do not constrict on exposure to low PO_2 levels, the concentration of oxygen in fetal blood can be reduced without altering the carbon dioxide concentration (fetal hypoxia) by decreasing the oxygen content of maternal inspired air (maternal hypoxia). Over time, as a result of a build-up in the end products of anaerobic metabolism, the pH decreases. Asphyxia is induced by decreasing gas exchange between the maternal and fetal circulations. This is accomplished by decreasing maternal or fetal perfusion of the placenta. Methods of reducing maternal uteroplacental perfusion have included compressing the abdominal aorta, clamping a hypogastric artery or a uterine artery, removing uterine tissue, inducing maternal hypotension, inducing uterine hyperactivity, and embolizing the maternal side of the placental circulation. Methods of reducing the fetal circulation through the placenta have included clamping the umbilical cord or an umbilical vessel, compressing the abdominal aorta, and inducing fetal hypotension.

In interpreting experimental results, it is necessary to consider species differences. There can be basic differences in the ways different species respond to stresses, and there are considerable differences in the rate of development of the nervous and endocrine systems among species and therefore in the ability to regulate the circulatory system and respond to stress at a particular point in gestation. Gestational age is also an important consideration within a species, as there are significant differences in the response to stress at different stages of development. It appears that more immature fetuses are not so vulnerable to brain damage due to hypoxia and asphyxia. Their cerebral vasculature is less developed, and therefore there is less to compromise. There are considerable differences in the responses of the adult and fetus to hypoxia. It is also necessary to consider the effects of additional stress: anesthesia, surgical intervention, and the method of study. Studies have been performed before proper recovery from surgery and while the effects of anesthesia are still present. There are substantial differences in the response to hypoxia of exteriorized fetuses and fetuses in utero and between anesthetized and unanesthetized fetuses. Moreover, differences in responses depend on the method of inducing hypoxia or asphyxia. If a hypoxic-asphyxic insult is severe and abrupt in onset, there may not be enough time for appropriate responses to manifest for compensation.

In the consideration of animal models of perinatal brain damage, species and gestational differences can become important:

1. The ratio of the volume of the brain to that of the total body. With a larger brain the ability to compensate for hypoxia and asphyxia could be limited.

2. The portion of cardiac output normally received by the brain.

3. Regional blood flow.

4. The rate of development, e.g., the degree of myelination.

5. Cerebral metabolic requirements.

6. Brain anatomy and physiology, e.g., basic structure, vasculature (state of development and basic architecture), and physiologic mechanisms.

It is important to search for and examine suitable animal models. A particular species may not be susceptible to a particular type of lesion, or a higher degree or different type of stress may be required to produce a particular lesion, or a lesion may not develop at a particular age.

Cardiovascular Responses

The cardiovascular response to hypoxia and asphyxia varies according to the animal model: possible species differences, method of producing hypoxia or asphyxia, gestational age, anesthetized or unanesthetized subject, acute or chronic preparation, exteriorized versus in utero. The basic response of adults is considerably different from that of fetuses.

Downing et al[16] suggested that fetal cardiac function is not depressed by acidosis unless there is accompanying hypoxemia. However, evidence suggests that even in the absence of a decreased PO_2, acidosis depresses the velocity of shortening, tension development, and responsiveness to norepinephrine.[11]

There is a demonstrated positive relationship between cardiac glycogen stores and the length of time fetal animals can survive anoxia.[17,18] The capacity of fetal and newborn animals to survive longer periods of anoxia than adults has been attributed to the greater reliance of their cardiac muscle on energy derived from glycolytic metabolism.[19,20]

Maternal Hypoxia

In the unanesthetized, chronically instrumented fetal lamb in utero, the arterial PO_2 and oxygen content can be reduced without altering the PCO_2 by having the ewe breathe low oxygen concentrations. Close to term (term = 146 or 147 days) the heart rate decreases and the arterial pressure increases in response to short-term hypoxia.[9,21-23] The response is different earlier in gestation. Walker et al[22] found no significant change in the heart rate and arterial pressure in response to hypoxia between 0.6 and 0.8 of gestation. Boddy et al[23] examined fetuses from days 97 to 145 of gestation. They found that the more immature fetuses responded with an initial increase in heart rate and no significant change in arterial pressure. As gestation increased, they found that the heart rate increased and arterial pressure progressively increased. They found, however, that over the time of exposure the heart rate gradually decreased. Jones and Robinson[24] found that a decreased heart rate persisted in fetuses if the fetal plasma catecholamine levels remained low. Combined ventricular cardiac output did not change significantly in response to mild hypoxia, but decreased significantly in response to more severe hypoxia combined with a decreased pH.[9] Maternal hypoxia in fetal lambs that is not too severe causes a decline in the umbilical venous oxygen content, but the umbilical blood flow is maintained. Despite a reduction in the oxygen content of the umbilical venous return and oxygen delivery to the entire fetus, oxygen delivery to an undeveloped organ can be maintained or even increased if the proportion of cardiac output to that organ is increased.

In response to short-term hypoxia there is a redistribution of the cardiac output to vital organs. Cohn et al[9] found that in response to short-term hypoxia, the percentage distribution of the combined ventricular cardiac output to the heart, brain, and adrenals was significantly increased, while that to the lungs, gut, spleen, and carcass was significantly reduced. They found that the responses were of greater magnitude when the hypoxia was more severe and combined with a decrease in pH. Peeters et al[21] found that as the fetal arterial oxygen content decreased from 6 to 1 mM the blood flow to the heart, brain, and adrenals progressively increased while that to the lungs progressively decreased. They did not find any consistent changes in the umbilical blood flow. Renal, gastrointestinal, and carcass blood flows decreased only when the arterial oxygen content was very low, when they declined sharply.

In addition to a redistribution of cardiac output, Reuss and Rudolph[25] investigated additional responses that compensate for decreased total oxygen and delivery. They found that during short-term maternal fetal hypoxia, the proportion of umbilical venous blood flow that passed through the ductus venosus and bypassed the liver significantly increased. Therefore, the amount of umbilical venous return distributed to the heart and brain increased as ductus venous flow was preferentially shunted across the foramen ovale.

They also investigated the response to maternal-fetal hypoxia of two fetal vascular shunts. One was umbilical venous return distributed back to the placenta without passing to the other fetal tissues, and the other was systemic venous return distributed back to the body without passing to the placenta. With hypoxia the umbilical blood flow did not change. They found that the proportion of cardiac output in these two shunts did not change with hypoxia, but that the portion recircu-lated to the placenta increased and the portion recirculated to the body decreased.

Peeters et al[21] found that during short-term hypoxia, oxygen delivery to the heart and brainstem was maintained while cerebral and cerebellar oxygen delivery declined.

Acute maternal hypoxia that produces a 40 percent reduction in the total fetal oxygen delivery results in a 100 percent increase in the oxygen delivery to the myocardium and a 40 percent increase to the brain. There is a reduction in oxygen delivery to the gut, carcass, and lungs of about 60 percent and a reduction of 40 percent to the renal circulation.[25]

In a study of the acutely prepared, anesthetized near-term fetal monkey, hypoxia was induced by causing the mother to breathe decreased oxygen. Behrman et al[26] found increases from the control values in the proportion of the cardiac output distributed to the heart, brain, and adrenals during hypoxia with mixed acidemia. (Maternal hypoxia in the monkey causes constriction of the uterine vessels, and therefore it is difficult to produce pure fetal hypoxia.) In their experiments only one set of measurements was made in each animal, and there was a separate group of control animals. They found a decrease in oxygen consumption, umbilical and pulmonary blood flow, and cardiac output. They also found an increase in the amount of superior vena cava return that crossed the foramen ovale and in the proportion of umbilical venous blood bypassing the liver through the ductus venosus. There was a selective redistribution of the cardiac output to the heart, brain, and adrenals, and blood flow to these organs was maintained despite a decrease in the cardiac output.

During spontaneous hypoxia in chronically instrumented fetal lambs, a small increase in the venous return from the superior vena cava crossing the foramen ovale has been noted.[14] Although this could be related to decreased umbilical blood flow due to umbilical cord compression, with experimentally induced hypoxia produced by maternal hypoxia this is not seen.[20]

Reduced Uterine Blood Flow

The near-term fetal lamb responds to short-term hypoxia and asphyxia induced by decreasing uterine blood flow by several methods, with a decrease in the heart rate.[27-35] The response of the fetal arterial pressure is variable. There may be little effect,[28-32] or it may increase significantly when the hypoxia or asphyxia is more severe.[33-36] The combined ventricular output may be maintained or decreased.[28,33] Brinkman et al[28] found that an acute reduction of the uterine blood flow slightly decreased the umbilical blood flow. The umbilical venous PO_2 was markedly decreased; resulting in a reduced arterial-venous oxygen content difference and a significant decrease in the total fetal oxygen consumption.

Umbilical Cord Compression

In the near-term fetal lamb, reducing the umbilical blood flow causes bradycardia and a variable response in the blood pressure. There is a reduction in the cardiac output associated with a reduction in the venous return.[36,37] There is a small increase in cerebral and myocardial blood flow and a marked rise in the adrenal flow. The pulmonary blood flow is reduced substantially and the flow to the gut, carcass, and kidneys is maintained or increased.[38]

Although umbilical cord compression reduces the umbilical blood flow, it does not alter the oxygen content of the umbilical venous blood.[36,37] Fetal oxygen consumption is maintained when the uterine blood flow is decreased by approximately 50 percent by umbilical cord compression. Further reduction, however, does compromise oxygen consumption.[37] Acute umbilical cord compression that produces a 50 percent reduction in the total fetal oxygen delivery results in a small reduction in the myocardial and cerebral oxygen delivery, about a 25 percent reduction to the gut, carcass, and kidneys, and a 70 percent reduction in the lung flow.[38]

Woods et al[39] examined the cardiovascular effects of complete umbilical cord occlusion in the exteriorized unanesthetized fetal sheep. A rapid decline in the PO_2 a more gradual rise in the PCO_2, and a decline in the pH were observed. The fetal heart rate declined, and arterial pressure increased for the first two minutes and then dropped below initial levels within about three minutes. With total asphyxia in the anesthetized term monkey fetus caused by complete umbilical clamping, there is an instantaneous rise in the arterial blood pressure. After the myocardium is perfused with essentially deoxygenated blood, depression occurs and the heart rate and blood pressure decline. The blood pressure stabilizes for a time and then circulatory collapse ensues.[40]

Special Circulations

Umbilical, Hepatic, and Ductus Venosus Blood Flow. When short-term hypoxia, induced in the near-term fetal lamb by maternal hypoxia, is not too severe, umbilical blood flow is maintained despite a reduction in the cardiac output.[9] The umbilical blood flow does not appear to demonstrate autoregulation,[41] and therefore the maintenance of flow is probably due to increased arterial pressure despite a decrease in cardiac output. Short-term maternal hypoxia also produces a reduction in the liver blood flow and an increase in the ductus venosus flow, while umbilical cord compression causes a reduction in the liver flow and a smaller reduction in the ductus venosus flow. The right hepatic blood flow is decreased more than the left hepatic flow in both situa-

tions.[42] In both situations there is also an increase in the proportion of umbilical venous flow that passes through the ductus venosus. This enhances the delivery of the most highly oxygenated blood to the heart and brain, since within the heart there is preferential streaming of the ductus venosus flow to these organs.[8,25] In the fetal lamb some portal venous blood is distributed to the ductus venosus and the rest to the right lobe of the liver.[4] During hypoxia there is no change in this distribution.[41]

Pulmonary and Ductus Arteriosus Blood Flow. Decreasing the fetal arterial PO_2 and oxygen content by inducing maternal hypoxia, umbilical cord compression, or decreasing uterine blood flow increases the pulmonary vascular resistance and decreases the pulmonary blood flow.[9,21,26,28,43] The response is greater as gestation progresses.[43] Brinkman et al[28] found that the ductus arteriosus flow increased markedly with a reduction in the uterine blood flow.

Shunting blood from the pulmonary circulation through the ductus arteriosus during hypoxia has at least two benefits. First, there is less desaturation of the combined ventricular cardiac output. Second, because less blood flows through the pulmonary circulation and into the left atrium, the left atrial pressure decreases, allowing more return from the inferior vena cava to cross from the right atrium through the foramen ovale into the left atrium. Therefore, more blood with a greater degree of oxygenation is distributed to the heart and brain.

Coronary Blood Flow. The fetal heart is preferentially perfused with the most highly oxygenated blood from the ascending aorta before mixture with ductus arteriosus blood.[26] The fetal lamb has a low PO_2 compared to the adult, but the myocardial blood flow per unit weight of tissue is about twice as high, and therefore both adult and fetal myocardiums have similar rates of oxygen delivery and consumption.[44] In the fetal lamb nearly all the myocardial oxygen consumption can be accounted for by the metabolism of carbohydrates, whereas in the adult sheep carbohydrate metabolism accounts for only about 40 percent of oxygen consumption. The rest can be accounted for by the metabolism of fatty acids.[44] Despite a relatively high resting level of myocardial blood flow, there is significant capacity for increase during hypoxia. Peeters et al[21] found that the coronary blood flow in the fetal lamb is a reciprocal function of the fetal ascending aortic oxygen content. Cohn et al[9] found that during a decline in the fetal arterial PO_2 from about 20 to 12 mm Hg induced by maternal hypoxia, fetal myocardial blood flow more than doubled from its normally high resting level.

Adrenal Blood Flow. In the fetal lamb near term, Peeters et al[21] found that the adrenal blood flow increases as a reciprocal function of the ascending aortic oxygen content. Cohn et al[9] found that adrenal blood flow was nearly tripled when the arterial PO_2 decreased from 20 to 12 mm Hg. Adrenal blood flow is also increased markedly during umbilical cord compression.[38]

Cerebral Blood Flow. The fetal brain, like the heart, is perfused with blood containing the highest oxygen saturation, because of preferential intracardiac streaming of blood from the inferior vena cava across the foramen ovale and to the ascending aorta.[26] The delivery of oxygen to the brain of the fetal lamb exceeds the level in the adult sheep by 70 percent relative to the amount of oxygen consumed by the brain.[45] In the normoxemic fetal lamb the brainstem and cerebellum receive a greater proportion of brain blood flow than the hemispheres.[21] A similar pattern of distribution has been observed in the primate fetus.[26,46]

In the fetal lamb the cerebral blood flow increases with increases in the arterial PCO_2 content.[47,48] The total cerebral blood flow appears to be less responsive to changes in the arterial PCO_2 than in the adult sheep, but regional brainstem blood flow in the fetus is more sensitive than in the adult.[48] During acute reductions in the fetal lamb arterial PO_2 and oxygen content due to maternal hypoxia, oxygen delivery to and oxygen consumption by the brain are maintained because blood flow to the brain is significantly increased.[9,21,25,49-51] It appears that the oxygen content is more important in determining the fetal cerebral blood flow than is the PO_2 level.[49] Peripheral chemoreceptors are more important than factors intrinsic to the brain in regulating the response of the cerebral blood flow to hypoxia.[52]

When acidemia is combined with hypoxia, the increase in blood flow to the brain is greater in magnitude.[9] In the acutely prepared, anesthetized fetal primate with hypoxia associated with mixed acidosis, Behrman et al[26] found a decreased cardiac output, but with redistribution, blood flow to the brain was maintained. The increase to the brainstem was significantly more than that to the cortex. There was no significant difference between the regional blood flows in other areas.

During acute hypoxia in the fetal lamb the regional blood flow in the brain is redistributed away from the hemispheres and cerebellum and to the brainstem.[21] Owing to the increased blood flow to the brain and the regional distribution, oxygen delivery to the brainstem is maintained, whereas it is decreased slightly to the hemispheres and cerebellum. Autoregulation of the cerebral circulation in fetal lambs has been described.[53]

Johnson et al[54] studied the effects of asphyxia on regional cerebral blood flow in the chronically catheterized, unanesthetized, near-term fetal lamb in utero. Asphyxia was produced slowly over one to two hours by partial compression of the umbilical cord. The fetal arterial PCO_2 value significantly increased, and the pH level was significantly reduced from 7.40 to 7.04. Fetal arterial oxygen saturation was reduced from 50 to 19 percent, but there was no significant change in the PO_2. A significant increase in the blood pressure occurred, but the heart rate response was variable. A marked increase in the cerebral blood flow was found in all areas of the brain, with the largest increase to deep cortical structures and the brainstem. The smallest increase occurred in flow to the cerebral cortex and cerebellum. Owing to decreased oxygen saturation but increased cerebral blood flow, oxygen delivery was essentially unchanged to deep cortical structures and the brainstem, whereas it was decreased to the cerebral cortex and cerebellum. Increased cerebral blood flow during asphyxia correlated closely with increased blood pressure but not with changes in the pH, PCO_2, PO_2, or oxygen saturation.

Ashwal et al[55] studied the effects of prolonged hypoxia on regional cerebral blood flow in the chronically instrumented, unanesthetized, near-term fetal lamb in utero. Hypoxia was produced by causing the ewe to inspire 10 percent oxygen for 90 minutes. The fetal arterial PO_2 was lowered to and maintained at 12 to 15 torr. The PCO_2 remained relatively constant, while the pH declined significantly. The fetal blood pressure was slightly elevated, and the heart rate initially declined but gradually returned toward the control level. Cardiac output remained relatively constant, but the portion of cardiac output going to the brain nearly doubled. During control and hypoxia, regional cerebral blood flow to the brainstem, deep cortical structures, and cerebellum was substantially greater than that to other regions, but hypoxia did not produce significant preferential shunting of blood to any particular region.

In a similar preparation Ashwal et al[56] examined the effects of several variables on the total and regional cerebral blood flows. Increases in the cerebral blood flow correlated with decreases in the fetal arterial PO_2 and oxygen content and increases in the PCO_2. The cerebral blood flow appeared to be independent of changes in the pH, arterial pressure, and cardiac output. In the fetal sheep Purves and James[51] found that the cerebral blood flow increased by 50 percent when the arterial PO_2 was reduced from 21 to 15 mm Hg.

Mechanisms of Response

Mild hypoxia results in fetal bradycardia through chemoreceptor stimulation, but bradycardia caused by severe hypoxia probably is also caused by a baroreflex and direct myocardial depression.

The acute hypoxia-asphyxia–induced increase in fetal arterial pressure appears to be due mainly to the action of aortic body chemoreceptors[57] and not the carotid body chemoreceptors.[58-60] Systemic vasoconstriction appears to occur as a result of sympathetic outflow.

The fetal heart rate response to acute hypoxia and asphyxia appears to be due primarily, to the action of peripheral chemoreceptors rather than to baroreceptors. With prolonged or severe hypoxia and asphyxia, baroreceptor-mediated bradycardia occurs as well as direct myocardial depression.

The duration of the reduction in uterine blood flow and the prior status of fetal oxygenation determine the fetal heart rate response to the reduced uterine blood flow. When sufficient, a reduction in the uterine blood flow in initially normoxemic fetal lambs causes bradycardia, apparently mediated through chemoreceptors. In chronically hypoxemic fetal lambs, bradycardia occurs apparently through the action of chemoreceptors, baroreceptors, and direct myocardial depression.[33,61] The fetal arterial pressure increases and is greater in the hypoxemic group whereas cardiac output falls.[33]

Parer et al[62] found increased heart rate variability while maintaining the umbilical arterial PO_2 at 11 mm Hg for 25 minutes in the fetal lamb. They contended that this might indicate a lack of cerebral depression with acute fetal hypoxemia.

Normally the cardiac output is closely related to the fetal heart rate. An exception seems to occur during acute hypoxia in which the cardiac output may be maintained or may decrease only slightly during bradycardia associated with increased arterial pressure. This could be related to increased ventricular contractility. Reductions in the cardiac output in response to hypoxia or asphyxia can be related to decreased heart rate, increased afterload (arterial pressure), decreased preload (venous return), and decreased contractility. Decreased contractility could be the result of direct myocardial depression. It is not a consequence of vagal stimulation, for this has little effect on ventricular contractility.

Endocrine and Metabolic Responses

Robinson et al[63] reviewed the endocrine and metabolic responses of fetal sheep to hypoxia.

Short-term hypoxia in the fetal lamb produces no consistent changes in the plasma concentrations of growth hormone, luteinizing hormone, prolactin, and oxytocin,[63,64] while the concentrations of vasopressin and adrenocorticotropic hormone significantly increase.[65-69] Despite elevated adrenocorticotropic hormone levels, there is no significant increase in the corticosteroid level in response to hypoxia until the fetal adrenal gland has sufficiently matured very near term.[69] Plasma concentrations of catecholamines increase rapidly in response to hypoxia in exteriorized fetal lambs and in chronically instrumented fetal lambs.[24,70,71] Hypoxia causes a considerable increase in the plasma concentration of glucagon. No significant change occurs in the plasma concentration of insulin.[63] Large increases in renin secretion do not accompany hypoxia in the fetal lamb.[72]

Infusion of vasopressin into the fetal lamb causes responses of heart rate and arterial pressure similar to those seen with hypoxia.[66,73] The heart rate, but not the arterial pressure response, is abolished by vagotomy.[66] However, atropine administration does not completely abolish the decrease in heart rate, suggesting that vasopressin may have a direct effect.[73] The arterial pressure response during hypoxia could be attributed to increased plasma vasopressin levels rather than sympathetic stimulation of alpha-adrenergic receptors, because it is not affected by phentolamine.[66]

As gestation nears completion, fetal sheep respond to short-term hypoxia with progressively increasing plasma concentrations of glucose.[74] This correlates with increasing fetal liver glycogen stores.[75] Short-term hypoxia in fetal sheep causes a substantial increase in the plasma concentration of lactate, which persists for several hours after the insult.[64,74,76] Fatty acid and ketone plasma concentrations begin to increase in response to hypoxia significantly after 130 days of gestation and increase considerably a few days before term.[74]

Behavioral Responses

In chronically instrumented, unanesthetized fetal lambs, short-term hypoxia induced by maternal hypoxia decreases the frequency of fetal breathing movements.[23,77] Increasing the fetal arterial PO_2 by inducing maternal hypercapnia or decreasing the fetal pH without altering the fetal arterial PCO_2 by infusing fixed acids in the fetus increases fetal breathing movement activity.[23,78,79] It appears that when the fetal arterial PCO_2 is increased, the effect of decreased arterial PO_2 on fetal breathing activity is diminished.[23,80] Mild or moderate asphyxia produced by reducing the uterine blood flow or briefly compressing the umbilical cord eliminates rhythmic fetal breathing activity.[34,35,81,82] In the chronically prepared fetal goat and sheep, severe asphyxia eliminates rhythmic breathing activity and causes fetal gasping to occur.[82,83]

Fetal breathing movements appear to occur only during rapid eye movement (REM) sleep activity.[84] Nathanielsz et al[85] found that small reductions in the fetal arterial PO_2 accompanying nonlabor uterine contractions of the last third of gestation in sheep were associated with a change in the fetal sleep state from REM to non-REM and with diminished fetal respiratory activity. Mild asphyxia in the fetal lamb produced by a brief reduction in the uterine blood flow also changed the fetal sleep state from REM to non-REM and eliminated fetal breathing activity.[35] Boddy et al[23] found that with the diminished respiratory movements in the fetal lamb that accompany hypoxia, there was also a decrease in the proportion of time occupied by low voltage electrocortical activity in the fetus. They also found that with the increased level of respiratory activity accompanying hypercapnia, there was also an increase in the proportion of time occupied by low level electrocortical activity in the fetus.

Natale et al[86] found that with a diminished arterial PO_2 in the fetal lamb there is a reduction of fetal forelimb movement. Bocking and Harding[81] found that accompanying a reduced uterine blood flow in the unanesthetized, chronically instrumented sheep preparation there was a decrease in fetal breathing movements and skeletal muscle activity. There was also a decrease in the proportion of time spent in low voltage electrocortical activity and a change in the sleep state from REM to non-REM.

Effects of Hypoxia and Asphyxia on the Fetal Brain

Animal Models

The etiology of perinatal brain damage is multifactorial, and the relative role of fetal hypoxia and asphyxia is unclear. It is difficult to choose appropriate animal models with relevance to human perinatal brain injury, and extrapolation of data from sheep or monkey fetus models to humans should be done cautiously. Studies of animal models using acute total asphyxia at birth were the first to examine the effects of fetal hypoxia and asphyxia on the brain. Resulting lesions were generally located in nuclei of the brainstem, thalamus, basal ganglia, and spinal cord, with cortical sparing.

Bailey and Windle[87] found that in the guinea pig, anoxia at birth produces damage to the brainstem and thalamic nuclei, with sparing of the cortex in survivors. Studies by Myers[88] in monkeys have revealed similar patterns of brain damage in survivors following birth asphyxia. Twelve to 13 minutes of total asphyxia is required to produce the first evidence of brain damage. Further periods produce progressive damage. Total asphyxia for 12 to 13 minutes or longer, which is compatible with survival, does not cause damage to the hemispheres, other than to the thalamic nuclei. Structures with the greatest blood flow, metabolic rates, and glycogen stores are most susceptible to damage.[88]

In many instances total asphyxia is not the appropriate model of perinatal brain damage. Partial asphyxia or prolonged hypoxia is more often implicated in perinatal brain damage in humans. Prolonged partial intrauterine asphyxia produces brain swelling, hemorrhagic or non-hemorrhagic necrosis of the cerebral cortex, basal ganglia, and thalamus, and ulegyria in the full-term newborn rhesus monkey.[89] There is cytotoxic edema with mitochondrial swelling.[90] Study of regional blood flow indicates ischemia in areas similar to those that are damaged.[91]

As Myers et al[92] have stated, it is well established that brain edema is a critical aspect of the damage from asphyxia to the term fetal monkey. Edema results when capillary permeability is increased as a result of damage from hypoxia and decreased pH. It is exacerbated by protein loss due to the increased capillary permeability and by brain compression from tissue expansion. The brain surface becomes flattened, blood vessels are compressed, ischemia results, and brain tissue is herniated.

In the anesthetized near-term sheep fetus in utero,

Lou et al[93] found that prolonged partial asphyxia causes a breakdown of the blood-brain barrier, particularly in the cortex and basal ganglia. Cerebral blood flow autoregulation was also noted to be impaired in this study.

It appears that the serum glucose concentration may be important in determining the neuropathologic effects of hypoxia. Myers and associates[92] found that fetuses of food-deprived mothers tolerate anoxia better than fetuses of fed mothers, and they hypothesized that the critical event that causes edema and injury to brain tissue is the accumulation of lactate.

Myers[94] has proposed that at levels above a critical concentration, lactate accumulation injures brain tissue by altering cell membrane permeability and causing cerebral edema. He suggests that diminished cerebral blood flow and perfusion pressure act to damage tissue by enhancing lactate accumulation, and that brain damage from hypoxia and asphyxia is subject to the availability of carbohydrates and the accumulation of lactate.

In anesthetized term monkey fetuses, decreases in the oxygen content from a normal level of 10 to 12 volumes percent to 3 to 4 volumes percent for even extended periods cause no observable cardiovascular or neurologic alterations. Below 3 to 4 volumes percent progressive cardiovascular changes occur. Between 0.8 and 1.5 volumes percent and about 0.5 volumes percent brain damage is observed after periods longer than about 30 minutes. Below 0.5 volumes percent there is rapid decline and death.[13] Therefore, the degree of hypoxia required to produce brain damage is very close to the level that causes death. A combination of low arterial oxygen content and cerebral blood flow leads to a decline in oxygen delivery to the brain.

With total asphyxia in the anesthetized term monkey fetus caused by complete umbilical clamping, there is an instantaneous rise in the arterial blood pressure. Shortly thereafter myocardial depression occurs, and the heart rate and blood pressure decline. The blood pressure stabilizes for a time, and then circulatory collapse ensues.[40,95]

Rapid cardiovascular collapse from total asphyxia, as occurs with umbilical cord occlusion, results in a "locked in" state in which lactate can be produced only from local stores of glycogen and glucose, according to Myers. This results in the accumulation of lactate above critical levels, particularly in the brainstem and thalamic nuclei where glycogen levels are generally higher. The extent of injury beyond these structures is determined by the serum glucose level at the time of the insult as well as the level of free glucose in the brain. With prolonged hypoxia, glycogenolysis and anaerobic metabolism are stimulated in both the brain and the liver, contributing to the lactate accumulation throughout the brain. Hypoxia-induced sympathetic stimulation enhances glycogen breakdown and glucose release by the liver. More diffuse damage may occur if the cerebral perfusion pressure and blood flow are also diminished. With acute total asphyxia preceded by a period of prolonged partial asphyxia, the prolonged partial asphyxia stimulates the liver to break down glycogen and release glucose. The serum glucose levels are increased. Because of hypoxia the level of anaerobic metabolism is increased and serum lactate levels increase. With the superimposition of total asphyxia there is circulatory collapse, and lactate levels are raised in many regions of the brain, resulting in more widespread damage.

There is a greater tolerance to asphyxia earlier in gestation and under anesthesia.[95,96] Earlier in gestation, fetuses are less vulnerable to hypoxia and asphyxia because the cerebral vasculature is less well developed and brain and liver glycogen stores are low. Anesthesia may be protective because of decreases in the metabolic requirements of the brain.

When the blood pressure is maintained above a critical level in spite of a period of hypoxia, the serum glucose level does not seem to influence the degree of brain damage, because brain lactate levels do not appear to be affected.[92] During prolonged partial asphyxia a high serum glucose concentration in association with a marked decline in the arterial blood pressure is required to produce brain lactate levels sufficiently high to cause injury.

During prolonged partial asphyxia in sheep fetuses, similar declines in the arterial PO_2 may be associated with different outcomes in different animals. Ting et al[97] observed intact survival, survival with widespread brain injury, or death in midgestational fetal lambs. Surviving fetuses experienced similar declines in the arterial PO_2. Myers and associates[40] found that the difference between these two surviving groups depends on whether there is a significant decline in the arterial blood pressure. They found that the serum glucose level was equivalent in both groups but that the serum lactate levels rose in the group in which a significant decline in arterial blood pressure and widespread brain damage occurred.

Myers[40] has characterized four patterns of brain damage and their conditions of occurrence in term rhesus monkeys:

1. Total asphyxia causes damage primarily to the brainstem and thalamic nuclei.
2. Prolonged hypoxia with mixed acidosis causes brain swelling and cortical hemorrhagic or nonhemorrhagic necrosis.
3. Prolonged hypoxia without significant acidosis causes hemispheral white matter damage. A similar pattern of damage has also been observed in sheep when fetal hypoxia is secondary to induced maternal hypoxemia.
4. Total asphyxia preceded by prolonged hypoxia with mixed acidosis causes, in addition to patterns 1 and 2, injury to the basal ganglia.

In an acute fetal lamb preparation, Mann et al[98] found that despite the lack of a significant decline in cerebral blood flow, asphyxia caused localized multifocal damage to the cerebral white matter. In the chronically instrumented fetal lamb preparation. Clapp et al[99] found selective multifocal damage to subcortical white matter following recurrent episodes of cardiovascular instability associated with persistent abnormal electrocortical activity and without systemic metabolic abnormalities. Hypoxia associated with cardiovascular deterioration, and progressive systemic metabolic acidosis and abnormal electrocortical activity, resulted in more extensive damage confined to the cerebral white matter. Following chronic intrauterine hypoxia due to progressive placental damage, brain weights at term were reduced but no brain damage was noted.

Effects in Humans

What is the role of fetal exposure to hypoxia and asphyxia in the etiology of perinatal brain damage in humans? From animal studies it is apparent that, in general, hypoxia must be rather severe to result in brain injury, although injury does not always occur, even with severe insults. Although caution must be exercised in extrapolating the results of animal experiments to obstetrical care, this information strongly suggests that short-term or mild asphyxia is unlikely to result in significant brain damage in the human fetus. In cases of perinatal brain damage attributed to fetal hypoxia or asphyxia there are often confounding factors, such as prematurity, low birth weight, and insults during the course of pregnancy.

The pattern of brain damage and the clinical course following acute total asphyxia at birth have been described.[100] The pattern of damage, which excludes the cerebral cortex, and the clinical course are similar to those seen in animal models. However, a fetal rhesus monkey model of prolonged partial asphyxia more closely approximates the outcome most generally seen in humans. Most often human perinatal insult is the consequence of a period of acute severe asphyxia preceded by prolonged partial hypoxia or asphyxia.[101]

The findings in animal studies after total asphyxia differ from the neuropathologic findings most often encountered in humans surviving perinatal brain insult. The models of prolonged partial asphyxia or total asphyxia preceded by prolonged partial asphyxia in utero appear to give a more accurate assessment of human perinatal brain damage.

The neuropathologic findings resulting from an insult late in pregnancy are likely to be different from those from an insult earlier in pregnancy, and lesions in infants born prematurely are likely to be different from those in infants born at term. In infants experiencing severe asphyxia at birth, those born prematurely are more likely to develop periventricular leukomalacia (softening of the white matter around the ventricles) and intraventricular hemorrhage. They are also more apt to incur brain damage during the neonatal period. In term infants there may be brain edema and swelling, with flattening of the cerebral convolutions and compression of the ventricles.

The neuropathologic result depends on the severity of the insult and the length of survival. Rapid death may result in no observable change. Brain swelling and necrosis of cortical and basal ganglia structures may be seen in infants who survive.[100,102,103]

Towbin[104] has asserted that spastic and athetoid types of cerebral palsy are due to damage to the basal ganglia and that such damage occurring as a result of hypoxic insult occurs before term. Observation of such damage in term infants therefore implies that the insult occurred prior to labor.

Chronic Intrauterine Hypoxia and Asphyxia

In general, chronic intrauterine asphyxia results in compensatory responses by the fetus that appear to be directed toward maintenance of vital organ blood flow and oxygen uptake. Alexander[105] surgically reduced the placental mass in sheep and found an increased frequency of intrauterine death, premature delivery, and a reduction in birth weight. Using this technique, Robinson et al[106] observed growth retardation in chronically hypoxic fetuses. Emmanouilides et al[107] produced chronic hypoxia in the fetal lamb by ligating a single umbilical artery and demonstrated reduced fetal weights at delivery. In fetal lambs Creasy and associates[108] produced chronic hypoxia with no significant change in pH by embolization of the maternal portion of the placenta with 15 μm microspheres. The hematocrit level was increased and fetal body and organ weights were decreased. In a subsequent study the fetal cardiac output was reduced by about one-third, and the proportion of the cardiac output distributed to the brain, heart, kidney, and gut was increased, at the expense of the pulmonary and umbilical flow.[109] Within the brain Clapp et al[110] found no significant alteration in the regional distribution of blood flow when experimental growth retardation was induced and the fetal PO_2 was decreased from 26 to 20 torr.

REFERENCES

1. Freeman J, ed. Prenatal and perinatal factors associated with brain disorders. Washington, DC: Department of Health and Human Service, National Institutes of Health, 1985: publication No. 85-1149.
2. Mincham P, et al. Antecedents and outcome of very early neonatal seizures in infants born at or after term. Br J Obstet Gynaecol 1987; 94:431.
3. Niswander K. Asphyxia in the fetus and cerebral palsy. In: Pitkin RM, Zlatnik FJ, eds. Year book of obstetrics and gynecology. Chicago: Year Book, 1983:107.
4. Edelstone DI, Rudolph AM, Heymann MA. Liver and ductus venosus blood flows in fetal lambs in utero. Circ Res 1978; 42:426.
5. Rudolph AM, Heymann MA. Circulatory changes during growth in the fetal lamb. Circ Res 1970; 26:289.
6. Bristow J, Rudolph AM, Itskovitz J. A preparation for studying liver blood flow, oxygen consumption, and metabolism in the fetal lamb in utero. J Dev Physiol 1981; 3:25.
7. Bristow J, Rudolph AM, Itskovitz J, et al. Hepatic oxygen and glucose metabolism in the fetal lamb. J Clin Invest 1983; 71:1.
8. Edelstone DI, Rudolph AM. Preferential streaming of ductus venosus blood to the brain and heart in fetal lambs. Am J Physiol 1979; 237:H724.
9. Cohn HE, Sacks E, Heymann M, et al. Cardiovascular responses to hypoxemia and acidemia in fetal lambs. Am J Obstet Gynecol 1974; 120:8174.
10. Friedman WF, Kirkpatrick SE. Fetal cardiovascular adaptation to asphyxia. In: Gluck L, ed. Intrauterine asphyxia and the developing fetal brain. Chicago: Year Book, 1977.
11. Friedman WF. The intrinsic physiologic properties of the developing heart. Prog Cardiovasc Dis 1972; 15:87.
12. Friedman WF, Pool PE, Jacobowitz D, et al. Sympathetic innervation of the developing rabbit heart: biochemical and histochemical comparisons of fetal, neonatal, and adult myocardium. Circ Res 1968; 23:25.
13. Barrett CT, Heymann MA, Rudolph AM. Alpha and beta adrenergic functions in fetal sheep. Am J Obstet Gynecol 1972; 112:1114.
14. Myers RE. Threshold values of oxygen deficiency leading to cardiovascular and brain and pathological changes in term monkey fetuses. In: Bruley DF, Bicher HI, eds. Oxygen transport to tissue: instrumentation, methods, and physiology. Vol 37B. New York: Plenum, 1973:1047.
15. Rudolph AM, Heymann MA. The circulation of the fetus in utero: methods for studying distribution of blood flow, cardiac output, and organ blood flow. Circ Res 1967; 21:163.
16. Downing SE, Talner NS, Gardner TH. Influences of arterial oxygen tension and pH on cardiac function in the newborn lamb. Am J Physiol 1966; 211:1203.
17. Dawes GS, Mott JC, Shelly HJ. The importance of cardiac glycogen for the maintenance of life in fetal lambs and newborn animals during anoxia. J Physiol 1959; 146:516.
18. Mott JC. The ability of young animals to withstand a total oxygen lack. Br Med Bull 1961; 17:144.
19. Opie LH. Metabolism of the heart and health and disease. Am Heart J 1969; 77:100.
20. Su JY, Friedman WF. Comparison of the responses of fetal and adult cardiac muscle to hypoxia. Am J Physiol 1973; 224:1488.
21. Peeters LLH, Sheldon RE, Jones MD, et al. Blood flow to systemic organs as a function of arterial oxygen content. Am J Obstet Gynecol 1979; 135:637.
22. Walker AM, Cannata JP, Dowling MH, et al. Age dependent pattern of autonomic heart rate control during hypoxia in fetal and newborn lambs. Biol Neonate 1979; 35:195.
23. Boddy K, Dawes GS, Fisher R, et al. Foetal respiratory movements, electrocortical and cardiovascular responses to hypoxemia and hypercapnia in sheep. J Physiol 1974; 243:559.
24. Jones CT, Robinson RO. Plasma catecholamines in foetal and adult sheep. J Physiol 1975; 248:15.
25. Reuss ML, Rudolph AM. Distribution and recirculation of umbilical and systemic venous blood flow in fetal lambs during hypoxia. J Develop Physiol 1980; 2:71.
26. Behrman RE, Lees MH, Peterson EN, et al. Distribution of the circulation in the normal and asphyxiated fetal primate. Am J Obstet Gynecol 1970; 108:956.
27. Kunzel W, Kastendieck E, Hohmann M. Heart rate and blood pressure response and metabolic changes in the sheep fetus following reduction of uterine blood flow. Gynecol Obstet Invest 1983; 15:300.
28. Brinkman CR, Mofid M, Assali NS. Circulatory shock in pregnant sheep. 3. Effects of hemorrhage on uroplacental and fetal circulation and oxygenation. Am J Obstet Gynecol 1974; 118:77.
29. Lucas WE, Kirschbaum TH, Assali NS. Effects of autonomic blockage with spinal anesthesia on uterine and fetal hemodynamics and oxygen consumption in the sheep. Biol Neonate 1966; 10:166.
30. Lander CN, Weston PV, Brinkman CR, et al. Effects of hydral-

azine on uteroplacental and fetal circulations. Am J Obstet Gynecol 1970; 108:375.

31. Bech-Jansen P, Brinkman CR, Johnson GH, et al. Circulatory shock in pregnant sheep. I. Effects of endotoxin on uteroplacental and fetal umbilical circulation. Am J Obstet Gynecol 1972; 112:1084.

32. Bech-Jansen P, Brinkman CR, Johnson GH. Circulatory shock in pregnant sheep. II. Effects of endotoxin on fetal and neonatal circulation. Am J Obstet Gynecol 1972; 113:37.

33. Itskovitz J, Goetzman BW, Rudolph AM. The mechanism of late deceleration of the heart rate and its relationship to oxygenation in normoxemic and chronically hypoxemic fetal lambs. Am J Obstet Gynecol 1982; 142:66.

34. Toubas PL, Monset-Couchard M, Rey P, et al. Fetal breathing and adaptation to maternal hemorrhage in the sheep. Am J Obstet Gynecol 1977; 127:505.

35. Harding R, Poore ER, Cohen GLP. The effect of brief episodes of diminished uterine blood flow on breathing movements, sleep states and heart rate in fetal sheep. J Develop Physiol 1981; 3:231.

36. Itskovitz J, LaGamma EF, Rudolph AM. Baroreflex control of the circulation in chronically-instrumented fetal lambs. Circ Res 1983; 52:589.

37. Itskovitz J, LaGamma EF, Rudolph AM. The effect of reducing umbilical blood flow on fetal oxygenation. Am J Obstet Gynecol 1983; 145:813.

38. Rudolph AM. The fetal circulation and its response to stress. J Dev Physiol 1984; 6:11.

39. Woods JR, Coppes V, Brooks DE, et al. Measurement of visual evoked potential in the asphyctic fetus and during neonatal survival. Am J Obstet Gynecol 1982; 143:944.

40. Myers RE. Four patterns of perinatal brain damage and their conditions of occurrence in primates. In: Meldrum BS, Marsden CD, eds. Advances in neurology. Vol 10. New York: Raven Press, 1975:223.

41. Berman W, Goodlin RC, Heymann MA, et al. Relationships between pressure and flow in the umbilical and uterine circulations in sheep. Circ Res 1976; 38:262.

42. Edelstone DI, Rudolph AM, Heymann MA. Effects of hypoxemia and decreasing umbilical blood flow on liver and ductus venosus blood flows in fetal lambs. Am J Physiol 1980; 238:H656.

43. Lewis AB, Heymann MA, Rudolph AM. Gestational changes in pulmonary vascular responses in fetal lambs in utero. Circ Res 1976; 39:536.

44. Fisher DJ, Heymann MA, Rudolph AM. Myocardial oxygen and carbohydrate consumption in fetal lambs in utero and in adult sheep. Am J Physiol 1980; 238:H399.

45. Jones MD, Rosenberg AA, Simmons MA, et al. Oxygen delivery to the brain before and after birth. Science 1982; 216:324.

46. Paton JB, Fisher DE, Peterson EN, et al. Cardiac output and organ blood flows in the baboon fetus. Biol Neonate 1973; 22:50.

47. Mann LI. Developmental aspects and the effect of carbon dioxide tension on fetal cephalic blood flow. Exp Neurol 1970; 26:336.

48. Rosenberg AA, Jones MD, Traystman RJ, et al. Response of cerebral blood flow to changes in PCO_2 in fetal, newborn, and adult sheep. Am J Physiol 1982; 242:H862.

49. Jones MD, Sheldon RE, Peeters LL, et al. Regulation of cerebral blood flow in the ovine fetus. Am J Physiol 1978; H162.

50. Sheldon BE, Peeters LL, Jones MD, et al. Redistribution of cardiac output and oxygen delivery in the hypoxemic fetal lamb. Am J Obstet Gynecol 1979; 135:1071.

51. Purves MJ, James JM. Observations on the control of cerebral blood flow in the sheep fetus and newborn lamb. Circ Res 1969; 25:651.

52. Vannucci RC, Hernandez MJ. Perinatal cerebral blood flow. In: Perinatal brain insult. Symposium on perinatal and developmental medicine, No. 17. Mead Johnson, 1981:17.

53. Heymann MA. Biophysical evaluation of fetal status: fetal cardiovascular physiology. In: Creasy RK, Resnik R, eds. Maternal-fetal medicine. Philadelphia: WB Saunders, 1984:259.

54. Johnson GN, Palahniuk RJ, Tweed WA, et al. Regional cerebral blood flow changes during severe fetal asphyxia produced by slow partial umbilical cord compression. Am J Obstet Gynecol 1979; 135:48.

55. Ashwal S, Majcher JS, Vain N, et al. Patterns of fetal lamb regional cerebral blood flow during and after prolonged hypoxia. Pediatr Res 1980; 14:1104.

56. Ashwal S, Dale PS, Longo LD. Regional cerebral blood flow: studies in the fetal lamb during hypoxia, hypercapnia, acidosis, and hypotension. Pediatr Res 1984; 18:1309.

57. Dawes GS, Duncan SLB, Lewis BV. Hypoxaemia and aortic chemoreceptor function in foetal lambs. J Physiol 1969; 201:105.

58. Itskovitz J, Rudolph AM. Denervation of arterial chemoreceptors and baroreceptors in fetal lambs in utero. Am J Physiol 1982; 242:H916.

59. Biscoe TJ, Purves MJ, Sampson SR. Types of nervous activity which may be recorded from the carotid sinus nerve in the sheep. J Physiol 1969; 202:1.

60. Dawes GS, Duncan SL. Lewis BV, et al. Cyanide stimulation of the sytemic arterial chemoreceptors in foetal lambs. J Physiol 1969; 201:117.

61. Martin CB, de Hahn J, van der Wilt B, et al. Mechanisms of late decelerations in the fetal heart. A study with autonomic blocking agents in fetal lambs. Eur J Obstet Gynecol Reprod Biol 1979; 9:361.

62. Parer JT, Dijkstra HR, Vredebregt PPM, et al. Increased fetal heart rate variability with acute hypoxia in chronically instrumented sheep. Eur J Obstet Gynecol Reprod Biol 1980; 10:393.

63. Robinson JS, Jones CT, Thorburn GD. The effects of hypoxaemia in fetal sheep. J Clin Pathol (Suppl 11) 1977; 30:127.

64. Alexander DP, Forsling ML, Martin MJ, et al. The effect of maternal hypoxia on fetal pituitary hormone release in the sheep. Biol Neonate 1972; 21:219.

65. Alexander DP, Forsling ML, Martin MJ, et al. Adrenocorticotrophin and vasopressin in foetal sheep and the response to stress. In: Pierrepoint CG, ed. The endocrinology of pregnancy and parturition: experimental studies in the sheep. Cardiff: Alpha Omega Alpha, 1973:112.

66. Rurak DW. Plasma vasopressin in foetal lambs. J Physiol 1976; 256:36P.

67. Rurak DW. Plasma vasopressin levels during hypoxemia and the cardiovascular effects of exogenous vasopressin in the fetal and adult sheep. J Physiol 1978; 77:341.

68. Boddy K, Jones CY, Mantell C, et al. Changes in plasma ACTH and corticosteroid of the maternal and fetal sheep during hypoxia. Endocrinology 1974; 94:588.

69. Jones CT, Ritchie JWK, Flint APF. Some experiments on the role of the foetal pituitary in the maturation of the foetal adrenal and the induction of parturition. J Endocrinol 1977; 72:251.

70. Comline RS, Silver M. The release of adrenaline and noradrenaline from the adrenal glands of the foetal sheep. J Physiol 1961 156:424.

71. Lewis AB, Evans WN, Sischo W. Plasma catecholamine responses to hypoxemia in fetal lambs. Biol Neonate 1982; 41:115.

72. Rudolph AM, Itskovitz J, Iwamoto H, et al. Fetal cardiovascular responses to stress. Semin Perinatol 1981; 5:109.

73. Iwamoto HS, Rudolph AM, Keil LC, et al. Hemodynamic responses of the sheep fetus to vasopressin infusion. Circ Res 1979; 44:430.

74. Jones CT! The development of some metabolic responses to hypoxia in the foetal sheep. J Physiol 1977; 266:743.

75. Dawes GS, Shelly HJ. Physiological aspects of carbohydrate metabolism in the foetus and newborn. In: Dickens F, Randle PJ, Whelan WJ, eds. Carbohydrate metabolism and its disorders. Vol 2. New York: Academic Press, 1968:87.

76. Britton HG, Hugget A St G, Nixon DA. Carbohydrate metabolism in the sheep placenta. Biochim Biophys Acta 1967; 136:426.

77. Maloney JE, Adamson TM, Brodecky V, et al. Modification of respiratory center output in the unanesthetized fetal sheep in utero. J Appl Physiol 1975; 39:423.

78. Molteni RA, Melmed MII, Sheldon RE, et al. Induction of fetal

breathing by metabolic acidemia and its effect on blood flow to respiratory muscles. Am J Obstet Gynecol 1980; 136:609.

79. Hohimer AR, Bissonette JM. Effects of metabolic acidosis on fetal breathing movements. Respir Physiol 1981. 43:99.

80. Bissonette JM, Hohimer AR, Cronan JZ, et al. Effect of oxygen and carbon dioxide tension on the incidence of apnea in fetal lambs. Am J Obstet Gynecol 1980; 135:575.

81. Bocking AD, Harding R. Effects of reduced uterine blood flow on electrocortical activity, breathing, and skeletal muscle activity in fetal sheep. Am J Obstet Gynecol 1986; 154:655.

82. Tchorbroutsky C, Monset-Couchard M, Dumez Y, et al. Fetal breathing during moderate asphyxia in sheep and in human related to outcome of pregnancy. Contrib Gynecol Obstet 1979; 6:80.

83. Towell ME, Salvador HS. Intrauterine asphyxia and respiratory movements in the fetal goat. Am J Obstet Gynecol 1974; 118:1124.

84. Dawes GS. Fox HE, Leduc BM, et al. Respiratory movements and rapid eye movement sleep in the foetal lamb. J Physiol 1972; 220:119.

85. Nathanielsz PW, Bailey A, Poore, et al. The relationship between myometrial activity and sleep state and breathing in the fetal sheep throughout the last third of gestation. Am J Obstet Gynecol 1980; 138:653.

86. Natale R, Clewlow F, Dawes GS. Measurement of fetal forelimb movement in the lamb in utero. Am J Obstet Gynecol 1981; 140:545.

87. Bailey CJ, Windle WF. Neurological, psychological, and neurohistological defects following asphyxia neonatorum in the guinea pig. Exp Neurol 1959; 1:467.

88. Myers R. Two patterns of brain damage and their conditions of occurrence. Am J Obstet Gynecol 1972; 112:246.

89. Brann AW, Myers RE. Central nervous system findings in the newborn monkey following severe in utero asphyxia. Neurology 1975; 25:327.

90. Bondareff W, Myers RD, Brann AW. Brain extracellular space in monkey fetuses subjected to prolonged partial asphyxia. Exp Neurol 1970; 28:167.

91. Revich M, Brann AW, Shapiro H, Meyers RE. Regional cerebral blood flow during intrauterine prolonged partial asphyxia. In: Meyer SS, Reivich M, Eickhorn O, eds. Research on the cerebral circulation. Fifth International Salzburg Conference. Springfield: CC Thomas, 1972:216.

92. Myers RE, de Courten-Myers GM, Wagner KR. Effect of hypoxia on fetal brain. In: Beard RW, Nathanielsz PW, eds. Fetal physiology and medicine: the basis of perinatology. 2nd ed. New York: Marcel Dekker, 1984:419.

93. Lou HC, Lassen WA, Tweed G, et al. Pressure passive cerebral blood flow and breakdown of the blood-brain barrier in experimental asphyxia. Acta Pediatr Scand 1979; 68:57.

94. Myers RE. Lactic acid accumulation as cause of brain edema and cerebral necrosis resulting from oxygen deprivation. In: Korobin R, ed. Advances in perinatal neurology. Vol 1. New York: Spectrum, 1979.

95. Myers RE. Experimental models of perinatal brain damage: relevance to human pathology. In: Gluck L, ed. Intrauterine asphyxia and the developing fetal brain. Chicago: Year Book, 1977:37.

96. Myers RE. Brain damage induced by umbilical cord compression at different gestational ages in monkeys. In: Goldsmith EI, Moor-Jankowski J, eds. Medical primatology 1970. Basel: S. Karger, 1971:394.

97. Ting P, Yamaguchi S, Bacher JD, et al. Hypoxic-ischemic cerebral necrosis in mid-gestational sheep fetuses: physiopathologic correlations. Exp Neurol 1983; 80:227.

98. Mann LI, Bhaktavathsalan A, Peress N, et al. Fetal brain function, metabolism and neuropathology following acute hypoxia. In: Longo LD, Reneau DD, eds. Fetal and newborn cardiovascular physiology. Vol 2. New York: Garland, 1978:313.

99. Clapp JF, Mann LI, Peress NS, et al. Neuropathology in the chronic fetal lamb preparation: structure-function correlates under different enviromental conditions. Am J Obstet Gynecol 1981; 141:973.

100. Banker BO. The neuropathological effects of anoxia and hypoglycemia in the newborn. Dev Med Child Neurol 1967; 9:544.

101. Brann AW. Neonatal hypoxic ischemic encephalopathy. In: Perinatal brain insult. Symposium on perinatal and developmental medicine. No. 17. Evansville, Indiana: Mead Johnson, 1981:49.

102. Terlan KL. Histopathologic brain changes in 1152 cases of the perinatal and early infancy period. Biol Neonate 1967; 11:348.

103. Towbin A. Central nervous system damage in the human fetus and newborn infant: mechanical and hypoxic injury incurred in the fetal-neonatal period. Am J Dis Child 1970; 119:259.

104. Towbin A. Obstetric malpractice litigation: the pathologist's view. Am J Obstet Gynecol 1986; 155:927.

105. Alexander DP. Studies on the placenta of the sheep. Effect of surgical reduction in the number of caruncles. J Reprod Fertil 1964; 7:307.

106. Robinson JS, Jones CT, Challis JRG, et al. Observations on experimental intrauterine growth retardation in sheep (Abstract). Pediatr Res 1976; 10:891.

107. Emmanouilides GC, Townsend DE, Bauer RA. Effects of single umbilical artery ligation in the lamb fetus. Pediatrics 1968; 42:919.

108. Creasy RK, Barret CT, de Swiet M, et al. Experimental intrauterine growth retardation in the sheep. Am J Obstet Gynecol 1972; 112:566.

109. Creasy RK, De Swiet M, Kahanpaa KV, et al. Pathophysiological changes in the foetal lamb with growth retardation. In: Comline KS, Cross KW, Dawes GS, et al, eds. Foetal and neonatal physiology. Cambridge: Cambridge University Press, 1973:398.

110. Clapp JF, McLaughlin MK, Gellis J, et al. Regional distribution of cerebral blood flow in experimental intrauterine growth retardation. Am J Obstet Gynecol 1984; 150:843.

7

Congenital Infections as Causes of Neurologic Sequelae: Prevention, Diagnosis, and Treatment

Charles G. Prober, M.D. and Ann M. Arvin, M.D.

Herpes Simplex Virus
    Transmission of Herpes Simplex Virus to the Fetus
      and Newborn
    Clinical Manifestations of Perinatal and
      Intrauterine Herpes Simplex Virus Infections
      and the Risk of Neurologic Sequelae
    Prevention
    Diagnosis and Treatment
Varicella Zoster Virus
    Transmission of Varicella Zoster Virus to the Fetus
      and Newborn
    Clinical Manifestations of Intrauterine and
      Perinatal Varicella Zoster Virus Infection and
      the Risk of Neurologic Sequelae
Cytomegalovirus
    Outcome in Infants Asymptomatic at Birth
    Outcome in Infants Symptomatic at Birth
Human Immunodeficiency Virus
Rubella
    Transmission of Rubella to the Fetus
    Clinical Manifestations of Intrauterine Rubella
      Infection and the Risk of Neurologic Sequelae
Toxoplasmosis
    Outcome in Infants Asymptomatic at Birth
    Outcome in Infants Symptomatic at Birth
Syphilis
    Early Congenital Syphilis
    Late Congenital Syphilis

Maternal infections, contracted during pregnancy, may be without fetal consequence, or they may have serious adverse effects on the fetus. These adverse effects may include fetal death, intrauterine growth retardation, stillbirth, or congenital infection. Congenitally infected neonates may be symptomatic or asymptomatic at birth. Those who are symptomatic at birth generally have substantial long-term sequelae. Those who are asymptomatic at birth may never manifest evidence of damage, or clinically evident sequelae may develop later in life. The overwhelming morbidity attributable to congenital infections is borne by the latter group.

This chapter discusses the neurologic consequences of congenital infections. The specific infectious agents to be discussed are varicella zoster virus, cytomegalovirus, human immunodeficiency virus, rubella, *Toxoplasma gondii*, and *Treponema pallidum*. Although the major clinical impact of herpes simplex virus results from exposure to the virus at delivery rather than in utero, discussion of the consequences of infection caused by this increasingly prevalent agent begins this chapter.

HERPES SIMPLEX VIRUS

Although herpes simplex virus (HSV) can cause encephalitis in older children and adults, this consequence of HSV infection is rare, whereas HSV infection in the newborn is likely to involve the central nervous system.

Transmission of Herpes Simplex Virus to the Fetus and Newborn

Neonatal infection with HSV can be caused by either HSV-1 or HSV-2, but two-thirds of these infections result from HSV-2.[1] The risk to the infant usually begins with exposure at the time of delivery to a mother with genital HSV-2 infection, although the maternal infection is asymptomatic in more than 70 percent of cases.[2,3] Asymptomatic HSV excretion by the mother can be a consequence of genital HSV infection at some time in the past, i.e., as the result of reactivation of latent virus, or it may represent acute primary genital herpes in the mother. Mothers who are shedding HSV asymptomatically at delivery often have no history of genital herpes; i.e., the initial infection was also silent. In our experience only 7 percent of women who had positive cultures for HSV at delivery had a history of genital herpes or contact with a partner who had known HSV infection.[4] Some perinatally acquired HSV infections result from close contact with individuals who have active HSV-1 infection. Transmission is probably rare under these circumstances, because many infants have acquired HSV-1 specific antibodies transplacentally, and the opportunity for and the duration of direct contact with the lesion are limited. Nosocomial transmission of HSV from infant to infant, apparently by personnel or fomites, has occurred in neonatal nurseries.

Regardless of the source or the type of the infecting virus, infants who acquire HSV infection are at risk for neurologic disease. Fortunately the incidence of HSV infection among infants whose mothers are experiencing recurrent HSV infection at delivery is low, probably because of the low virus inoculum, the localization of infectious virus to external genital sites, and the fact that these infants usually have transplacentally acquired serum HSV antibodies capable of mediating virus neutralization and antibody-dependent cellular cytotoxicity.[5-7] The theoretic maximal incidence was less than 8 percent in a study of 34 infants born to mothers with known recurrent genital herpes who were inadvertently exposed to HSV by vaginal delivery. In contrast, the incidence of infection among infants born to mothers with primary genital herpes at delivery has been estimated to be more than 50 percent. Primary genital herpes in women is associated with viral infection of the cervix and prolonged excretion of HSV in high titers. The risk of infection may also be greater because the infant whose mother has primary genital herpes late in gestation may be born before HSV antibodies have crossed the placenta.

A few infants who have had intrauterine HSV infection have been identified.[8] The risk factors for HSV infection before birth have not been determined. Affected infants have been born to mothers with both primary and recurrent HSV infection during pregnancy and to mothers who have had no history of symptomatic HSV infection. These infections have been caused by HSV-2 in the cases documented by viral culture. Given the prevalence of HSV in the general population, this HSV transmission to the fetus in utero appears to be rare.

Clinical Manifestations of Perinatal and Intrauterine Herpes Simplex Virus Infections and the Risk of Neurologic Sequelae

Infants with neonatal HSV infection are classified according to the manifestations of the disease at the time of the onset of symptoms. These infants present with mucocutaneous infection only, disseminated HSV, or HSV encephalitis. For each category of disease the risk of neurologic sequelae can be altered by early diagnosis and antiviral therapy with acyclovir or vidarabine.

The mucocutaneous form of the infection consists of vesicular lesions, which may occur singly or as a cluster of lesions on the skin or scalp, e.g., around a fetal scalp monitor site, or on the mucous membranes of the eye or mouth. The mucocutaneous lesions can be difficult to distinguish from staphylococcal or other types of rash by clinical appearance, but must be identified as herpetic as soon as possible, using specific viral diagnostic methods. Without treatment the disease progresses to the disseminated or encephalitic form of neonatal herpes in more than 75 percent of these infants. In addition, before the antiviral drug era, more than 25 percent of the infants who were thought to have mucocutaneous disease only in the neonatal period had evidence of neurologic damage at later evaluation. With early antiviral treatment the chance that the infant will escape neurologic sequelae is 90 percent.[9] An assessment of the risk of late sequelae among infants with mucocutaneous HSV is part of the continuing evaluation of antiviral therapy for neonatal HSV by the National Institute of Allergy and Infectious Diseases (NIAID) Collaborative Antiviral Study group. There is a small risk that infants treated for localized superficial HSV infections will develop HSV encephalitis within a few weeks. Frequent recurrences of mucocutaneous lesions are common among infants who have had mucocutaneous HSV infection in the newborn period. The significance of these recurrences with regard to the risk of late neurologic sequelae is also being investigated by the Antiviral Study Group.

Infants with disseminated herpes usually present during the first seven to 10 days of life with fever and signs indistinguishable from those of bacterial sepsis in the newborn.[10] Disseminated HSV infection is often fulminant and is associated with severe hepatitis, thrombocytopenia and bleeding diatheses, pneumonia, and encephalitis. The diagnosis is made by isolating the virus from the oropharynx of the infant, from the blood, and occasionally from the cerebrospinal fluid (CSF).

Disseminated neonatal herpes has a mortality incidence of more than 70 percent if untreated. Because of the rapid progression of the infection in many of these infants, the mortality approaches 50 percent even with acyclovir or vidarabine therapy. Infants who have had central nervous system infection in the course of the disease usually have neurologic sequelae if they survive. However, despite the severity of the acute illness, many of the survivors who have not had encephalitis are developmentally normal.

Herpes encephalitis usually occurs in infants who are about two weeks old (range, one to six weeks). Some infants have active or resolving mucocutaneous lesions, but the majority do not. The signs of neonatal HSV encephalitis include fever, lethargy, poor feeding, and seizures. The seizures often begin as focal unilateral tonic-clonic movements, which then become generalized; apnea is common. The CSF can be normal at the onset of symptoms but usually shows a mild pleocytosis (20 to 100 cells) and an elevated protein level (more than 100); the glucose level may be normal or slightly low. The electroencephalogram is usually diffusely abnormal. A computed tomographic (CT) brain scan may be normal or may show diffuse enhancement. Histologically, extensive hemorrhagic necrosis of the brain is often evident immediately after the onset of symptoms. HSV is isolated from the CSF of infants with a meningitic presentation but is seldom recovered from the CSF except late in the clinical course of those with HSV-2 encephalitis. Unless the infant has superficial lesions as well, a brain biopsy is required to establish the diagnosis of herpes encephalitis.

The treatment of these infants with antiviral drugs reduces the mortality, but few infants with HSV encephalitis escape serious neurologic consequences. The few infants who present with meningitis as opposed to meningoencephalitis, many of whom have positive CSF cultures initially, seem to respond well to antiviral therapy. In general, HSV-1 central nervous system infection carries a much better prognosis than HSV-2 disease in infants.

The mortality in HSV encephalitis is approximately 15 to 20 percent regardless of whether infants receive vidarabine or acyclovir. Unlike HSV-1 encephalitis in older children and adults, acyclovir is not clearly superior to vidarabine in its effect on morbidity and mortality in neonatal HSV encephalitis. The severity of the neurologic sequelae in some infants with neonatal HSV-2 encephalitis is such that the life expectancy of the child is reduced to only a few months or years. Death often follows from respiratory complications due to aspiration pneumonia. Some infants develop progressive hydrocephalus. Other infants survive for longer periods, but many have hemiparesis, spasticity, and severe psychomotor retardation. The extent of the central nervous system insult is often obvious in these children because of the failure of the head circumference to increase beyond its size in infancy. Later CT scans demonstrate severe cerebral atrophy, often with large cystic areas of tissue destruction.

Infants with intrauterine HSV infection usually are diagnosed because of the appearance of widespread cutaneous HSV lesions at birth. At birth these infants typically have evidence of intrauterine infection of the central nervous system, including severe microcephaly with cerebral atrophy, hydranencephaly, and chorioretinitis. Most of these infants survive but exhibit profound psychomotor retardation as a consequence of intrauterine encephalitis.

Prevention

Since most neonatal disease is acquired from maternal genital infection at the time of delivery, the first problem is to identify women with active genital HSV infection at the onset of labor. If the mother has obvious genital herpes lesions, exposure of the infant can be avoided by cesarean delivery before or within a few hours after rupture of the membranes. Approximately 1 to 2 percent of women with a history of recurrent genital herpes show HSV excretion without any lesions at the time of delivery. Because of the brief duration of asymptomatic shedding and the time required to process an HSV culture, these women cannot be identified by antepartum screening cultures.[11] Nevertheless, cesarean delivery for every woman with a history of genital herpes is not reasonable. The combined low risk of exposure to HSV and the low incidence of infection in these infants are not greater than the maternal and neonatal morbidity of cesarean delivery. Women who have had symptomatic primary genital herpes late in pregnancy may constitute a special subpopulation at greater risk of asymptomatic shedding.[12]

Since most mothers of infants with neonatal herpes have no history of genital herpes, the infant's risk of HSV exposure will not be known. The maternal history may be absent because the past HSV-2 infection was asymptomatic and was not associated with clinically obvious recurrences, or because the mother had primary genital HSV infection late in gestation that was not diagnosed or was asymptomatic. Fortunately the frequency of asymptomatic shedding among women with serologic evidence of past HSV-2 infection who have never had symptoms appears to be equivalent to the 1 to 2 percent incidence among women with a history of genital herpes, and the incidence of infection for their infants also seems to be low.

At present there is no standard serologic method for identifying women who may have had silent genital HSV-2 infection. Research serologic techniques that can detect antibodies to the HSV-2 specific glycoprotein G reveal that 20 to 30 percent or more of women of childbearing age have had past HSV-2 infection.[4,13] Studies are now in progress to determine whether HSV cultures should be carried out routinely in all women at the time of delivery on the basis of the hypothesis that exposed infants could be monitored carefully and treated immediately if signs of neonatal HSV infection occurred.

Diagnosis and Treatment

Direct immunofluorescence and viral cultures provide the only means of making the diagnosis of HSV infection in the symptomatic infant. Serologic tests are not helpful, because the majority of newborn infants have passive HSV antibodies owing to prior maternal infection with HSV-1, HSV-2, or both. A negative titer does not rule out herpes, because the infant may have acquired the infection as a result of primary maternal HSV infection or from a nonmaternal source. None of the standard commercial assays for HSV antibodies can distinguish between HSV-1 and HSV-2, nor is there a reliable method for HSV IgM detection. In addition, the IgM response in infants with proved HSV infection occurs very late or not at all.

Since the maternal history of herpes is not a reliable clue, infants with neonatal herpes can be recognized only if pediatricians include viral diagnostic procedures in the evaluation of those with suspicious mucocutaneous lesions, those with apparent sepsis, and those with unexplained intractable seizures. The optimal management of these infants is still being investigated by the Collaborative Antiviral Study Group, but infants with HSV infection are clearly most likely to benefit if acyclovir or vidarabine is administered early, while the infection is localized to superficial sites. Any infant who has had a neonatal HSV infection should have continued follow-up through childhood, because the extent to which the neurologic sequelae of neonatal HSV infections can be prevented with current regimens and antiviral drugs has not yet been fully determined.

VARICELLA ZOSTER VIRUS

Primary infection with varicella zoster virus (VZV) causes varicella (chickenpox), whereas reactivation of the latent infection results in herpes zoster (shingles). Although pregnant women occasionally contract varicella, this virus is an unusual cause of intrauterine or perinatal infection, because more than 90 percent of the women of childbearing age who live in temperate climates have had varicella in childhood.

Transmission of Varicella Zoster Virus to the Fetus and Newborn

The transmission of VZV transplacentally, resulting in obvious fetal damage, occurs in fewer than 5 percent of the infants born to mothers who have had varicella during pregnancy.[14,15] Almost all the cases of the congenital varicella syndrome that have been reported have followed maternal infection in the first trimester.[16] Immunologic evidence of intrauterine VZV infection can be found in some asymptomatic infants.

Maternal varicella during the last few weeks or days of pregnancy can result in transplacental infection, presumably because of maternal viremia, or the infant may be infected because of exposure to the virus in the mother's lesions at delivery.[17] Infants whose mothers contract varicella more than one week before delivery can be expected to escape infection or to have an uncomplicated illness, probably because the interval between the onset of maternal infection and birth provides enough time for transplacental transmission of VZV antibodies.[18] In contrast, infants who are born within four days after or 48 hours before the onset of maternal varicella are at risk for fatal varicella. The incidence of perinatal infection under these circumstances is approximately 20 percent and the incidence of fatal infection is 30 percent. Nosocomial exposure of high risk infants also can result in neonatal varicella.[19]

Herpes zoster, due to the reactivation of latent VZV, occurs during pregnancy, but has not been associated with the classic features of the congenital varicella syndrome. Viremia is not known to be associated with herpes zoster in the otherwise healthy host; thus transplacental transmission is not likely. Infants whose mothers experience herpes zoster late in pregnancy or immediately post partum are not at risk for serious illness because VZV reactivation occurs in women who have had primary infection sometime in the past; therefore the infant will have acquired VZV antibodies transplacentally. If the zosteriform eruption is in the lumbosacral dermatomes, maternal HSV infection should be excluded, since as many as 15 percent of patients with apparent herpes zoster in this distribution have HSV.

Clinical Manifestations of Intrauterine and Perinatal Varicella Zoster Virus Infection and the Risk of Neurologic Sequelae

Neurologic damage is a prominent finding in the congenital varicella syndrome among affected infants. Symptomatic infants have characteristic cicatricial cutaneous scars, limb atrophy, rudimentary digits, chorioretinitis, and microcephaly. Autonomic disorders, such as gastroesophageal reflux, which causes recurrent aspiration pneumonia, and neurogenic bladder with hydronephrosis, are common. Cerebral atrophy can be observed on the CT scan even if the infant is normocephalic. The few infants with intrauterine exposure to VZV who have immunologic evidence of intrauterine infection but are otherwise asymptomatic and those who present with herpes zoster during infancy do not appear to be at risk for late neurologic sequelae.

With respect to perinatal infection, the infant born to a mother whose rash started more than one week before delivery will be asymptomatic or may have cutaneous varicella lesions at or shortly after birth. Severe VZV infection was very unusual in these infants even before prophylaxis and antiviral therapy were available. In contrast, infants born to mothers who acquire varicella in the last few days of pregnancy may develop clinical signs of varicella and are at risk for disseminated infection, including encephalitis. The infants at greatest risk for serious varicella are well until after the first five to 10 days of life.

The infection begins with the typical cutaneous exanthem. The diagnosis is usually obvious because of the characteristic vesicular lesions and the recognition of recent maternal varicella. The clinical diagnosis can be confirmed by viral culture of the lesions or by direct immunofluorescence staining of cells from the base of a cutaneous lesion using VZV specific antibody. Progressive cutaneous infection is associated with life-threatening illness resulting from VZV pneumonia, encephalitis, hepatitis, and bleeding diatheses. Encephalitis is diagnosed because of the onset of seizures, the presence of leukocytes and an elevated protein level in the CSF, and electroencephalographic abnormalities. Because of the limited number of cases of infants with perinatal VZV infection that have been reported, the risk of neurologic involvement has not been established.

If a pregnant woman presents with acute varicella, the parents should be counseled that the risk of the congenital varicella syndrome is very low even with maternal varicella during the first trimester. Although transplacental infection does occur and can produce devastating effects on the fetus, investigation of pregnancies complicated by varicella has not demonstrated that the risk of fetal damage is higher than the expected frequency of congenital malformations in the population.

Because of the risk of maternal complications, pregnant women with varicella should be followed carefully. Although the experience with acyclovir administration during pregnancy is limited, the treatment of a potentially life-threatening infection (e.g., varicella pneumonia) in the mother may require giving acyclovir intravenously. The low risk of intrauterine VZV infection, even during the first trimester, and the unknown consequences of exposing the fetus to acyclovir early in gestation argue against treating pregnant women who have mild varicella with acyclovir on the assumption that fetal damage will be prevented.

Although the administration of varicella zoster immune globulin (VZIG) is a familiar strategy for modifying the severity of varicella in immunocompromised patients, passive antibody prophylaxis is rarely an issue for pregnant women exposed to VZV, because only a very few adult women are susceptible. There is no evidence to suggest that the fetus can be protected by administering VZIG to the susceptible pregnant woman who has been exposed to VZV. Nevertheless, VZIG prophylaxis should be considered if the mother is proved to be susceptible by a sensitive serologic test for VZV antibodies (e.g., immunofluorescence or enzyme-linked immunosorbent assay) in order to modify the severity of the maternal infection. VZIG prophylaxis must be given within 72 to 96 hours after the exposure and is not useful after symptoms appear.

VZIG should always be given to infants with perinatal exposure to maternal varicella either immediately after birth, if the mother has acute varicella beginning less than four days before delivery, or at the first signs of maternal rash if the mother develops varicella within 48 hours after delivering.

Perinatal VZV infection among infants in the group identified as high risk, i.e., those with a late onset of symptoms, who were born to mothers whose illness began four days before or within 48 hours after delivery, should be treated with intravenous doses of acyclovir. Although the clinical experience with acyclovir treatment of infants with perinatal varicella is lacking, the drug prevents progressive VZV infection among other immunodeficient patients. Acyclovir therapy should be given if an infant develops extensive cutaneous lesions even if VZIG was administered at birth.

No intervention is required for infants who are exposed to maternal herpes zoster. These infants will have transplacentally acquired VZV antibodies and can be expected to have mild varicella or, more often, no disease.

CYTOMEGALOVIRUS

Cytomegalovirus (CMV) is the most common cause of congenital infection; the incidence of in utero transmission ranges from 0.2 to 2.2 percent among all live births.[20] Over 90 percent of infected neonates are asymptomatic at birth. However, as will be detailed, approximately 10 percent of these asymptomatic infants may have later-appearing sequelae, which may include sensorineural hearing loss and learning and behavioral abnormalities.[29-31] In contrast, most of the unfortunate minority of congenitally infected neonates who are symptomatic at birth manifest severe developmental deficits and mental retardation.[32,33] Unlike the other congenital infections discussed in this chapter, congenital CMV infection may result from a primary maternal infection or from reactivation of a maternal infection that preceded conception.[34] With few exceptions, neonates with clinically apparent disease have been born to women who have had a primary CMV infection during gestation.[34] Preliminary data also suggest that primary infections that occur earlier in pregnancy (before the 27th week of gestation) are more likely to be associated with a poor outcome for the infant than primary infections occurring later in pregnancy.[35-38]

Outcome In Infants Asymptomatic At Birth

The majority of neonates with congenital CMV infections are asymptomatic at birth. These infants are likely to be detected only if routine viral cultures are performed in newborns. Several longitudinal studies have been conducted to assess the possible long-term effects of these "silent" congenital CMV infections.[20-31] The sequelae identified have included sensorineural hearing loss and possible impairment of intellectual development. It is apparent that hearing loss is the most common irreversible sequela of congenital CMV infection; the incidence of hearing loss in children assessed between three and seven years of age has ranged from 13 to 17 percent.[25,26,32] Like rubella, hearing loss caused by CMV may be progressive.[27,39] A study published in 1984, which included a literature summary of 31 children with hearing impairment following asymptomatic congenital CMV infection, revealed that 55 percent had moderate to profound hearing loss and 58 percent had bilateral disease.[30] Considering the incidence of congenital CMV infection in the United States and the frequency of consequent hearing loss, it has been estimated that approximately 2,000 children are born each year with CMV-induced sensorineural hearing loss.[40] Therefore CMV is one of the major nonhereditary causes of congenital deafness.

Several studies have attempted to address the issue of possible intellectual deficits in neonates with congenital CMV who are asymptomatic at birth. Interpretation of the results of some of the studies is hampered by relatively short periods of follow-up, a lack of appropriately matched controls, and a failure to control for the presence of hearing loss. The most recently published study evaluated intellectual development in 18 prospectively followed school-age children with asymptomatic congenital CMV infection and normal hearing.[31] The results in testing these children were compared with the results in 18 control subjects matched for age, sex, race, school grade, and socioeconomic status. All children were evaluated between 6.5 and 12.5 years of age using the Wechsler Intelligence Scale for Children (Revised), the Kaufman Assessment Battery for Children, and the Wide Range Achievement Test. No differences were observed between the infected and uninfected children on intelligence scores or subscales, achievement scores, or incidence of learning disabilities.

It remains plausible that hearing-impaired, congenitally infected infants will eventually manifest intellectual dysfunction. Hearing impairment per se is associated with a lower than average performance on traditional language-dependent intelligence tests,[41] and hearing impairment in CMV-infected infants may be evidence that the virus has grown in and damaged at least some central nervous system tissue. Indeed, on the basis of a combination of IQ, behavioral, neurologic, and auditory test data, a several-fold increase in the "predicted"

school failure incidence has been noted in children of lower socioeconomic classes who were congenitally infected with CMV and asymptomatic at birth.[26] In the same study infected children of middle and higher socioeconomic classes did not have increased predicted school failure incidences when compared with appropriately matched controls. Therefore it seems that the expression of adverse outcomes in asymptomatic CMV infections may be multifactorial. Future studies must attempt to control for all relevant contributing factors.

In addition to the possibility of overt intellectual dysfunction, behavioral problems have been noted in a cohort of prospectively followed children with asymptomatic congenital CMV infections.[28] The authors "had a clinical impression, confirmed by parent questionnaires," that behavioral problems were more common in infected children than in the matched controls. The conclusions of this study were confounded by the infected children living in economically deprived, less stimulating environments with exposure to "more readily implemented discipline and punishment."[28]

Outcome in Infants Symptomatic at Birth

The majority of neonates who are symptomatic as a result of congenital CMV infection have been exposed, in utero, to a primary maternal infection.[34] Japanese investigators have hypothesized that, in their country, symptomatic congenital infection "is not an unusual complication" of recurrent maternal CMV infection.[42] However, the numbers of well-documented cases in the literature supporting this premise are few.[43] The clinical abnormalities found most frequently in neonates with symptomatic congenital CMV infection include hepatomegaly, splenomegaly, jaundice, microcephaly, chorioretinitis, and petechiae.[44] The cerebral abnormalities that have been recognized in association with congenital CMV infection have been summarized and extensively referenced.[45] In addition to microcephaly, these abnormalities include microgyria, periventricular calcifications, spongiosis of the brain, encephalomalacia, calcification of the cerebral arteries, parietal lobe cyst, cerebral cortical immaturity, cerebellar aplasia, and dolichocephaly. A recent report that assessed four congenitally infected neonates with real-time ultrasonography described previously unreported intracranial lesions—paraventricular cysts and intraventricular strands.[46]

Although less than 10 percent of congenitally infected neonates manifest overt signs of congenital infection, their ease of identification and the poor long-term prognosis underscore the importance of this group.[21,22,32,33,38] Central nervous system sequelae that have been attributed to congenital CMV infection include microcephaly, mental retardation and developmental delays, learning and behavioral disorders, seizures, and neuromuscular disorders, including facial asymmetry, spasticity, quadriparesis, diplegia, and hemiatrophy and hemiparesis.[47] Defects in hearing and vision are also common after symptomatic congenital infection.

The largest prospective study of symptomatic neonates was published in 1980.[33] In that study 34 patients who had clinically evident disease at birth were followed for a mean duration of four years. Twenty-nine percent died and more than 90 percent of the survivors developed central nervous system or auditory handicaps; 70 percent had microcephaly, 61 percent mental retardation, 35 percent neuromuscular disorders, 30 percent hearing loss, and 22 percent chorioretinitis or optic atrophy. Although the extent of disease apparent at birth was not entirely predictive of central nervous system sequelae, all children with IQ's less than 50 or neuromuscular disorders were clearly abnormal by one year of age.[33]

Another longitudinal study evaluated 17 patients with symptomatic infection for a mean of 5.5 years.[32] All the children had developmental disorders that necessitated special education; more than half performed in the retarded range.

It must be recognized that although the estimated risk of permanent neurologic sequelae after a CMV infection with symptoms in the neonatal period is high, in a given case development may be more favorable than expected.[38]

Congenital CMV infection should be considered in any newborn with unexplained prematurity, growth retardation, hepatomegaly, splenomegaly, jaundice, microcephaly, chorioretinitis, or petechiae. This diagnosis can be proved or ruled out by attempting to isolate the virus from a urine or salivary culture obtained during the first weeks of life.

Any infant with a congenital CMV infection, whether symptomatic or asymptomatic at birth, should undergo careful audiometric examinations. These evaluations should be repeated over the first several years of the child's life to assess for late-appearing, progressive abnormalities. Defects, including language difficulties, should be corrected as soon as possible.

Currently there is no known effective antiviral therapy for infants with congenital CMV infections. Trials to be initiated by the NIAID Antiviral Treatment group will be evaluating an antiviral drug known as 9-(1,3-dihydroxy-2-propoxymethyl)guanine (DHPG) in unfortunate neonates who are symptomatic at birth. The results of these trials will not be available for several years.

HUMAN IMMUNODEFICIENCY VIRUS

The acquired immunodeficiency syndrome (AIDS) was first described in 1981.[48] It was initially reported in homosexual men, but high risk groups now include Haitians, addicts who use illicit drugs intravenously, heterosexual prostitutes, patients with hemophilia and other recipients of transfused products, and infants born to mothers in one of the at-risk groups.[49] The etiologic agent of AIDS is a retrovirus referred to as human immunodeficiency virus (HIV). Most neonates who have contracted AIDS have been born to mothers who use illicit drugs intravenously.[50] The neurologic evaluations of their infants potentially are confounded by factors other than infection with HIV.

Most neonates infected with HIV develop signs and symptoms during the first year of life; often by three months of age. The most frequent manifestations are failure to thrive, chronic interstitial pneumonitis, hepatosplenomegaly, diffuse lymphadenopathy, recurrent or persistent oral candidiasis, protracted or recurrent diarrhea, thrombocytopenia, and recurrent severe infections caused by bacteria and opportunistic pathogens.[49] Neurologic complications in patients with AIDS may result from neoplasms or opportunistic infections of the central nervous system, or from direct infection with HIV. Evidence suggests that HIV may be responsible for subacute encephalopathy-dementia, polyneuropathy of axonal or demyelinating types, vacuolar myelopathy, and acute and chronic meningitis.[51,52] Both adults and children may manifest neurologic disease before clinical manifestations of immunodeficiency are evident.[52,53] Viral DNA or RNA has been isolated directly from the brains of patients who have died of subacute encephalopathy and from the CSF of patients with AIDS with a variety of neurologic syndromes; virus has been isolated from the CSF of patients even before neurologic symptoms develop.[52,54-58]

The encephalopathy caused by HIV occurs in about one-third of the adults and more than half the children with AIDS.[54,59-61] In adults the disease characteristically begins with impaired concentration and memory loss and progresses to severe dementia. In children with AIDS, development during the first several months of life is usually normal, but developmental regression is noted thereafter.[61-63] The predominant developmental delays are in motor milestones, perceptual motor abilities, and expressive speech. In one series of 36 children with AIDS, time to the onset of progressive encephalopathy ranged from two months to five years.[61] Hyperreflexia, increased tone, and spasticity often accompany the cognitive impairment.[59-61,63] Some patients develop paraparesis, bilateral pyramidal tract signs, a spastic-ataxic gait, or seizures.[60] Acquired microcephaly associated with cerebral atrophy is common in children.[61] Progression usually occurs over several weeks to months. Typical pathologic findings in the brain include diffuse calcification of the cerebrum, cerebellum, and pons, reduced brain volume, and ventriculomegaly.[52,59,60] Vacuolar degeneration of the spinal cord occurs in about one-fifth of patients with AIDS.[64] It results in paraparesis, ataxia, and incontinence.

Any infant known to be or suspected of being infected with HIV and any infant at risk for developing such an infection should be monitored for the development of neurologic sequelae. It is important to recognize that infection of the central nervous system is part of the spectrum of HIV infection in children. Brain infection usually occurs early and is persistent and progressive. As antiviral drugs active against HIV are introduced, the importance of their distribution into the central nervous system must be considered in view of the frequent involvement of the nervous system.

In a recent study, the continuous intravenous infusion of the antiviral drug zidovudine (AZT) resulted in improvement in neurodevelopmental abnormalities in all of 13 children who had presented with AIDS-associated encephalopathy. If these results are verified, AZT will become an important part of the management of these children.[64a]

RUBELLA

The rubella virus is an RNA virus, classified as a togavirus, that is unrelated to any other human viral pathogen. Before the introduction of childhood immunization for rubella, the virus caused major epidemics once or twice every decade in the United States.[65] During rubella epidemics many individuals were infected without any associated illness, while others had the classic diffuse exanthem and other signs. Because most children in the United States are now immunized during the second year of life, widespread epidemics of rubella have disappeared. Nevertheless, many young adult women remain susceptible to rubella, and thus the introduction of rubella into a local community is still associated with the risk of congenital rubella syndrome.

Transmission of Rubella to the Fetus

Rubella produces viremia in the susceptible host during primary infection. This viremic phase in the pregnant woman often results in placental infection, with or without subsequent infection of the fetus. The risk of fetal infection is related to the week of gestation at which maternal infection occurs, the highest risk occurring during the first eight weeks. Serologic studies show that the frequency of fetal infection at this stage of gestation is above 50 percent with a decline to about 10 percent by 24 weeks.[65,66] Viral transmission to the fetus also can occur in the last trimester. Because of the limitations of serologic diagnosis, the true risk of fetal infection associated with maternal rubella at varying intervals after conception has not been defined with precision. Some studies using viral culture to prove intrauterine infection suggest incidences of transmission that are greater than 90 percent in the first eight weeks of gestation.[65]

Clinical Manifestations of Intrauterine Rubella Infection and the Risk of Neurologic Sequelae

Intrauterine rubella infection can be proved most reliably by obtaining a viral culture from the oropharynx of the infant; the shedding of the virus at this site persists for six months or longer after birth. The virus also can be found by culturing the rectum, urine, and CSF, and persistent viral infection of peripheral blood cells can be demonstrated. Although efforts have been made to develop a rubella IgM antibody assay for the diagnosis of congenital rubella infection, many infants with infection proved by culture do not have detectable rubella IgM antibodies, even with optimal methodology.

Despite the extent of the viral infection, fewer than 5 to 10 percent of infants with intrauterine rubella have signs of the congenital rubella syndrome at birth. As is true of the attack incidence, the clinical manifestations of intrauterine rubella are related directly to the fetal age at the time of maternal infection.[67] Infants infected with rubella virus at the earliest stages of development have pulmonary artery and aortic stenosis caused by damage to the vascular endothelium along with patent ductus arteriosus, in addition to the hearing and ocular abnormalities characteristic of later infection. The estimated risk of defects detectable in the first four years of life among infected infants is 85 percent following maternal rubella at eight weeks, 52 percent at nine to 12 weeks, and 16 percent at 13 to 20 weeks.[66] Maternal infection after 20 weeks' gestation can cause fetal infection, but these infants are asymptomatic in the newborn period and the risk of late sequelae is low.

Infants with congenital rubella who are microcephalic can be expected to have neurologic sequelae, but many infected infants do not present with microcephaly and should not be presupposed to have central nervous system damage.[68] In some cases central nervous system involvement can present as active encephalitis, with elevated CSF protein levels with or without pleocytosis in the newborn period. Extensive meningoencephalitis is one of the reasons for early postnatal death from congenital rubella. However, the neurologic sequelae of congenital rubella are much more likely to be subtle and therefore may be recognized only later as hearing deficits and delays in language and psychomotor development. In these infants it is always difficult to determine the extent to which delayed development is due to primary central nervous system damage as opposed to the severe communication problems that result from deafness and impaired vision related to cataracts, microphthalmia, and glaucoma. Many infants with no other evidence of symptomatic intrauterine rubella have severe hearing impairment, which must be recognized early in infancy in order to provide optimal intervention.

The persistence of the infectious virus may allow the intrauterine infection to progress postnatally with continuing pathologic changes identified in many tissues, including the central nervous system, in some children. The progressive nature of intrauterine rubella infection was demonstrated in a group of nonretarded children who were followed for nine to 12 years by Desmond et al.[69] An increase in the percentage of the population with hearing loss, motor incoordination, and behavioral disturbances was observed with increasing age. A late follow-up, 86 percent of the children had hearing deficits, 52 percent had learning problems, 48 percent had behavioral problems, and 61 percent had poor balance or muscle weakness. Ocular disease can also worsen if the chorioretinitis of congenital rubella results in neovascularization of the retina or if glaucoma progresses. Chess et al[70] described the psychiatric and behavioral consequences of congenital rubella among 205 children examined at eight to nine years of age; 25 percent of the children were retarded, 18 percent had a reactive behavior disorder, and 6 percent were autistic.

As children with congenital rubella were followed for prolonged periods of time, a few patients were identified who developed a syndrome of progressive encephalitis, comparable to the subacute sclerosing panencephalitis caused by the measles virus.[71] These children had progressive deterioration after 10 years of age, which was associated with diminished intellectual and motor function and with elevated IgG levels in the CSF; rubella virus was recovered from brain biopsy specimens in one case. Fortunately this syndrome has been a rare consequence of intrauterine rubella.

The evaluation of a pregnancy potentially complicated by rubella remains a difficult diagnostic problem. The interval required to isolate the virus interferes with the use of tissue culture as a diagnostic method. If the pregnant woman has not had a previous rubella titer, it often is impossible to determine whether a seroconversion has occurred, because rubella antibodies as measured by hemagglutination inhibition are present within a few days after the onset of infection. The detection of rubella IgM antibodies can be helpful, but the method can yield false positive results, and the absence of an IgM response does not exclude a recent rubella infection. A high titer of rubella antibodies in a single serum sample does not establish a diagnosis of recent infection, since many individuals maintain persistently high rubella titers. Rubella titers are also generally higher with the newer serologic tests (e.g., latex agglutination and enzyme immunoassay). In some cases a recent infection can be proved by demonstrating rubella antibodies by hemagglutination inhibition or other sensitive methods in a serum that is negative by the rubella complement fixation assay.[65] Finally, a properly documented past immunization with rubella vaccine can be considered to reduce the likelihood that a nonspecific exanthem was rubella and therefore alters the assessment of the potential risk to the fetus.

If an exposure to rubella is identified in a pregnant woman whose immune status is not known, she should be tested for rubella antibodies immediately. A positive rubella titer at the time of exposure eliminates any concern. If the titer is negative, the determination should be repeated two weeks and six weeks after the exposure to be certain that subclinical infection has not occurred. Transplacental transmission of the virus is possible if seroconversion is demonstrated regardless of whether the pregnant woman has had symptoms.

Congenital rubella can be eliminated by preventing the exposure of susceptible pregnant women to the virus. The rubella vaccination program has reduced the annual number of cases of rubella by 99 percent from the incidence during the prevaccine era.[72] However, localized rubella outbreaks continue to occur, followed by cases of congenital rubella syndrome, as was noted in New York City in 1985 to 1986.[73]

A vaccine strategy designed only to immunize children at 15 months takes 10 to 30 years to produce a highly immune cohort of women of childbearing age. Current rubella vaccination programs must take into account the fact that 10 to 20 percent of postpubertal women remain susceptible. Susceptible young women should be encouraged to receive the rubella vaccine. Although 4.5 percent of adult women given rubella vaccine have experienced vaccine-associated arthropathy, this complication is self-limited and also has been reported in 30 percent of adult women with natural rubella. Although candidates for rubella vaccine should be advised that pregnancy is a contraindication to rubella immunization, inadvertent rubella vaccination in early pregnancy has not been associated with the congenital rubella syndrome.[74] Finally, the experience in New York showed that half the mothers of infants with congenital rubella had had a previous live birth, suggesting the significant potential for postpartum immunization in eliminating cases of congenital rubella.

TOXOPLASMOSIS

The etiologic agent of toxoplasmosis, *Toxoplasma gondii*, was first demonstrated in the brain of a newborn infant with encephalomyelitis in 1939.[75] The incidence of congenital toxoplasmosis in the United States is approximately 1 in 1,000 live births.[2] The clinical spectrum of congenital toxoplasmosis is broad.[76] As with congenital CMV infection, the majority of infants infected in utero with *T. gondii* are asymptomatic at birth. Some of these infants may manifest sequelae, especially ophthalmologic dysfunction and intellectual impairment, at a later age. The small number of congenitally infected infants who have clinically evident disease at birth may be severely injured, either dying shortly after birth or surviving with serious cerebral damage.[76]

Outcome in Infants Asymptomatic at Birth

Although congenital toxoplasmosis is not so prevalent as congenital CMV, it is potentially more dangerous for the individual patient. Subclinical infection with *T. gondii* is more frequently associated with impaired intellectual performance and chorioretinitis than is subclinical infection with CMV.[76-78] The intellectual and ocular sequelae of congenital toxoplasmosis may not be clinically obvious until nine to 10 years of age.[76]

The most recent study published in the United States, which evaluated the long-term outcome in 24 infants born with subclinical congenital toxoplasmosis, concluded that nearly all such children have adverse sequelae.[78] This study, however, was not controlled, and assessments were made prospectively only for the 13 children identified at birth. Eight of these 13 neonates were detected as a result of routine screening of cord serum for IgM antibodies specific for *T. gondii*, and five were detected either because acute toxoplasmosis was diagnosed during pregnancy or at term in the mother (two children) or because the neonates were screened for nonspecific findings (three children). The remaining 11 children included in this study were asymptomatic at birth and were identified by the authors only after the first ocular sign developed. Thus, there are limitations to the data. The frequency with which sequelae develop in children born with subclinical infection is probably overestimated as a result of the means of data collection. Eleven of the 13 children (85 percent) prospectively followed from birth developed chorioretinitis. Severe permanent neurologic sequelae were noted in one of the 13 infants (8 percent) followed from birth and in three of the 11 children (27 percent) followed from the time of initial presentation with eye disease. Considering all four children with severe neurologic sequelae, all had seizures, three had severe psychomotor retardation, which was diagnosed when major motor dysfunction was identified by an IQ less than 70, two had microcephaly, and one had hydrocephaly.

In addition to the severe sequelae noted in these 24 congenitally infected children, seven (29 percent) developed minor sequelae. Six infants had minor cerebellar signs and four had transiently delayed psychomotor development. In 16 of the 24 infected children skull roentgenography was performed during the first year of life. Five (31 percent) had intracranial calcification; all five developed neurologic sequelae—three suffered major sequelae, and two suffered minor sequelae. Nineteen of the 24 congenitally infected children were evaluated for sensorineural hearing loss. Some degree of hearing loss was noted in five (26 percent)—moderate (hearing reception threshold, 51 to 80 db) in two children and mild (hearing reception threshold, 25 to 50 db) in three.

Outcome in Infants Symptomatic at Birth

Only about 20 percent of neonates congenitally infected with *T. gondii* are symptomatic at birth. The infection is rarely fulminant but it is often severe. Symptoms and signs of generalized infection are prominent, and signs referable to the central nervous system are invariably present.[76] The "classic triad" in these unfortunate neonates is hydrocephalus, chorioretinitis, and diffuse intracranial calcifications. The most frequent extraneural signs associated with symptomatic congenital toxoplasmosis include hepatosplenomegaly, fever, anemia, and jaundice.[76] The overall mortality in these infants is 10 to 15 percent. Approximately 85 percent of the survivors are mentally retarded, 75 percent experience convulsions, spasticity, and palsies, and 50 percent have severe visual impairment.[76] Deafness, a prominent sequela of congenital viral infections (e.g., CMV and rubella), occurs less frequently after congenital toxoplasmosis; its approximate incidence is 10 to 15 percent.

Infants identified at birth as being congenitally infected with *T. gondii* must be recognized as being at high risk for the development of ophthalmologic or intellectual dysfunction. Because the onset of sequelae can be markedly delayed, serial ophthalmologic and intellectual assessments must be performed until the child is at least 10 years of age. Preliminary evidence from uncontrolled nonrandomized studies suggests that treatment may decrease the frequency or severity of adverse sequelae.[76,78,79] On the basis of these imperfect data, treatment with sulfadiazine and pyrimethamine should be initiated as soon as the diagnosis is made or highly suspected. There may be some advantage to prescribing alternating courses of these antifolate antibiotics with courses of the macrolide antibiotic spiramycin.[76] Clearly there is a need for controlled randomized trials to determine the effects of different treatment regimens on the development of sequelae in children born with congenital toxoplasmosis.

SYPHILIS

Congenital infections caused by *Treponema pallidum*, the etiologic agent of syphilis, are declining but continue to occur in the United States. The disease is estimated to occur in 0.05 percent of live-born children.[80] In 1984, 326 cases of congenital syphilis in all age groups were reported by the Centers for Disease Control in Atlanta.[81] This undoubtedly represents a gross underestimate owing to deficiencies in the diagnosis and reporting of this infection. Manifestations of syphilitic infections in the perinatal period are similar in many ways to those of other infectious diseases acquired in utero. The outcome may be stillbirth, prematurity, intrauterine growth retardation, or neonatal death. Survivors with infection are usually asymptomatic at birth, but they frequently develop later-appearing symptoms.[82] When symptoms appear within the first two years of life, the cases are designated as early congenital syphilis; cases in which symptoms develop thereafter are designated as late congenital syphilis.[83]

Early Congenital Syphilis

The older literature reported that more than 60 percent of the neonates with congenital syphilis had abnormal findings on CSF examination.[84] In the referenced study CSF was regarded as abnormal if it contained five or more white blood cells per cubic millimeter and had a protein content higher than 45 mg per deciliter. We now recognize that these definitions of abnormal CSF may not be appropriate for newborn infants.[85,86] Indeed a recent study of 78 newborn infants, born to mothers with serologic evidence of syphilis, found that none of the neonates had CSF abnormalities. The criteria for normal CSF in this study were fewer than 32 white blood cells per cubic millimeter and less than 170 mg per deciliter of protein.[87]

Neurologic manifestations of congenital syphilis, evident in the first two years of life, now are reported infrequently. In a recent series of 78 cases of congenital syphilis there were no clear cases of central nervous system sequelae.[87] When reported, the most common clinical types of central nervous system involvement in early congenital syphilis are acute leptomeningitis and chronic meningovascular syphilis.[83] Leptomeningitis usually becomes evident between three and six months of age. It is clinically indistinguishable from other bacterial causes of meningitis. The CSF typically contains 100 to 200 mononuclear cells per cubic millimeter, shows an increase in the protein level, and shows a positive serologic test for syphilis. This form of neurosyphilis responds to antisyphilitic therapy. Chronic meningovascular syphilis tends to follow a protracted and progressive course, starting late in the first year of life. It usually results in communicating hydrocephalus and cranial nerve palsies. Cerebral infarctions from syphilitic endarteritis may also result in a variety of cerebrovascular syndromes, paresis and seizures being the most consistent features.

Late Congenital Syphilis

Neurologic involvement in late congenital syphilis was frequently reported in the older literature.[84] Such involvement is currently reported only infrequently.[87,88] Neurologic manifestations that have been reported include hydrocephalus, seizures, mental retardation, paresis, paralysis, blindness, and deafness. The deafness is caused by progressive labyrinthitis with symptoms beginning about the time of puberty. Hearing loss usu-

ally starts in the higher frequencies, and coincident vertigo is common.

The diagnosis of congenital syphilis should be considered in any neonate born to a mother with a reactive serologic test for syphilis. It also should be considered in neonates with unexplained prematurity or low birth weight, bullous skin lesions, maculopapular rashes, "snuffles," skeletal lesions, jaundice, splenomegaly, or lymphadenopathy. As part of the diagnostic evaluation, especially if the neonate has clinical features compatible with syphilis, a CSF specimen should be obtained and analyzed.[87] If the CSF is abnormal, a 10-day course of aqueous or procaine penicillin therapy is indicated to insure adequate spirocheticidal concentrations of penicillin in all tissues.[89] All infants with suspected or proven congenital syphilis, regardless of whether central nervous system involvement is present at diagnosis, must undergo careful long-term evaluations of mental and motor function, hearing and vision.

REFERENCES

Herpes Simplex

1. Nahmias AJ, Keyserling HL, Kerrick GM. Neonatal herpes simplex virus infections. In: Remington JS, Klein JO, eds. Infectious diseases of the fetus and newborn infant. Philadelphia: WB Saunders, 1983:636.
2. Whitley RJ, Nahmias AJ, Visintine AM, et al. The natural history of herpes simplex virus infection of mother and newborn. Pediatrics 1980; 66:489.
3. Yeager AS, Arvin AM. Reasons for the absence of a history of recurrent genital infections in mothers of neonates infected with herpes simplex virus. Pediatrics 1984; 73:188.
4. Prober CG, Hensleigh PA, Boucher FD, et al. Identification of neonates exposed to herpes simplex virus: the value of routine viral cultures at delivery. N Engl J Med 1987; 318:887.
5. Prober CG, Yasukawa LL, Au DS, et al. Low risk of herpes simplex virus infections in neonates exposed to virus at the time of vaginal delivery to mothers with recurrent genital herpes simplex virus infections. N Eng J Med 1987; 316:240.
6. Brown ZA, Vontver LA, Benedetti J. Genital herpes in pregnancy: risk factors associated with recurrences and asymptomatic viral shedding. Am J Obstet Gynecol 1985; 153:24.
7. Sullender WM, Miller JL, Yasukawa LL, et al. Humoral and cellular immunity in neonates with herpes simplex virus infection. J Infect Dis 1987; 55:28.
8. Hutto C, Arvin A, Jacobs R, et al. Congenital herpes simplex virus infections. J Pediatr 1987; 110:97.
9. Whitley RJ, et al. Vidarbine versus acyclovir therapy of neonatal herpes simplex virus infection (abstract). Soc Pediat Res May 1986.
10. Arvin AM, Yeager AS, Bruhn F, Grossman M. Neonatal herpes simplex infection in the absence of mucocutaneous lesions. J Pediatr 1982; 100:715.
11. Arvin AM, Hensleigh PA, Prober CG, et al. Failure of antepartum maternal cultures to predict the infant's risk of exposure to herpes simplex virus at delivery. N Engl J Med 1986; 315:796.
12. Brown ZA, Vontver LA, Benedetti J, et al. Effects on infants of a first episode of genital herpes during pregnancy. N Engl J Med 1987; 317:1246.
13. Coleman RM, Pereira L, Bailey PD, et al. Determination of herpes simplex virus type specific antibodies by enzyme-linked immunosorbent assay. J Clin Microbiol 1983; 18:287.

Varicella Zoster Virus

14. Paryani SG, Arvin AM. Intrauterine infection with varicella-zoster virus after maternal varicella. N Engl J Med 1986; 314:1542.
15. Enders G. Varicella-zoster virus infection in pregnancy. Prog Med Virol 1984; 29:166.
16. Borzyskowski M, Harris RF, Jones RWA. The congenital varicella syndrome. Eur J Pediatr 1981; 37:335.
17. Myers JD. Congenital varicella in term infants: risk reconsidered. J Infect Dis 1974; 129:215.
18. Gershon AA, Raker R, Steinberg S, et al. Antibody to varicella-zoster virus in parturient women and their offspring during the first year of life. Pediatrics 1976; 58:692.
19. Gustafson TL, Shehab Z, Brunell PA. Outbreak of varicella in a newborn intensive care nursery. Am J Dis Child 1984; 138:548.

Cytomegalovirus

20. Stagno S, Pass RF, Alford CA. Perinatal infections and maldevelopment. Birth Defects 1981; 17:31.
21. McCracken GH Jr, Shinefield HR, Cobb K, et al. Congenital cytomegalic inclusion disease: a longitudinal study of 20 patients. Am J Dis Child 1969; 117:522.
22. Berenberg W, Nankervis G. Long-term follow-up of cytomegalic inclusion disease of infancy. Pediatrics 1970; 46:403.
23. Kumar ML, Nankervis GA, Gold E. Inapparent congenital cytomegalovirus infection: a follow-up study. N Engl J Med 1973; 288:1370.
24. Melish ME, Hanshaw JB. Congenital cytomegalovirus infection: developmental progress of infants detected by routine screening. Am J Dis Child 1973; 126:190.
25. Reynolds DW, Stagno S, Stubbs KG, et al. Inapparent congenital cytomegalovirus infection with elevated cord IgM levels: causal relation with auditory and mental deficiency. N Engl J Med 1974; 290:291.
26. Hanshaw JB, Scheiner AP, Mozley AW, et al. School failure and deafness after "silent" congenital cytomegalovirus infection. N Engl J Med 1976; 95:468.
27. Stagno S, Reynolds DW, Amos CA, et al. Auditory and visual defects resulting from symptomatic and subclinical congenital cytomegalovirus and *Toxoplasma* infections. Pediatrics 1977; 59:669.
28. Saigal S, Lunyk O, Larke B, Chernesky MA. The outcome in children with congenital cytomegalovirus infection: a longitudinal follow-up study. Am J Dis Child 1982; 136:896.
29. Preece PM, Pearl KN, Peckham CS. Congenital cytomegalovirus infection. Arch Dis Child 1984; 59:1120.
30. Kumar ML, Nankervis GA, Jacobs IB, et al. Congenital and postnatally acquired cytomegalovirus infections: long-term follow-up. J Pediatr 1984; 104:674.
31. Conboy TJ, Pass RF, Stagno S. Intellectual development in school-aged children with asymptomatic congenital cytomegalovirus infection. Pediatrics 1986; 77:801.
32. Williamson WD, Desmond MM, LaFevers N, et al. Symptomatic congenital cytomegalovirus. Disorders of language, learning, and hearing. Am J Dis Child 1982; 136:902.
33. Pass RF, Stagno S, Myers GJ, et al. Outcome of symptomatic congenital cytomegalovirus infection: results of long-term longitudinal follow-up. Pediatrics 1980; 66:758.
34. Stagno S, Reynolds DW, Huang ES, et al. Congenital cytomegalovirus infection: occurrence in an immune population. N Engl J Med 1977; 296:1254.
35. Stagno S, Pass RF, Cloud G, et al. Primary cytomegalovirus infection in pregnancy: incidence, transmission to fetus, and clinical outcome. JAMA 1986; 256:1904.
36. Stern H, Tucker SM. Prospective study of cytomegalovirus infection in pregnancy. Br Med J 1973; 2:268.
37. Monif GRG, Egan A, Held B, et al. The correlation of maternal cytomegalovirus infection during varying stages in gestation with neonatal involvement. J Pediatr 1972; 80:17.
38. Ahlfors K, Forsgren M, Ivarsson SA, et al. Congenital cytomegalovirus infection: on the relation between type and time of maternal infection and infant's symptoms. Scand J Infect Dis 1983; 15:129.
39. Dahle A, McCollister FP, Stagno S, et al. Progressive hearing impairment in children with congenital cytomegalovirus infection. J Hearing Speech Dis 1979; 44:220.
40. Hanshaw JB. On deafness, cytomegalovirus, and neonatal screening. Am J Dis Child 1982; 136:886.
41. Rainer JD, Altshuler KZ. A psychiatric program for the deaf: experiences and implications. Am J Psychiatry 1971; 127:103.
42. Chiba S, Kamada M, Yoshimura H, et al. Congenital cytomegalovirus infection in Japan. N Engl J Med 1984; 310:50.
43. Ahlfors K, Harris S, Ivarsson S, et al. Secondary maternal cytomegalovirus infection causing symptomatic congenital infection. N Engl J Med 1981; 305:284.
44. Weller TH, Hanshaw JB. Virologic and clinical observations on cytomegalic inclusion disease. N Engl J Med 1962; 266:1233.
45. Hanshaw JB. Developmental abnormalities associated with congenital cytomegalovirus infection. Adv Teratol 1970; 4:64.
46. Butt W, Mackay R, de Crespigny LC, et al. Intracranial lesions of congenital cytomegalovirus infection detected by ultrasound scanning. Pediatrics 1984; 73:611.
47. Virnig NL, Balfour HH. Hemiatrophy and hemiparesis in a patient with congenital cytomegalovirus infection. Am J Dis Child 1975; 129:1359.

Human Immunodeficiency Virus

48. Gottlieb MS, Schroff R, Schanker HM, et al. *Pneumocystis carinii* pneumonia and mucosal candidiasis in previously healthy homosexual men: evidence of a new acquired cellular immunodeficiency. N Engl J Med 1981; 305:1425.
49. Shannon KM, Ammann AJ. Acquired immune deficiency in childhood. J Pediatr 1985; 106:332.
50. Rogers MF. AIDS in children: a review of the clinical, epidemiologic and public health aspects. Pediatr Infect Dis 1985; 4:230.
51. Snider WD, Simpson DM, Nielsen S, et al. Neurologic complications of acquired immune deficiency syndrome: analysis of 50 patients. Ann Neurol 1983; 14:403.
52. Ho DD, Rota TR, Schooley RT, et al. Isolation of HTLV-III from cerebrospinal fluid and neural tissues of patients with neurologic syndromes related to the acquired immunodeficiency syndrome. N Engl J Med 1985; 313:1493.
53. Davis SL, Halsted CC, Levy N, et al. Acquired immune deficiency syndrome presenting as progressive infantile encephalopathy. J Pediatr 1987; 110:884.
54. Shaw GM, Harper ME, Hahn BH, et al. HTLV-III infection in brains of children and adults with AIDS encephalopathy. Science 1985; 227:177.
55. Levy JA, Kaminsky LS, Morrow WJW, et al. Infection by the retrovirus associated with the acquired immunodeficiency syndrome: clinical, biological, and molecular features. Ann Intern Med 1985; 103:694.
56. Levy JA, Shimabukuro J, Hollander H, et al. Isolation of AIDS-associated retrovirus from cerebrospinal fluid and brain of patients with neurological symptoms. Lancet 1985; 2:586.
57. Hollander H, Levy JA. Neurologic abnormalities and recovery of human immunodeficiency virus from cerebrospinal fluid. Ann Intern Med 1987; 106:692.
58. Ragni MV, Urbach AH, Taylor S, et al. Isolation of human immunodeficiency virus and detection of HIV sequences in the brain of an ELISA antibody-negative child with acquired immune deficiency syndrome and progressive encephalopathy. J Pediatr 1987; 110:892.
59. Nielsen S, Petito CK, Urmacher CD, et al. Subacute encephalitis

in acquired immune deficiency syndrome: a postmortem study. Am J Clin Pathol 1984; 82:678.

60. Epstein LG, Sharer LR, Joshi VV, et al. Progressive encephalopathy in children with acquired immune deficiency syndrome. Ann Neurol 1985; 17:488.

61. Epstein LG, Sharer LR, Oleske JM, et al. Neurologic manifestations of human immunodeficiency virus infection in children. Pediatrics 1986; 78:678.

62. Oleske J, Minnefor A, Cooper R, et al. Immune deficiency syndrome in children. JAMA 1983; 249:2345.

63. Belman AL, Ultmann MH, Horoupian D, et al. Neurological complications in infants and children with acquired immune deficiency syndrome. Ann Neurol 1985; 18:560.

64. Petito CK, Navia BA, Cho ES, et al. Vacuolar myelopathy pathologically resembling subacute combined degeneration in patients with the acquired immunodeficiency syndrome. N Engl J Med 1985; 312:874.

64a. Pizzo PA, Eddy J, Falloon J, et al. Effect of continuous intravenous infusion of Zidovudine (AZT) in children with symptomatic HIV infection. N Engl J Med 1988; 319:889.

Rubella

65. Alford CA. Rubella. In: Remington JS, Klein JO, eds. Infectious diseases of the fetus and newborn infant. Philadelphia: WB Saunders, 1983:69.

66. Peckham GS. Clinical and laboratory study of children exposed in utero to maternal rubella. Arch Dis Child 1972; 47:571.

67. Ueda K, Nishida Y, Oshima K, Shepard TH. Congenital rubella syndrome: correlation of gestational age at time of maternal rubella with type of defect. J Pediatr 1979; 94:763.

68. Macfarlane DW, Boyd RD, Dodrill CB, Tufts E. Intrauterine rubella, head size and intellect. Pediatrics 1975; 55:797.

69. Desmond MM, Fisher ES, Borderman AL, et al. The longitudinal course of congenital rubella encephalitis in non-retarded children. J Pediatr 1978; 93:584.

70. Chess S, Fernandez P, Korn S. Behavioral consequences of congenital rubella. J Pediatr 1978; 93:699.

71. Weil ML, Itabashi HH, Cremer NE, et al. Chronic progressive panencephalitis due to rubella virus simulating subacute sclerosing panencephalitis. N Engl J Med 1975; 292:994.

72. Bart KJ, Orenstein WA, Preblud SR, et al. Elimination of rubella and congenital rubella from the United States. Pediatr Infect Dis 1085; 4:14.

73. Rubella and congenital rubella syndrome—New York City. MMWR, December 19, 1986.

74. Rubella vaccination during pregnancy—United States, 1971–86, July 24, 1987.

Toxoplasmosis

75. Wolf A, Cowen D, Paige BH. Toxoplasmic encephalomyelitis. III. A new case of granulomatous encephalomyelitis due to a protozoon. Am J Pathol 1939; 15:657.

76. Remington JS, Desmonts G. Toxoplasmosis. In: Remington JS, Klein JO, eds. Infectious diseases of the fetus and newborn infant. Philadelphia: WB Saunders, 1983:143.

77. Stagno S, Reynolds DW, Amos CS, et al. Auditory and visual defects resulting from symptomatic and subclinical congenital cytomegaloviral and toxoplasma infections. Pediatrics 1977; 59:669.

78. Wilson CB, Remington JS, Stagno S, et al. Development of adverse sequelae in children born with subclinical congenital toxoplasma infection. Pediatrics 1980; 66:767.

79. Couvreur J, Desmonts G. Toxoplasmosis. In: Vinken PJ, Bruyn GW, eds. Handbook of clinical neurology. Vol 35. Infections of the nervous system. Amsterdam: North-Holland, 1978:115.

Syphilis

80. Grossman J. Congenital syphilis. Teratology 1977; 16:217.

81. Centers for Disease Control. Annual summary 1984: reported morbidity and mortality in the United States 1984; 33:59.

82. Brown RJ, Moore MB Jr. Congenital syphilis in the United States. Clin Pediatr 1963; 2:220.

83. Ingall D, Musher D. Syphilis. In: Remington JS, Klein JO, eds. Infectious diseases of the fetus and newborn infant. Philadelphia: WB Saunders 1983:335.

84. Platou RV. Treatment of congenital syphilis. Adv Pediatr 1949; 4:39.

85. Naidoo BT. The cerebrospinal fluid in the healthy newborn infant. S Afr Med J 1968; 42:933.

86. Sarff L, Platt L. McCracken G. Cerebrospinal fluid examination in high risk neonates without meningitis. J Pediatr 1966; 88:473.

87. Srinivasan G, Ramamurthy RS, Bharathi A, et al. Congenital syphilis: a diagnostic and therapeutic dilemma. Pediatr Infect Dis 1983; 2:436.

88. Fiumara NJ, Lessell S. Manifestations of late congenital syphilis. An analysis of 271 patients. Arch Dermatol 1970; 102:78.

89. Speer ME, Mason EO, Scharnberg JT. Cerebrospinal fluid concentrations of aqueous procaine penicillins in the neonate. Pediatrics 1981; 67:387.

Management of the Depressed or Neurologically Dysfunctional Infant

8

Immediate Management

William E. Benitz, M.D., Lorry R. Frankel, M.D., and
David K. Stevenson, M.D.

Objectives of Neonatal Resuscitation
Anticipation
Preparation
Immediate Assessment and Initiation of Resuscitation
Drug Therapy in Neonatal Resuscitation
   Routes of Drug Administration
   Restoration of Metabolic Homeostasis
      Glucose
      Oxygen
      Bicarbonate
   Enhancement of Cardiac Output
      Methods of Increasing the Heart Rate
         Epinephrine and Isoproterenol
         Atropine
         Cardioversion and Defibrillation
      Drugs that Increase Preload
         Crystalloid and Colloid Solutions
         Inotropic Drugs
         Calcium

Management of the infant during the immediate postpartum period is often subject to rigorous scrutiny by malpractice attorneys and their medical consultants. Although recent studies suggest that postpartum events account for only a fraction of untoward outcomes, such as cerebral palsy, mental retardation, and chronic seizure disorders, the potential for cerebral injury during the postpartum period is real, and there is no doubt that skillful resuscitation can spare many distressed infants from exposure to potentially injurious circumstances. The approach to diagnosis and imme-

This work was supported in part by a grant from the General Clinical Research Centers Program of the Division of Research Resources, National Institutes of Health (RR-00081), and the Christopher Taylor Harrison Research Fund. Dr. Benitz is the recipient of a Clinician-Scientist Award from the American Heart Association.

diate management of the distressed neonate should reflect practical and well-coordinated procedures for facilitating the transition from fetal to neonatal cardio-respiratory function, as outlined in a recent review by Stevenson and Benitz.[1] Although extended intensive care may not be possible in level I or even level II nurseries, the current standard of care for any hospital that provides obstetrical delivery services requires availability of personnel who can provide competent resuscitation, emergency stabilization, and preparation for transport by a highly trained neonatal team to the nearest level III facility, if necessary.

OBJECTIVES OF NEONATAL RESUSCITATION

The objectives of neonatal resuscitation must include not only survival of the distressed infant but also mitigation of prepartum or intrapartum injuries and prevention of subsequent cerebral injury. The latter objectives, even more so than the first, require careful attention to each of the factors that affect utilization of metabolic substrates, especially oxygen and glucose, by the brain. Optimal substrate utilization depends on adequate delivery of these materials to the brain, which cannot occur if the infant is hypoxemic or hypoglycemic or if cerebral perfusion is inadequate. Even with normal substrate delivery, however, utilization may be compromised by metabolic disturbances. For example, severe acidosis may impair even anaerobic glucose utilization by inhibiting the activity of phosphofructokinase. The practical goals for neonatal resuscitation may therefore be summarized as follows: Ensure adequate blood levels of oxygen and glucose, ensure adequate cerebral perfusion, primarily by promoting sufficiency of cardiac output, and correct conditions that may impair substrate utilization, such as acidosis or hypothermia.

Effective pursuit of these goals requires recognition of several circumstances that are unique to the fetus who suddenly has become a newborn infant. In utero the placenta serves as the primary organ of gas exchange and the major source of glucose and other nutrients. The establishment of independent respiration, which becomes essential for survival immediately upon separation from the placenta, constitutes the most abrupt and dramatic set of physiologic adjustments required at any stage of life. Adequate gas exchange requires stable gaseous distention of the lungs, markedly increased pulmonary perfusion, and regular and effective respiratory effort. Delay or impairment of these processes represents the most common maladaptation requiring immediate management by a physician or other health care personnel. In addition, the apparently "paradoxical" pressor response of the neonate's pulmonary vasculature to hypoxemia, hypercarbia, and acidosis (the handmaidens of asphyxia) may confound resuscitation attempts. This seemingly "maladaptive" response of the pulmonary vasculature to these stimuli is best understood by reference to the immediately previous fetal state of the neonate.

In the fetus, pulmonary vasoconstriction in response to hypoxemia, hypercarbia, or acidosis results in diversion of a greater proportion of the right ventricular output across the ductus arteriosus into the descending aorta, and hence back to the placenta for gas exchange. Simultaneously, reduced venous return from the lungs to the left atrium may allow an increased flow of blood returning from the placenta across the foramen ovale, effectively increasing the proportion of this oxygenated and "ventilated" blood that is available for perfusion of the brain and heart. The neonate, who no longer has access to a placenta but does have potentially patent fetal circulatory pathways (the foramen ovale and the ductus arteriosus), may exhibit similar vascular responses to asphyxia, resulting in the shunting of blood through fetal pathways (toward umbilical arteries that are no longer connected to a placenta), which may lead paradoxically to serious injury or death rather than correction of the metabolic crisis.[2] For the neonate the "appropriate" response of the fetus becomes an "inappropriate" response, contributing further to hypoxemia, hypercarbia, and acidosis.

This "vicious circle" of physiologic responses often does not break spontaneously until injury has occurred or even until death approaches. Fortunately correction of the "handmaidens of asphyxia" usually can be achieved by assisted ventilation and the administration of oxygen (although administration of sodium bicarbonate also may be required occasionally). Similarly, because the responsibility for maintenance of normoglycemia must be assumed by the neonatal liver immediately after birth, the distressed infant may be at risk for hypoglycemia if hepatic glycogen stores are inadequate

or cannot be mobilized. Removal of the infant from the protected thermal environment of the uterus also mandates markedly increased thermogenesis, which poses a particular challenge for the small wet infant in a cool delivery room. Superimposition of these dramatic physiologic adaptations on any pathologic processes leading to neonatal distress dictates that neonatal resuscitation must incorporate facilitation of the transition from fetus to neonate, as well as restoration of the prior state of homeostasis, which is the predominant feature of resuscitation efforts in older children and adults.

ANTICIPATION

Traditional methods of obstetrical assessment during pregnancy and labor allow diagnosis of many conditions for which neonatal resuscitation may be indicated, including prematurity, placental abruption, vasa or placenta previa, polyhydramnios, and possible sepsis. Recent advances in obstetrical practice have allowed both antenatal detection of fetal distress and antenatal diagnosis of specific fetal anomalies. Whenever these assessment tools provide evidence of any maternal or fetal abnormality that potentially compromises the adaptive response of the newly born infant, a resuscitation team should be in attendance at the delivery. (A partial listing of such conditions has been presented elsewhere.[3]) Some maternal complications, such as preeclampsia or vaginal bleeding, may place the infant at risk for prepartum or intrapartum asphyxia. Others, such as polyhydramnios, oligohydramnios, or poor fetal growth, may suggest intrinsic fetal abnormalities. Meconium staining of the amniotic fluid, aberrant fetal heart rate patterns, or a depressed pH level of the fetal blood (obtained from the scalp) may indicate that fetal homeostasis is compromised; these changes may reflect underlying disease, such as congenital infection, which causes the infant to be intolerant to the stress of normal labor, as well as intercurrent problems, such as cord compression or impaired placental perfusion, which may accentuate this stress. Prenatal screening of isoimmunization, elevated maternal alpha-fetoprotein levels, glucose intolerance, and the like may reveal fetal diseases or conditions that are likely to result in fetal malformations or maladaptation. The increasing use of fetal ultrasonography, both routinely and in evaluation of other risk factors, has substantially increased the number of fetal abnormalities diagnosed early in gestation. More extensive discussion of these methods is provided elsewhere in this volume.

If delivery is not impending and the infant is not in acute distress, referral to a tertiary center should be considered when significant fetal abnormalities are diagnosed. Ideally detection of one of these conditions also should lead to a concerted effort to identify its underlying cause, which often requires collaboration between the obstetrician (or perinatologist) and the pediatrician (or neonatologist). Thus, polyhydramnios should prompt examination for evidence of abnormalities of the fetal gastrointestinal tract or nervous system (by ultrasonography, for example); preterm labor should prompt evaluation for fetal infection, especially if the membranes are ruptured; and so on. These additional investigations often provide specific diagnostic information that allows initiation of specific treatment by the resuscitation team immediately after delivery. In many cases this can be of critical importance. For instance, prenatal diagnosis allows prompt drainage of pleural effusions, which otherwise might thwart resuscitation attempts. Responsibility for the exchange of information relating to fetal distress or fetal abnormalities, which should be a routine part of preparation for neonatal resuscitation, is shared by the obstetrical and pediatric staffs.

PREPARATION

Personnel trained to resuscitate distressed newborn infants must be readily available, 24 hours a day, in any hospital that offers obstetrical services. Training and supervision of these personnel should be the responsibility of a physician or group of physicians, who are designated to prepare, review, and periodically revise protocols for resuscitation of infants in the delivery rooms. The composition of the resuscitation team may vary, depending on the personnel available in each hospital. In general, this team must have at least two members, one of whom is skilled in immediate assessment, initiation of resuscitation, and stabilization of the infant prior to transport to the nursery. He must be able to provide endotracheal intubation, assisted ventilation, umbilical catheter placement, and drug administration, as required. These tasks often are assigned to an anesthesiologist, pediatrician, or another physician. If a physician is not always available, these responsibilities may be assumed by a nurse or respiratory therapist. In teaching hospitals they may be shared by the house staff but should be delegated only to those who have learned the techniques and principles of resuscitation under supervision. It is never appropriate to expect an inexperienced individual to resuscitate a potentially sick neonate.

When delivery of a distressed infant is anticipated, responsibility for various aspects of the resuscitation should be clearly delegated to each team member prior to delivery. These tasks depend on the problems anticipated. One team member should attend to the airway and assist breathing, if necessary. Another should palpate the cord or auscultate the heart to assess the heart rate, provide this information to the team, and initiate chest compressions, if required. A third should be responsible for other procedures, such as umbilical vessel cannulation or thoracentesis. If necessary, others should prepare and administer drugs and record the progress of the resuscitation. Ideally the individual directing the resuscitation should not be responsible for any of these

tasks so that he or she can give full attention to overseeing the work of the entire team.

Items of equipment required for resuscitation are listed in Table 8–1. This equipment must be checked periodically to ensure that all items are readily available and in working order. If the nursery is not adjacent to the delivery room, additional equipment may be needed in the delivery room or resuscitation room to allow more thorough stabilization of the infant prior to transfer to the nursery, as indicated in Table 8–1. Ready access to equipment for blood gas and hematocrit determinations is also essential. In addition to these items, which should be routinely available, there are often occasions when other materials are required. For example, blood products (preferably cross matched against maternal blood) should be available for infants with severe isoimmune hemolytic disease or blood loss due to placenta or vasa previa, and large bore intravenous catheters should be available to drain large pleural or pericardial effusions.

IMMEDIATE ASSESSMENT AND INITIATION OF RESUSCITATION

Immediate assessment of the distressed infant by experienced personnel is of critical importance. This process should begin with immediate observation of the infant's tone, color, heart rate, respiratory effort, and response to the stimulation of being dried with a towel or warm blanket for 10 to 20 seconds. Continuous observation of these physiologic parameters throughout the resuscitation should allow continuing evaluation of

TABLE 8–1   Equipment for Neonatal Resuscitation

Resuscitation table with radiant heat
Overhead illumination (100 foot-candles minimum)
Wall clock with sweep second hand
Compressed air and oxygen sources
Gas blender and heated humidifier
Bulb syringes and DeLee suction catheters
Adjustable suction and sterile suction catheters
Infant stethoscope
Face masks (Bird or Bennett sizes 1 to 4 or Ambu sizes
  O and OA)
Laryngoscopes with infant blades (e.g., Miller 0 and 1)
Endotracheal tubes (2.5, 3.0, 3.5, and 4.0 mm ID) with stylets
Anesthesia-ventilation bags, 500 ml, with adjustable pop-off
  valves and pressure manometers (non-self-inflating type
  preferred)
Nasogastric tubes, 5 and 8 French
Sterile syringes and needles
Umbilical catheters (3.5 and 5 French)
Intravenous catheters, infusion sets, and tubing
Intravenous fluid solutions (D5W, D10W, heparin 1 U/ml in
  normal saline)
Resuscitation medications

Additional equipment for extended resuscitation and stabilization
  Sterile umbilical catheterization trays
  Pressure transducers and monitors
  Transcutaneous oxygen tension or saturation monitors
  Thoracostomy trays and tubes (10 and 12 French)

the efficacy of the resuscitation measures and the need for continued or more vigorous resuscitation. The traditional use of these criteria for assignment of the Apgar score at one and five minutes should not discourage earlier assessment of the infant's condition. Similarly, if the neonate does not respond promptly to resuscitation, Apgar scores should be assigned and recorded every five minutes up to 20 minutes of age or until the infant achieves two consecutive scores of 8 or more.

Most neonates respond quickly to standard resuscitative maneuvers, which should follow the same protocol regardless of the setting or cause of distress (Table 8–2). The first priority is establishment of airway patency. Positioning of the head and neck to attain the "sniffing" position, with slight extension of the neck and jaw thrust, is usually adequate to obtain an open airway. Endotracheal intubation provides definitive control of the airway, which is much easier to maintain during application of other resuscitation procedures, such as chest compressions, and should not be delayed if the infant does not respond promptly to bag-mask ventilation. If spontaneous respiration is inadequate by visual inspection or auscultation, breathing should be assisted, even before hypoventilation is documented by measuring the PCO_2 in arterial blood. If the heart rate cannot be auscultated or the pulse is not palpable or is weak in the context of poor peripheral perfusion, or if the heart rate remains below 100 beats per minute, circulation should be supported by immediate initiation of external cardiac compressions. If these maneuvers do not effect prompt recovery of the heart rate, color, and respiratory effort, drug administration is usually required (to be described). The cardiac electrical rhythm electrocardiogram should be monitored continuously, as soon as possible after birth. Failure to improve should suggest that the FIO_2 is insufficient; this most commonly occurs when self-inflating ventilation bags entrap room air because the oxygen reservoir is improperly connected or the oxygen flow rate is inadequate.

Glucose also should be administered as soon as venous access is attained, because hypoglycemic infants may be refractory to all resuscitative efforts. Radiant heat should be provided to prevent hypothermia, which increases metabolic requirements, impairs myocardial performance, and increases vascular resistance. Systematic application of a well-defined protocol is essential to ensure effective resuscitation and allows the resuscitation team to proceed with confidence that critical interventions are not being neglected. The optimal application of these protocols requires continuous reevaluation of the infant and adjustment of resuscitation measures as the infant's condition changes.

For infants with a vigorous cry, a heart rate greater than 120 beats per minute, and good tone, color, and reflex irritability (i.e., an Apgar score of 8 to 10), no resuscitation (beyond routine suctioning and observation) is required. If the infant has a good heart rate (more than 120 beats per minute) but has poor air exchange, shallow or intermittent respiratory effort, and pallor or cyanosis (an Apgar score of 5 to 7), oxygen should be administered by mask and airway patency should be ensured by head and jaw positioning and suctioning of the oropharynx. If the infant responds quickly, no further resuscitation may be needed. If the respiratory effort does not improve or if the heart rate decreases, assisted ventilation should be initiated immediately. More severely depressed infants who are apneic or have only occasional gasps and little tone or irritability but have heart rates greater than 120 beats per minute (an Apgar score of 2 to 4) should receive immediate assisted ventilation with 100 percent oxygen. Most infants respond rapidly to this intervention with an increased heart rate, color, and respiratory effort. If such a response is not observed within 15 to 30 seconds, the airway should be secured by intubating the trachea, and assisted ventilation should be continued. If the infant has an initial heart rate less than 120 beats per minute (an Apgar score of 0 to 1), or if the heart rate decreases during resuscitation, assisted ventilation with 100 percent oxygen by mask may be attempted briefly (10 to 20 seconds) but is usually not sufficient. Unless there is a virtually instantaneous improvement, prompt initiation of endotracheal intubation, ventilation with 100 percent oxygen, and chest compressions are necessary. Failure to improve after these measures should prompt consideration of drug therapy to correct metabolic disorders or other conditions that impair cardiac output, such as hypovolemia. Identification and treatment of underlying diseases, such as pneumothorax, congenital heart disease, or pulmonary malformations (e.g., diaphragmatic hernia), also become critically important in this circumstance. Inadvertent deviations from optimal resuscitation techniques, such as esophageal or endobronchial intubation or ventilation with air rather than oxygen also must be considered.

DRUG THERAPY IN NEONATAL RESUSCITATION

The pharmacology of neonatal resuscitation is the subject of a recent review, which is included here with some modification.[4,5] Drugs used in neonatal resuscitation may be classified as agents that restore or maintain

TABLE 8–2   The ABCs of Neonatal Resuscitation

Airway	Electrocardiogram
Breathing	FIO_2
Circulation	Glucose
Drugs	Heat

From Benitz WE, Frankel LR, Stevenson DK. The pharmacology of neonatal resuscitation and cardiopulmonary intensive care. Part I. Immediate resuscitation. West J Med 1986; 144:704.

metabolic homeostasis, increase cardiac output, alter the distribution of the circulation, alter pulmonary function or gas exchange, or treat the underlying condition. Those in the first two of these categories are discussed in this chapter; the remaining three groups are addressed in Chapter 9.

Routes of Drug Administration

Drugs such as epinephrine and atropine can be administered into the endotracheal tube prior to the establishment of vascular access. However, vascular access is virtually always possible within minutes by cannulation of the umbilical vein.[6] Only the presence of an omphalocele or another major anomaly involving the umbilical anatomy precludes easy access. Although passage of a catheter through the ductus venosus into the vena cava or right atrium is usually easy during the transitional period immediately after birth, it may not be possible after a very short time and generally is difficult after 12 hours of age. Under emergency conditions it usually can be assumed that the tip of the catheter is above the diaphragm if it has been advanced 10 cm into the vessel (6 to 8 cm in the premature infant) and blood can be withdrawn freely, and drugs may be administered through the catheter. If the catheter tip is in the portal venous system, there is a risk of hepatic or intestinal injury, but such injury is uncommon and the danger is outweighed by the risks of cardiopulmonary dysfunction necessitating the drug therapy. Radiographic documentation is necessary to confirm appropriate placement of the catheter before it can be used for drug administration after the emergency has resolved, however. Insertion of the umbilical arterial catheter requires greater skill and usually should not be attempted during the first few minutes of a resuscitation, unless the resuscitation team is prepared for this procedure with designated personnel assigned to the task.

These measures ultimately provide access for measuring the blood pressure and sampling for blood gas determinations. However, intense splanchnic, renal, and peripheral vasoconstriction may occur after administration of catecholamines into arterial catheters, which should be avoided. Thus, the early placement of an umbilical venous catheter into a central position is advisable for the administration of vasopressor drugs, both early in resuscitation and in the extended care of the distressed infant. The distressed infant often has poor peripheral perfusion, making percutaneous venous cannulation for peripheral infusions or placement of a central venous catheter very difficult. Under emergency conditions in which no access is available, a 16 or 18 gauge needle can be placed into the tibial or femoral marrow cavity for the administration of fluids and drugs.[7] As a last resort, administration of drugs via direct cardiac puncture is possible, but this poses serious hazards, including intramyocardial injection, with necrosis, pneumopericardium or hemopericardium, or pneumothorax.

Restoration of Metabolic Homeostasis

Drug therapy in neonatal resuscitation is directed primarily at correction of metabolic abnormalities. Glucose, oxygen, and bicarbonate can restore or maintain metabolic homeostasis by providing substrates for cellular metabolism or correcting abnormalities that impair the capacity of cells to utilize substrate.

Glucose

The infant depends on glucose as a major energy substrate during the transitional period. The cessation of glucose delivery via the placenta at the time of birth predisposes the neonate to hypoglycemia. Under normal circumstances the term neonate can easily mobilize hepatic glycogen stores to maintain blood glucose levels as well as begin gluconeogenesis. Premature infants and intrauterine growth-retarded infants may have minimal glycogen stores and sometimes impaired gluconeogenesis, making them more vulnerable to hypoglycemia. Infants of diabetic mothers have abnormal metabolism, with inability to mobilize hepatic glycogen and impaired gluconeogenesis. Some premature infants who have been exposed to beta-mimetic drugs may have exhausted hepatic glycogen stores as well as enhanced insulin release. Moreover, glucose consumption may be increased by such conditions as hypoxia, hypothermia, hyperthermia, or infection. These factors account for the occurrence of hypoglycemia in most cases.[8] Hypoglycemia can be rapidly documented in the neonate by using any of several bedside colorimetric methods (Chemstrip bG, Dextrostix) and should be confirmed by measurement of the blood glucose level by the glucose oxidase method. During resuscitation, therapy for suspected hypoglycemia often has to be initiated without the benefit of these diagnostic tests, however.

If the clinical circumstances suggest hypoglycemia or if the blood glucose level is less than 40 mg per deciliter, intravenous administration of glucose (100 to 200 mg per kilogram or 1 to 2 ml per kilogram of 10 percent dextrose solution in water) should be followed by a continuous infusion of glucose at 6 to 8 mg per kilogram per minute. Except when glucose utilization is increased, as in the infant of a diabetic mother or a premature infant exposed prenatally to beta-mimetic drugs, the administration of glucose at that rate is usually sufficient to maintain euglycemia. Infants of diabetic mothers, and sometimes infants with hypoxia, hypothermia, hyperthermia, or sepsis, may require infusions exceeding this rate, and therapy should be started at a rate of 8 to 10 mg per kilogram per minute. Infants with adequate hepatic glycogen stores, such as infants of diabetic mothers, can be treated with glucagon (300 μg per kilogram, up to a total of 1 mg), administered intramuscularly, in order to transiently correct hypoglycemia while venous access is established. Although serious cerebral injury may not result from periods of hypoglycemia in excess of one hour, hypoglycemia represents a medical emergency, which should be corrected within minutes. To state it bluntly, the physician should not leave the infant unattended until the problem is corrected or the threat to the infant from hypoglycemia is considered resolved. Frequent measurement of the blood glucose level and repeated administration of glucose boluses until stable euglycemia is documented are requirements in standard care.

Oxygen

A physiologic classification of hypoxic conditions is presented in Table 8–3. The administration of oxygen is the most straightforward approach to correcting tissue hypoxia in many of these conditions. Hypotonic hypoxemia (group I, Table 8–3) is most likely to be responsive. Ventilation-perfusion mismatching, due to pneumonia or aspiration, or impaired oxygen diffusion, due to retained fluid or the respiratory distress syndrome, is likely to respond to supplemental oxygen alone. Other conditions usually require more specific therapies, such as assisted ventilation for hypoventilation. If there is fixed right to left shunting, as in cyanotic congenital heart disease, the administration of oxygen will not correct hypoxemia, but the lack of response may be of diagnostic importance.

During resuscitation in the delivery room, the administered oxygen concentration should be 100 percent. Until the nature of the hypoxia is delineated, it is appropriate to administer oxygen to any infant with cyanosis or respiratory distress. As the infant responds to resuscitation, the FIO_2 value may be decreased but should be maintained at levels sufficient to relieve distress and keep the infant pink. As soon as possible, arterial blood gas measurements should be carried out to guide further adjustments of the FIO_2 level. In the premature infant a PaO_2 level of 50 to 60 mm Hg is usually adequate, but a PaO_2 level of 100 to 120 mm Hg is more desirable in an infant with persistent pulmonary hypertension. Whether oxygenation is adequate depends on other factors, including oxygen carrying capacity and cardiac output (to be discussed). Failure to respond to oxygen administration should initiate a search for mechanical problems in the delivery system, such as kinked tubing, air entrainment, or disconnection of the oxygen source.

Oxygen should be considered as a drug, for it is potentially toxic as well as therapeutic. It has been associated with bronchopulmonary dysplasia, adult respiratory distress syndrome, and retinopathy of prematurity. Although concerns about toxicity warrant close attention to titration of the FIO_2 to the minimal level compatible with adequate arterial oxygenation, the withholding of oxygen from any distressed infant cannot be justified.

Bicarbonate

Correction of acidemia can result in improved cardiac output, tissue perfusion, and substrate utilization by reversing numerous detrimental effects, including impaired myocardial function, increased systemic and pulmonary vascular resistance, reduced response to catecholamines, and inhibition of oxidative glucose metabolism. During cardiorespiratory arrest or following severe asphyxia, bicarbonate may be given empirically at a dose of 1 mEq per kilogram followed by additional doses of 0.5 to 1 mEq per kilogram about every 10 minutes. Arterial blood gas measurements should be used to guide the bicarbonate dosage as soon as possible. Unless the pH is less than 7.2, bicarbonate administration is usually unnecessary. Metabolic acidosis caused by the accumulation of lactic acid after a short period of asphyxia usually corrects spontaneously, as lactate is converted in the liver to pyruvate and oxidative metabolism is reestablished. Persistent metabolic acidosis, resulting from the accumulation of organic acids, suggests inadequate delivery of substrate to tissues (decreased cardiac output, severe anemia), toxic hypoxia (sepsis, severe asphyxia), localized tissue infarction (necrotizing enterocolitis, intracranial hemorrhage, pulmonary hemorrhage), or inborn errors of metabolism. In these conditions bicarbonate administration is useful only as a

TABLE 8–3   Physiologic Classification of Hypoxic Conditions

Physiologic Category	Group I Hypotonic Hypoxemia	Group II Normotonic Hypoxemia	Group III Hypodynamic Hypoxia	Group IV Histotoxic Hypoxia
Arterial O₂ tension	↓	↔	↔	↔
Arterial O₂ content	↓	↓	↔	↔
Arterial O₂ saturation	↓	↔	↔	↔
O₂ carrying capacity	↔	↓	↔	↔
Mixed venous O₂ saturation	↓	↓	↓	↑
Cardiac Output	↔,↑	↑	↓	↔,↑
Tissue O₂ use	↓,↔	↓,↔	↓,↔	↓

↓ = decreased; ↑ = increased, ↔ = unchanged

From Benitz WE, Frankel LR, Stevenson DK. The pharmacology of neonatal resuscitation and cardiopulmonary intensive care. Part I. Immediate resuscitation. West J Med 1986; 144:704.

transitional measure to allow survival until the underlying problem can be corrected.

Expeditious documentation of adequate alveolar ventilation is essential, because bicarbonate administration is contraindicated by inadequate ventilation.[9] In fact, the blood pH does not increase and the cerebrospinal fluid pH *decreases* after bicarbonate administration unless adequate alveolar ventilation ensures excretion of the carbon dioxide generated by the buffer reaction.[10] Overcorrection of the pH to near 7.4 early in resuscitation also may be detrimental, because subsequent metabolism of endogenous acids may lead to significant metabolic alkalosis, which impairs the dissociation of oxygen from hemoglobin and may impede oxygen delivery. Rapid infusion of hypertonic solutions should also be avoided.[11] The drug should be infused over five to 10 minutes, and the concentration should never exceed 0.5 mEq per milliliter (1,000 mOsm per liter). Catecholamines are inactivated by bicarbonate and calcium salts cause precipitation.

Enhancement of Cardiac Output

Clinical signs of decreased cardiac output include pallor, mottling, prolonged capillary filling times (more than three to four seconds), and cool or cyanotic extremities. Because of immature autonomic regulation of vascular tone, these findings are variably observed in very low birth weight infants of less than 28 weeks' gestation, even when cardiac output is severely compromised. Hypotension and tachycardia may be manifestations of decreased cardiac output, but the absence of these findings does not rule out impaired cardiac output; sick newborn infants may not mount an adequate sympathetic response (and thus no tachycardia), and the blood pressure may be maintained by increased systemic vascular resistance, even with a substantially impaired systemic blood flow. Nonetheless the arterial blood pressure in the neonate should be measured immediately on admission to the nursery, if not in the delivery room, because a low systemic blood pressure can be the sole cause of persistent cyanosis and imposes a clear risk of inadequate perfusion of vital tissues. If a low arterial blood pressure persists despite initiation of cardiorespiratory support with 100 percent oxygen and assisted ventilation, supportive therapy should be undertaken immediately. Urine output, although useless early in resuscitation, later becomes another indicator of cardiac output. A urine output of less than 1 ml per hour, a urine sodium concentration of less than 10 to 15 mEq per liter (20 mEq per liter in the premature infant), or a fractional sodium excretion of less than 1 percent suggests that renal perfusion or intravascular volume is inadequate. Unfortunately urine flow and sodium excretion may be maintained in the immature infant because of immature renal function. Inappropriate diuresis can also result

from acute renal failure. Metabolic acidosis (see foregoing) is a late sign of severely compromised cardiac output. Doppler echocardiography may provide semiquantitative information in a given individual,[12] but more classic techniques such as thermodilution are unreliable because of shunting through fetal pathways. Assessment of the cardiac output in the neonate therefore still depends primarily on the physical examination.

In general, the drugs that affect cardiac output exert their action through the following effects on the primary determinants of cardiac output: improvement of cardiac rate and rhythm (chronotropy), increasing ventricular end diastolic volume (preload), enhancement of myocardial contractility (inotropy), and reduction of vascular resistance (afterload). Drugs that primarily affect heart rate and preload are discussed in the following sections; those used for their inotropic or vasodilatory effects are discussed in Chapter 9.

Methods of Increasing the Heart Rate

Unlike the adult, the newborn infant does not respond to bradycardia with an increased stroke volume, because the volume of the relatively noncompliant ventricles in the neonate is not significantly increased by increased end diastolic pressures resulting from longer diastolic intervals. Cardiac output in the infant is therefore virtually a linear function of heart rate, and is substantially compromised by even modest bradycardia.[13] A heart rate between 120 and 160 beats per minute in term infants or 140 to 180 beats per minute in preterm infants is usually sufficient to sustain an adequate cardiac output.

Although the heart rate generally responds to the administration of 100 percent oxygen and assisted ventilation, there are other causes of bradycardia in the neonate. The correction of bradycardia is generally nonspecific, although there may be specific causes, including increased vagal tone (often because of visceral distention), central nervous system dysfunction (associated with the postasphyxial state), congenital heart block (which may be associated with maternal systemic lupus erythematosus), and maternal medication (such as propranolol). Low birth weight infants occasionally may have low heart rates because of hypocalcemia. Thus, besides decompression of a distended organ, such as the intestine or bladder, persistent bradycardia can be treated with atropine, calcium administration in the low birth weight infant, or chronotropic drug support (to be discussed).

Epinephrine and Isoproterenol. Epinephrine (0.1 ml per kilogram of a 1/10,000 solution) can be administered intravenously or intratracheally in infants with bradycardia or asystole and may help restore myocardial contractility in infants with electromechanical dissociation. The dose may be repeated every three to five minutes until an adequate cardiac rhythm is obtained. The drug has both beta- and alpha-adrenergic effects[14] and remains the primary choice for managing bradycardia in the neonate. If repeated doses are required to maintain a heart rate of greater than 120, an isoproterenol infusion (0.1 to 1.5 μg per kilogram per minute, titrated to achieve the desired heart rate) can be started. If alpha-adrenergic effects are desirable, epinephrine can be infused continuously (0.1 to 1 μg per kilogram per minute). The latter drug is better for maintaining systemic arterial pressure, for hypotension commonly complicates infusion of isoproterenol at higher doses. Isoproterenol is a pure beta-adrenergic agonist. Notably epinephrine is ineffective if the systemic pH is less than 7.1 and is inactivated by admixture with alkaline solutions. Tachycardia can occur, and excessive doses may impair renal, splanchnic, or peripheral perfusion. Extravasation of the drug peripherally or intramyocardial injection may cause local tissue necrosis.

Atropine. The dosage of atropine is 0.01 to 0.04 mg per kilogram every two to five minutes, as indicated for bradycardia with compromised cardiac output or for second or third degree heart block. It also may be effective for asystole refractory to epinephrine and calcium, but this circumstance is encountered infrequently. Because the response is dependent on vagolytic effects mediated by peripheral blockade of the muscarinic effects of acetylcholine, the degree of vagal tone is an important determinant of the efficacy of atropine. Vagal blockade usually is complete after cumulative doses of 0.1 mg per kilogram; thus doses in excess of this amount are unlikely to be beneficial. Atropine can cause tachyarrhythmias and increases myocardial oxygen consumption at therapeutic doses.

Cardioversion and Defibrillation. Electrical stimulation of the heart is rarely indicated during neonatal resuscitation in the delivery room, because infants who might require this therapy usually already have sustained an overwhelming injury. The dose is 1 to 2 watts per second per kilogram using pediatric paddles, which occasionally may restore a normal cardiac rhythm in infants with ventricular fibrillation, ventricular tachycardia, or asystole.

Drugs That Increase Preload

Because the cardiac ventricles of the neonate are less compliant than those of adults,[15] increased cardiac output does not result from expansion of an already adequate vascular volume. Nonetheless inadequate end diastolic pressures due to decreased intravascular volume is one of the most common correctable causes of decreased cardiac output in the neonate, and hypovolemia always should be suspected in an infant who appears to be poorly perfused in spite of an adequate heart rate and assisted ventilation. This condition also should be expected in several clinical circumstances, such as placenta or vasa previa and severe hydrops fetalis. Hypovolemia may masquerade as respiratory distress, presenting with grunting respiration in the absence of apparent pulmonary disease, arterial spasm associated with an umbilical artery catheter, or refractory hypoxemia in an infant who is easily ventilated.

If hypovolemia is suspected, the best diagnostic procedure is also therapeutic: administration of 10 to 20 ml per kilogram of blood or plasma. In the acute resuscitation situation, the clinical response (improved color and perfusion) may be the only indicator of efficacy. Later, invasive measurement of the central venous pressure, which is most readily achieved by catheterization of the umbilical vein, may serve as a guide to the adequacy of the intravascular volume. Positioning of the catheter tip must be documented, because crossing into the left atrium is not uncommon. Central venous pressures as high as 8 to 10 mm Hg or left atrial pressures of 12 to 15 mm Hg may be required to achieve an optimal cardiac output in a sick infant. End diastolic pressures are slightly lower. However, isolated measurement of the central venous pressure is of little value unless considered in a clinical context; no reliance should be placed on absolute numbers without establishing their relationship to the clinical condition of the neonate. The intravascular volume may be adequate or excessive with a high central venous pressure, which simply may reflect a reduced capacity of the ventricles to accommodate and pump the quantity of blood returning to the heart (heart failure). If the central venous pressure is subnormal, the effects of transfusion of blood or plasma should be assessed. If blood or colloid solution is not available, the administration of crystalloid solution will temporarily increase the intravascular volume and cardiac output. If transfusion results in a sustained increase in the central venous or left atrial pressure, it can be assumed that the intravascular volume is adequate, especially if blood pressure and peripheral perfusion also improve. If filling pressures are not increased after volume administration, or rapidly decline to pretransfusion levels, the infant is hypovolemic, and additional volume expansion is indicated. A single transfusion may not be adequate for sustaining the blood pressure, necessitating continuous monitoring and repeated small transfusions as indicated by the clinical condition of the neonate. In septic or severely asphyxiated infants, surprisingly large quantities of volume expanders may be required to achieve an intravascular volume sufficient to maintain a cardiac output adequate for vital organ metabolism. Occasionally the fluid needed to maintain the intravascular volume may exceed the infant's blood volume.

Crystalloid and Colloid Solutions. Normal saline solution is always readily available, inexpensive, and well tolerated when used empirically. The dosage is 20 ml per kilogram, which may be given in two doses of 10 ml per kilogram. After administration, complications such as hyponatremia, hypervolemia, and metabolic acidosis are highly unlikely. Albumin or plasma protein fractions are readily available and easily stored. The dosage is 10 ml per kilogram. Although these drugs are distributed primarily into the vascular space, these effects are short lived, and the protein may be distributed extravascularly into the periphery or pulmonary tissues, exacerbating anasarca and pulmonary edema. The products are also expensive. The preferred product is fresh frozen plasma, because it contains more high molecular weight components as well as immunoglobulins, complement, and clotting factors. The mainstay of volume expansion, particularly when blood loss is suspected, is packed erythrocytes diluted to the desired hematocrit level with fresh frozen plasma. Cytomegalovirus seronegative, type specific or type O Rh negative blood cross-matched against the mother's blood is ideal and should be available if delivery of a severely ill infant is anticipated. Non-cross-matched type O Rh negative blood also can be used in emergencies, but transfusion reactions sometimes occur. The hematocrit level should be measured within four hours after administration to determine whether additional transfusions may be required.

Inotropic Drugs. Impaired myocardial function can result from many conditions that require specific treatment, such as sepsis (especially due to group B streptococcus, which produces a cardiotoxin), metabolic derangements, including acidemia, hypoglycemia, and hypocalcemia, and intrinsic disorders of the myocardium, such as hypertrophic cardiomyopathy (infants of diabetic mothers) or myocardial edema (hydrops fetalis). Cardiotonic therapy is indicated only after correction of the heart rate and intravascular volume (combined with exclusion of anatomic heart disease and cardiogenic persistent pulmonary hypertension of the newborn) has failed to correct systemic hypotension and other signs of poor cardiac output, including poor peripheral perfusion, low urine output, and hypoxemia. During acute resuscitation, inotropic therapy consists primarily of calcium administration (to be described). As the infant is stabilized, administration of catecholamines (dopamine or dobutamine) may also be required; these drugs are discussed in Chapter 9. Such cardiotonic therapy should be undertaken by the primary care physician only in preparation for transport of the infant to a level III nursery, in consultation with the neonatologist who will be caring for the infant in the level III facility.

Calcium. Calcium has been shown to increase the heart rate, cardiac contractility, and blood pressure in premature infants with hypocalcemia[16,17] and may be useful in infants with low ionized calcium levels, as may occur after massive transfusions. During resuscitation, calcium chloride (20 mg per kilogram per dose, given intravenously over several minutes) is the preferred salt. It may be useful in the management of cardiac arrest or electromechanical dissociation. The dose can be repeated every 10 minutes as required. Extravasation of calcium results in rapid tissue necrosis. For nonemergency situations calcium gluconate (50 to 100 mg per kilogram every four to six hours) is a better choice, because it is less toxic to tissues.

Neonatal resuscitation is among the most frequently criticized medical activities in medicolegal litigation. The practitioner is both obligated and well-advised to ensure that resuscitation of the neonate is consistently performed skillfully and expeditiously. Optimal resuscitation requires anticipation and preparation, which demand collaboration between the obstetrician and pediatrician. Resuscitation should begin as soon as possible after delivery and should follow a specific and well-designed protocol for infant assessment and intervention. The practitioner responsible for resuscitation must be prepared to secure the airway, by endotracheal intubation if necessary, provide positive pressure breathing with a ventilation bag, cannulate umbilical vessels, and administer appropriate resuscitation drugs. Measures to address underlying conditions must not be neglected. Most important, this individual must take charge of the situation and direct the activities of the other health care personnel assisting in the resuscitation, to ensure that it is carried out well. Skillful resuscitation should minimize postnatal cerebral injury, by ensuring adequate delivery of substrate to the brain, but cannot be expected to alter the nature or severity of injury that has occurred prior to delivery.

REFERENCES

1. Stevenson DK, Benitz WE. A practical approach to diagnosis and immediate care of the cyanotic neonate. Clin Pediatr 1987; 26:325.
2. Smith CA, Nelson NM. The physiology of the newborn infant. Springfield, Illinois: Charles C Thomas, 1976:61.
3. Brann AW Jr, Cefalo RC, eds. Guidelines for perinatal care. Elk Grove, Illinois: American Academy of Pediatrics, 1983:260.
4. Benitz WE, Frankel LR, Stevenson DK. The pharmacology of neonatal resuscitation and cardiopulmonary intensive care. Part I. Immediate resuscitation. West J Med 1986; 144:704.
5. Benitz WE, Frankel LR, Stevenson DK. The pharmacology of neonatal resuscitation and cardiopulmonary intensive care. Part II. Extended intensive care. West J Med 1986; 145:47.
6. Kitterman JA, Phibbs RH, Tooley WH. Catheterization of umbilical vessels in newborn infants. Pediatr Clin North Am 1970; 17:895.
7. Berg RA. Emergency infusion of catecholamines into bone marrow. Am J Dis Child 1984; 138:810.
8. Cornblath M, Schwartz R. Hypoglycemia in the neonate. In: Disorders of carbohydrate metabolism in infancy. Philadelphia: WB Saunders, 1976:155.
9. Bishop RL, Weisfeldt ML. Sodium bicarbonate administration during cardiac arrest—effect on arterial pH, PCO_2 and osmolality. JAMA 1976; 235:506.
10. Berenyi KJ, Work M, Killip T. Cerebrospinal fluid acidosis complicating therapy of experimental cardiopulmonary arrest. Circulation 1975; 52:319.
11. Papile L, Burnstein J, Burnstein R, et al. Relationship of intravenous sodium bicarbonate infusions and cerebrospinal intraventricular hemorrhage. J Pediatr 1978; 93:834.

12. Alverson DC, Eldridge M, Dillon T, et al. Noninvasive pulsed Doppler determination of cardiac output in neonates and children. J Pediatr 1982; 101:46.

13. Rudolph AM, Heymann MA. Circulatory changes during growth in the fetal lamb. Circ Res 1970; 26:289.

14. Zaritsky A, Chernow B. Use of catecholamines in pediatrics. J Pediatr 1984; 105:341.

15. Romero T, Fridman WF. Limited left ventricular response to volume overload in the neonatal period: a comparative study with the adult animal. Pediatr Res 1979; 13:910.

16. Salsburey DJ, Brown DR. Effect of parenteral calcium treatment on blood pressure and heart rate in neonatal hypocalcemia. Pediatrics 1982; 69:605.

17. Mirro R, Brown DJ. Parenteral calcium treatment shortens the left ventricular systolic time intervals of hypocalcemic neonates. Pediatr Res 1984; 18:71.

9

Extended Management

William E. Benitz, M.D., Lorry R. Frankel, M.D., and David K. Stevenson, M.D.

Supporting Ventilation
Sustaining Cardiac Output
   Inotropic Drugs
      Dopamine
      Dobutamine
   Afterload Reduction
      Nitroprusside
Management of Anemia
Evaluation and Management of Refractory Hypoxemia
   Hyperoxia Test
   Detection of Ductal Shunting
   Hyperoxia-Hyperventilation Test
   Severe Pulmonary Parenchymal Disease
   Pulmonary Arterial Disease
   Cyanotic Congenital Heart Disease
Consultation and Referral

The events that comprise the period of extended intensive care of the depressed neonate are subject to medicolegal challenge less frequently than are those of the immediate resuscitation and prenatal periods. In part this may be the case because infants requiring extended intensive care are among the most critically ill and usually are transferred to level III intensive care nurseries where their management can be supervised by board-certified neonatologists. The range of therapies that can be undertaken in these well-equipped facilities, with sub-specialist consultants and specifically trained nurses and other personnel, is quite broad and encompasses a variety of treatments that address specifically identified disabilities or dysfunctions. Within this spectrum of medical practice are many different management schemes that may be acceptable. It is not the intent in this chapter to review all the management protocols used for the numerous conditions encountered in neonatal intensive care. Rather we focus on the early transitional period following birth and resuscitation, during which the condition of a depressed infant can be substantially improved by expert care.

Failure to provide competent care, optimizing the opportunity for cerebral recovery, while the infant is prepared for referral to a level III intensive care nursery, is frequently the basis for litigation. As is the case with the initial resuscitation, the condition of the infant during this period may have been determined by factors whose effects were incurred prior to or during the delivery and initial resuscitation, many of which are beyond the control of the obstetrician and neonatologist. It is also important to recognize that significant neurologic or physiologic compromise is not always evident in poor Apgar scores; thus significant problems may become apparent only after an infant with good initial Apgar scores has left the intensive care environment. Nonetheless it is possible to identify many infants who require continuing intensive care after the initial resuscitation, including all those who remain depressed, require vigorous resuscitation, or remain dependent on supplemental oxygen, assisted ventilation, or drug administration. The roles of pharmacologic therapy in extended intensive care and in the management of refractory neonatal hypoxemia have been reviewed recently in detail.[1] In this chapter we provide an overview of the aspects of extended intensive care that address maintenance of cerebral integrity and preparation for transfer to a level III facility, and provide recommendations for the implementation of these interventions by the primary care

Study supported by a grant (RR81) from the General Research Centers Program of the Division of Research Resources, National Institutes of Health, and the Christopher Taylor Harrison Research Fund. Dr. Benitz is the recipient of a Clinician-Scientist Award from the American Heart Association.

practitioner.[2] These interventions consist of sustaining ventilation, supporting cardiac output, correcting anemia, and evaluating and initiating therapy for hypoxemia.

SUPPORTING VENTILATION

Assisted ventilation should be provided for any infant who is not able to maintain acceptable arterial blood gas levels without such assistance, or who does so only with extreme effort. The range of desired arterial oxygen tensions depends on the clinical circumstances, as indicated in Chapter 8. In the premature infant a PaO_2 level of 50 to 60 mm Hg is usually adequate, but a PaO_2 of 100 to 120 mm Hg is more desirable in an infant with persistent pulmonary hypertension. In some situations extremely vigorous support (with a concomitant risk of adverse effects, such as pneumothorax, adult respiratory distress syndrome, or bronchopulmonary dysplasia) may be required to achieve these "ideal" arterial oxygen tensions. In this setting it may be preferable to accept lower oxygen tensions (35 to 50 mm Hg) if this allows less vigorous utilization of positive pressure ventilation or greatly reduced inspired oxygen concentrations, as long as both the oxygen carrying capacity of the blood and the cardiac output are good. These compromises should be made only after consultation with a neonatologist at the level III nursery, however.

Similarly, the target range for the $PaCO_2$ level depends on the diagnosis. Although the "normal" range is 35 to 45 mm Hg, higher values are often accepted as long as the arterial pH level is not excessively depressed, because these values may be achieved with less aggressive mandatory ventilation, especially in patients with pulmonary parenchymal disease, such as hyaline membrane disease. On the other hand, infants with persistent pulmonary hypertension are often hyperventilated in order to achieve elevated arterial pH values (7.55 or higher) and decreased $PaCO_2$ values (30 mm Hg or less). Some have advocated hyperventilation of infants after episodes of apparent asphyxia, but few centers routinely employ this practice, and there have been no systematic trials to evaluate its efficacy. Extreme hyperventilation should be used with caution, because alkalosis shifts the hemoglobin-oxygen dissociation curve to the left, which is unfavorable for oxygen delivery to tissues. Somatic metabolism may not be compromised with hyperventilation, but the effects on cerebral metabolism are not fully understood.[3] Moreover, attempts to hyperventilate the infant with pulmonary disease using conventional mechanical ventilation entail significant risks of pulmonary injury, including pneumothorax and pulmonary interstitial emphysema. The primary care physician should not undertake such procedures routinely during stabilization in preparation for transport.

Occasionally large vigorous infants cannot be helped by mechanically assisted ventilation administered with pressure limited machines. Asynchrony between the infant's respiratory effort and cycling of the mechanical ventilator or a large contribution of chest wall muscle tone to the total pulmonary resistance may make it virtually impossible to achieve adequate gas exchange safely. To facilitate safe and effective ventilatory management, paralysis with pancuronium or metocurine may be required when such circumstances are recognized. The administration of pancuronium bromide (0.1 mg per kilogram per dose) or metocurine iodide (0.2 mg per kilogram per dose) every two to four hours may allow maintenance of neuromuscular relaxation, produce significant improvement in gas exchange, and reduce the risk of barotrauma.[4,5] Both these drugs have weak atropine-like and histamine-releasing effects, which may cause a reduction in blood pressure, tachycardia, and an apparent increase in skin perfusion. It is also possible that these drugs may increase the risk of intracranial hemorrhage. We also recommend sedation with morphine sulfate (0.05 to 0.1 mg per kilogram every one to two hours) during neuromuscular blockade.

SUSTAINING CARDIAC OUTPUT

If the cardiac output remains impaired after correction of bradycardia (by assisted ventilation or the administration of epinephrine, isoproterenol, or atropine), hypovolemia, and metabolic disorders (acidemia, hypoglycemia, and hypocalcemia), as described in Chapter 8, inotropic or vasodilator drug therapy may be required.

Inotropic Drugs

It is important for the clinician to remember that the absence of bradycardia by auscultation does not necessarily ensure an adequate cardiac output because inotropy has an important role in this context. Some infants may have myocardial injury and dysfunction because of sepsis or severe asphyxia. Less commonly myocardial edema, as with hydrops, may compromise myocardial contractility. Administration of beta-mimetic catecholamines may increase the stroke volume and cardiac output under such conditions. Such drugs may not increase the cardiac output in infants with structural abnormalities of the heart, such as endocardial fibroblastosis or congenital cardiac malformations (especially ventricular hypoplasia). Infants of poorly controlled diabetic mothers may have a temporary congenital defect characterized by hypertrophic cardiomyopathy. These infants may have a reduced cardiac output when treated with such drugs because of narrowing of the right ventricular infundibulum. Knowledge of this condition would contraindicate the use of such drugs, or at least require weighing of the risks and benefits in the context of a particular case. Finally, administration of these drugs is also unlikely to result in beneficial changes in the circulation if the heart rate or diastolic ventricular volume is inadequate, the pH is below 7.1, or they are inactivated by admixture with alkaline solutions for infusion.

Dopamine

Dopamine is the cardiotonic drug most frequently used in the level III nursery. Its effects are dose dependent and are similar to those seen in adult patients. However, a recent report suggests that measurable beneficial effects may occur at doses as low as 0.8 μg per kilogram per minute.[6] Typically, however, the initial dose is 2 to 5 μg per kilogram per minute. At this rate of administration the effect is predominantly dopaminergic receptor-mediated dilation of renal and splanchnic vessels, causing an increase in the glomerular filtration rate, urine output, and urinary sodium excretion. Beta-adrenergic effects result in improved cardiac contractility, a moderate increase in the heart rate, and mild peripheral vasodilatation, all contributing to an increased cardiac output. Such effects are observed with doses up to 15 μg per kilogram per minute, but any increases above the 5 μg per kilogram per minute range may be associated with increasing alpha-adrenergic effects. These effects may result in increased systemic vascular resistance and arterial blood pressures, with a reduction in cardiac output and renal perfusion. The effects on the pulmonary vascular resistance and pulmonary artery pressure may be less pronounced under some conditions, and the alpha-adrenergic effects of dopamine may be useful in establishing a favorable ratio of systemic to pulmonary vascular resistance, leading to decreased right to left shunting in infants with hypoxemia refractory to mechanical ventilation. This differential systemic vasoconstriction may be observed at doses between 10 to 25 μg per kilogram per minute, particularly when combined with vasodilator infusion. A rapid method of preparing and calculating infusion rates is the following:

Dilute 15 mg of dopamine per kilogram of body weight to 250 ml in 5 or 10 percent dextrose in water. This provides a solution for which the dose in micrograms per kilogram per minute equals the rate of infusion in milliliters per hour.

Despite its frequent use in newborn intensive care, dopamine is not a harmless medicine. It should be used only for appropriate indications, and its use requires continued monitoring. Even when used properly, it can increase myocardial oxygen demands and sometimes causes tachyarrhythmias. In unusual infants it also can cause intensive vasoconstriction and hypertension at doses that would be considered dopaminergic. This phenomenon is most common with excessive doses. Tissue necrosis, because of severe local ischemia following extravasation, can be prevented by prompt infiltration with phentolamine mesylate (0.5 to 1 mg) into the affected area. In general, peripheral administration of the drug should be avoided, but this can be done for short periods of time in larger full-term or near-term infants.

Dobutamine

This selective beta-adrenergic drug can increase cardiac contractility and cardiac output but has minimal effects on heart rate and vascular tone.[7] It has been used primarily for cardiac shock refractory to dopamine infusion and often is used in conjunction with dopamine. It should be administered at a dose between 2.5 and 15 μg per kilogram per minute, titrated to achieve the desired improvement in cardiac performance. In the context of sepsis it must be used with great caution, because hypotension can occur. There is generally less experience with the use of dobutamine in infants younger than 12 months, and it must be used with caution, particularly if it is used alone.

For cardiogenic shock unresponsive to other catecholamines, epinephrine infusion (0.5 to 1.5 μg per kilogram per minute) may have to be used.[7] However, the benefits of increased contractility are often balanced against the adverse effects of increased vascular resistance.

Afterload Reduction

Another strategy for the management of severely compromised myocardial function is to decrease the systemic vascular resistance (afterload). This should be attempted only after aggressive management of the heart rate, preload, and inotropic therapy have maximized the cardiac output. Administration of a vasodilator may improve the Frank-Starling relationship between cardiac output and end diastolic ventricular volumes, moving the curve upward and to the left,[8] without affecting myocardial function itself. Dilatation of arterioles and precapillary sphincters may reduce the systemic vascular resistance, resulting in increased cardiac output. However, cardiac output may *decrease* because of reduced preload due to increased venous capacitance, or it may be unchanged if these effects are balanced. Therefore, use of these drugs requires frequent assessment of cardiac output and continuous invasive monitoring of systemic arterial and central venous pressures. The intravascular volume must be at least normal and supported by judicious expansion of the vascular volume in preparation for vasodilator therapy. Blood or plasma should always be immediately available when vasodilator infusion is initiated.

Nitroprusside

Infusion of this vasodilator should begin at a dose of 0.25 to 0.5 μg per kilogram per minute, which can be doubled every 15 to 20 minutes, until the cardiac output and systemic perfusion improve, hypotension or excessive tachycardia supervenes, or the dose reaches 6 μg per kilogram per minute.[9] After 12 to 24 hours of hemodynamic stability, the dose can be decreased as tolerated, in decrements of 15 to 25 percent at intervals of four to six hours, until it is reduced to 0.25 to 0.5 μg per kilogram per minute, when the infusion can be discontinued. Occasionally rebound hypertension during weaning may necessitate moving in small decrements at more frequent intervals. Nitroprusside in combination with dopamine, accompanied by appropriate support of the intravascular volume, may provide the opportunity to maximize cardiac inotropy and achieve a balance of systemic to pulmonary vascular resistance favoring pulmonary perfusion. This compound may be especially beneficial in premature infants with severe respiratory distress syndrome refractory to conventional or high frequency ventilation who are too small to be eligible for extracorporeal membrane oxygenation. Although cyanide and thiocyanate may accumulate during prolonged infusion of nitroprusside, we have not encountered toxic effects from therapeutic doses in the neonate.[9] The possibility of toxicity necessitates persistent attempts to reduce nitroprusside infusions, which cannot be justified unless a beneficial effect is demonstrable, even if metabolite levels are low.

MANAGEMENT OF ANEMIA

The oxygen carrying capacity of the blood is especially important for the newborn infant. Hemoglobin F interacts less well with 2,3-diphosphoglycerate, thus limiting any compensatory response to hypoxia by a shift in the hemoglobin-oxygen dissociation curve. Practically, an oxygen carrying capacity of at least 16 ml of oxygen per deciliter may provide a margin of safety for oxygenation in the asphyxiated infant with a normal cardiac output. This translates to a hemoglobin concentration of 12 mg per deciliter, because 1 gm of hemoglobin can bind 1.34 ml of oxygen. The "magic" number of 40 percent for a minimal desirable hematocrit level in a distressed neonate is thus derived. In infants in whom optimal oxygen tensions cannot be achieved, the increased oxygen carrying capacity imparted by elevation of the hematocrit level to 50 percent may ensure adequate tissue oxygen delivery, allowing marginal oxygen tensions to be better tolerated. These objectives can be realized by transfusion of packed erythrocytes (10 ml per kilogram), as described in Chapter 8; several transfusions may be necessary, depending on the hematocrit level prior to treatment.

EVALUATION AND MANAGEMENT OF REFRACTORY HYPOXEMIA

The infant who remains hypoxemic in spite of ventilation with 100 percent oxygen is at risk for cerebral injury, depending on the severity and duration of the hypoxemic episode. Although the metabolic hallmark of severe hypoxemia is metabolic acidosis, it is better to suspect hypoxemia and initiate therapy than to identify its late consequences. A physiologic classification of hypoxemic conditions is given in Table 8–3. The practitioner should recognize that hypoxemia may be present despite a normal arterial oxygen tension (PaO_2 level greater than 50 mm Hg) or hemoglobin saturation (greater than 90 percent). In particular, severe anemia (physiologic group 1) is a common and easily correctable problem, which may have consequences as serious as those created by a low oxygen tension. In fact, infants with severe anemia may present with respiratory distress despite having normal arterial oxygen tensions and oxygen saturations. A normal PaO_2 value with an arterial blood gas sample may be falsely reassuring in the presence of pallor caused by anemia or acidosis. Thus, the practitioner should remember that cyanosis may not always be observed with clinically significant hypoxemia. Conversely, a PaO_2 level as low as 40 mm Hg may be associated with an oxygen saturation exceeding 90 percent and adequate oxygen delivery to tissues, especially if hemoglobin F is the predominant hemoglobin and the oxygen carrying capacity (red cell mass) is normal.

Conditions included in group 2 (methemoglobinemia, hemoglobinopathies) are uncommon causes of hypoxemia in the newborn. From a practical perspective most infants with reduced arterial oxygen contents have arterial oxygen tensions below 50 mm Hg and present with respiratory difficulties. The physiologic processes contributing to this syndrome include alveolar hypoventilation, impaired diffusion of oxygen from alveoli into blood, ventilation-perfusion mismatching, and right to left shunting. Studies useful in evaluation of the neonate with hypotonic hypoxemia (PaO_2 less than 50 mm Hg), listed in Table 9–1, are to be discussed. In addition, the medical record should include a careful history and physical examination, which may contribute to the diagnosis suggested by those studies. Metabolic disorders (acidosis, hypoglycemia, hypocalcemia) and rheologic abnormalities (hyperviscosity) always should be ruled out before this evaluation is initiated.

Hyperoxia Test

By definition, infants with refractory hypoxemia have already been subjected to the hyperoxia test, which consists simply of determining the PaO_2 level during the administration of 100 percent oxygen. Most infants who

TABLE 9-1 Evaluation of the Neonate with Hypotonic Hypoxemia

Test	Result	Probable Diagnosis	Potential Causes of Error	Additional Studies
Hyperoxia test	$PaO_2 > 150$ mm Hg	Pulmonary parenchymal disease	Reactive pulmonary hypertension	Consider pre- and postductal PaO_2 or echocardiography
	PaO_2 100–150 mm Hg		All diagnoses possible	
	$PaO_2 < 100$ torr	Right to left shunting	Severe pulmonary parenchymal disease	Compare pre- and postductal PaO_2 consider trial of continuous positive airway pressure
Preductal and postductal PaO_2	Preductal < postductal	Transposition of great arteries	Venous preductal sample	Echocardiogram
	Preductal = postductal	Intracardiac or intrapulmonary right to left shunting	May result from cardiac disease, severe parenchymal disease, or severe pulmonary hypertension	Hyperventilation-hyperoxia test, echocardiogram, electrocardiogram
	Preductal > postductal	Ductal right to left shunting	Must distinguish pulmonary hypertension from reduced left ventricular output	Hyperventilation-hyperoxia test, assess systemic blood pressure and cardiac output
Hyperventilation-hyperoxia test	$PaO_2 > 100$ mm Hg	Pulmonary hypertension	Hypoplastic left heart, interrupted aortic arch with ventricular septal defect, total anomalous pulmonary venous return	Consider echocardiogram
	$PaO_2 < 100$ mm Hg	Fixed right to left shunting	Must distinguish heart disease from intrapulmonary shunting	Echocardiogram, electrocardiogram

From Stevenson DK, Benitz WE. A practical approach to diagnosis and immediate care of the cyanotic neonate. Clin Pediatr 1987; 26:325.

have low arterial oxygen tensions under these conditions have right to left shunting as a result of congenital heart disease or pulmonary vascular disease. However, some infants with severe pulmonary parenchymal disease may have persistently low PaO_2 levels owing to diffusion block or ventilation-perfusion mismatching. Those with the latter conditions often respond well to administration of continuous positive airway pressure at 5 to 6 cm of water, with a significant increment in the PaO_2 value. On the other hand, infants with pulmonary hypertension or congenital heart disease usually do less well during such administration and require additional evaluation.

Detection of Ductal Shunting

Simultaneous measurement of preductal (temporal or right radial artery) and postductal (umbilical, dorsalis pedis, or posterior tibial artery) oxygen tensions can be performed by the clinician while the infant is breathing 100 percent oxygen. If the postductal PaO_2 level exceeds the preductal value, transposition of the great arteries can be suspected clinically. Right to left ductal shunting is present if the preductal PaO_2 level exceeds the postductal value by more than 15 to 20 mm Hg. If both the preductal and postductal PaO_2 values are low, the absence of such a difference does not exclude ductal shunting. Shunting at other levels (foramen ovale, intra-

pulmonary) cannot be either excluded or detected by this test. Measurement of the systemic blood pressure and assessment of the systemic cardiac output are essential in interpreting this observation, because right to left shunting may result from a decrease in the systemic arterial pressure or cardiac output, as well as increased pulmonary arterial pressures. These hemodynamic abnormalities must be corrected before evaluation of the cause of refractory hypoxemia can be completed, using the studies to be described.

Hyperoxia-Hyperventilation Test

This test consists of measurement of the PaO_2 level during manual hyperventilation with 100 percent oxygen to achieve a $PaCO_2$ value less than 20 mm Hg or a pH greater than 7.6. There is little evidence that such marked hyperventilation, when applied for a short period as a diagnostic procedure, is deleterious to the neonatal brain.[3] However, if adequate oxygenation (PaO_2 greater than 80 mm Hg) can be achieved with less severe hypocarbia ($PaCO_2$ 20 to 25 mm Hg), this is preferable. If the arterial oxygen tension increases to a value greater than 100 mm Hg in response to hyperventilation, the diagnosis of pulmonary arterial hypertension, at least in part related to pulmonary arterial vasoconstriction, can be made. Unfortunately the absence of a response does not exclude this diagnosis. Moreover, other diagnoses, including hypoplastic left heart syndrome, aortic arch interruption with ventricular septal defect, and anomalous pulmonary venous return, cannot be excluded by this test alone. If pulmonary venous obstruction is present, hyperventilation usually does not improve oxygenation.

Information obtained from these diagnostic maneuvers must be combined with that obtained from other studies, including chest radiography and echocardiography. These data often do not correspond precisely to a description of a typical infant with any of the conditions listed in Table 9–2 and may appear to be contradictory or confusing. Thoughtful synthesis of all available information, including that from the history, physical examination, and laboratory studies, is required. All diagnostic information must be reevaluated regularly, because it frequently becomes apparent that the infant's condition has changed or that the initial diagnostic impression was wrong or incomplete.

The primary care physician should have a clear understanding of the priorities in the management of neonatal hypoxemia. These priorities are summarized in

TABLE 9–2   Pathophysiologic Categories of Refractory Hypoxemia

Category	Characteristics
Reduced systemic pressure	Ductal or intracardiac right to left shunting Usually no improvement in PaO_2 during hyperventilation Reduced systemic blood pressure or cardiac output
Pulmonary hypertension	Ductal or intracardiac right to left shunting Hyperventilation produces $PaO_2 > 100$ mm Hg in those conditions associated with partially reversible pulmonary arterial constriction If the cause of pulmonary hypertension is not associated with reversible arterial constriction, diagnosis depends upon recognition of prolonged right ventricular systolic time intervals and exclusion of intrapulmonary right to left shunting, cardiac malformations, and systemic hypotension
Congenital heart disease	Ductal or intracardial right to left shunting No improvement in PaO_2 during hyperventilation Echocardiogram usually diagnostic
Intrapulmonary shunting	No demonstrable ductal shunt Modest or no improvement in PaO_2 during hyperventilation Usually no evidence for pulmonary hypertension

From Stevenson DK, Benitz WE. A practical approach to diagnosis and immediate care of the cyanotic neonate. Clin Pediatr 1987; 26:325.

TABLE 9–3   Priorities in Management of Neonatal Hypoxemia*

Promote oxygenation by administering 100% oxygen and assisting ventilation to achieve modest hyperventilation.
Correct hypotension and/or anemia by correcting bradycardia and administering plasma and/or blood.
Correct metabolic acidosis by administering bicarbonate (after adequate alveolar ventilation is confirmed by arterial blood gas analysis).
Correct hypoglycemia with intravenous glucose.
Correct hypocalcemia with intravenous calcium gluconate.
Correct polycythemia by partial exchange transfusion.
Obtain cultures and treat potential infection with antibiotics.
Request consultation from the neonatologist at the nearest tertiary care nursery for any infant who does not improve promptly in response to these interventions.

* Although these interventions are listed sequentially, it is imperative that they be carried out as expeditiously as possible; it is not appropriate to delay subsequent items while observing the response to initial measures.
From Stevenson DK, Benitz WE. A practical approach to diagnosis and immediate care of the cyanotic neonate. Clin Pediatr 1987; 26:325.

Table 9–3. However, the ventilatory approaches and the pharmacologic management of infants with this syndrome surpass the capabilities of the facilities in which most primary care physicians practice, and it is invariably necessary to refer these infants to the regional level III nursery. The management of any infant with the syndrome of refractory hypoxemia should be discussed with the neonatologist at the regional level III nursery while transport is being arranged. The details of this management depend on the diagnosis, the facilities available, and the preferences of the consulting neonatologist. Most of these infants require attention to maintenance of the cardiac output, using volume expansion and inotropic drugs, as already described. A comprehensive discussion of the management of conditions that cause refractory hypoxemia is beyond the scope of this work; a brief review of three common categories of disease is given in the following section. In addition to the therapies discussed, a variety of innovative therapies, including high frequency ventilation and extracorporeal membrane oxygenation, are becoming available. To a large extent, the application of these therapies remains limited, and their places in the standard of care have not been fully defined.

Severe Pulmonary Parenchymal Disease

Pulmonary parenchymal disease, such as bacterial pneumonia or severe hyaline membrane disease, that is refractory to the administration of 100 percent oxygen and assisted ventilation at low to moderate pressures and rates is most commonly treated by increasingly aggressive mechanical ventilation. This can be achieved in a variety of ways, including the use of an increased peak inspiratory pressure, increased end expiratory pressure, longer inspiratory times, higher gas flow rates, or higher ventilation rates. In some instances these maneuvers succeed in improving arterial oxygenation. They must be used with caution, however, because they increase the risk of air leak complications (e.g., pneumothorax, pneumopericardium, interstitial emphysema). In addition, excessive distending pressures may compromise pulmonary perfusion, resulting in increased extrapulmonary right to left shunting and exacerbation of hypoxemia. Neuromuscular blocking drugs may be useful in improving ventilator management in large vigorous infants, as discussed already.

Diuretic therapy may help improve pulmonary gas exchange, especially if there is significant pulmonary edema. Diuretics are most effective in patients with hypervolemia or pulmonary overperfusion, but should be used with great caution in infants with pulmonary edema due to increased capillary permeability (e.g., in postasphyxial or septic infants), in whom intravascular volumes may already be diminished. The effects of diuretics result primarily from the decrease in vascular volume achieved by diuresis, but furosemide also increases venous capacitance, allowing translocation of pulmonary interstitial fluid into the venous system. Prolonged use of furosemide may lead to hypokalemia, hyponatremia, hypochloremia, and metabolic alkalosis. Moreover, long-term furosemide use may be associated with renal calculi, related to hypercalciuria. Thus the use of other diuretics, such as chlorothiazide, may be preferable.

Persistent patency of the ductus arteriosus beyond the first 48 hours of life often is associated with the shunting of blood from the aorta into the pulmonary artery (left to right), causing pulmonary congestion, increased interstitial lung fluid, and congestive heart failure. Such patency can exacerbate pulmonary disease in premature infants, leading to a requirement for increased mechanical ventilatory support and consequent complications. This complication is managed most effectively by closure of the ductus arteriosus. There is no uniform agreement regarding the optimal approach in selection of infants for therapy, choice of medical versus surgical intervention, or the protocol for medical management. In most centers active intervention is reserved for selected infants with demonstrable respiratory compromise due to left to right shunting through the ductus arteriosus. In most cases initial management can consist of fluid restriction and diuretic therapy. Such procedures can eliminate the duct as an important clinical factor in 25 percent of the infants with hemodynamic abnormalities.

If ductal patency and significant pulmonary hyperperfusion persist, attempted closure of the ductus with indomethacin is appropriate, if there are no contraindications to administration of the drug. Indomethacin is most effective if given in the first few days of life and soon after ductal patency becomes clinically apparent. Closure is achieved most consistently in premature infants with a birth weight greater than 1,000 gm. Prophylactic use is recommended at some institutions[10] but is not uniformly practiced. The incidence of clinically significant ductus arteriosus, in fact, varies greatly among institutions, reflecting differences in fluid management and ventilator management. Indomethacin is used at a dose of 0.2 to 0.25 mg per kilogram, given intravenously two to three times at 12 to 24 hour intervals. Other dose schedules may be preferable if drug levels can be monitored. Surgical ligation may be required in infants who do not improve after treatment with indomethacin.

Glomerular filtration, urinary sodium excretion, and urine output can be affected adversely (decreased) after treatment with indomethacin, especially in infants who already have compromised renal function because of a large ductus arteriosus.[11] Administration of furosemide concurrently with indomethacin may ameliorate these adverse effects, but theoretically also may reduce the efficacy of indomethacin in blocking prostaglandin synthesis. Indomethacin should not be given to an infant with impaired renal function (a blood urea nitrogen level more than 30 mg per deciliter or a creatinine level greater than 1.8 mg per deciliter or oliguria (urine output less than 0.6 ml per kilogram per hour in the preceding eight hours). Because platelet function also may be compromised (decreased aggregability), indomethacin should not be used in infants with a bleeding diathesis or a platelet count less than 60,000 per microliter. Because necrotizing enterocolitis and focal gastrointestinal perforation have been associated with oral indomethacin use, the drug should not be used in infants with clinical or radiographic evidence of gastrointestinal dysfunction. Intracranial hemorrhage, detected by echoencephalography, also may be a relative contraindication to treatment with indomethacin.

The standards of care in this area of practice continue to evolve rapidly. The advent of surfactant replacement therapy promises to significantly reduce the incidence of severe respiratory distress syndrome and is likely to alter the clinical course in infants who develop this disorder in spite of surfactant therapy. We recently have found that vasodilator infusion (nitroprusside as a dose of 1 to 1.5 μg per kilogram per minute) is effective in improving both oxygenation and carbon dioxide excretion in neonates with severe hyaline membrane disease. The role of these and other novel approaches to the management of severe pulmonary parenchymal disease remains to be delineated.

Pulmonary Arterial Disease

Intrinsic disease of the pulmonary arteries is encountered most frequently in cases of persistent pulmonary hypertension of the newborn, which is often associated with meconium aspiration. Infants with this disorder have both structural and functional abnormalities of the pulmonary arteries, typified by excessive muscularity and hyperreactivity to a variety of stimuli, including hypoxia and acidemia. The primary therapeutic strategies for these infants include sedation, oxygen administration, and achievement of an alkaline pH of arterial blood. The latter objective may be achieved by either hyperventilation or bicarbonate administration, or a combination of these methods. As already noted, this condition may be exacerbated by a poor systemic cardiac output; thus judicious volume expansion and inotropic drug infusion are often utilized. In severely affected infants the use of vasopressor infusion to increase systemic arterial pressures may be useful. In particular, dopamine, which may affect the pulmonary circulation to a lesser extent than the systemic vascular bed, has been widely used.[12]

If these methods fail to secure an acceptable PaO_2 level, vasodilators are frequently administered, even though no carefully controlled studies have verified the efficacy of this therapeutic modality. Nitroprusside (2 to 6 μg per kilogram per minute) has become the drug of first choice for us, because it is easily titrated and has a very short half-life. We also have found it to be better tolerated than tolazoline. However, some infants with pulmonary hypertension do not respond to nitroprusside and seem to require infusion of tolazoline, which has both histamine-like and alpha-adrenergic blocking effects, causing both pulmonary and systemic vasodilation. Tolazoline can be administered as a continuous infusion (1 mg per kilogram per hour) or as a bolus (0.5 to 1 mg per kilogram) because of its longer half-life. Recent reports suggest that these recommended doses may be too high.[13] Much lower infusion rates probably could be used. More extensive use of tolazoline levels (which are not yet widely available) may allow for refinement of the therapeutic use of this drug. Severe hypotension unresponsive to volume expansion may follow tolazoline infusion, especially in premature infants with the respiratory distress syndrome and infants with relative hypovolemia.[14] Other complications with tolazoline include gastrointestinal and pulmonary hemorrhage, thrombocytopenia, and tachyarrhythmias.

Cyanotic Congenital Heart Disease

In a variety of congenital cardiac malformations, including those in which pulmonary blood flow must be derived from the aorta via the ductus arteriosus (because of obstruction of the right heart), those in which systemic perfusion is dependent on blood flow from the pulmonary artery to the aorta via the ductus arteriosus (due to left-sided heart obstruction), and those in which

admixture of blood from the systemic and pulmonary circulations is essential for maintaining systemic arterial oxygen content (Table 9-4), maintaining patency of the ductus arteriosus may be life-saving. This can be accomplished with the administration of prostaglandin E$_1$ with a loading dose of 50 to 100 ng per kilogram (0.05 to 0.1 μg per kilogram) followed by infusion at 50 to 100 ng per kilogram per minute. Once patency of the ductus is established, the dose can be gradually decreased to 10 to 20 ng per kilogram per minute.[15] Infusion at higher doses may cause pulmonary and systemic vasodilatation, but other drugs (already discussed) may be more desirable for these purposes. Higher doses of prostaglandin E$_1$ can be associated with diarrhea, fever, tachyarrhythmias, and systemic hypertension. Apnea also can be life-threatening, especially if the patient is not intubated. Because most community hospitals are not equipped to undertake definitive diagnostic (echocardiography, cardiac catheterization) or therapeutic (cardiac or vascular surgery) procedures for the newborn infant, this treatment should be initiated only in consultation with the neonatologist at a center capable of providing these services, where the infant should be transferred as soon as possible.

CONSULTATION AND REFERRAL

Attempts to manage critically ill neonates beyond the initial stabilization (in preparation for transfer to level III facilities) may contribute to unnecessary additional risk and possible compromise of the neonate. Even though a particular physician has been appropriately trained to do so, the temptation to care for such neonates in a level I or II nursery should be resisted, because these facilities rarely include all appropriate equipment and sufficient specially trained personnel to support the diagnostic and therapeutic undertakings required to

TABLE 9-4   Ductus Dependent Cardiac
Malformations

Right-sided heart obstruction
  Tricuspid atresia
  Pulmonary atresia or severe stenosis
  Truncus arteriosus with ductus-dependent pulmonary arteries
  Tetralogy of Fallot

Left-sided heart obstruction
  Coarctation of the aorta (preductal or juxtaductal)
  Interruption of the aortic arch
  Severe aortic stenosis

Mixing dependent lesions
  Transposition of the great arteries with an intact ventricular septum

From Benitz WE, Frankel LR, Stevenson DK. The pharmacology of neonatal resuscitation and cardiopulmonary intensive care. Part II. Extended intensive care. West J Med 1986; 145:47.

confirm the diagnosis of cyanotic congenital heart disease (echocardiography) or treat persistent pulmonary hypertension of the newborn (special procedures for the implementation and monitoring of hyperventilation and vasodilator therapy). Thus, consultation always should be obtained with an experienced neonatologist, usually from the level III facility to which the infant will be transported, if special procedures are judged to be necessary immediately, such as the use of prostaglandin in an infant suspected of having a ductus-dependent congenital cardiac defect. However, encountering the syndrome of hypoxemia (PaO_2 level less than 50 mm Hg) refractory to 100 percent oxygen and assisted ventilation should not lead to automatic abandonment by the primary care physician and, in fact, mandates the physical attendance by the latter until the arrival of the transport team.

Because of the high medicolegal hazard to all physicians involved in the care of a depressed infant, all easily treated conditions contributing to the infant's disorder should be treated immediately after birth by the physician in attendance. As a minimum, the practitioner should be able to insert an umbilical venous catheter and ideally also should be able to insert an arterial catheter (usually through an umbilical artery) for direct measurement of the blood pressure and administration of crystalloid, colloid, or drugs to support the blood pressure. The infant requiring stabilization and preparation for transport by a highly trained neonatal transport team has most often failed to improve in response to 100 percent oxygen and assisted ventilation. The practitioner should initiate specific therapies to correct cardiac dysfunction in the context of hypoxemia refractory to assisted ventilation. In addition, there may be many correctable problems that can contribute to the syndrome of hypoxemia. Such treatment should also constitute preparation of the infant for transport to the nearest level III facility, if necessary. Nonetheless, complete characterization of and appropriate treatment for cyanotic congenital heart disease are not expected of the primary care physician at a level I or II nursery. Clearly, what is expected of the practitioner at such a nursery is different from what is expected of the neonatologist at a level III facility, where a variety of special diagnostic and therapeutic procedures might be attempted to correct or ameliorate the problem after the patient's arrival.

When the problem is considered in the medicolegal context, generalization about the extended intensive care of depressed infants should be considered a disservice to the legal as well as the medical community. With the presentation of certain clinical facts in retrospect, some comments can be made about therapeutic options and the application of therapies. However, it is inappropriate to guess about the reasoned decision making of a physician involved with the care of such an infant without that physician's supplying the context in which the decision was made. Moreover, it undermines the trust of the public in the health care professionals who have dedicated their lives to caring for such infants. Most important, the clinical determinant of standard of care must remain the response of the patient to the therapies selected and should be independent of individual preferences.

REFERENCES

1. Benitz WE, Frankel LR, Stevenson DK. The pharmacology of neonatal resuscitation and cardiopulmonary intensive care. Part II. Extended intensive care. West J Med 1986; 145:47.
2. Stevenson DK, Benitz WE. A practical approach to diagnosis and immediate care of the cyanotic neonate. Clin Pediatr 1987; 26:325.
3. Bruce DA. Effects of hyperventilation on cerebral blood flow and metabolism. Clin Perinatol 1984; 11:673.
4. Crone RK, Favorito J. The effects of pancuronium bromide on infants with hyaline membrane disease. J Pediatr 1980; 97:991.
5. Goudsouzian NG, Liu MPL, Savarese JJ. Metocurine in infants and children: neuromuscular and clinical effects. Anesthesiology 1978; 49:266.
6. Padbury J, Agata Y, Ludlow J, et al. Dopamine pharmacokinetics in critically ill newborns (abstract). Clin Res 1986; 34:146.
7. Zaritsky A. Chernow B. Use of catecholamines in pediatrics. J Pediatr 1984; 103:341.
8. Friedman WF, Georgew BL. Treatment of congestive heart failure by altering loading conditions of the heart. J Pediatr 1985; 106:697.
9. Benitz WE, Malachowski N, Cohen RS, et al. Use of sodium nitroprusside in neonates: efficacy and safety. J Pediatr 1985; 105:102.
10. Mahony L, Carrero V, Brett C, et al. Prophylactic indomethacin therapy for patent ductus arteriosus in very-low-birth-weight infants. N Engl J Med 1982; 306:506.
11. Gleason C, Clyman RI, Heymann MA, et al. PDA and indomethacin: effects on renal function (abstract). Clin Res 1986; 34:143.
12. Drummond WH, Webb IB, Purcell KA. Cardiopulmonary response to dopamine in chronically catheterized neonatal lambs. Pediatr Pharmacol 1981; 1:347.
13. Ward RM, Daniel CH, Kendig JW, et al. Oliguria and tolazoline pharmacokinetics in the newborn. Pediatrics 1986; 77:307.
14. Stevenson DK, Kasting DS, Darnall RA, et al. Refractory hypoxemia associated with neonatal pulmonary disease: the use and limitations of tolazoline. J Pediatr 1979; 95:595.
15. Heymann MA. Pharmacologic use of prostaglandin E_1 in infants with congenital heart disease. Am Heart J 1981; 837.

10 Hypoxic-Ischemic Encephalopathy

Edward J. Novotny Jr., M.D.

Pathophysiology
    Biochemical Aspects
    Cerebral Blood Flow
Neuropathology
Clinical Features and Management
    General Evaluation
    Clinicopathologic Syndromes
Future Prospects

Hypoxic-ischemic encephalopathy is a well-recognized clinical syndrome and the most common cause of acute neurologic impairment and seizures in the neonatal period.[1-3]. Hypoxic ischemic brain injury secondary to birth asphyxia can result in the development of "cerebral palsy," but study of the recent literature has shown that only a small percentage of children with cerebral palsy had intrapartum asphyxia as a possible etiology.[4-6] More emphasis has been placed on antenatal events as having a greater association with cerebral palsy.[7] The pathophysiology, neuropathology, clinical features, and management of hypoxic-ischemic encephalopathy in the newborn are presented in this chapter.

PATHOPHYSIOLOGY

Biochemical Aspects

Knowledge of the biochemical alterations that occur in hypoxic-ischemic encephalopathy is necessary to understand the structural and functional defects that result from this disorder. It is even more important when one considers carrying out specific therapeutic interventions. The biochemical changes can be grouped into variations in the metabolism of substrates, alterations in the metabolism of high energy compounds, fluctuations in neurotransmitters, and changes in ion gradients. The majority of this information is derived from both in vitro and in vivo biochemical studies in different animal species. Nonetheless these investigations have provided important information about the pathophysiology of this disorder. The recent development of new techniques such as positron emission tomography, Doppler ultrasonography, nuclear magnetic resonance spectroscopy, and near infrared spectrophotometry has permitted noninvasive in vivo measurements of the regional metabolism of substrate analogues, cerebral blood flow, alterations in cerebral high energy compounds, lactate, amino acids and intracellular pH levels, and cerebral oxygenation in both animals and humans with hypoxic-ischemic encephalopathy.[8-11]

Neurophysiologic measures of cerebral function such as the electroencephalogram show the earliest changes in ischemia and asphyxia.[12,13] These changes occur within the first 10 to 60 seconds after the insult. Also, abnormalities often persist after metabolic recovery.[14]

The major changes in ion gradients occur within the first 20 to 30 minutes after the insult. Microelectrode techniques have been utilized to measure the fluctuations of specific ions in the extracellular space.[15,16] A marked increase in the extracellular potassium level is accompanied by a decrease in the levels of sodium, chloride, and calcium ions. There is also a contraction of the extracellular volume during this period. The accumulation of intracellular calcium ions is thought to play a crucial role in the mechanisms leading to cell death.[17,18]

The accumulation of lactic acid secondary to increased anaerobic glycolysis and glycogenolysis is the earliest alteration observed in substrate utilization pathways. This occurs in the first three to 10 minutes following an asphyxic insult.[19] A decline in brain glucose and glycogen levels accompanies this increase in the lactate level. In one study five minutes of ischemia produced no changes in the total brain glutamate, aspartate, glutamine, or asparagine levels but resulted in a marked increase in gamma-aminobutyric acid (GABA) and alanine levels.[20]

Recent investigations utilizing a dialysis tube inserted into the extracellular space have shown a marked increase in GABA, glutamate, aspartate, and taurine levels in this compartment.[21] During the first 30 minutes of ischemia, there is a rise in the tissue concentrations of free fatty acids, which is mediated by the increase in cytosolic calcium by activation of phospholipases.[22] Arachidonic acid is an important free fatty acid that accumulates. During recirculation it is metabolized to prostaglandins and leukotrienes by the cyclooxygenase and lipoxygenase enzyme systems. These metabolites lead to alterations in the cerebral microcirculation and the production of free radicals, which ultimately lead to cell damage.[23]

The immature animal has been shown to be particularly sensitive to the availability of glucose at the time of insult.[24,25] Animals who were hypoglycemic prior to anoxia had a poorer outcome than those who were normoglycemic. It remains to be confirmed that hyperglycemia is as deleterious to the immature brain as it has been shown to be in the mature nervous system.[26,27]

Recent studies utilizing positron emission tomography in newborns and infants have shown that the subcortical gray matter has a much higher rate of glucose utilization than the cortex.[28,29] This metabolic pattern may explain why a significant portion of the cases of neuropathologic disease in the asphyxiated newborn occur in the subcortical regions.

The initial change in high energy phosphate compounds is observed in the phosphocreatine level, which decreases inversely with the rise in the lactate concentration. Over the next 10 to 30 minutes the adenosine triphosphate (ATP) level decreases, and there is an increase in the inorganic phosphate, adenosine diphosphate (ADP), adenosine monophosphate (AMP), and cyclic AMP levels.[13] The latter compounds act as activators of glycolytic regulatory enzymes to further increase glucose utilization and lactate production. Energy failure alone is unlikely to result in cell injury because there is a poor correlation with the degree of energy failure and neuropathologic damage.[17]

Phosphorus nuclear magnetic resonance (NMR) spectroscopic studies in human newborns with asphyxia have shown several important changes in high energy phosphate compounds.[10,30-32] NMR spectroscopy can measure the concentrations of high energy phosphates, since the naturally abundant ^{31}P nucleus has magnetic properties. The metabolites that can be measured are shown in Figure 10-1. The intracellular pH also can be measured by determining the chemical shift of the inorganic phosphorus peak or phosphomonoester peak.[33,34] These studies were performed on small groups of infants, but they demonstrated that this technique can be applied in critically ill newborns. An important observation in the earlier reports was that several asphyxiated infants initially had normal phosphorus NMR spectroscopic study results, which deteriorated over the next 24 to 48 hours.[31] This suggests that there may be a period immediately after an hypoxic ischemic insult during which therapeutic interventions may be of value. In the same study it was suggested that the ratio of phosphocreatine to inorganic phosphorus was predictive of outcome, yet this was not compared with other prognostic indicators. A more recent study in premature infants

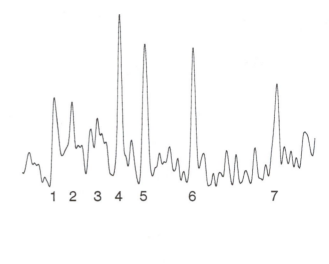

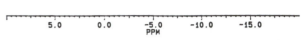

Figure 10-1 Phosphorus nuclear magnetic resonance spectrum of a rabbit brain obtained on a 4.7 Tesla, Bruker/ORS spectrometer with a 16 mm surface coil placed over the cranium. The spectrum represents the sum of 512 scans acquired over 12 minutes. The peak assignments are as follows: 1, phosphomonoesters; 2, inorganic phosphorus; 3, phosphodiesters; 4, phosphocreatine; 5–7, gamma-, alpha-, and beta-nuclei of nucleotide phosphates (primarily ATP).

with echodense lesions on ultrasound examination suggested that phosphorus NMR imaging could be used to predict the infants who would develop cystic lesions, cerebral atrophy, and neurologic handicaps.[10]

The alterations in neurotransmitters during cerebral hypoxia-ischemia include changes in the putative amino acid neurotransmitters, already described, and changes in catecholamines and acetylcholine. In one study an acute decrease in the striatal dopamine concentration was observed with ischemia.[35] Three weeks following recovery there was a decrease in the number of striatal dopaminergic, GABAergic, and cholinergic markers. The number of cholinergic markers, however, was considerably more reduced than the other two. It was suggested that the vulnerability of certain neuronal populations is dependent on the stage of development.

The role of the putative excitatory amino acid neurotransmitters in neuronal death has been an area of intense research and holds much promise for potential therapeutic interventions.[36,37] Most work with this neurotransmitter system has been in cell culture systems, but recent animal investigations have demonstrated a decrease in neuronal cell death after pretreatment with excitatory neurotransmitter antagonists.[38-40]

Cerebral Blood Flow

Cerebral blood flow in perinatal asphyxia has been investigated in many experimental systems.[41-43] The major findings from these studies are that asphyxia produces an alteration in cardiac output such that there is a two-fold increase in the proportion delivered to the brain. This is associated with an initial increase in cerebral blood flow and a loss in autoregulation. Later in the course one observes a decrease in cerebral blood flow associated with decreased cardiac output. In addition to these general changes there are important differences in regional cerebral blood flow, the greatest increase in flow occurring in the brainstem and thalamus and a relative decrease in flow observed in the white matter.

Investigations of cerebral blood flow in the human neonate have provided important insight into the pathogenesis of brain injury. Early studies using radio-isotope techniques and jugular venous occlusion plethysmography have shown that autoregulation is very labile, especially in the preterm infant.[44-46] This feature has important clinical implications, since the cerebral blood flow varies passively with systemic circulation. Episodes of systemic hypotension therefore may lead to impairment of cerebral blood flow. In the preterm infant this may lead to a decrease in flow in the periventricular white matter and in the term infant to a decrease in flow in the parasagittal regions. The latter has been demonstrated in the human infant by positron emission tomography using ^{15}O-labeled water.[8] Doppler ultrasound techniques can be used to measure cerebral blood flow velocity. Several studies have described important alterations in flow velocity in different clinical settings.[8,47] The determination of brain death and the management of infants at risk for intraventricular hemorrhage are two clinical applications of this technique. Future studies using these new methods of determining cerebral blood flow undoubtedly will provide further important information regarding the pathogenesis of brain injury in the human newborn.

NEUROPATHOLOGY

The neuropathologic lesions resulting from a hypoxic ischemic insult have been reviewed extensively.[48-51] The specific type of lesion varies with the gestational age of the infant, the characteristics of the primary insult, and the subsequent management. Over the past century several specific patterns of brain injury have been well characterized, and more recent neuroimaging studies have identified the neuropathologic alterations in the neonatal period, allowing the designation of specific clinicopathologic syndromes. Recognition of these disorders provides an understanding of the mechanisms leading to their development and allows prediction of possible neurologic disabilities.

The neuropathologic changes can be divided into lesions that are the result of primary damage to specific types of cells and structures and those due to hemorrhage, which is the most common lesion associated with hypoxic-ischemic encephalopathy.[50] The pathologic change observed in the term infant is different from that seen in the premature infant (Table 10-1).

The term infant most commonly is observed to have neuropathologic changes involving primarily the gray matter and specific neuroanatomic structures in both the cortical and subcortical regions. Intraventricular hemorrhage occurs in the term infant, but the pathogenetic mechanisms are different from those in the preterm infant. On the contrary, periventricular or intraventricular hemorrhage is the most common neuropathologic finding in the premature infant. Pathologic changes in the white matter are the next most common disorder, followed by lesions involving selected neuronal populations.

The patterns of brain injury observed in the newborn can be categorized into lesions involving four major areas of the central nervous system: the cortex, deep gray matter nuclei, brainstem, and cerebellum. There is often an overlap of these pathologic processes, but primary involvement of one of these regions results in specific clinical characteristics both acutely and over the long term.

Cortical injury may result from occlusion of either the venous or arterial vasculature. Trauma, coagulopathy, and congenital heart disease are common associated disorders. Venous occlusions often involve the sinuses or major veins, leading to superficial cortical infarcts, which are frequently hemorrhagic. Arterial occlusions occur most often in the term infant and have been observed in 5 to 9 percent of autopsy series.[52,53] The middle cerebral artery is most frequently involved. Another form of cortical injury resulting from a general decrease in the cerebral blood flow is referred to as the watershed infarction, since the disorder involves the border zones of the three major arterial supply zones. Ulegyria, a term describing cortical gyri that are atrophic, particularly at the depth of sulci, is the chronic lesion resulting from this particular brain injury (Fig. 10-2). In one autopsy series of neurologically handicapped

TABLE 10-1 Neuropathologic Lesions Associated with Neonatal Hypoxic Ischemic Encephalopathy

Full-Term Newborn	Preterm Newborn

Cortical infarctions
  Arterial occlusion
  Venous occlusion
  "Watershed" lesions
	Periventricular or intra-
	  ventricular hemorrhage
	
	White matter disease

Necrosis of deep gray nuclei
  Basal ganglia
  Thalamus
  Diencephalon
	Necrosis of deep gray nuclei
	  Basal ganglia
	  Thalamus
	  Diencephalon

Brainstem necrosis
  Pontosubicular necrosis
  Selective nuclei
	Brainstem necrosis
	  Pontosubicular necrosis
	  Selective nuclei

Cerebellar necrosis	Cerebellar necrosis
Intraventricular hemorrhage	Cortical infarctions
White matter disease	

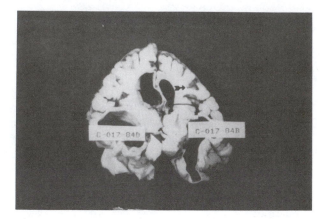

Figure 10-2 Coronal section of the brain of a five-year-old child with severe mental retardation and a spastic quadriparesis following cardiopulmonary arrest as a newborn. Microencephaly (brain weight, 215 gm), cystic degeneration of basal ganglia, ventriculomegaly, ulegyria (arrow), and atrophy of white matter are depicted.

children 30 of 153 subjects had this lesion in the parasagittal watershed region.[54]

Lesions in the deep gray nuclei (thalamus, basal ganglia, and diencephalon) have been described for nearly a century in children with presumed birth injury who exhibited choreoathetosis and dystonia.[51] Recently infants with this pathologic lesion have been identified in the neonatal period by neuroimaging studies.[55] Early in the course there is often hemorrhage and infarction in these structures. Eventually cystic changes develop, particularly in the neostriatum (caudate and putamen; Figs. 10-2, 10-3). The neurons and penetrating vessels become calcified (see Fig. 10-3). The basal ganglia and thalamus develop a chronic pathologic lesion termed "status marmoratus." This lesion was observed in 173 of 198 cases of presumed perinatal birth injury.[56] The lesions are probably the result of both impairment of blood flow through the penetrating arteries and the high level of metabolic activity of this structure.

Pathologic changes of the brainstem are rarely isolated, and other structures, especially the thalamus, are also involved. Brainstem injury usually occurs in the setting of acute hypotension.[57] One particular brainstem lesion, termed pontosubicular necrosis by Friede,[58] involves necrosis of neurons in the pons and subiculum of the hippocampus. Friede suggested that these neurons were particularly vulnerable to anoxia, but more recently hyperoxemia was noted to be associated with this lesion.[59] Selective necrosis of specific brainstem nuclei has been observed, and the nuclei adjacent to the floor of the fourth ventricle are more often affected. These nuclei include the inferior colliculi, fifth and seventh cranial nerve nuclei, and nucleus ambiguus (ninth and tenth cranial nerves).

The cerebellum is especially vulnerable to hypoxic ischemic insult, and the Purkinje cells are the most vulnerable type of cell. The cerebellum is often affected

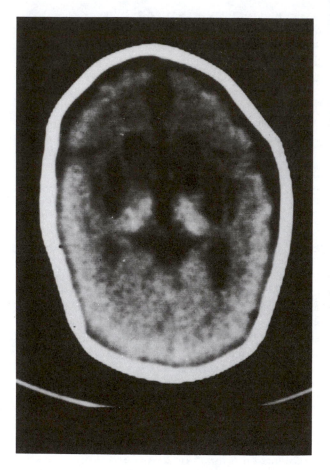

Figure 10-3 Noncontrast CT scan of a six-week-old male infant born at 34 weeks' gestation with severe hypoxic ischemic encephalopathy secondary to abruptio placentae. Cystic degeneration of the basal ganglia, thalamic calcification, and ventriculomegaly are depicted.

by bilateral lesions at the boundaries of the superior and inferior cerebellar arterial zones or by lesions of the foliar cortex. White matter edema and small hemorrhages accompany the neuronal loss. Chronic lesions are referred to as cerebellar sclerosis. In this condition there is a loss of Purkinje cells and an increase in Bergmann's astrocytes. The folia are narrowed and there is an increased space between them.

There are three types of white matter lesions observed most commonly in the preterm infant. The first, referred to as glial fatty metamorphosis by Leech and Alvord,[60] is due to deposition of lipid in the white matter. These authors regard this as an abnormal response of immature glia to hypoxia. Others regard this as a normal feature in myelin formation.[51]

The second lesion, characterized by increased reactive astrocytes within the white matter, also has been referred to as perinatal telencephalic leukoencephalopathy.[61] This lesion has been observed in 15 to 40 percent of autopsy cases and ultimately may lead to retardation of myelin development.[50,61] Many other factors, such as infectious diseases, hyperbilirubinemia, and nutritional deficiencies, are thought to play a role in the development of this disorder.

The third lesion, characterized by necrosis of the white matter, may include hemorrhage. Periventricular leukomalacia is the term frequently used to describe this disorder.[62] The lesion is readily identified by ultrasonography, and recent prospective studies have determined that the incidence is 4 to 26 percent in low birth weight infants.[63-65] The acute lesion is characterized by white spots in the periventricular regions, which occasionally may show hemorrhagic infiltration (Fig. 10–4). Focal coagulative necrosis is observed on microscopic examination. These areas often develop into cystic lesions and later contract into gliotic scars. The lesions are observed most frequently in the corona radiata, occipital and temporal horns of the lateral ventricles, and just anterior to the anterior horn of the lateral ventricles. In the term infant the lesions are usually hemorrhagic and are associated with a coagulopathy or congenital heart disease.

Periventricular or intraventricular hemorrhage is the most common neuropathologic change observed in the premature infant. It is observed in 31 to 43 percent of low birth weight infants in prospective neuroimaging studies.[66,67] The hemorrhage arises from the germinal matrix at the ventromedial angle of the lateral ventricle. Cerebral hypoxic ischemia leads to impaired autoregulation of cerebral blood flow and injury to the germinal matrix and capillary endothelium, which have a high level of oxidative metabolism. Changes in the systemic blood pressure, platelet and coagulation disturbances, and increased cerebral venous pressure also contribute to the pathogenesis of this lesion.

The pathologic findings include subarachnoid hemorrhage with blood in the basal and pontine cisterns and cisterna magna. The hemorrhage may range from a small area of bleeding in the subependymal matrix zone to massive distention of the ventricular system associated with extension of blood into the centrum semiovale. Hydrocephalus may be a complication in infants with this disorder. The hydrocephalus is often secondary to an obstruction at the aqueduct or the foramina exiting from the fourth ventricle or may be due to impairment of reabsorption of cerebrospinal fluid over the convexities.

Intraventricular hemorrhage in the term infant often arises from the choroid plexus, and trauma is thought to be an important pathogenetic factor.[68,69] In 25 percent of term infants with this disorder there is no identifiable cause for the hemorrhage.[68]

CLINICAL FEATURES AND MANAGEMENT

The clinical features in the infant with hypoxic ischemic encephalopathy are presented here by first des-

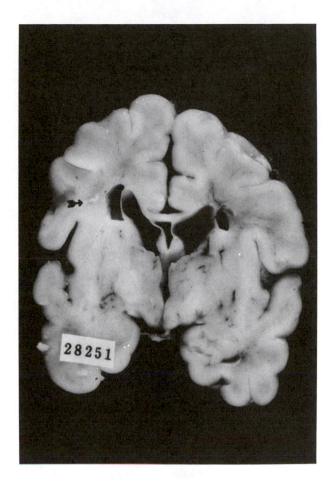

Figure 10–4   Coronal section of the brain of a three-week-old infant (estimated gestational age, 35 weeks) depicting the "white spots" of periventricular leukomalacia (arrow) and cystic lesions at angles of lateral ventricles noted at two days of age on ultrasound examination.

cribing a general approach to the evaluation. Then the specific clinical features, diagnostic studies, prognosis, and management of infants with the previously described neuropathologic disorders are described.

General Evaluation

The initial assessment of the infant with suspected hypoxic-ischemic encephalopathy relies on obtaining a thorough history and carrying out a careful physical examination. The history should be directed toward determining whether there were any specific antenatal factors that might account for the disorder. Review of the maternal history, fetal monitoring studies, fetal ultrasonographic findings, and fetal acid-base measurements is essential. Information regarding examination of the placenta should also be obtained.

A general physical examination is required to establish the infant's gestational age, cardiopulmonary status, presence of congenital anomalies, and growth parameters. A carefully performed neurologic examination is essential to obtain information about the infant's current status. This information is used to determine the supplementary evaluations that are indicated and is critical in establishing a prognosis. Many studies have shown that the neonatal neurologic examination is a valuable predictor of outcome.[2,70]

A detailed neurologic examination provides the most information in regard to the localization and severity of the encephalopathy, but a clinical staging examination, used in several studies of asphyxiated newborns, should be performed initially.[70] The clinical stages of hypoxic-ischemic encephalopathy are divided into three categories. The major clinical features to assess are the infant's level of consciousness, cranial nerve findings, muscle tone, deep tendon reflexes, neonatal reflexes, spontaneous motor activity, and autonomic function.

Infants with a mild degree of encephalopathy often have variable levels of consciousness in which periods of lethargy alternate with periods of irritability and "hyper-alertness." They often feed poorly, have disturbed sleep-wake cycles with a preponderance of active sleep, and are described as "jittery." Jitteriness is best described as a spontaneous or stimulus-induced myoclonus. Findings on the cranial nerve examination are normal. Muscle tone is normal or increased, with exaggerated deep tendon reflexes. The Moro reflex is often exaggerated and other neonatal reflexes are normal. Pupillary dilation and tachycardia are frequently observed.

Infants with a moderate degree of encephalopathy are lethargic and can be aroused with auditory and tactile stimuli. Feeding is extremely poor. Muscle tone is decreased, with a prominent head lag, a positive scarf sign, and a poor response to the Landau maneuver. Exaggerated deep tendon reflexes with clonus are elicited, and clonus of the jaw may be observed. The results of cranial nerve examination are normal except for a decreased gag reflex. Spontaneous motor activity is decreased, and the observed movements may include spontaneous myoclonus or show signs of extrapyramidal dysfunction. Pupils are often constricted, and periodic breathing associated with bradycardia may be present. Seizures may occur and must be differentiated from other abnormal movements and behavior.

The infant with severe encephalopathy is comatose, unresponsive to noxious stimuli, and flaccid. Deep tendon and neonatal reflexes are absent. The pupils are poorly reactive or fixed, and the oculocephalic reflex is absent. The infant often has bradycardia, systemic hypotension, and irregular respirations or apnea.

Laboratory investigations of the asphyxiated infant should include measurements of arterial blood gas and pH levels, serum electrolyte levels (including calcium and magnesium), and serum glucose, blood urea nitrogen, and creatine levels. A lumbar puncture with measurements of cerebrospinal fluid (CSF) pressure, cell count, and protein and glucose levels should be per-

formed. Measurements of several other metabolic indicators of the degree of insult could be carried out, including blood and CSF lactate levels, various serum enzyme levels, and CSF GABA and serum catecholamine levels.[71-73] The majority of these parameters reflect the severity of the systemic asphyxic insult rather than the severity of the insult to the brain. Creatine kinase isoenzyme determinations with either CSF or blood show particular promise for both diagnostic and prognostic measures of brain injury.[74,75] However, further studies are required to determine the sensitivity and specificity of this and the other metabolic parameters.

The electroencephalogram (EEG) is a valuable measure of cerebral function that can be performed at the bedside. It complements the clinical examination in establishing the severity of the encephalopathy and in determining the prognosis. The diagnosis of seizures in this age group is dependent on this study, since a significant number of abnormal behavior patterns thought to represent seizures actually represent other phenomena.[1] Its application to the evaluation of the encephalopathic newborn is described in detail in Chapter 15. Other neurophysiologic measures of nervous system function, such as somatosensory, brainstem, and visual evoked responses, have only recently been applied to evaluating the asphyxiated newborn and are not recommended as part of the general evaluation.[76-78]

Neuroimaging studies are an essential component of the assessment of the newborn with hypoxic-ischemic encephalopathy. Ultrasonography has proven to be a valuable technique in the diagnosis of intraventricular hemorrhage and periventricular leukomalacia. This study should be carried out in all infants with evidence of encephalopathy. However, when one is concerned about disease involving the cortex or posterior fossa, other imaging modalities are required. Computed tomography (CT) continues to be the procedure of choice when there is concern about hemorrhagic lesions. Magnetic resonance imaging (MRI) has been demonstrated to provide better anatomic detail in the newborn, especially when there is suspicion of disease in the posterior fossa. Information relating to normal and abnormal development of myelination also can be obtained by use of this neuroimaging technique.[79] Further details about the use of neuroimaging studies in the newborn are discussed in Chapter 17.

The most important aspect of managing the infant with hypoxic-ischemic encephalopathy is supportive care. In the asphyxiated newborn there is involvement of multiple systems, all of which require intervention. Maintenance of adequate ventilation is a critical component of the infant's care. Prevention of further episodes of hypoxemia and hypercarbia may play an important role in determining the ultimate neurologic outcome. Hyperoxemia may also be deleterious to the nervous system.[59] Maintenance of adequate cerebral perfusion is also critical; this is best achieved by maintaining normal systemic arterial pressure and avoiding excessive fluctuations. The fluid and electrolyte status requires close observation, since the asphyxiated infant has a higher risk of developing hypocalcemia, hyponatremia, hypoglycemia, and fluid overload.

Treatment directed toward the control of cerebral edema is controversial. Most pathologic studies suggest that cerebral edema rarely develops to the extent that herniation is observed at autopsy.[80] The role of brain edema in causing further brain injury is unknown. There have been no studies that demonstrate that the drugs used to decrease edema diminish the degree of neuronal injury. Nevertheless it is important to avoid fluid overload, realizing that the asphyxiated infant is at higher risk for developing the syndrome of inappropriate antidiuretic hormone secretion and may also have compromised renal function. The use of corticosteroids or osmotic diuretics is rarely indicated.

No other therapeutic modalities have been shown to be effective in altering the course of the encephalopathy. High dose barbiturate therapy has been used in the neonate and showed no benefit.[81] These drugs often cause further systemic complications.

Clinicopathologic Syndromes

The majority of information about infants with cortical infarcts secondary to vascular occlusion is derived from retrospective studies and case reports. Therefore the exact incidence of various clinical features in this population is unknown. However, several clinical features have been observed frequently.

The infants may have variable degrees of encephalopathy. A more severe encephalopathy is noted with venous occlusion because of frequently associated hemorrhage. Seizures are recurrently described in infants with this disorder.[82,83] Focal clonic seizures are often exhibited, and these seizures can be readily diagnosed by clinical criteria.[1] Focal findings are noted on neurologic examination, but they may be subtle. The EEG usually demonstrates lateralized abnormalities and allows assessment of the severity of the encephalopathy in other cortical regions. CT and MRI are essential investigations to determine the number, size, and location of the lesions. MRI is particularly useful in the diagnosis of infarcts due to venous occlusions. Infants may develop "congenital hemiplegia" as long-term sequelae. The extent and location of the pathologic lesion are important factors in determining whether intellectual impairment and epilepsy will also develop.[84]

Cortical infarcts in the watershed regions are difficult to diagnose in the neonatal period. Radioisotope studies and positron emission tomography have identified infants with decreased cerebral blood flow in the parasagittal cortex,[8,85] but there are few neuroimaging studies describing permanent lesions.[86] This is most likely because CT does not visualize this region well. Many cases of "atrophy" diagnosed by CT may be examples of this lesion. MRI potentially can identify these infants earlier in the course, especially when coronal images are obtained. These newborns often have a moderate encephalopathy in the neonatal period and may show evidence of weakness involving the proximal extremities. Seizures can be observed, especially in more severely affected infants. The neurologic sequelae often include a spastic quadriparesis with varying degrees of intellectual impairment. The latter is frequently noted, since the parietal, posterior temporal, and occipital cortices are often affected by this lesion. Research is needed to determine the spectrum of the acute clinical syndrome and long-term outcome in newborns with this disorder.

Infants with disease involving the deep gray matter nuclei, brainstem, and cerebellum usually have moderate to severe encephalopathy in the neonatal period. A history of maternofetal hemorrhage, hypotension, or congenital heart disease is often described.

Neurologic examination reveals brainstem dysfunction, flaccid quadriparesis, and respiratory abnormalities. The majority of infants require mechanical ventilation. As the encephalopathy evolves, the infants are described as having clinical seizures, the brainstem signs persist, and temperature instability may be observed. Bilateral facial weakness, gaze abnormalities, and tongue fasciculations have been described in an infant with brainstem involvement.[87] Infants with more extensive brainstem involvement may require prolonged ventilatory support. Ultrasonography is adequate to diagnose thalamic disease, but MRI allows better definition of thalamic and brainstem involvement.[55] Cerebellar involvement is often observed concurrently. Impairment of the posterior circulation due to hyperextension of the neck at the time of delivery has been suggested as being a factor in the pathogenesis of this lesion.[50]

These children usually have a poor long-term outcome. They often develop choreoathetosis, dystonia, and quadriparesis if there is greater involvement of the basal ganglia. The movement disorder has a delayed onset and may deteriorate over a one- to two-year period. Infants with brainstem involvement have bulbar dysfunction associated with poor feeding, failure to thrive, and recurrent aspiration. Hypotonia and ataxia are observed as sequelae of cerebellar involvement. Intellectual impairment is common and may be severe.

The clinical characteristics of infants with necrotic white matter lesions have only recently been described, but the spectrum of the clinical features during the acute phase still requires further definition.[88] Neonates usually are described as having evidence of increased tone in the lower extremities associated with increased neck extensor tone. Apnea, pseudobulbar palsy with poor feeding, and irritability have been described. Clinical seizures without electroencephalographic confirmation have been reported in 10 to 30 percent of the infants. EEGs have been described as having variable degrees of background abnormalities with a high correlation with positive rolandic sharp waves.[89] The diagnosis is made by ultrasonography, but MRI in later infancy better defines the extent of the disease and the associated abnormalities of myelination.[79] Spastic diplegia with varying degrees of intellectual impairment, especially visuomotor dysfunction, is the usual sequela. The latter may be predicted in the neonatal period by testing visual evoked responses.[80]

Periventricular or intraventricular hemorrhage often is clinically silent in the preterm neonate. Severe hemorrhage may present with an acute syndrome, with rapid deterioration of the level of consciousness, brainstem dysfunction, decerebrate posturing, and clinical tonic seizures. The latter events are unlikely to be epileptic seizures, since recent EEG-video monitoring studies have demonstrated that less than 10 percent of these events are accompanied by an electrographic seizure.[1] A subacute presentation is more common, with intermittent neurologic symptoms superimposed on slowly progressive encephalopathy. The newborn may have episodes of abnormal eye movements, hypotonia, and decreased spontaneous motor activity. A fall in the hematocrit level is often an important sign. Ultrasonography is the diagnostic procedure of choice.

The prognosis is extremely variable and many infants have no sequelae. The prognosis is most closely correlated with the degree of parenchymal involvement rather than the extent of the hemorrhage. The EEG has been demonstrated to be a valuable prognostic indicator in this population.[90]

FUTURE PROSPECTS

The management of the asphyxiated newborn requires early identification, assessment, and stabilization of the cardiopulmonary status and a detailed neurologic evaluation. The identification of infants with specific clinicopathologic syndromes allows prediction of both acute and long-term problems. It is important to identify newborns with these various syndromes early in the course when considering various treatment protocols.

Further insight into the pathophysiology of hypoxic-ischemic encephalopathy will undoubtedly be obtained through the application of positron emission tomography, near infrared spectrophotometry, and Doppler ultrasonography in the human neonate. An NMR spectroscopic technique utilizing the proton (^1H) nucleus (which is also used in imaging) has yet to be applied to the neonate. This noninvasive technique potentially can answer many critical questions regarding this disorder.

With this technique, measurement of brain concentrations of glutamate, glutamine, lactate, and GABA have already been achieved in animal studies of hypoxia and hypoglycemia (Fig. 10–5).[91,92] Phosphorus spectros-

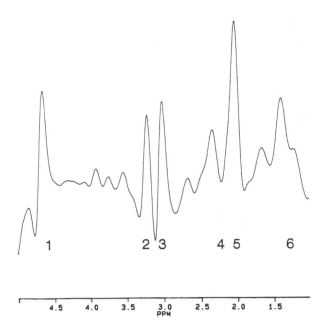

Figure 10-5 Proton nuclear magnetic resonance spectrum of a rabbit brain obtained on a 4.7 Tesla, Bruker/ORS spectrometer with a 16 mm surface coil. The spectrum represents the sum of 256 scans acquired over five minutes. The peak assignments are as follows: 1, water; 2, choline-phosphocholine; 3, creatine-phosphocreatine; 4, glutamate and glutamine; 5, N-acetyl aspartate and sialic acid; 6, lipid and proteins.

copy also can be performed concurrently so that both high energy phosphate compounds and these metabolites can be measured. Measurements can be made serially so that information regarding the kinetics of enzyme reactions can be obtained in vivo. Application of this technique to animals and yeast has demonstrated that canonical views determined by in vitro methods relating to metabolism need to be reconsidered.[93]

Proton NMR spectroscopy just recently has been applied to the adult brain.[94] Its application to investigation of the neonatal brain is anticipated. Issues regarding prognosis, efficacy of therapeutic interventions, and, most important, the regulation of metabolism under both normal and pathologic conditions will be addressed.

REFERENCES

1. Mizrahi EM, Kellaway P. Characterization and classification of neonatal seizures. Neurology 1987; 37:1837.
2. Finer NN, Robertson CM, Richards RT, et al. Hypoxic-ischemic encephalopathy in term neonates: perinatal factors and outcome. J Pediatr 1981; 98:112.
3. Brown JK, Purvis RJ, Forfar JO, Cockburn F. Neurological aspects of perinatal asphyxia. Dev Med Child Neurol 1974; 16:567.
4. Blair E, Stanley FJ. Intrapartum asphyxia: a rare cause of cerebral palsy. J Pediatr 1988; 112:515.
5. Nelson KB. What proportion of cerebral palsy is related to birth asphyxia? J Pediatr 1988; 112:572.
6. Nelson KB, Ellenberg JH. Antecedents of CP: multivariate analysis of risk. N Engl J Med 1986; 315:81.

7. Naeye RL, Peters EC. Antenatal hypoxia and low IQ values. Am J Dis Child 1987; 141:50.

8. Volpe JJ, Herscovitch P, Perlman JM, et al. Positron emission tomography in the asphyxiated term newborn: parasagittal impairment of cerebral blood flow. Ann Neurol 1985; 17:287.

9. Bada HS, Miller JE, Menke JA, et al. Intracranial pressure and cerebral arterial pulsatile flow measurements in neonatal intraventricular hemorrhage. J Pediatr 1982; 100:291.

10. Hamilton PA, Cady EB, Wyatt JS, et al. Impaired energy metabolism in brains of newborn infants with increased echodensities. Lancet 1986; 1:1242.

11. Wyatt JS, Delpy DT, Cope M, et al. Quantification of cerebral oxygenation and hemodynamics in sick newborn infants by near infrared spectrophotometry. Lancet 1986; 2:1063.

12. Rossen R, Kabat H, Anderson JP. Acute arrest of cerebral circulation in man. Arch Neurol Psychiatry 1943; 50:510.

13. Vannucci RC, Duffy TE. Cerebral metabolism in newborn dogs during reversible asphyxia. Ann Neurol 1977; 1:528.

14. Kleihaus P, Hossmann K-A, Pegg AE, et al. Resuscitation of the monkey brain after 1 hour of complete ischemia. III. Indicators of metabolic recovery. Brain Res 1975; 95:61.

15. Nicholson C. Measurement of extracellular ions in the brain. Trends Neurosci 1980; 3:216.

16. Harris RJ, Symon L, Branston NM, Bayhan M. Changes in extracellular calcium activity in cerebral ischemia. J Cereb Blood Flow Metab 1981; 1:203.

17. Siesjo BK. Cell damage in the brain: a speculative synthesis. J Cereb Blood Flow Metab 1981; 1:155.

18. Hossmann K-A. Treatment of experimental cerebral ischemia. J Cereb Blood Flow Metab 1982; 2:275.

19. Vannucci RC, Duffy TE. Carbohydrate metabolism in fetal and neonatal rat brain during anoxia and recovery. Am J Physiol 1976; 230:1269.

20. Folbergrová J, Ljunggren B, Norberg K, Siesjo BK. Influence of complete ischemia on glycolytic metabolites, citric acid cycle intermediates, and associated amino acids in the rat cerebral cortex. Brain Res 1975; 80:265.

21. Hagberg H, Lehmann A, Sanberg M, et al. Ischemia-induced shift of inhibitory and excitatory amino acids from intra- to extracellular compartments. J Cereb Blood Flow Metabol 1985; 5:413.

22. Gardiner M, Nilsson B, Rehncrona S, Siesjo BK. Free fatty acids in the rat brain in moderate and severe hypoxia. J Neurochem 1981; 36:1500.

23. Cheung JY, Bonventre JV, Malis CO, Leaf A. Calcium and ischemic injury. N Engl J Med 1986; 314:1670.

24. Himwich HE, Bernstein AO, Herrlich H, et al. Mechanisms for maintenance of life in the newborn during anoxia. Am J Physiol 1942; 135:387.

25. Voorhies TM, Rawlinson D, Vannucci RC. Glucose and perinatal hypoxic-ischemic brain damage. Neurology 1986; 36:1115.

26. Vannucci RC, Vasta F, Vannucci SJ. Cerebral metabolic response of hyperglycemic immature rats to hypoxia-ischemia. Pediatr Res 1987; 21:524.

27. Myers RE, Yamaguchi S. Nervous system effects of cardiac arrest in monkeys. Arch Neurol 1977; 34:65.

28. Chugani HT, Phelps ME, Mazziotta JL. Positron emission tomography study of human brain functional development. Ann Neurol 1987; 22:487.

29. Doyle LW, Nahmias C, Firnau G, et al. Regional cerebral glucose metabolism of newborn infants measured by positron emission tomography. Dev Med Child Neurol 1985; 25:143.

30. Cady EB, Dawson MJ, Hope PL, et al. Noninvasive investigation of cerebral metabolism in newborn infants by phosphorus nuclear magnetic resonance spectroscopy. Lancet 1983; 1:1059.

31. Hope PL, Cady EB, Tofts PS, et al. Cerebral energy metabolism studied with phosphorus NMR spectroscopy in normal and birth asphyxiated infants. Lancet 1984; 2:366.

32. Younkin DP, Delivoria-Papadopoulas M, Leonard JC, et al. Unique aspects of cerebral metabolism evaluated with phosphorus nuclear magnetic resonance spectroscopy. Ann Neurol 1984; 16:581.

33. Petroff OAC, Prichard JW, Behar KL, et al. Cerebral intracellular pH by ^{31}P nuclear magnetic resonance spectroscopy. Neurology 1985; 35:781.

34. Corbett RJT, Laptook AR, Nunnally RL. The use of the chemical shift of the phosphomonoester P-31 magnetic resonance peak for the determination of intracellular pH in the brains of neonates. Neurology 1987; 37:1771.

35. Johnston MV. Neurotransmitter alteration in a model of perinatal hypoxic-ischemic brain injury. Ann Neurol 1983; 13:511.

36. Rothman SM, Olney JW. Glutamate and the pathophysiology of hypoxic-ischemic brain damage. Ann Neurol 1986; 19:105.

37. Schwarcz R, Meldrum B. Excitatory amino acid antagonists provide a therapeutic approach to neurological disorders. Lancet 1985; 2:140.

38. Ozyurt E, Graham DI, Woodruff GN, McCulloch J. Protective effect of the glutamate antagonist MK-801 in focal cerebral ischemia in the cat. J Cereb Blood Flow Metab 1988; 8:138.

39. McDonald J, Silverstein FS, Johnston MV. The glutamate antagonist MK-801 attenuates perinatal hypoxic-ischemic brain injury. Ann Neurol 1987; 22:407.

40. Ford LM, Rogelson HM, Norman A, Sanberg P. MK-801 protects hippocampal neuronal function from neonatal hypoxic-ischemic damage. Neurology 1988; 30(Suppl 1):158.

41. Ashwal S, Dale PS, Longo LD. Regional cerebral blood flow: studies in the fetal lamb during hypoxia, hypercapnia, acidosis and hypotension. Pediatr Res 1984; 18:1309.

42. Young RSK, Hernandez MJ, Yagel SK. Selective reduction of blood flow to white matter during hypotension in newborn dogs: a possible mechanism of periventricular leukomalacia. Ann Neurol 1982; 12:445.

43. Laptook AR, Stonestreet BS, Oh W. Brain blood flow and O_2 delivery during hemorrhagic hypotension in the piglet. Pediatr Res 1983; 17:77.

44. Lou HC, Lassen NA, Friis-Hansen B. Impaired autoregulation of cerebral blood flow in the distressed newborn infant. J Pediatr 1979; 94:118.

45. Ment LR, Ehrenkranz RA, Lange RC, et al. Alterations in cerebral blood flow in preterm infants with intraventricular hemorrhage. Pediatrics 1981; 68:763.

46. Milligan DW, Bryan MH. Failure of autoregulation of the cerebral circulation in the sick newborn infant. Pediatr Res 1979; 13:527.

47. McMenamin JB, Volpe JJ. Doppler ultrasonography in the determination of cerebral brain death. Ann Neurol 1983; 14:302.

48. Norman MG. Perinatal brain damage. In: Rosenberg HS, Bolande RP, eds. Perspectives in pediatric pathology. Vol 4. Chicago: Year Book, 1978:41.

49. Urich H. Malformations of the nervous system, perinatal damage and related conditions in early life. In: Blackwood W, Corellis JAN, eds. Greenfield's neuropathology. 3rd ed. London: Edward Arnold, 1976:361.

50. Rorke LB. Pathology of perinatal brain injury. New York: Raven Press, 1982.

51. Friede RL. Developmental neuropathology. New York: Springer-Verlag, 1975:24.

52. Barmada MA, Moosy J, Shuman RM. Cerebral infarcts with arterial occlusion in neonates. Ann Neurol 1979; 6:495.

53. Banker BQ. Cerebral vascular disease in infancy and childhood. I. Occlusive vascular disease. J Neuropathol Exp Neurol 1961; 20:127.

54. Myer JE. Uber die Lokalisation Frühkindlicher Hirnshäden in arterial Grenzgebieten. Arch Psychiatry Z Neurol 1953; 190:328.

55. Voit T, Lemburg P, Neuen E, Lumenta C, Stork W. Damage of thalamus and basal ganglia in asphyxiated full-term neonates. Neuropediatrics 1987; 18:176.

56. Malamud N, Hirano A. Atlas of neuropathology. 2nd ed. Berkeley: University of California Press, 1974.

57. Gilles FH. Hypotensive brain stem necrosis: selective symmetrical necrosis of tegmental neuronal aggregates following cardiac arrest. Arch Pathol 1969; 88:32.

58. Friede RL. Pontosubicular lesions in perinatal anoxia. Arch Pathol 1972; 94:343.

59. Barmada MA, Moosy J, Painter M. Pontosubicular necrosis and hyperoxemia. Pediatrics 1980; 66:840.

60. Leech RW, Alvord EC. Glial fatty metamorphosis: an abnormal response of premyelin glia frequently accompanying periventricular leukomalacia. Am J Pathol 1974; 74:603.

61. Gilles FH, Murphy SF. Perinatal telencephalic leucoencephalopathy. J Neurol Neurosurg Psychiatry 1969; 32:404.
62. Banker BQ, Larroche JC. Periventricular leukomalacia of infancy. Arch Neurol 1962; 7:386.
63. Guzzetta F, Shackleford GD, Volpe S, et al. Periventricular intraparenchymal echodensities in the premature newborn: critical determination of neurologic outcome. Pediatrics 1986; 78:995.
64. Fawer CL, Calame A, Perentes E, Anderegg A. Periventricular leukomalacia: a correlation study between real-time ultrasound and autopsy findings. Neuroradiology 1985; 27:292.
65. Trounce JQ, Rutter N, Levene MI. Periventricular leukomalacia and intraventricular haemorrhage in the preterm neonate. Arch Dis Child 1986; 16:1196.
66. Enzmann D, Murphy-Irwin K, Stevenson D, et al. The natural history of subependymal germinal matrix hemorrhage. Am J Perinatol 1985; 2:123.
67. Dolfin T, Skidmore MB, Fong KW, et al. Incidence severity and timing of subependymal and intraventricular haemorrhage in preterm infants born in a perinatal unit as detected by serial real-time ultrasound. Pediatrics 1983; 71:541.
68. Volpe JJ. Neurology of the newborn. 2nd ed. Philadelphia: WB Saunders, 1987.
69. Seher MS, Wright FS, Lockman LA, Thompson TR. Intraventricular haemorrhage in the full-term neonate. Arch Neurol 1982; 39:769.
70. Levene MI, Grindulis H, Sands C, Moore JR. Comparison of two methods of predicting outcome in perinatal asphyxia. Lancet 1986; 1:67.
71. Fernandez F, Verdu A, Quero J, et al. Cerebrospinal fluid lactate levels in term infants with perinatal hypoxia. Pediatr Neurol 1986; 2:35.
72. Hedner T, Iversen K, Lundborg P. γ-Aminobutyric acid concentrations in the cerebrospinal fluid of newborn infants. Early Hum Dev 1982; 7:53.
73. Nylund L, Dahlin I, Lagercrantz H. Fetal catecholamines and the Apgar score. J Perinat Med 1987; 15:340.
74. Hollander PI, Wright L, Nagey DA, et al. Indicators of perinatal asphyxia. Am J Obstet Gynecol 1987; 157:839.
75. Ezitis J, Finnstrom O, Hedman G, Rabow L. CK_{BB}-enzyme activity in serum in neonates born after vaginal delivery and cesaerean section. Neuropediatrics 1987; 18:146.
76. Majnemer A, Rosenblatt B, Riley P, et al. Somatosensory evoked response abnormalities in high-risk newborns. Pediatr Neurol 1987; 3:350.
77. Stockard JE, Stockard JJ, Kleinberg F, Westmoreland BF. Prognostic value of brainstem auditory evoked responses in neonates. Arch Neurol 1983; 40:360.
78. Whyte HE, Taylor MJ, Menzies R, et al. Prognostic utility of visual evoked potentials in term asphyxiated neonates. Pediatr Neurol 1986; 2:220.
79. DeVries LS, Connell JA, Dubowitz LMS, et al. Neurological, electrophysiological and MRI abnormalities in infants with extensive cystic leukomalacia. Neuropediatrics 1987; 18:61.
80. Pryse-Davies J, Beard RW. A necropsy study of brain swelling in the newborn with special reference to cerebellar herniation. J Pathol 1973; 109:51.
81. Eyre JA, Wilkinson AR. Thiopentone induced coma after severe birth asphyxia. Arch Dis Child 1986; 61:1084.
82. Clancy R, Malin S, Laraque D, et al. Focal motor seizures heralding stroke in full-term neonates. Am J Dis Child 1985; 139:601.
83. Wong VK, LeMesuier J, Franceschini R, et al. Cerebral venous thrombosis as a cause of neonatal seizures. Pediatr Neurol 1987; 3:235.
84. Levine SC, Huttenlocher P, Banich MT, Duda E. Factors affecting cognitive function of hemiplegic children. Dev Med Child Neurol 1987; 29:27.
85. Volpe JJ, Pasternak JF. Parasagittal cerebral injury in neonatal hypoxic-ischemic encephalopathy: clinical and neuroradiological features. J Pediatr 1979; 91:472.
86. Pasternak JF. Parasagittal infarction in neonatal asphyxia. Ann Neurol 1987; 21:202.
87. Rolande EH, Hill A, Norman MG, et al. Selective brainstem injury in an asphyxiated newborn. Ann Neurol 1988; 23:89.
88. Trounce JQ, Shaw DE, Leverne MI, Rutter N. Clinical risk factors and periventricular leucomalacia. Arch Dis Child 1988; 63:17.
89. Novotny EJ, Tharp BR, Coen RW, et al. Positive rolandic sharp waves in the EEG of the premature infant. Neurology 1987; 37:1481.
90. Clancy RR, Tharp BR, Enzmann D. EEG in premature infants with intraventricular hemorrhage. Neurology 1984; 34:583.
91. Behar KL, den Hollander JA, Stromski ME, et al. High-resolution 1H nuclear magnetic resonance study of cerebral hypoxia in vivo. Proc Natl Acad Sci USA 1983; 80:4945.
92. Behar KL, den Hollander JA, Petroff OAC, et al. The effect of hypoglycemic encephalopathy upon amino acids, high energy phosphates, and pH$_i$ in the rat brain in vivo: detection by sequential 1H and 31P NMR spectroscopy. J Neurochem 1985; 44:1045.
93. Shulman RG. High resolution NMR in vivo. Trends Biochem Sci 1988; 13:37.
94. Hanstock CC, Rothman DL, Prichard JW, et al. Spatially localized 1H NMR spectra of metabolites in the human brain. Proc Natl Acad Sci 1988; 85:1821.

11

Neonatal Seizures

Robert R. Clancy, M.D.

What Types of Clinical Events are Called Seizures?
The Electrographic Seizure
   Clinical Electroencephalographic Recording:
     Characteristics of a Neonatal Seizure
   Morphology
   Spatial Distribution
   Temporal Profile
   Caveats
   The Interictal Electroencephalographic Background
Failure to Capture an Electrographic Seizure
   The "Classic" Interictal Tracing
   Do "Epileptiform" Sharp Waves Always Imply
     Seizures?
The Uncoupling of Clinical and Electrographic Seizures
Occult Neonatal Seizures
Long-Term Electroencephalographic Monitoring
The Significance of Neonatal Seizures
   High Incidence
   Etiology: Acute Seizures
   Case Studies
   Prognosis for Death and Neurologic Morbidity
     Recent Trends
     Influence of Etiology
     Measures of Seizure Severity
   Direct Ictal Injury
Medicolegal Pitfalls
   Establishing the Diagnosis of Neonatal Seizures
   Etiology of Seizure
   The Neonatal Electroencephalogram

> "The Fallyng Euyll called in the Greke Tonge Epilepsia: Not only other ages but also lytle chyldren, are oftentimes afflicted with this greuouse syckenes...and than it is impossible, or difficile to cure...whereupon this infirmity procedeth, whiche if it be in one that is young and tender, it is very hard to be removed.... Thomas Phaire (d.1560): *The Boke of Chyldren*[1]

It has been known since antiquity that newborn infants may be subject to "seizures," "fits," or "convulsions." The term *seizure* is derived from the Greek implying a sudden "attack" of disease. The invention of electroencephalography (EEG) by Hans Berger provided clinical investigators with the necessary tool to discover the epileptic mechanism that underlies the clinical phenomena of grand mal and petit mal seizures. As the electrophysiologic basis for seizures in older children and adults came to be better understood, it was assumed that clinical seizures in neonates were similarly founded on an epileptic mechanism—the abnormal, excessive, paroxysmal electrical discharges arising from hypersynchronous, repetitive neuronal firing in the cerebral cortex.

The study of epilepsy in adults gradually evolved with the implementation and revision of classification schema proposed to organize the clinically observed phenomena of seizures. Gradually electroclinical correlates were recognized and epileptic syndromes defined. Unfortunately progress in the nosology of neonatal seizures met many obstacles owing to the precarious medical conditions of afflicted babies and the unique features of the immature developing central nervous system.[2] Although it was clear that some neonatal seizures were accompanied by simultaneous epileptic discharges demonstrated by EEG, it generally was assumed that neonatal seizures closely paralleled adult epilepsy. It is now clear that not every clinical event in a neonate that appears as an abrupt "attack" is epileptic in nature and that the relationship between neonatal seizures and the conventional connotations of the term *epilepsy* demands careful scrutiny.[3]

This chapter first reviews the protean types of paroxysmal events that have been called seizures by clinical observers. Next the epileptic basis of some neonatal seizures is discussed in the context of the EEG—the "gold standard" for determining the electrophysiologic basis of epileptic behavior. The electroclinical correlates of neonatal seizures are then addressed, emphasizing that many abnormal attacks in sick infants are not founded on a specific epileptic mechanism and, conversely, that many electrographic seizures may be clinically occult. Finally the significance of neonatal seizures is emphasized, stressing the notion that neonatal seizures are a potent sign of acute neurologic disease, which requires immediate recognition and treatment and which frequently presages an adverse neurologic outcome.

WHAT TYPES OF CLINICAL EVENTS ARE CALLED SEIZURES?

Clinical observation of the behavior of the neonate reveals that healthy babies have a definite but limited repertoire of mental and motor skills. Arousal, behavior, feeding, and sleep are continuously cycled. During quiet wakefulness the infant's eyes are open, and spontaneous conjugate eye movements scan the environment. Brief visual fixation and following of a close target are reproducibly observable. However, the content of consciousness is impossible to infer. Motor activity appears to be random and purposeless. Indeed some developmental pediatricians regard the newborn motor system as resembling a physiologic "cerebral palsy" in which purposeful volitional motor acts are not possible since the infant cannot control the body, involuntary movements of the trunk and limbs appear to represent subcortically directed activity, the infant is dominated by primitive and postural reflexes that exert a net influence defining their ultimate tone and posture, and "pathologic reflexes" such as the Babinski sign are common. Observation of the awake infant reveals a rich collection of abundant movements, startles, postures, and tremors that collectively compose the infant's motor and behavioral repertoire.

The historical use of the diagnosis "seizure" denoted a distinctive dramatic "fit" or "convulsion"—forceful, involuntary, unnatural contractions of the somatic musculature. In the past, hypocalcemia accounted for many instances of convulsions. The signs of central nervous system hyperirritability then were often evidenced by the appearance of latent or active tetany. Latent signs became manifest only after the appropriate provocation elicited Chvostek's and Trousseau's signs. Active signs arose spontaneously as tonic contractions of the hands or feet (carpopedal spasms) and "convulsions." Although distinctive convulsions were the prototype of the neonatal seizure described in the period 1950 to 1970, the actual clinical characteristics of the attacks were often poorly described in the medical literature. For example, Keen and Lee's study of neonatal seizures included patients observed to have "generalized clonic movements with or without a tonic phase."[4] (The inclusion of generalized tonic-clonic activity is notable, since the modern use of video-EEG telemetry indicates that the "grand mal seizure" probably does not exist in the neonate.) Nevertheless the description of seizures as "generalized" has persisted even into recent times. In another study the seizure population was composed of those infants with attacks such that "any event thought to be a convulsion by a person experienced in the care of newborns [was] considered to be so."[5]

There was, however, a gradual appreciation that neonatal seizures need not be dramatic, forceful, violent convulsions. Freeman[6] suggested that "any type of bizarre or unusual transient event" should raise the suspicion of a neonatal seizure. Attacks of repeated stereotyped unnatural tonic stiffening, posturing, clonic jerking, or more complex, integrated limb activity such as swimming or bicycling motions might be the clinical expression of a neonatal seizure. The bulbar signs of seizures expanded to include nystagmus, eye rolling, staring, tongue thrusting, and lip smacking.

In the early 1970s Volpe[7] suggested a scheme to organize the protean clinical manifestations of neonatal seizures. In that classification the predominant expression of the attacks could be characterized as focal clonic, multifocal clonic, tonic, myoclonic, or subtle seizures (Table 11-1). Subtle seizures implied an abnormal constellation of behavior and movements whose unnatural, repetitive, obligatory, stereotyped choreography signified a "nonconvulsive" seizure. The implications of such classification schemes are that the epileptic process underlies the clinical ictal activity, that the movements and patterns of the tonic posturing or subtle seizure explicitly guarantee coincident epileptic discharges on the EEG and that antiepileptic drugs such as phenobarbital, phenytoin, and diazepam are the appropriate pharmacotherapy.

Unfortunately the use of this clinical classification opened the door to diagnosing virtually any paroxysmal behavior as a subtle seizure; e.g., sucking movements may indeed be one facet of a genuine subtle seizure in a sick neonate. However, other sick intubated infants may innocently suck on the endotracheal tube or tongue thrust without exhibiting other features of a seizure. Too often the latter are overdiagnosed as neonatal seizures.

Newborn infants exhibit many behavior patterns that the anxious or inexperienced observer may erroneously interpret as having an epileptic basis and label as a subtle seizure. During dream sleep (rapid eye movement or active sleep), infants may suck, grimace, squirm, posture, tremble, or display bursts of "nystagmoid" eye movements. Infants who are tremulous or jittery for any reason can be mistakenly thought to have "clonic seizures." Apnea, hiccups, cyanotic spells, and gastroesophageal reflux are collectively common events that could be mistakenly labeled as "neonatal seizures" with

TABLE 11-1   Clinical Classification of Neonatal Seizures

Clonic	These movements appear as repeated jerking or twitching of a body part with a characteristic rapid contraction phase and a slower relaxation phase. Clonic jerking lacks the rhythmic oscillation of tremor and is not abolished by holding or repositioning the affected parts.
Tonic	The abrupt onset of sustained contraction of a group of muscles causes an alteration in tone that produces a sudden change in posture. The term "posturing" is often used synonymously with "tonic attack." The abrupt tone change can affect a single limb (focal tonic seizure) or all muscles of the trunk and limbs (generalized tonic seizure).
Myoclonic	A myoclonic movement implies a sudden shocklike muscle twitch. The involved part displays a single jolt that can repeat erratically and recur arrhythmically.
Subtle	The term embraces a wide spectrum of complex, semi-integrated movements such as oral-buccal-lingual automatisms or pedaling-swimming gestures of the limbs.

the implication of an underlying epileptic process.[8] The implications of such instances of overdiagnosis are many and include an unwarranted search for the cause of the seizures (unnecessary diagnostic testing such as lumbar puncture or computed tomographic [CT] scanning) and the needless administration of anticonvulsant drugs. Such a diagnostic overreaction also clouds the issue of future neurologic prognosis and unnecessarily generates fear of brain damage. Furthermore, it provides unfounded medicolegal "ammunition," which assumes the existence of acute encephalopathy that in fact may not exist.

Although the term *seizure* can be applied in a general sense to any sudden "attack," most physicians assume that the diagnosis automatically implies the presence of an epileptic abnormality. In infants some seizures may be dramatic and obvious, but many are subtle and diagnostic inaccuracies that may occur easily. It is likely that interobserver agreement in regard to the diagnosis of seizures by different bedside clinical observers will be poor. Thus, the older medical literature relating to neonatal seizures (especially those lacking any EEG confirmation) probably describes a heterogeneous mixture of patients, including those with genuine epileptic seizures grouped with those with innocuous tremors, mild posturing, activities of dream sleep, and other paroxysms. The contemporary low threshold of the diagnosis of "subtle seizure" probably has inflated the apparent incidence of seizures, since many children with a few tongue thrusts or peculiar eye movements are suspected of exhibiting subtle seizures. Unaided clinical inspection of the patient is invaluable in order to first note unusual motor activity or behavioral changes consistent with pathologic, epilepsy-based seizures, but confirmation of the diagnosis rests on the objective findings on the electroencephalogram.

THE ELECTROGRAPHIC SEIZURE

At the very heart of the epileptic process is the abnormal excessive repetitive electrical firing of neurons. Affected neurons lose their autonomy and independent behavior and are engulfed by the synchronized bursts of repeated electrical discharges. Sustained trains of action potentials arise in the affected nerve cells, which repeatedly fire and eventually propagate beyond their site of origin. At the conclusion of the ictus, inhibitory influences materialize, terminate the microscopic cascade, and bring the seizure to an end.

Epileptic seizures have been studied in several animal species including the newborn rat, kitten, rabbit, dog, and chimpanzee, and such studies provide important insights into seizure mechanisms in the immature cortex of human neonates. For example, neurons in the immature hippocampus may be provoked to seizure activity with greater ease than pyramidal cells in the neocortex.[9] However, both types of cells exhibit consistent electrophysiologic differences from the behavior of their mature counterparts and are inherently less apt to initiate and sustain ictal discharges.[10]

The epileptic seizure is an electrophysiologic event that begins with characteristic changes in a small nest of abnormal neurons—the epileptic "focus." Although normal immature cortex has a relatively high seizure threshold, cortical injury enhances its susceptibility to seizures. Once initiated, the activity of the focus propagates beyond its original boundaries and subverts the behavior of neurons in neighboring cortex. Immature neurons apparently possess only weak refractoriness following a seizure compared to stronger postictal suppression in mature cortex. Consequently repeated seizures can arise in immature cortex owing to feeble postictal seizure immunity.[9] Although the barrier to the first neonatal seizure may be relatively high, it is fragile and easily overwhelmed permitting repetitive seizures to arise.

Clinical Electroencephalographic Recording: Characteristics of a Neonatal Seizure

The pathophysiologic events of a seizure arise locally within the synapses and cell bodies of individual neurons. In clinical neonatal medicine intraneuronal recordings are never obtained. Instead scalp-surface tracings are recorded, which reflect the summated extracellular potentials generated by many thousands of underlying nerve cells. The clinical EEG thus reflects the collective behavior of large populations of neurons and is the "gold standard" for demonstrating unequivocally the presence of epileptic activity in the sick neonate.

Morphology

An electrographic seizure is a discrete abnormal event with a definite beginning and end. There is no single morphology of EEG patterns that constitutes a seizure (Fig. 11-1). Indeed, even in the same patient the morphology of the ictal EEG activity may appear pleomorphic. The "typical" neonatal seizure begins as low amplitude, rhythmic, or sinusoidal wave forms or spike-sharp waves. In the course of the evolution of the seizure, the amplitude of the ictal activity increases while its frequency slows (Fig. 11-2). It must be emphasized that spikes or sharp waves are not necessarily present. Instead evolving rhythmic activity of any frequency (delta, theta, alpha, or beta) can make up the ictal patterns observable at the scalp surface.

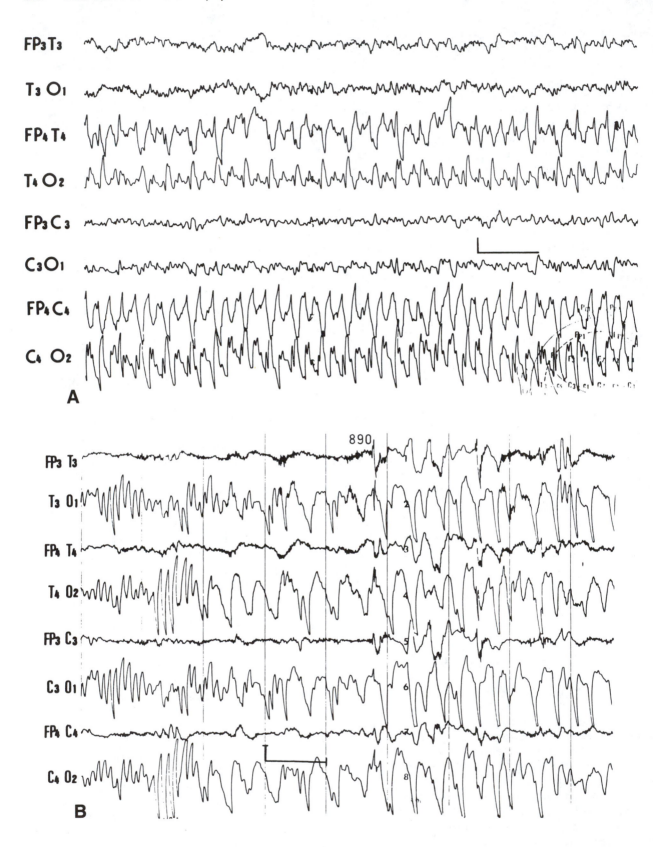

Figure 11–1   The appearance of electrographic seizures is diverse and reflects the variable morphology of the patterns that constitute the ictus. *A*, A portion of continuing seizure involving the right central-temporal region (channels 3, 4, 7, and 8) is seen consisting of repetitive sharp waves. *B*, The ictus appears in both occipital regions (channels 2, 4, 6, and 8) as hypersynchronous rhythmic 5 Hz activity, which rapidly evolves to stereotyped delta patterns. *Figure continues.*

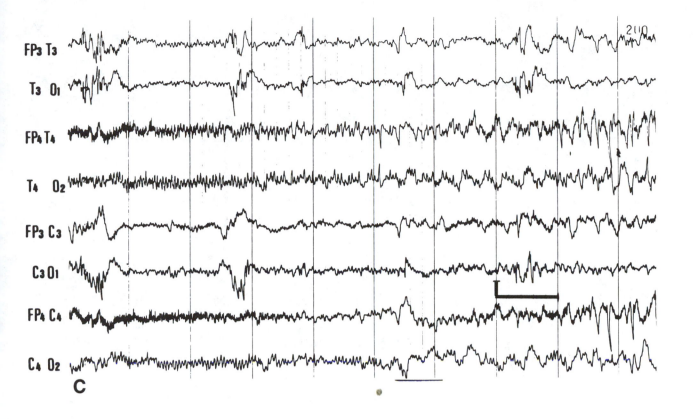

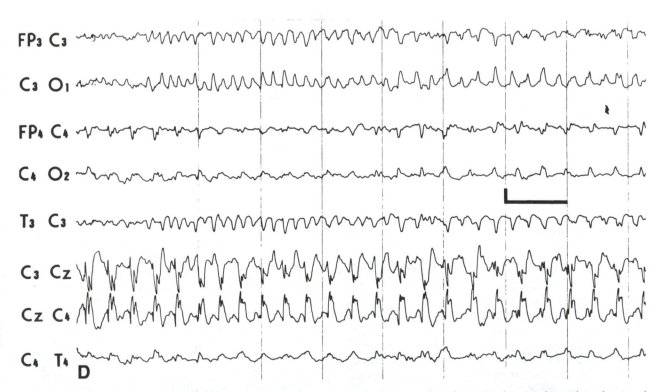

Figure 11-1 Continued   C, The seizure begins as low amplitude, rhythmic, fast activity in the right temporal-occipital area (channels 3, 4, and 8) which evolves to a different morphology, including repetitive spikes. D, The seizure comprises repetitive spike slow waves at the central vertex (channels 6 and 7). However, in the adjacent central region (channels 1, 2, and 5) the same seizure has a different appearance in the form of rhythmic delta activity. (Calibration in these and all subsequent EEG segments: 50 microvolts, two seconds.) (Reprinted with permission from Clancy RR, Legido A. The exact ictal and interictal duration of electroencephalographic neonatal seizures. Epilepsia 1987; 28:537.)

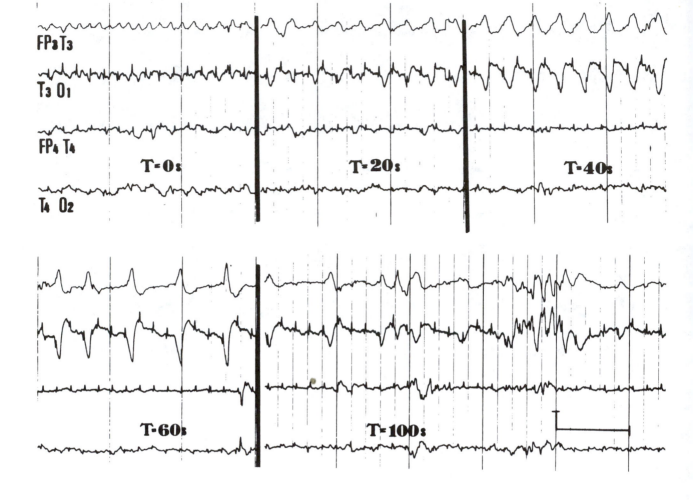

Figure 11-2   Electrographic seizures unfold as an evolving process. At the beginning of the ictus (T = 0 s), low amplitude, rhythmic, 3 to 4 Hz, sinusoidal patterns arise in the left temporal area (channels 1 and 2). There is a gradual metamorphosis of the ictal wave forms so that by time 60 seconds, higher amplitude, 2 Hz sharp waves constitute the seizure. The seizure finally terminates after 100 seconds. Note the electrocardiographic artifact on channels 3 and 4, which does not evolve.

Spatial Distribution

In older individuals generalized seizures may arise that appear simultaneously, synchronously, and symmetrically in both hemispheres. This well-orchestrated organization requires a physiologic maturity and harmony that are wanting in the neonatal brain. In contrast to this sophisticated ictal activity, individual neonatal seizures always arise focally. For example, an individual focal seizure might first appear in the left temporal region (T_3)* and eventually migrate to adjacent electrode sites $(FP_3, C_3,$ or $O_1)$ and then engage the entire hemisphere. The seizure might later spread to the opposite hemisphere. Occasionally simultaneous focal seizures may arise that appear to behave in an independent autonomous manner (Fig. 11-3). A single focal seizure may spread to all brain regions and superficially masquerade as a "generalized seizure." However, the morphology of those ictal patterns does not resemble that of the truly generalized seizure, which usually is composed of spike—or polyspike—slow wave discharges.

---

*The international 10-20 system employs an abbreviated notation to designate different scalp regions. In that scheme the following key applies: T = temporal, C = central, O = occipital, F = frontal, FP = frontal polar, P = parietal. Odd number subscripts refer to the left hemisphere; even number subscripts refer to the right hemisphere.

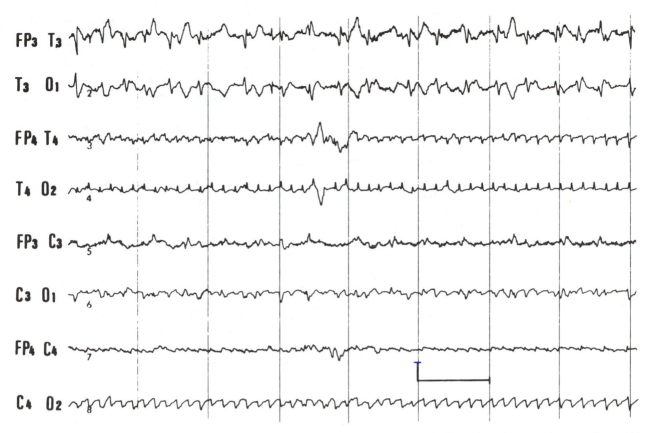

Figure 11-3 A true generalized neonatal seizure, with bilateral synchronous and symmetrical spike or sharp slow waves is extremely rare, if it occurs at all. However, simultaneous independent seizures can be recorded that affect multiple scalp locations. In this example, note that one seizure is occurring in the left temporal region (channels 1 and 2) and is composed of 1 to 1.5 Hz sharp and slow waves. An entirely different seizure evolves in the right temporal-occipital region (channels 3, 4, and 8) and is composed of 3 Hz spikes, which are independent of the left temporal ictal activity.

Neonatal seizures begin focally regardless of the specific etiology. Although one might expect diffuse causes of encephalopathy (such as meningitis, hypoglycemia, or hypoxia-ischemia) to produce generalized seizures, they do not. Rather each seizure arises from a restricted area of cortex. However, if multiple seizures are recorded, each may arise from a different scalp region and they are then designated as "multifocal onset" seizures. In contrast, if multiple seizures are recorded, all of which arise from the same scalp location, the seizures are designated as "unifocal onset." This raises the suspicion of a localized structural abnormality reflecting the restricted functional disturbance.[11]

Different brain regions possess distinctive diatheses for epileptogenesis. Thus, although any brain region can be the site of origin of an electrographic seizure, some regions appear to foster ictal activity more than others. One study reported that the majority of neonatal seizures arose from the temporal or central region, followed in frequency by the frontal, occipital, and vertex loci (Table 11-2).[12]

During some electrographic seizures it occasionally may be observed that the ictal activity does not completely replace the underlying background rhythms. The morphology may appear to be a blend of commingled ictal and background patterns. This suggests that there are two populations of neurons recorded at one location: a group of neurons that supports the epileptic process and its nonictal neighbors. For example, in a child with a severe diffuse encephalopathy whose basic interictal background pattern is burst suppression, the EEG recorded at a single site may simultaneously demonstrate the electrographic seizure and the patterns of burst suppression. These observations imply that at times only a subset of neurons participate in the electrophysiologic activity of the seizure.

Temporal Profile

An account of the temporal behavior of electrographic seizures highlights their recurrence as relatively brief attacks. A typical seizure lasts about two minutes and is followed by an interictal period of variable duration. These characteristics describe seizure duration recorded during relatively brief tracings randomly

TABLE 11-2   Sites of Origin of Electrographic Seizures in 41 Neonates

Multifocal onset seizures	18
Unifocal onset seizures	23
Temporal-occipital	6
Temporal-central	6
Central	4
Frontal-temporal-central	3
Frontal-temporal	2
Midline vertex	2

selected during a variety of acute encephalopathies.[13] There are no studies that comprehensively describe the natural history of electrographic seizures during extended periods (e.g., 72 hours) of continuous monitoring from the onset of the acute neurologic illness.

Solitary prolonged electrographic seizures are rare in newborn infants. Over 97 percent of the seizures recorded in one study lasted less than 30 minutes (Fig. 11-4).[13] Whereas in mature cortex a generalized seizure can persist uninterrupted for many hours, this is not the usual case with the neonatal cortex. Repeated serial seizures are much more characteristic. Some clinical observers have suggested a different temporal profile for the duration of neonatal seizures. For example, in the National Collaborative Perinatal Project (NCPP), Holden and Mellits[14,15] suggested that neonatal seizures not uncommonly last longer than 30 minutes. It is a difficult task to judge accurately the duration of an electrographic seizure by unaided clinical inspection of the patient.

Caveats

Several common recording artifacts can generate EEG patterns that superficially resemble the evolving wave forms of an electrographic seizure. An inex-

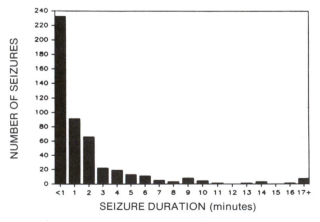

Figure 11-4   The temporal behavior of neonatal seizures is profiled in this histogram, which describes the distribution of duration of 487 electrographic seizures recorded in 42 neonates. The typical neonatal seizure is relatively brief, with an average duration of about two minutes. (Reprinted with permission from Clancy RR, Legido A. The exact ictal and interictal duration of electroencephalographic neonatal seizures. Epilepsia 1987; 28:537.)

perienced electroencephalographer could mistakenly interpret some artifacts as signalling a seizure. For example, the central vertex electrode (C_Z) sometimes can detect the cardiac pulse under the fontanelle, which simulates an electrographic seizure (Fig. 11-5). Faulty application of a single electrode may produce "electrode pop" artifacts; even soothing gestures such as patting the baby can create convincing replicas that mimic genuine electrographic seizures.

The Interictal Electroencephalographic Background

The continuing cerebral electrical activity is the stage on which the brief drama of the episodic electrographic seizure unfolds. In many ways the integrity of the EEG background is more critical than the mere presence or absence of the seizures themselves. For example, with or without electrographic seizures, an extremely abnormal background (e.g., a burst suppression or isoelectric tracing) inherently conveys a sense of profound electrophysiologic disruption and realistically forecasts a risk of death or an adverse neurologic outcome.[16-19] Conversely, a nearly normal interictal EEG background suggests relatively preserved neurologic health despite the intrusion of the unwanted seizures. The interictal background also occasionally can offer clues to seizure etiology. Hypocalcemia is suggested in the setting of a well-maintained background with excessive bilateral rolandic spikes. Some inborn errors of metabolism (e.g., maple syrup urine disease) cause the display of distinctive vertex wicket spikes (Fig. 11-6). Pseudoperiodic discharges raise the suspicion of herpes simplex virus encephalitis. A grossly abnormal EEG that was not expected in the absence of any obvious acquired disease suggests cerebral dysgenesis. Persistent focal slowing or spatially restricted sharp waves raise the question of a localized acquired injury such as contusion, subarachnoid hemorrhage, or stroke.

FAILURE TO CAPTURE AN ELECTROGRAPHIC SEIZURE

By their nature, seizures are brief episodic events. After the physician witnesses a clinical event that is suspected to represent a genuine epileptic seizure, a routine EEG examination is requested, which samples 30 or 40 minutes of cerebral electrical activity. If an actual electrographic seizure is captured during the test, the presence of epilepsy-based seizures is unequivocally confirmed. However, definite epileptic seizures can be missed in some infants if randomly scheduled routine EEG fails to coincide with an actual seizure.

What are the features of the interictal tracing that support an epileptic basis for the clinical attacks?

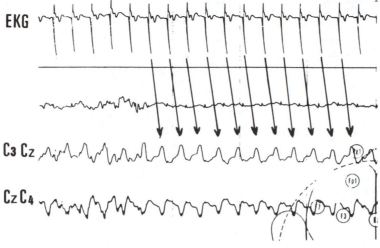

Figure 11-5 Cardiac pulsations generate an artifact at the central vertex (bottom two channels), which mimics the appearance of an electrographic seizure.

Although this question appears obvious, clear answers are hard to find. Several studies have described the interictal neonatal EEG.[16-18,20-22] However, most investigators have selected their seizure population on the basis of clinically diagnosed attacks. These studies are probably contaminated by the inclusion of babies who were misdiagnosed as having epileptic seizures. One study included only babies whose seizures were unequivocally confirmed by capturing at least one electrographic seizure on a randomly recorded tracing.[23] Although this guarantees that all subjects have unquestionably suffered epileptic seizures, the study group is biased to include sicker infants who displayed seizures with sufficient frequency to be captured by a randomly recorded routine tracing.

The unique physiologic signature of the epileptic process is the sharp transient, which announces a sudden, rapid voltage fluctuation. The EEG voltage instability connotes the tendency for uncontrolled transmembrane potentials in individual neurons and the consequent predilection for seizures. In older individuals various "sharp" wave forms may mimic pathologic spikes or sharp waves, which are highly associated with epileptogenesis. Examples include artifacts from eye blinking, electrocardiography, the mu rhythm, temporal wicket spikes, and small sharp spikes.

A similar interpretative problem exists in neonatal EEG (Table 11-3), since normal healthy babies also display a variety of expected sharp EEG transients that could mislead the inexperienced electroencephalographer into erroneously reporting an "abnormally low seizure threshold" (Fig. 11-7). For example, encoche frontales are normal, high amplitude, synchronous, stereotyped sharp waves that appear in the bifrontal regions in infants between conceptional ages 34 and 45 weeks.[24] They are sometimes confused with pathologic cerebral potentials.

In healthy babies solitary, randomly distributed sharp EEG transients appear commonly and are more abundant in the temporal than in the central regions (Figs. 11-8).[21,22,24-26] Sharp waves and occasional spikes occur with a typical frequency of one transient per minute of active sleep. A nonspecific diffuse enhancement of

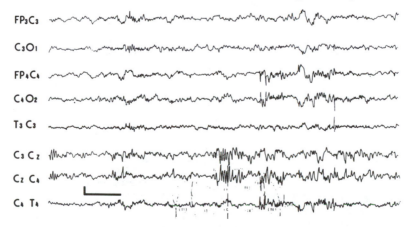

Figure 11-6 The interictal EEG sometimes can offer valuable clues suggesting the specific etiology of the seizures. This segment was recorded in a full-term newborn infant who developed lethargy, feeding intolerance, and hypotonia at three days of age. The distinctive central vertex wicket spikes (midportion of segment on channels 6 and 7) correctly suggested an inborn error of metabolism before clinical laboratory testing confirmed the diagnosis of maple syrup urine disease.

TABLE 11-3 Examples of Sharp Electroencephalographic Transients

I. Normal transients

Encoches frontales
Solitary, occasional temporal sharp waves (negative or polyphasic polarity)
Low amplitude, positive, temporal sharp waves in premature babies
Synchronous, bicentral, monophasic, negative sharp waves in premature babies
Sharply contoured fragments of rhythmic temporal theta activity in the premature baby
"Spikey" trace alternant

II. Artifactual transients

Sucking and electromyographic artifact
Electrocardiography
Electrode capacitance discharge
Hiccups
"Patting the baby"

III. Abnormal transients

Excessive atypical or unilateral encoches frontales
Paroxysmal or bizarre beta activity
Excessive runs of negative or polyphasic spikes or sharp waves
Positive rolandic or vertex sharp waves
Positive temporal sharp waves in some term infants

fast or sharp activity may confer a "spikey" quality to the bursts of normal trace alternant. Finally, recording artifacts can be encountered, especially in the electronically contaminated atmosphere of an intensive care unit, that simulate pathologic EEG potentials.

A unique feature of the EEG in premature infants is the pathologic positive polarity sharp wave.[27-29] The positive vertex sharp wave and positive rolandic sharp wave do not imply a "lower seizure threshold" but rather connote the presence of deep cerebral white matter injury that usually occurs with periventricular leukomalacia, intraventricular hemorrhage, hydrocephalus, and some inborn errors of metabolism (Fig. 11-9). The presence of frequent positive sharp waves in the central and vertex regions thus signifies a cerebral abnormality but does not support the notion of epileptic seizures. The significance of positive temporal sharp waves is less clear.

The "Classic" Interictal Tracing

If no seizure is captured during a routine EEG recording, what findings should be sought to help sup-

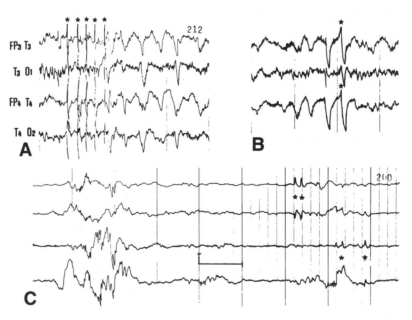

Figure 11-7 A variety of normal neonatal EEG patterns are "sharply contoured" but bear no connotation of abnormality or epilepsy. *A*, Prominent myogenic "spikes" (stars) are recorded during the infant's sucking. *B*, Notched, synchronous, symmetrical frontal sharp waves (encoches frontales, stars) are seen in a healthy term baby. *C*, Low amplitude, positive, bitemporal sharp waves (stars) are identified in the interburst portion of a discontinuous tracing recorded during quiet sleep in a healthy premature infant.

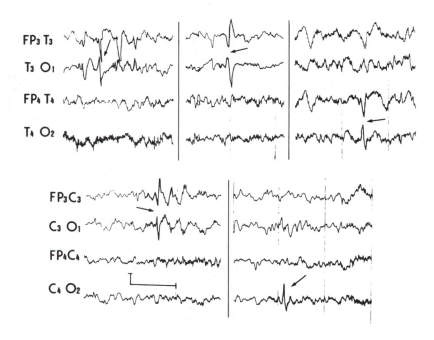

Figure 11-8   Sharp EEG transients (arrows) are commonly recorded in the temporal or central scalp region of healthy babies. Less frequently occipital sharp waves may be seen. Inexperienced electroencephalographers sometimes misinterpret these benign transients as evidence of potential epileptogenicity.

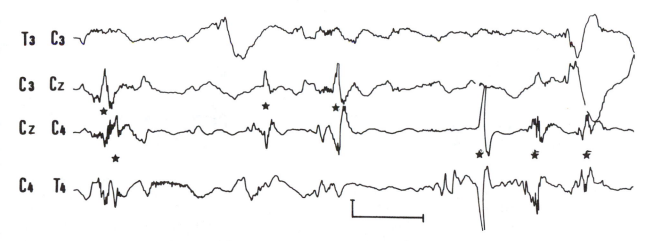

Figure 11-9   Some sharp waves recorded in the neonatal EEG indicate cerebral disease but are not correlated with a "lowered seizure threshold." This EEG was recorded in a premature baby and shows frequent positive vertex and right rolandic sharp waves (stars), which reflect the presence of periventricular leukomalacia but do not imply epileptic seizures.

port the suspicion of an epileptic basis for the infant's seizure? In contemporary neonatal neurology most seizures are provoked by significant neurologic illness such as trauma, hemorrhage, or hypoxic ischemic encephalopathy.[17] Consequently the interictal EEG frequently shows a background abnormality reflecting the underlying acute illness that provoked the seizures. The abnormal background is often punctuated by an excessive abundance of sharp EEG transients, which may cluster into brief trains with a greater than expected proportion of spikes rather than sharp waves (Fig. 11–10).[23] This con-

trasts with the benign sharp EEG transients recorded in healthy neonates, which are fewer, randomly dispersed spatially, and typically not spikes.[26] Unfortunately, the full blown constellation of abnormal background, excessive abundance of sharp EEG transients, spikes rather than sharp waves, trains or runs or sharp waves instead of solitary transients, and an unusually restricted spatial distribution of sharp transients occurs in only about one-third of the babies with unequivocally demonstrated electrographic seizures.[23] Consequently uncertainty will exist about the epileptic basis for many infants' seizures

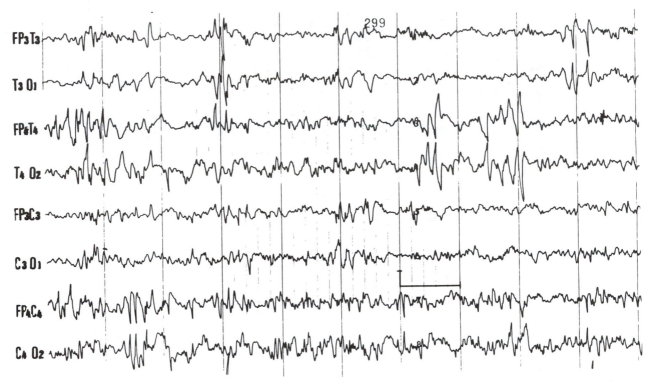

Figure 11-10   This EEG was obtained following clinically witnessed seizures in a term infant with meningitis. The record helps support the clinical diagnosis of epileptic seizures, since the tracing shows an abnormal background and an excessive abundance of temporal and central spikes, and sharp waves, some of which recur in brief runs. (Reprinted with permission from Clancy RR. Interictal sharp EEG transients in neonatal seizures. J Child Neurol, in press.)

even after a careful skillful analysis of the standard clinical bedside neonatal EEG.

Do "Epileptiform" Sharp Waves Always Imply Seizures?

Although there is a natural connection between pathologic sharp EEG transients and epileptic seizures, the correlation is not perfect. Some infants with acute encephalopathy display an excessive abundance of sharp EEG transients even though there is no clinical suspicion of seizures and no recorded EEG seizures. The immoderate presence of sharp EEG transients does not necessarily herald the appearance of epileptic seizures. It is unknown whether such infants have a substantially greater risk of clinical seizures than comparably ill neonates whose EEGs lack excessive sharp transients.

THE UNCOUPLING OF CLINICAL AND ELECTROGRAPHIC SEIZURES

In the past most physicians have probably assumed that there is a close analogy between the traditional concept of seizures in mature individuals and sick neonates, i.e., that each clinical neonatal seizure is coupled with an electrographic seizure[3,30-32]. Each time an observer visually witnesses a clinical "seizure," the

patient has also suffered an electrographic seizure. Some early studies of neonatal seizures hinted that the marriage between clinical and electrographic seizures was flawed. Some babies had "typical clinical convulsions" without coincident ictal EEG patterns.[20]

One way to examine this problem is to ask the question, How specific is visual inspection (clinical diagnosis) in the recognition of ictal EEG activity? The answer to this question is furnished by the technique of simultaneous video-EEG monitoring, which permanently captures simultaneous clinical events (seizures) with the coincident EEG activity. The most recent comprehensive studies have been reported by Kellaway, Hrachovy, and Mizrahi.[33-35] They stress that not all paroxysmal neonatal behavior patterns generally considered to be "seizures" require simultaneous ictal EEG activity. Thus, infants can have either epileptic or nonepileptic "seizures." Focal clonic seizures most consistently correlate with simultaneous ictal EEG activity. However, both subtle and tonic "seizures" bear a weak and inconsistent relationship to epileptic discharges. Indeed 85 percent of generalized tonic attacks in sick neonates arise without coincident ictal EEG discharges.[33] The majority of subtle "seizures" are also uncoupled from electrographic discharge.[34,35] Thus, for some types of clinical "seizures," visual inspection provides a very nonspecific tool to identify ictal EEG activity.

Mizrahi and Kellaway[35] have proposed that such nonepileptic "seizures" are fragments of behavior or

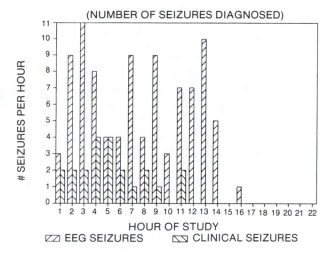

(NUMBER OF SEIZURES DIAGNOSED)

HOUR OF STUDY

▨ EEG SEIZURES   ◇ CLINICAL SEIZURES

Figure 11-11 Although visual inspection of the patient first alerts caregivers to the presence of suspected neonatal seizures, unaided clinical diagnosis is an insensitive tool to quantify measures of seizure abundance in some babies. This is illustrated by one neonate who experienced birth trauma and a subdural hemorrhage with repeated seizures. Continuous video-EEG telemetry monitoring was conducted for 22 hours. During each hour of the study the numbers of clinically visible and electrographic seizures were contrasted. Altogether there were 94 electrographic seizures, but only 22 of these provoked a coincident clinical seizure. Thus only 23 percent of the electrographic seizures were diagnosable by visual inspection alone.

motor patterns released by subcortical structures such as the brainstem. The acute encephalopathy disrupts the normal braking influence that the healthy cortex exercises over subcortical structures. The loss of normal cortical inhibition permits the episodic release of automatisms or posturing that the unaided eye interprets as an "epileptic seizure." However, Moshe[9] cautions that in animals some bona fide electrographic seizures may remain buried in the depths of the limbic structures where routine surface scalp recordings fail to register ictal activity. Whether similar ictal confinement occurs in the human newborn is unknown.

OCCULT NEONATAL SEIZURES

If the clinical diagnosis of epilepsy-based seizures can be nonspecific in some neonates, the corollary issue of sensitivity must also be examined: How sensitive is visual inspection of the patient in the accurate recognition of electrographic seizures? Can electrographic seizures be missed by unaided clinical inspection? If the patient does not appear to be clinically "seizing," can the clinician be assured that there are not "occult," "subclinical," or "silent" electrographic seizures? (Fig. 11-11).

Early neonatal seizure studies suggested that some typical electrographic seizure patterns might arise without distinctive clinical signs.[20] How commonly does this occur? Only a few studies have specifically quantified the sensitivity of clinical diagnosis during electrographic seizures. One study found that only 10 percent of electrographic seizures recorded in nonparalyzed infants

produced definite concurrent clinical seizures.[18] Others reported that only 20 percent of electrographic seizures were accompanied by distinctive clinical seizures.[36] During the other 80 percent of EEG seizures, no clinical seizure activity was observed or the activity was not distinct from behavior displayed before or after the ictus. Occult neonatal seizures occurred with or without a depressed level of consciousness, EEG background abnormality, and antiepileptic medication. Other investigators have also reported relatively high proportions of seizures that were subclinical, including electrographic status epilepticus![37-40]

LONG-TERM ELECTROENCEPHALOGRAPHIC MONITORING

Unaided clinical inspection of sick infants for "seizures" is extremely valuable but suffers from the limitations of nonspecificity and insensitivity. Consequently EEG monitoring has been conducted in a variety of investigational formats to document more objectively and follow the cerebral electrical patterns over extended periods and to substantiate more accurately the abundance of electrographic seizures.[41] The most sophisticated technique is simultaneous video-EEG monitoring, which has been successfully employed by several investigators.[33-35] Ambulatory EEG cassette recording has been used but is limited in that record review is delayed by 12 to 24 hours.[42] Information regarding seizure abundance must be made available to the physician in a timely fashion if prompt therapeutic intervention is desired. The use of continuous computer-assisted EEG analysis by compressed spectral array is another technique that may assist in the recognition of seizures (Fig. 11-12).[37,43]

THE SIGNIFICANCE OF NEONATAL SEIZURES

High Incidence

Although the physiologic threshold for provoking a seizure in the immature cerebral cortex is formidable, the incidence of neonatal seizures is very high and far exceeds that of any other six-week period of life. The frequency of neonatal seizures largely reflects the ample opportunities for potent neuropathologic disease to endanger the newborn infant.[8]

Etiology: Acute Seizures

Most contemporary accounts of neonatal seizures describe an extremely high incidence of symptomatic cause(s) of neonatal seizures.[17] This differs sharply from the situation in older children in whom seizures fre-

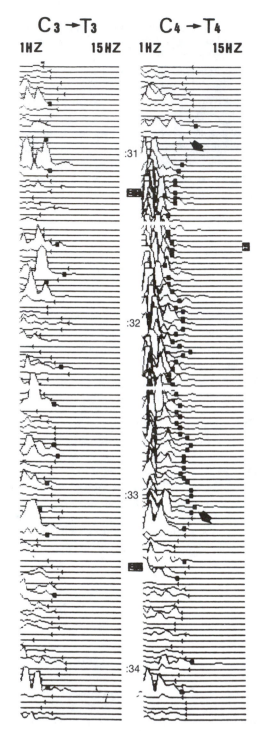

$C_3 \rightarrow T_3$ $C_4 \rightarrow T_4$

1HZ   15HZ   1HZ   15HZ

:31

:32

:33

:34

Figure 11-12 Long-term monitoring is desirable in some neonates to evaluate cortical function more objectively and to quantify the number of seizures. Most electrographic seizures appear different from the interictal background, since they introduce higher voltage patterns with a different frequency composition. Computer assisted EEG analysis displays the frequency-power characteristics of the EEG signal in a compressed spectral array format. Each of the two channels reflects the output of electrical power in the band width: 1 Hz (left side of each channel) to 15 Hz (right side of each channel). Each line of the compressed spectral array corresponds to a two second epoch of signal analysis. The left channel was recorded from the left hemisphere and the right channel was recorded from the right hemisphere. During an electrographic seizure (arrows) a distinctive change occurs in the compressed spectral array, which can be exploited for long-term seizure monitoring of the sick neonate by a cerebral function monitor.

quently occur without visible provocation. A careful search for the cause(s) of seizures is warranted in every infant. Serious underlying etiologies often can be undercovered by a diligent search, including a careful history and physical examination and ancillary testing, which may include CT scanning, lumbar puncture, EEG, and appropriate blood and urine studies. Nevertheless a definite cause cannot be assigned in a significant fraction of neonatal seizure patients. In some infants with "idiopathic" seizures, careful inquiry may reveal the presence of familial neonatal seizures.[44,45]

Hypoxic ischemic encephalopathy remains the single most common cause of seizures in the full-term newborn.[17] This has an important medicolegal corollary: hypoxia-ischemia that is sufficiently severe to provoke acute encephalopathy and neonatal seizures is probably severe enough to cause "with a reasonable degree of medical certainty" a subsequent chronic static encephalopathy such as cerebral palsy with mental retardation. Consider the following two examples:

Case Studies

Case 1

Baby A was conceived uneventfully by healthy parents. Intrauterine growth and development unfolded flawlessly. Spontaneous rupture of the membranes occurred at term while the mother was at home. She noted the pulsating umbilical cord protruding through the vagina and immediately summoned help. She was rushed to the hospital and promptly evaluated by the obstetrical staff. They found that the umbilical cord pulsations had stopped. External fetal monitoring revealed a heart rate of 80 beats per minute. An emergency cesarean section delivered an acutely asphyxiated male with a heart rate of 80, no respiratory effort, and minimal reflex grimacing. He was immediately intubated, ventilated, and administered fluids and bicarbonate. Despite vigorous resuscitation, he remained hypotonic and obtunded with sluggishly reactive pupils. Eight hours after birth the nurses saw the first of numerous stereotyped attacks, which included repetitive arm jerking, eye blinking, and nystagmus. An EEG showed a burst suppression background and frequent multifocal onset seizures. The child survived the immediate acute encephalopathy due to the hypoxia-ischemia but later demonstrated a chronic static encephalopathy with spastic quadriparesis and mental retardation.

Case 2

Baby B was conceived uneventfully by physically healthy parents. There were minor problems during the gestation, including maternal obesity, excessive weight gain, and mild hypertension. The infant was stressed during a prolonged labor, and two late decelerations registered during fetal heart rate monitoring. At birth he was large for dates and mildly depressed, with Apgar scores of 4 at one minute and 6 at five minutes. He looked well after revival in the delivery room. There was no immediate clinical neurologic signs of acute encephalopathy. Routine monitoring of the blood sugar level showed an equivocal low value of 20 to 40 mg per deciliter. An inexperienced nurse observed the infant to be "jittery" but misinterpreted the tremors as neonatal seizures. The diagnosis "neonatal seizures" persisted in the infant's medical record. A normal EEG was recorded, but an inexperienced electroencephalographer overread the normal benign temporal-central sharp waves and used the phrase "burst suppression" to describe the expected discontinuity of trace alternant sleep. The official report declared this objective test finding to be "abnormal." Phenobarbital was administered intravenously with a 5 percent glucose solution. As the hypoglycemic jitteriness abated, the physicians concluded the phenobarbital terminated the neonatal seizures.

Following discharge from the hospital the infant's psychomotor development was slow. The family initiated litigation because it was a high risk pregnancy, there were signs of intrapartum distress revealed by fetal heart rate monitoring, the infant had low Apgar scores and required delivery room resuscitation, there was an immediate acute encephalopathy in the form of neonatal seizures supported by the "objective" abnormality of the electroencephalogram, and there was an undesired final outcome that they believed could be causally connected to perinatal events.

A neurologic evaluation was undertaken to examine independently the possible relationship between the perinatal events and the infant's delayed development. The family history was notable for mental retardation in the mother's brother. It was noted that except for the tremors (misinterpreted as seizures), there was no depression of consciousness, hypotonia, or disturbance of sucking or swallowing. The neonatal EEG was retrieved and correctly reinterpreted by a knowledgeable electroencephalographer. The "burst suppression" was nothing more than normal quiet sleep trace alternant activity. Physical examination revealed a retarded child without signs of cerebral palsy. A blood sample then confirmed the real cause of the child's mental retardation: the fragile X chromosome syndrome.

Prognosis for Death and Neurologic Morbidity

Recent Trends

The prognosis in infants with seizures in the neonatal period has improved over the past two decades. In reports of 1,667 patients with neonatal seizures gathered from several published series, Bergman et al[46] noted a mortality of 24.7 percent before 1969 and 18 percent after 1970. Volpe[47] reported that the mortality was 39 percent before 1969 and 15 percent after 1970. Lombroso[17] found that mortality decreased modestly from about 20 percent previously to 16 percent in the early 1980s. These improvements probably relate to better obstetrical management and modern neonatal intensive care. All these studies relied on seizure diagnosis by clinical criteria and did not require EEG confirmation. In one study that included only patients with confirmed electrographic seizures, the mortality was 32.5 percent.[19] Despite the reduced mortality, the incidence of neurologic sequelae in the form of mental retardation, cerebral palsy and epilepsy has changed less and remains approximately 30 to 35 percent. With confirmed seizures, the incidence of handicapping neurologic sequelae exceeded 55 percent.

Despite the limitations of earlier, less sophisticated studies of neonatal seizures, it was still clear that infants ill enough to definitely "seize" (regardless of whether they were actually confirmed by EEG) faced a significantly higher risk of an unfavorable neurologic outcome. Certainly there were many examples of "benign" neonatal seizures after which the survivors were free of neurodevelopmental defects, but neonatal seizures were rightfully regarded as an ominous sign of brain damage.[48] Indeed, in the NCPP population the presence of neonatal seizures was a potent independent marker, which forecast an exaggerated risk for combinations of severe disabilities such as mental retardation coupled with cerebral palsy.[49]

Influence of Etiology

The principal determinant of outcome following neonatal seizures is probably the underlying etiology itself.[50] Whereas most babies with relatively innocuous conditions such as hypocalcemia do well despite the seizures, those with more serious conditions such as hypoxic-ischemic encephalopathy and intracranial hemorrhage experience greater morbidity. Seizure etiology is the main determinant of outcome but not the only one: Gestational age (premature infants fare worse than full-term babies), time of seizure onset (infants with seizures on the first day of life have a poorer outcome than those with later onset seizures), and severity of seizures all relate statistically to the neurologic outcome.

Measures of Seizure Severity

Descriptions of seizure abundance are relevant to predicting the neurologic prognosis. Infants with status epilepticus or frequent seizures can reasonably be expected to fare worse than those with infrequent seizures.[39] In the NCPP population a seizure lasting longer than 30 minutes or seizures persisting for several days were considered prognostically unfavorable.[14,15] However, the reliability of these observations based on clinical criteria alone are unknown because of the shortcomings of unaided visual diagnosis.

In a homogeneous group of asphyxiated babies, those with more frequent EEG seizures (more than 10 seizures per hour) had a significantly higher incidence of handicaps than those with less frequent seizures.[19] However, when Lombroso[17] compared outcome with seizure duration, he found no difference if the seizures lasted longer or less than four minutes.

Direct Ictal Injury

There has been a long-standing suspicion that neonatal seizures are not innocent markers signaling the presence of a serious encephalopathy but may actively participate in the genesis of brain damage following the primary inciting injury.[34] There is no direct evidence that neonatal seizures are inherently harmful in humans. The demonstration of direct ictal injury of the immature cortex has been the product of research investigations in newborn laboratory animals.[51,52] Newborn animals that are well preserved physiologically (by maintaining normal oxygenation and blood pressure with artificial life support) and provoked to "seize" show definite neuronal damage as the result of repeated electrographic seizures.[51-53] Similar concerns are raised in human newborn infants who experience repeated seizures. There are several potential avenues leading to the production of ictal brain damage:

1. The physiologic effects of the seizure itself can disturb vital functions, including blood pressure, pulse, carbon dioxide tension, oxygenation, and respirations.[26,54]
2. Ictal metabolic effects arise that divert high energy metabolic currency from the mainstream of normal neuronal function to fuel the ravenous demands of the epileptic process.[55-57]
3. Epileptic seizures promote the release of neurotoxic substances such as glutamate, which can generate neuronal damage at distant sites.[58]

Although the fundamental prognosis is contingent upon the underlying etiology, the presence, frequency, duration, and spatial distribution of seizures could exert a modifying influence such that a milder original injury could be transformed into a more serious one by frequent seizures. It therefore seems justified to attempt energetically to reduce or terminate electrographic seizures by the judicious administration of antiepileptic drugs.[34,36]

MEDICOLEGAL PITFALLS

Establishing the Diagnosis of Neonatal Seizures

The diagnosis of neonatal seizures is still largely a clinical one in the contemporary practice of neonatal medicine. Individual observers possess different skills and experience in their ability to recognize neonatal seizures and distinguish them from other "paroxysmal" behavior patterns displayed by the healthy or sick neonate. Too often an inexperienced nurse or physician mistakenly reports the presence of "seizures." Once the diagnosis is officially recorded in the medical records, it can become a powerful medicolegal weapon. It might be preferable to designate the clinician's concerns as "suspected seizure" or "possible seizure" until the diagnosis is clarified.

Etiology of Seizure

Most babies with definite neonatal seizures have a demonstrable cause for the condition (see Chapter 18). However, in some series as many as 25 percent of affected patients have no clear definable cause for the seizures.[17] It is then preferable to describe the etiology as "neonatal seizures of undetermined cause" rather than assume that the infant must have had some "lack of oxygen at birth" to account for the condition. An infant who is sufficiently asphyxiated to develop neonatal seizures will not appear neurologically well between seizures but should show definite signs of acute encephalopathy such as hypotonia, lethargy, inactivity, and a poor suck. It is also important to inquire about other family members who may have had neonatal seizures.

The Neonatal Electroencephalogram

The obtaining and interpretation of a neonatal EEG reflects the skill and experience of the individual laboratory and electroencephalographer. Although it is widely regarded as an "objective" test, the interpretation is inherently subjective. The official typed report declaring the presence of an EEG abnormality should not be automatically accepted as a cold analytical fact. It might be desirable in some medicolegal circumstances to retrieve the actual tracing for independent review by an experienced neonatal electroencephalographer.

The topic of neonatal seizures has maintained a prominent position among the classic neurologic signs of the high risk neonate. Unaided visual observation of the patient has been complemented recently with more sophisticated diagnostic methods intended to substantiate and quantify the epileptic basis of suspected neonatal seizures. This is achieved by prolonged EEG monitoring and ambulatory cassette or video-EEG technology. Much has been learned about the nature of neonatal seizures, including the realization that clinical observation is a limited, imperfect diagnostic tool. As a result, it is probable that in the past many earnest observers erroneously mislabeled innocent activity and behavior as a "subtle" seizure. Some repetitive, stereotyped, unnatural appearing attacks may be pathologic but nonepileptic in origin, since they are not founded on a simultaneous ictal EEG. True epileptic neonatal seizures are probably less frequent than clinically diagnosed and inherently require confirmation by EEG. Although interictal EEGs may offer evidence of a "lowered seizure threshold" in some infants, substantial interpretive difficulties remain. This is accentuated by the fact that many practicing electroencephalographers have had inadequate opportunity to interpret neonatal tracings and may misread a variety of expected healthy background patterns and sharp transients. Definite clinical seizures should always compel the physician to launch an immediate investigation to discover and possibly remove their causes. However, not every neonatal seizure has a definable etiology, and it should not be assumed that perinatal factors were the cause. Safe levels of antiepileptic drugs are given to reduce or eliminate electrographic seizures to help prevent secondary ictal injury. Unfortunately, despite the most careful and immediate attention, many affected infants do not survive and those who do face a high risk of serious future neurologic handicap.

REFERENCES

1. Phayer T. The boke of chyldren. London: E & S Livingstone, 1957:28.
2. Purpura DP. Factors contributing to abnormal neuronal development in the cerebral cortex of the human infant. In: Berenberg SR, ed. Brain: fetal and infant. The Hague: Martinus-Nijhoff, 1977:54.
3. Camfield PR, Camfield CS. Neonatal seizures: a commentary on selected aspects. J Child Neurol 1987; 2:244.
4. Keen JH, Lee D. Sequelae of neonatal convulsions: study of 112 infants. Arch Dis Child, 1973; 48:542.
5. Dennis J. Neonatal convulsions: aetiology, late neonatal status and long-term outcome. Dev Med Child Neurol 1978; 20:143.
6. Freeman JM. Neonatal seizures—diagnosis and management. J Pediatr 1970; 77:701.
7. Volpe JJ. Neonatal seizures. N Engl J Med 1973; 289:413.
8. Clancy R. Neonatal seizures. In: Polin R, Berg F, eds. Workbook of Neonatology. Philadelphia: WB Saunders, 1983:125.
9. Moshe SL. Epileptogenesis and the immature brain. Epilepsia 1987; 28 (Suppl 1):S3.
10. Prince DA, Gutnick MJ. Neuronal activities in epileptogenic foci of immature cortex. Brain Res 1972; 45: 455.
11. Clancy RR, Malin S, Laraque D, et al. Focal motor seizures heralding stroke in full term neonates. Am J Dis Child 1985; 139: 601.
12. Fischer RA, Clancy R. Midline sagittal epileptogenic foci in children. J Child Neurol 1987; 2:224.
13. Clancy RR, Legido A. The exact ictal and interictal duration of electroencephalographic neonatal seizures. Epilepsia 1987; 28:537.
14. Holden KR, Mellits ED, Freeman JM. Neonatal seizures. I. Correlation of prenatal and perinatal events with outcomes. Pediatrics 1982; 70:165.
15. Mellits ED, Holden KR, Freeman JM. Neonatal seizures. II. A multivariate analysis of factors associated with outcome. Pediatrics 1982; 70:177.
16. Rose AL, Lombroso CT. A study of clinical, pathological and electroencephalographic features in 137 full term babies with a long-term follow-up. Pediatrics 1970; 45:404.
17. Lombroso CT. Prognosis in neonatal seizures. In: Delgado-Escueta AV, Wasterlain CG, Freiman DM, Porter RJ, eds. Advances in neurology. Vol 34. Status epilepticus. New York: Raven Press, 1983: 101.
18. Rowe JC, Homes GI, Hafford J, et al. Prognostic values of the electroencephalogram in term and preterm infants following neonatal seizures. Pediatr Res 1987; 21:489A (abstract). 60:183.
19. Clancy RR, Legido A. Neurologic outcome after EEG proven neonatal seizures. Pediatr Res 1987; 21:489A.
20. Monod N, Pajot N, Guidasci S. The neonatal EEG: statistical studies and prognostic value in full-term and preterm babies. Electroencephalogr Clin Neurophysiol 1972; 32:529.
21. Hughes JR, Fino J, Gagnon L. The use of electroencephalogram in the confirmation of seizures in premature and neonatal infants. Neuropediatrics 1983; 14:213.
22. Watanabe K, Hara K, Miyazaki S, et al. Electroclinical studies of seizures in the newborn. Folia Psychiatr Neurol Jap 1977; 31:383.
23. Clancy RR. Interictal sharp EEG transients in neonatal seizures. J Child Neurol, in press.
24. Tharp BR. Neonatal electroencephalography. In: Korobkin R, Guilleminault C, eds. Progress in perinatal neurology. Baltimore: Williams & Wilkins, 1981:31.
25. Karbowski K, Nencka A. Right mid-temporal sharp EEG transients in healthy newborns. Electroencephalogr Clin Neurophysiol 1980; 48:461.
26. Clancy R, Spitzer A. Cerebral cortical function in infants at risk for sudden death syndrome. Ann Neurol 1985; 18:41.
27. Novotny EJ, Tharp BR Coen RW, et al. Positive rolandic sharp waves in the EEG of the premature infant. Neurology 1987; 37:1481.
28. Marret S, Parain D, Samson-Dollfus D, et al. Positive rolandic sharp waves and periventricular leukomalacia in the newborn. Neuropediatrics 1986; 17:199.
29. Clancy R, Tharp B. Positive rolandic sharp waves in the electroencephalograms of premature neonates with intraventricular hemorrhage. Electroencephalogr Clin Neurophysiol 1984; 57:395.
30. Fenichel GM, Fitzpatrick JE. Difficulty in clinical identification of neonatal seizures: an EEG monitor study. Electroencephalogr Clin Neurophysiol 1984; 58:33P.
31. Shewmon DA. Dissociation between cortical discharges and ictal movements in neonatal seizures. Ann Neurol 1983; 14:368 (abstract).
32. Sarnat HG. Pathogenesis of decerebrate "seizures" in the premature infant with intraventricular hemorrhage. J Pediatr 1975; 87:154.
33. Kellaway P, Hrachovy RA. Status epilepticus in newborns: a perspective on neonatal seizures. In: Delgado-Escueta AV, Wasterlain CG, Treiman DM, Porter RJ, eds. Status epilepticus. Advances in neurology. New York: Raven Press, 1983:93.
34. Mizrahi EM. Neonatal seizures: problems in diagnosis and classification. Epilepsia 1987; 28 (Suppl l):S46.
35. Mizrahi EM, Kellaway P. Characterization and classification of neonatal seizures. Neurology 1987; 37:1837.
36. Clancy RR, Legido A, Lewis D. Occult neonatal seizures. Epilepsia 1988; 29:256.
37. Hellstrom-Westas L, Rosen I, Swenningsen NW. Silent seizures

in sick infants in early life. Acta Paediatr Scand 1985; 74:741.

38. Olmos-Garcia de Alba G, Mora EU, Valdez JM, et al, Neonatal status epilepticus. II: Electroencephalographic aspects. Clin Electroencephalogr 1984; 15:197.

39. Dreyfus-Brisac C, Monod N. Neonatal status epilepticus. In: Remond A, ed. Handbook of electroencephalopathy and clinical neurophysiology. Vol 15. Amsterdam, Elsevier, 1972:38.

40. Watanabe K, Negoro T, Inokuma K, Yamazaki T. Subclinical delta status in the newborn: an unfavorable prognostic sign. Clin Electroencephalogr 1984; 15:125.

41. Tharp BR. Intensive video/EEG monitoring of neonates. In: Gumnit RJ, ed. Intensive neurodiagnostic monitoring. Advances in neurology. Vol 46. New York: Raven Press, 1989:107.

42. Bridgers SL, Ebersole JS, Ment LR, et al. Cassette electroencephalography in the evaluation of neonatal seizures. Arch Neurol 1986; 43:49.

43. Clancy RR, DiMario FJ. Detection of electrographic neonatal seizures by compressed spectral array. Ann Neurol (abstract) 1988; 24:345.

44. Kaplan RE, Lacey DJ. Benign familial neonatal-infantile seizures. Am J Med Genet 1983; 16:595.

45. Pettit RE, Fenichel GM. Benign familial neonatal seizures. Arch Neurol 1980; 37:47.

46. Bergman I, Painter MJ, Hirsch RP, et al. Outcome in neonates with convulsions treated in an intensive care unit. Ann Neurol 1983; 14:642.

47. Volpe JJ. Neonatal seizures. In: Volpe JJ, ed. Neurology of the newborn. 2nd Ed. Philadelphia: WB Saunders, 1987:129.

48. Plouin P. Benign neonatal convulsions (familial and non-familial).

In: Roger J, Dravet C, Bureau M, Dreifuss FE, Wolf P, eds. Epileptic syndromes in infancy, childhood and adolescence. John Libbey, 1985:2.

49. Nelson KB, Broman SH. Perinatal risk factors in children with serious motor and mental handicaps. Ann Neurol 1979; 2:371.

50. Legido A, Clancy RR, Berman PH. Recent advances in the diagnosis, treatment and prognosis of neonatal seizures. Pediatr Neurol 1988; 4:79.

51. Wasterlain CG, Duffy TE. Status epilepticus in immature rats. Arch Neurol 1976; 33:821.

52. Wasterlain CG, Plum F. Vulnerability of developing rat brain in electroconvulsive seizures. Arch Neurol 1973; 29:38.

53. Dwyer BE, Wasterlain CG. Neonatal seizures in monkeys and rabbits: brain glucose depletion in the face of normoglycemia, prevention of glucose loads. Pediatr Res 1985; 19:992.

54. Perlman JM, Volpe JJ. Seizures in the preterm infant: effects on cerebral blood flow velocity, intracranial pressure and arterial blood pressure. J Pediatr 1983; 102:288.

55. Younkin DP, Delivoria-Papadopoulos M, Maris J, et al. Cerebral metabolic effects of neonatal seizures measured with in vivo ^{31}P NMR spectroscopy. Ann Neurol 1986; 20:513.

56. Young RSK, Briggs RW, Yagel SK, Gorman I. ^{31}P nuclear magnetic resonance study of the effects of hypoxemia on neonatal status epilepticus. Pediatr Res 1986; 20:581.

57. Young RSK, Petroff OAC, Chen B, et al. ^{31}P and ^{1}H nuclear magnetic resonance study of the effects of diazepam on neonatal seizures. Ann Neurol 1987; 22:420.

58. Collins RC, Olney JW. Focal cortical seizures cause distant thalamic lesion. Science 1982; 218: 177.

12

Hypoglycemia and Brain Injury

Ronald S. Cohen, M.D. and David K. Stevenson, M.D.

Brain Energy Metabolism
Mechanism of Hypoglycemic Brain Injury
Clinical Picture
Treatment
Outcome of Neonatal Hypoglycemia

The definition of hypoglycemia generally is accepted to be a plasma glucose level less than 30 mg per deciliter in a term infant on the first day of life, or less than 45 mg per deciliter thereafter.[1,2] For the preterm infant the definition is somewhat less settled; a "cut-off" of 25 mg per deciliter in the first 24 hours has been suggested.[2] Earlier studies document that premature infants have blood glucose levels somewhat lower than those in term neonates during the first several days of life.[3] However, for very low birth weight premature infants, the picture is even less clear; indeed the "range of normal glucose values in neonates <1000 gm has not been determined and may never be known."[4]

Unfortunately the available numbers only address the question of "What is the mean ±2 SI) blood of plasma glucose level for newborn infants of a certain gestational age, weight, and postnatal age?" but do not deal with the real issue; i.e., "What is the blood or plasma glucose level below which deleterious effects occur in the newborn of a given gestational age, weight, and postnatal age?" Unfortunately this issue is hard to address in the human model. The clinical findings commonly attributed to hypoglycemia are non-specific, and may or may not appear in a given infant at any given glucose level, such that clinicians are handicapped by "the lack of a universal threshold below or above which symptoms can be expected."[2] Similarly, the degree of hypoglycemia necessary to cause brain injury is poorly defined at best.

BRAIN ENERGY METABOLISM

Neurologic injury from hypoglycemia commonly is believed to be due to inadequate energy for intracellular metabolism, for glucose is believed to be the major fuel for brain cell metabolism. However, recent data indicate that alternative energy sources for the fetal and neonatal brain exist, such as ketone bodies,[5,6] which may serve as a protective mechanism during short periods of low glucose availability. However, prolonged dependence on ketone bodies for brain metabolism may be deleterious to brain growth owing to the inhibition of pyrimidine synthesis.[7] Additionally, some debate remains about the availability of ketone bodies during the neonatal period. A marked increase in circulating levels of ketone bodies has been reported in suckled neonatal rat pups, the so-called suckling ketosis.[8-10] However, the picture is less clear in the human neonate, some investigators reporting ketosis and others not.[11,12] This may reflect differences in feeding styles, because feeding an artificial formula to rat pups resulted in lower levels of ketone bodies.[13]

An additional potential energy source for the fetal and neonatal brain is lactate, which has been demonstrated to be a significant source of energy for the fetal myocardium.[14] The permeability of the blood-brain barrier to lactate is inversely related to age in rats, such that lactate crosses readily in the newborn but not in the adult.[15] Lactate also has been shown to reverse symptoms due to insulin-induced hypoglycemia in young mice.[16]

MECHANISM OF HYPOGLYCEMIC BRAIN INJURY

Hypoglycemia was first linked to brain injury in neonates by Hartmann and Jaudon[17] in 1937. Thirty years later the associated pathologic changes in the central nervous system were described and compared with those caused by hypoxia.[18] Over time, human and animal data demonstrated the different pathologic pictures that these two insults cause.[19-21] Basically the injury is selective neuronal necrosis, not unlike that seen with hypoxia but with a different distribution, such as an affinity for more superficial layers in the cortex and greater spinal involvement. Animal research has shown that 30 to 60 minutes of hypoglycemia-induced electroencephalographic changes is needed to cause discernible cell injury.[20,21] Repetitive insulin-induced hypoglycemia in rat pups resulted in decreased brain levels of DNA, protein, lipids, and glycogen and overall brain weight.[22]

However, the mechanism of brain injury in hypoglycemia is not as straightforward as thought originally and is probably not due merely to a lack of energy. The level of brain ATP during profound hypoglycemia is significantly higher than that seen after ischemia,[23,24] suggesting that something other than energy depletion is responsible for neuronal death. The pattern of injury also goes against the energy depletion hypothesis, for metabolically active glial cells are spared and the neuronal injury does not seem to be affected by alterations in blood flow distribution.[24] Indeed, in the adult animal at least, the data suggest strongly that the injury is secondary to an excitotoxin produced in the central nervous system during hypoglycemia.[24-26]

Although there is convincing evidence for an excitotoxin-mediated mechanism of neuronal injury in adult animals, newborn animals in fact may be quite different. Auer[24] clearly states that, "Neonatal hypoglycemia in all probability constitutes an entirely different situation from the adult with regard to hypoglycemic brain damage." He postulates that the additional fuel sources available to the neonatal animal may prevent the production of excitotoxin. Furthermore, excitotoxin-mediated neuronal injury would require a degree of developmental maturity of neurotransmitter systems and dendritic receptors that might not be present in the immature brain.

CLINICAL PICTURE

As stated previously, the clinical signs and symptoms of acute neonatal hypoglycemia are nonspecific. They include such findings as jittery or tremulous movements; a high-pitched cry and irritability; lethargy and poor feeding; respiratory distress, apnea, and cyanosis; hypothermia; and seizure activity. These findings are not diagnostic, but in the appropriate clinical setting they should raise a suspicion of hypoglycemia. Clearly, screening for blood glucose levels should be a common procedure in newborn units.

The common clinical situations in which hypoglycemia is likely to be found can be divided etiologically into inadequate glucose production, exaggerated glucose consumption, or a mixture of the two (Table 12–1). These categories encompass a great variety of neonatal patients, from the smallest to the largest. It is also important to determine whether the hypoglycemia is transient or persistent, as this has significant diagnostic and prognostic implications. The majority of cases of neonatal hypoglycemia are of the transient type.

Low birth weight infants are at risk for hypoglycemia as a result of inadequate glucose production. Prema-

TABLE 12–1   Etiology of Neonatal Hypoglycemia

Inadequate glucose production
  Prematurity
  Intrauterine growth retardation
  Perinatal stress, asphyxia
  Hypopituitarism
  Glycogen storage disorders
  Other inborn errors of metabolism
  Maternal beta-blocker therapy
Increased glucose consumption
  Infant of diabetic mother
  Nesidioblastosis
  Beckwith-Wiedemann syndrome
  Erythroblastosis fetalis
  Maternal tocolytic therapy
Mixed and idiopathic
  Infant large for gestational age
  Sepsis

ture infants may have inadequate fat and glycogen stores. Those who are small because of intrauterine growth retardation, i.e., small-for-gestational-age babies, have limited glycogen stores and potentially a decreased gluconeogenic capability too.[27]

Very large infants are also at increased risk for hypoglycemia. Infants of diabetic mothers frequently are large for gestational age and have increased glucose consumption secondary to hyperinsulinemia. Other causes of congenital hyperinsulinism, such as the Beckwith-Wiedemann syndrome and nesidioblastosis, also place large infants at risk for profound hypoglycemia. Furthermore, large-for-gestational-age infants of obese nondiabetic women appear to be at an increased risk for hypoglycemia, although the exact etiology remains unclear.[28]

Neonates of any gestational age or birth weight who have suffered significant stress (e.g., hypoxia or hypothermia) may deplete their available metabolic stores and thus come to be at risk for hypoglycemia if an adequate source of exogenous glucose is not made available. Sepsis, probably because of its effects on catechols and steroids, may cause either hypoglycemia or hyperglycemia in infants of any size.

Intrauterine exposure to any of a number of drugs can be associated with neonatal hypoglycemia in infants of any size. Premature infants may be placed at additional risk if their mothers have been treated with beta-adrenergic agonists for tocolysis.[29,30] The theoretical mechanisms include direct stimulation of hepatic glucose production and pancreatic insulin secretion in the fetus, and indirect effects secondary to increased maternal blood glucose levels and uterine vasodilation.[31,32] Hypoglycemia has been related to tocolytic therapy as long as five days after discontinuation, but the greatest risk is probably in patients who are delivered within two days after the last dose of maternal beta-agonist treatment.[30] Maternal treatment with beta-blocking drugs such as propranolol has also been associated with hypoglycemia, thought to be due to decreased catechol-mediated glucose production.[27]

Another unusual cause of neonatal hypoglycemia needs to be mentioned specifically. Although its incidence has greatly decreased since the advent of Rhogam, erythroblastosis fetalis (Rh incompatibility) causes hyperinsulinism, which may result in hypoglycemia.[33] It is therefore important to monitor these patients closely, especially during and after exchange transfusions.[34,35] These procedures are risky because, on one hand, the infusion of large amounts of glucose-containing packed red blood cells may stimulate further insulin secretion, whereas, on the other hand, there may be intermittent interruptions of glucose delivery during blood removal. It therefore is advisable to monitor these patients closely and provide alternate routes for glucose delivery if umbilical catheters are being used for exchange transfusion.

Hypopituitarism, with or without associated central nervous system defects, also can cause neonatal hypoglycemia secondary to growth hormone deficiency.[36] Infants born with panhypopituitarism may have midfacial anomalies or, in males, a micropenis.[37] Neonates with seemingly idiopathic but persistent hypoglycemia should be examined with this in mind, and in patients with either or both of these physical findings the blood sugar level should be checked.[38] One brief British report indicated that of 6,627 live-born infants, 43 had hypoglycemia; of these, two had pituitary dysfunction as the probable underlying cause.[39] In addition to the endocrinopathies already discussed, many inborn errors of metabolism may result in persistent or recurrent hypoglycemia presenting in the newborn period. These include, among others, glycogen storage disorders, galactosemia, fructose-1,6-diphosphatase deficiency, and several aminoacidopathies.[40]

TREATMENT

The key to the treatment of neonatal hypoglycemia is early detection. Because the signs and symptoms of a low blood sugar level are nonspecific, it is important to maintain a high degree of vigilance. A blood or plasma glucose determination should be part of the admission evaluation of practically every high risk infant brought to the neonatal intensive care unit, for it may be either the source of the patient's symptoms or a complication of the primary problem. It is important to remember that blood glucose measurements are about 15 percent below plasma levels, that samples left without ice for any length of time may be falsely low owing to continuing metabolism, and that some types of "dipstick" determinations may be inaccurate at lower glucose levels. Nevertheless, in most clinical situations a screening method involving a whole blood laboratory stick is, and should

be, employed for expediency. If the results of the screen are low, a "stat" blood or plasma glucose level should be determined. In the interim, treatment for presumed hypoglycemia should begin, because the theoretical risks of undertreatment, with prolongation of the possible hypoglycemic exposure, far outweigh the concerns about overtreatment.

In otherwise well term infants, oral treatment often is appropriate. Gavage feeding of 5 percent dextrose in water (1 or 2 oz) should be adequate. In infants who are symptomatic, low birth weight, premature, or in another known high risk group (as already mentioned), intravenous treatment usually is preferable, because these patients are at greater risk for feeding intolerance and continuing increased glucose demand. Most agree that the so-called minibolus treatment is the appropriate initial management: 200 mg per kilogram (2 cc per kilogram of 10 percent dextrose in water) given over one minute, followed immediately by a constant infusion of glucose at about 8 mg per kilogram per minute (about 120 cc per kilogram per day or 5 cc per kilogram per hour of 10 percent dextrose in water) (Fig. 12–1).[41] No matter what treatment is begun, it is imperative that blood glucose levels be followed closely thereafter until adequate maintenance of euglycemia can be demonstrated. Generally this requires blood glucose determinations every 15 to 30 minutes until the level is stable in the 60 to 100 mg per deciliter range.

Persistent or recurrent hypoglycemia requires treatment by continuous intravenous infusion (Table 12–2). The minibolus may be repeated and the infusion rate increased by about 2 mg per kilogram per minute (about 1 cc per kilogram per hour) until the desired results are achieved. If glucose infusion rates greater than about 12 to 15 mg per kilogram per minute are required,

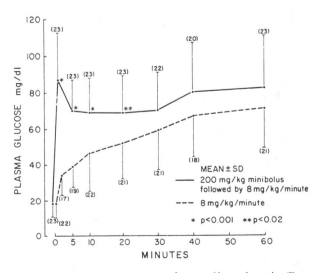

Figure 12-1   Minibolus treatment of neonatal hypoglycemia. (From Lilien LD, Srinivasan G, et al. Treatment of neonatal hypoglycemia with minibolus and intravenous glucose infusion. J Pediatr 1980; 97:295.)

TABLE 12-2   Practical Approach to Treatment of Hypoglycemia in the Neonate

Plasma Glucose	Therapy*	Comment
≤25 mg/dl	A. 200 mg/kg/min (D10W, 2 cc/kg) IV push stat	Draw sample to recheck glucose but start treatment
	B. Follow with 8 mg/kg/min (D10W, 4.8 cc/kg/hr) and recheck glucose in 10–20 min	Use volumetric pump only Determine etiology and correct if possible
Repeat glucose: >40 mg/dl	C. Maintain IV at 8 mg/kg/min D10W for 12–24 hr unless glucose >100 mg/dl/min	Monitor glucose hourly until stable; start feeds if tolerated
Repeat glucose: >25 mg/dl <40 mg/dl	D. Increase dextrose by 2 mg/kg/min increments (maximum 12 mg/kg/min)	Maintain 2 IV sites; start feeds if tolerated
Repeat glucose: ≤25 mg/dl	E. Repeat A and proceed to D; recheck glucose	Monitor glucose hourly till stable; check for signs of fluid overload
Intractable hypoglycemia (glucose ≤40 after E)	Hydrocortisone IV or IM 5 mg/kg BID for 3–5 days	
Recovery phase (glucose >70 mg)	Decrease dextrose by 2 mg/kg/min decrements q 6–12 hr Discontinue hydrocortisone when glucose requirement normalizes	Recheck glucose q 4–6 hr; increase enteral feeds

*From Pildes RS, Pyati SP. Hypoglycemia and hyperglycemia in tiny infants. Clin Perinatol 1986; 13:351.

additional pharmacologic treatment should be considered. Generally the next step would be hydrocortisone, 5 to 10 mg per kilogram per day divided into two doses. Treatment usually needs to be maintained for a few days to allow achievement of a stable blood glucose level; thereafter the dosage should be tapered over about one week. Should the addition of steroid treatment not prove efficacious, generally the next line of treatment would be diazoxide, a thiazide antihypertensive, which also inhibits insulin secretion by the pancreas. Unlike the usual procedure when given to decrease blood pressure, the intravenous diazoxide dose should be given slowly to increase the protein binding of the drug and therefore decrease its hypotensive effect. The dosage is 5 mg per kilogram every eight hours. Treatment with glucagon (0.3 mg per kilogram intravenously or intramuscularly) is controversial. It clearly would be contraindicated in a patient with inadequate metabolic stores, such as small-for-gestational-age, very low birth weight, and premature infants. Although glucagon might increase glucose production transiently in some other instances, such as

large-for-gestational-age term infants and term infants of diabetic mothers, it would not be a substitute for intravenous treatment, but might serve as a temporary measure while the intravenous line is being started. Epinephrine, too, has been used, but because of its variable effects on the blood glucose level, it is not recommended.[27]

Patients with hypoglycemia persistent enough to require pharmacotherapy should be evaluated for possible metabolic and endocrine causes of persistent hyperinsulinemia. This generally entails a pediatric endocrinology consultation and the determination of serum levels of insulin and other homeostatic hormones. Neonates with persistent hyperinsulinemia may require partial pancreatectomy.

OUTCOME OF NEONATAL HYPOGLYCEMIA

There is a distinct dearth of human data regarding pure hypoglycemic brain insults over clearly defined periods of time, for obvious reasons. There are, however, some data available for extrapolation. Haworth et al[42] reported six infants with symptomatic hypoglycemia in the first three days of life. Treatment was erratic, with oral feedings, glucose infusions (rate unknown), glucagon, and steroids used in some of the cases. The glucose delivery rate was probably low by today's standards. Three of the patients were also diagnosed as being hypocalcemic. The follow-up period was short (two to 13 months), but two of the six patients were pronounced "mentally retarded." No blood gas levels were obtained although both of the "mentally retarded" patients were described as being cyanotic at times, and one was placed in oxygen; this patient was also quite likely small for gestational age. Little of relevance to current nursery practice can be gleaned from this article.

Koivisto et al[43] presented data relating to the outcome in 151 hypoglycemic infants. Blood glucose levels were determined thrice daily during the first two to four days of life and apparently when indicated by symptoms. Their patients were divided into three groups—symptomatic-convulsion, symptomatic-nonconvulsion, and asymptomatic. They concluded that there was a high incidence (50 percent) of central nervous system damage in the group with convulsions. However, these patients were not diagnosed until a mean age of 39 hours, their therapy was not begun for an additional four hours, and the mean duration of hypoglycemia was 105 hours! Even the patients in the symptomatic-nonconvulsion group had a mean duration of hypoglycemia of 49 hours, with an 11 hour delay between diagnosis and treatment. The asymptomatic infants were diagnosed and treated earlier, with a mean duration of hypoglycemia of 37 hours. The outcome in these patients was not significantly different from that in the control subjects. From this, it was concluded that "asymptomatic hypoglycemia, regardless of how low the blood glucose values may be, probably does not damage the brain." In regard to the prolonged duration of hypoglycemia in their patients, they also stated that "There is obviously a long latent period between the beginning of hypoglycaemia and the appearance of the severe symptoms, convulsions. Since it is evident that asymptomatic hypoglycaemia does not have a damaging effect, and that symptomatic hypoglycaemia with convulsions can cause severe damage, the indications for treatment must be weighed accordingly."

Pildes et al[44] reported follow-up data in 39 infants diagnosed with hypoglycemia between 1960 and 1964. These infants were largely small for gestational age (72.2 percent had a birth weight and 37.5 percent had a head circumference less than the 10th percentile for gestational age) and had a high incidence of seizures (20.5 percent), sepsis (10.3 percent), and central nervous system bleeding (13.8 percent). The hypoglycemic infants also had more respiratory problems and a higher incidence of meconium staining than did their retrospectively matched controls. It is important to note that these infants were diagnosed by daily blood glucose determinations from one to four days of age, except when symptoms prompted blood glucose determinations, such that they defined the "early diagnosis" of hypoglycemia as being within 12 hours after onset; even so, over 30 percent of the patients were not diagnosed until even later. Somewhat surprisingly, their outcome was very reassuring. The investigators concluded that "Only three had moderately severe neurological handicaps that could have been the result of neonatal hypoglycemia and one had not been given any therapy for several days." All these patients had seizures in the neonatal period. These investigators, like Koivisto,[43] noted the prognostic significance of seizures: "Neonatal seizures associated with symptomatic hypoglycemia were the only clinical manifestation that could be correlated with outcome." Although there was some decrease in the IQ in the hypoglycemic infants, there were too many confounding factors in the study population to ascribe this to low blood sugar levels.

Several studies have reported the long-term outcome in infants with neonatal hypoglycemia related to maternal diabetes. Persson and Gentz[45] reported no obvious relationship between plasma glucose determined at two to four hours after birth and IQ at follow-up and Haworth and co-workers[46] found "no statistically significant differences between the hypoglycaemic and the non-hypoglycaemic infants." Cummins and Norrish[47] could find no significant difference in the IQs of the hypoglycemic and nonhypoglycemic infants, including one case of prolonged hypoglycemia related to maternal chlorpropamide treatment. These are all relatively recent studies, demonstrating perhaps the significance of improved obstetrical and neonatal care more than the insignificance of hypoglycemia. However, it would seem safe to surmise that in infants of diabetic mothers, transient hypoglycemia, treated while still asymptomatic, apparently poses relatively little risk of long-term central nervous system morbidity.

The exact mechanism of brain injury in hypoglycemic neonates remains unsettled. It continues to be a fairly commonly encountered clinical problem, although patients today usually have few or no symptoms and are treated very early. Clearly it is no longer possible ethically to perform studies of untreated prolonged hypoglycemia in the human infant. However, the data available strongly suggest that unless there is a profound and prolonged hypoglycemic insult, the outcome is likely to be good. For infants with seizures and hypoglycemia, the picture is more worrisome. Intravenous treatment with dextrose by minibolus and adequate continuous infusion seems to be effective in most cases, except in those with persistent hyperinsulinism due to congenital pancreatic conditions, which may necessitate partial pancreatectomy. With careful monitoring of patients at risk, which would include virtually all neonatal intensive care unit patients, hypoglycemic brain injury should be very rare indeed. To ascribe brain injury to hypoglycemia alone would be very difficult given the fact that it so frequently is a complication of other disorders that in and of themselves are more likely causes of long-term morbidity.

REFERENCES

1. Heck LJ, Ehrenberg A. Serum glucose levels (G) during the first 48 hours (R) of life in the healthy full term neonate. Pediatr Res 1983; 17:317A.
2. Cowett RM, Stern L. Carbohydrate homeostasis in the fetus and newborn. In: Avery GB, ed. Neonatology: pathophysiology and management of the newborn. 3rd ed. Philadelphia: JB Lippincott 1987:691.
3. Cornblath M, Reisner SH. Blood glucose in the neonate and its clinical significance. N Engl J Med 1965; 273:378.
4. Pildes RS, Pyati SP. Hypoglycemia and hyperglycemia in tiny infants. Clin Perinatol 1986; 13:351.
5. Adam PAJ, Raiha N, Rahaila EL, Kekomaki M. Oxidation of glucose and D-β-OH-butyrate by the early human fetal brain. Acta Paediatr Scand 1975; 64:17.
6. Kraus H, Schlenker S, Schwedesky D. Developmental changes of cerebral ketone body utilization in human infants. Hoppe-Seyler Z Physiol Chem 1974; 355:164.
7. Bhasin S, Shambough GE III. Fetal fuels. V. Ketone bodies inhibit pyrimidine biosynthesis in fetal rat brain. Am J Physiol 1982; 243:E234.
8. Robles-Valdes C, McGarry JD, Foster DW. Maternal-fetal carnitine relationships and neonatal ketosis in the rat. J Biol Chem 1976: 251:6007.
9. Drahota Z, Hahn P, Kleingeller A, Kostolanska A. Acetoacetate formation by liver slices from adult and infant rats. Biochem J 1964; 93:61.
10. Page MA, Krebs HA, Williamson DH. Activities of enzymes of ketone-body utilization in brain and other tissues of suckling rats. Biochem J 1971; 121:49.
11. Persson B, Gentz J. The pattern of blood lipids, glycerol and ketone bodies during the neonatal period, infancy and childhood. Acta Paeditr Scand 1966; 55:353.

12. Anday EK, Stanley CA, Baker L, Delivoria-Papadopoulos M. Plasma ketones in newborn infants: absence of suckling ketosis. J Pediatr 1981; 98:628.
13. Sonnenberg N, Bergstrom JD, Ha YH, Edmond J. Metabolism in the artificially reared rat pup: effect of an atypical rat milk substitute. J Nutr 1982; 112:1506.
14. Fisher DJ, Heymann MA, Rudolph AM. Myocardial oxygen and carbohydrate consumption in fetal lambs in utero and in adult sheep. Am J Physiol 1980; 238:H399.
15. Cremer JE, Cunningham VJ, Pardridge WM, et al. Kinetics of blood-brain barrier transport of pyruvate, lactate and glucose in suckling, weanling and adult rats. J Neurochem 1979; 33:439.
16. Thurston JH, Hauhart RE, Schiro JA. Lactate reverses insulin-induced hypoglycemic stupor in suckling-weanling mice: biochemical correlates in blood, liver, and brain. J Cereb Blood Flow Metabol 1983; 3:498.
17. Hartmann AF, Jaudon JC. Hypoglycemia. J Pediatr 1937; 11:1.
18. Anderson JM, Milner RDG, Stritch SJ. Effects of neonatal hypoglycaemia on the nervous system: a pathological study. J Neurol Neurosurg Psychiatr 1967; 30:295.
19. Griffiths AD, Laurence KM. The effect of hypoxia and hypoglycemia on the brain of the newborn human infant. Develop Med Child Neurol 1974; 16:308.
20. Agardh CD, Kalimo H, Olsson Y, Siesjo BK. Hypoglycemic brain injury. I. Metabolic and light microscopic findings in rat cerebral cortex during profound insulin-induced hypoglycemia and in the recovery period following glucose administration. Acta Neuropathol 1980; 50:31.
21. Auer RN, Wieloch T, Olsson Y, Siesjo BK. The distribution of hypoglycemic brain damage. Acta Neuropathol 1984; 64:177.
22. Chase HP, Marlow RA, Dabierre CS, Welch NN. Hypoglycemia and brain development. Pediatrics 1973; 52:513.
23. Mayman CI, Tijerina ML. The effect of hypoglycemia on energy reserves in adult and newborn brain. Clin Develop Med 1971; 39/40:242.
24. Auer RN. Progress review: hypoglycemic brain damage. Stroke 1986; 17:699.
25. Wieloch T. Hypoglycemia-induced neuronal damage prevented by an N-methyl-D-aspartate antagonist. Science 1985; 230:681.
26. Lindvall O, Auer RN, Siesjo BK. Selective lesions of neostriatal dopamine neurons ameliorate hypoglycemic damage in the caudate-putamen. Exp Brain Res 1986; 63:382.
27. Ogata ES. Carbohydrate metabolism in the fetus and neonate and altered neonatal glucoregulation. Pediatr Clin North Am 1986; 33:25.
28. Kleigman R, Gross T, Morton S, et al. Intrauterine growth and postnatal fasting metabolism in infants of obese mothers. J Pediatr 1984; 104:601.
29. Brazy JE, Pupkin MJ. Effects of maternal isoxsuprine administration on preterm infants. J Pediatr 1979; 94:444.
30. Epstein MF, Nicholls E, Stubblefield PG. Neonatal hypoglycemia after beta-sympathomimetic tocolytic therapy. J Pediatr 1979; 94:449.
31. Tenenbaum D, Cowett RM. Mechanism of beta-sympathomimetic action on neonatal glucose homeostasis in the lamb. J Pediatr 1982; 101:588.
32. Procianoy RS, Pinheiro CEA. Neonatal hyperinsulinism after short-term maternal beta sympathomimetic therapy. J Pediatr 1982; 101:612.
33. Barrett CT, Oliver TK Jr. Hypoglycemia and hyperinsulinism in infants with erythroblastosis fetalis. N Engl J Med 1968; 178:1260.
34. Schiff D, Aranda JV, Chan G, et al. Metabolic effects of exchange transfusions. I. Effect of citrated and of heparinized blood on glucose, nonesterified fatty acids, 2-(4-hydroxybenzeneazo) benzoic acid binding, and insulin. J Pediatr 1971; 78:603.
35. Schiff D, Aranda JV, Colle E, Stern L. Metabolic effects of exchange transfusion. II. Delayed hypoglycemia following exchange transfusion with citrated blood. J Pediatr 1971; 79:589.
36. Johnson JD, Hansen RC, Albritton WL, et al. Hypoplasia of the anterior pituitary and neonatal hypoglycemia. J Pediatr 1973; 82:634.
37. Lovinger RD, Kaplan SL, Grumbach MM. Congenital hypopituitarism associated with neonatal hypoglycemia. J Pediatr 1975; 87:1171.
38. Stanhope R, Brook CGD. Neonatal hypoglycaemia: an important early sign of endocrine disorders. B Med J 1985; 291:728. 39. Sutton AM, Kingdom JCP. Neonatal hypoglycaemia: an important early sign of endocrine disorders. B Med J 1985; 291:1046.
39. Sutton AM, Kingdom JCP. Neonatal hypoglycaemia: an important early sign of endocrine disorders. B Med J 1985; 291:1046.
40. Cornblath M, Schwartz R. Disorders of carbohydrate metabolism in infancy. Philadelphia: WB Saunders, 1976.
41. Lilien LD, Pildes RS, Srinivasan G, et al. Treatment of neonatal hypoglycemia with minibolus and intravenous glucose infusion. J Pediatr 1980; 97:295.
42. Haworth JC, Coodin FJ, Finkel KC, Weidman ML. Hypoglycemia associated with symptoms in the newborn period. Can Med Assoc J 1963; 88:23.
43. Koivisto M, Blanca-Sequeiros M, Krause U. Neonatal symptomatic and asymptomatic hypoglycaemia: a follow-up study of 151 children. Dev Med Child Neurol 1972; 14:603.
44. Pildes RS, Cornblath M, Warren I, et al. A prospective controlled study of neonatal hypoglycemia. Pediatrics 1974; 54:5.
45. Persson B, Gentz J. Follow-up of children of insulin-dependent and gestational diabetic mothers: neuropsychological outcome. Acta Paediatr Scand 1984; 73:349.
46. Haworth JC, McRae KN, Dilling LA. Prognosis of infants of diabetic mothers in relation to neonatal hypoglycaemia. Develop Med Child Neurol 1976; 18:471.
47. Cummins M, Norrish M. Follow-up of children of diabetic mothers. Arch Dis Child 1980; 55:259.

13 Hematologic Disorders: Anemia, Polycythemia, and Hyperbilirubinemia

David K. Stevenson, M.D. and Herbert C. Schwartz, M.D.

Anemia in the Neonate
Hemorrhage
Hemolysis
Bleeding Disorders
Polycythemia and the Hyperviscosity Syndrome
Heavy Maternal Smoking
Pre-eclampsia
Hemorheologic Profiles in Infants Born to Smoking or
    Pre-eclamptic Mothers
Polycythemia and Hyperviscosity as Epiphenomena
Anemia Caused by Hemolysis and Polycythemia Linked
    to Hyperbilirubinemia.

Many hematologic disorders can contribute to fetal or neonatal brain injury. Most of them contribute to such injury because there are too few circulating red cells capable of carrying oxygen and delivering it to tissues (anemia) or too many red cells (polycythemia) so that tissue perfusion is compromised. Hyperbilirubinemia is another clinical syndrome that is closely linked with anemia and polycythemia that still occasionally threatens the neonate with brain injury. Although classic kernicterus appears to be a syndrome of the past, more subtle bilirubin encephalopathy in premature infants may contribute to intellectual impairment, motor dysfunction, dyslexia and learning disabilities, and hearing problems, which are difficult to attribute to bilirubin toxicity or to other confounding perinatal factors, such as asphyxia and birth trauma.

As a preface to this discussion, it is important to acknowledge that normal hematologic values can be consistent with acute blood loss, even though the blood volume and red cell mass may be deficient, and inadequate delivery of oxygen to tissues results because of compromised oxygen carrying capacity (Tables 13–1, 13–2). Moreover, acute blood gain, as with placental overtransfusion, may be manifested only as a circulatory overload syndrome in the early transitional period before hemoconcentration has taken place.

Normal hematologic values at birth can be affected by several variables, the most important being the site of sampling and the time of cord clamping. This topic has been expertly reviewed elsewhere.[1] In brief, capillary hemoglobin and hematocrit values typically exceed venous values, but the differences vary greatly among individuals and over time. The time of cord clamping and the position of the infant relative to the introitus also have a profound effect on the placental transfusion and thus hematologic values at birth, including blood volume and red cell mass. Relevant to the risk of anemia, the shorter the time from birth to clamping and the higher the elevation of the infant above the introitus during the time before cord clamping, the more likely it is that placental transfusion will be compromised or that blood loss will occur (retrograde flow back into the placenta).

ANEMIA IN THE NEONATE

A complete review of the erythrocyte and its disorders in the fetus and newborn is beyond the scope of this analysis.[2] Because the syndrome of anemia in the neonate has been reviewed a number of times,[3-5] the purpose of this presentation is to reemphasize the three major categories of anemia with their respective differential diagnoses, to delineate a unifying rationale for the treatment of anemia in the neonate, and to outline a diagnostic and therapeutic approach in order to avoid brain injury.

Study supported by a grant (RR81) from the General Research Centers Program of the Division of Research Resources, National Institutes of Health, and the Christopher Taylor Harrison Research Fund.

147

TABLE 13-1   Normal Cord Blood Hemoglobin Values

Author(s)	Mean Hemoglobin (gm/dl)	Range (gm/dl)	Number of Observations
Mollison (1951)	16.6		134
Dochain et al (1952)	17.9	14.4–21.6	40
Walker et al (1953)	16.5		145
Marks et al (1953)	16.9	12.3–22.0	221
Guest et al (1957)	17.1	13.0–25.0	59
McKay (1957)	17.4		60
Booth et al (1957)	16.7	11.2–26.6	414
Mean	16.8		

From Nathan DE, Oski FA, eds. Hematology of infancy and childhood. 3rd ed. Philadelphia: WB Saunders, 1987:17.

Blood loss, hemolysis, and deficient red cell production are three mechanisms that can contribute to anemia at the time of birth or in the first 28 days of life (the neonatal period). From a practical perspective, abnormalities of red cell production are infrequent causes of anemia at birth. Although the practitioner should be aware of the Diamond-Blackfan syndrome (pure red cell anemia), it is a rare recessive condition that usually appears later in infancy as an anemia of insidious onset. This primary failure of erythropoiesis is often (30 percent) associated with physicial anomalies.[6,7] Congenital infections, particularly cytomegalic inclusion virus infection, may also lead to anemia at the time of birth, but conditions such as rubella are much less common today than in the past. A new cause is the human immunodeficiency virus. Other diseases, such as congenital leukemia and osteopetrosis, are also exceedingly rare. Thus, blood loss and hemolysis are the predominant hematologic disorders threatening the neonate with brain injury in the transitional period.

TABLE 13-2   Red Cell Values on First Postnatal Day

Gestational Age (Weeks)	24-25 (7)*	26-27 (11)	28-29 (7)	30-31 (25)	32-33 (23)	34-35 (23)	36-37 (20)	Term (19)
RBC × 10^6	4.65 ±0.43	4.73 ±0.45	4.62 ±0.75	4.79 ±0.74	5.0 ±0.76	5.09 ±0.5	5.27 ±0.68	5.14 ±0.7
Hb (gm/dl)	19.4 ±1.5	19.0 ±2.5	19.3 ±1.8	19.1 ±2.2	18.5 ±2.0	19.6 ±2.1	19.2 ±1.7	19.3 ±2.2
Hematocrit (%)	63 ±4	62 ±8	60 ±7	60 ±8	60 ±8	61 ±7	64 ±7	61 ±7.4
MCV (μm^3)	135 ±0.2	132 ±14.4	131 ±13.5	127 ±12.7	123 ±15.7	122 ±10.0	121 ±12.5	119 ±9.4
Reticulocytes (%)	6.0 ±0.5	9.6 ±3.2	7.5 ±2.5	5.8 ±2.5	5.0 ±1.9	3.9 ±1.6	4.2 ±1.8	3.2 ±1.4
Weight (gm)	725 ±185	993 ±194	1174 ±128	1450 ±232	1816 ±192	1957 ±291	2245 ±213	

* Number of infants
Mean values ±SD
From Zaizov R, Matoth Y. Red cell values on the first postnatal day during the last 16 weeks of gestation. Am J Hematol 1976; 1:276.

HEMORRHAGE

There are many types of blood loss in the newborn. They include occult hemorrhage prior to birth, obstetrical accidents, malformations of the placenta and cord, and internal hemorrhage. The types of hemorrhage in the newborn are listed in Table 13-3. With respect to occult hemorrhage, fetal-to-maternal hemorrhage may occur in as many as 50 percent of all pregnancies,[8] but a volume of blood loss large enough to contribute to serious anemia (more than 40 ml) probably is found in 1 percent or fewer pregnancies. The latter circumstance is most likely to occur in association with traumatic diagnostic amniocentesis or external cephalic version prior to delivery. A Kleihauer-Behtke procedure for detecting fetal (HbF) cells in the maternal circulation is helpful,[9] but may miss evidence of fetal-to-maternal hemorrhage if the mother and infant are incompatible for the ABO blood group because the infant's A or B cells may be rapidly cleared from the maternal circulation. Evidence of erythrophagocytosis in smears of the maternal buffy coat or a rise in maternal immune anti-A or anti-B titers in the weeks following delivery also may suggest the diagnosis if this is important in distinguishing the cause of anemia. It is also important to acknowledge the possibility that blood loss may not be acute, but chronic, therefore presenting a different clinical syndrome at the time of birth, as well as requiring a different therapeutic approach (Table 13-4).

TABLE 13-3   Types of Hemorrhage in the Newborn

Occult hemorrhage prior to birth
　Fetal-maternal
　　Traumatic amniocentesis
　　Spontaneous
　　Following external cephalic version
　Twin-to-twin

Obstetrical accidents, malformations of the placenta and cord
　Rupture of a normal umbilical cord
　　Precipitous delivery
　　Entanglement
　Hematoma of the cord or placenta
　Rupture of an abnormal umbilical cord
　　Varices
　　Aneurysm
　Rupture of anomalous vessels
　　Aberrant vessel
　　Velamentous insertion
　　Communicating vessel in multilobed placenta
　Incision of placenta during cesarean section
　Placenta previa
　Abruptio placentae

Internal hemorrhage
　Intracranial
　Giant cephalohematoma, caput succedaneum
　Retroperitoneal
　Ruptured liver
　Ruptured spleen

From Nathan DG, Oski FD, eds. Hematology of infancy and childhood. 3rd ed. Philadelphia: WB Saunders, 1987:17.

TABLE 13-4   Characteristics of Acute and Chronic Blood Loss in the Newborn

Characteristics	Acute Blood Loss	Chronic Blood Loss
Clinical	Acute distress; pallor; shallow, rapid, and often irregular respiration; tachycardia; weak or absent peripheral pulses; low or absent blood pressure; no hepatosplenomegaly	Marked pallor disproportionate to evidence of distress; on occasion signs of congestive heart failure may be present, including hepatomegaly
Venous pressure	Low	Normal or elevated
Laboratory		
Hemoglobin concentration	May be normal initially; then drops quickly during first 24 hours of life	Low at birth
Red cell morphology	Normochromic and macrocytic	Hypochromic and microcytic; anisocytosis and poikilocytosis
Serum iron	Normal at birth	Low at birth
Course	Prompt treatment of anemia and shock necessary to prevent death	Generally uneventful
Treatment	Intravenous fluids and whole blood; iron therapy later	Iron therapy; packed red cells may be necessary on occasion

From Nathan DE, Oski FA, eds. Hematology of infancy and childhood. 3rd ed. Philadelphia: WB Saunders, 1987:17.

For example, a large acute blood loss represents a medical emergency, requiring prompt treatment of anemia and shock in order to prevent brain injury or death. In contrast, chronic blood loss represents a threat to adequate delivery of oxygen to tissues because of a decreased oxygen carrying capacity, but compensatory mechanisms, such as an increased cardiac output and respiratory rate, may diminish the immediate threat to well-being unless congestive heart failure or respiratory failure is a complication. Chronic blood loss is invariably associated with a low hemoglobin concentration and hematocrit level at birth, whereas acute blood loss may be associated with a normal hemoglobin concentration and hematocrit level initially, dropping quickly during the first two to four hours of life. The treatment of acute blood loss requires the immediate transfusion of whole blood or reconstituted packed cells (hematocrit, 60 to 70 percent) mixed with saline or fresh frozen plasma to increase the intravascular volume and reestablish the cardiac output as well as to increase the oxygen carrying capacity. Chronic blood loss can be treated more conservatively using iron therapy (or if distress is present, packed red cells) transfused over a long interval of time (four hours). Slow transfusion of packed cells is recommended in order to avoid the precipitation of congestive heart failure. Diuretic therapy usually is not required. A decrease in the cardiac output would be an appropriate response to increasing oxygen carrying capacity.

Fetus-to-fetus transfusions are observed only in monozygotic multiple births with monochorial placentas. The latter circumstance exists in approximately 70 percent of monozygotic twin pregnancies,[10] and up to 33 percent of such pregnancies are complicated by a twin-to-twin transfusion.[11,12] The donor twin may be anemic and the recipient twin, polycythemic and threatened by the hyperviscosity syndrome. Similar to fetal-to-maternal hemorrhage, the transfusion may be acute or chronic. The treatment of anemia caused by fetus-to-fetus transfusion, in principle, does not differ from that for maternal-to-fetal transfusion. Whereas the Kleihauer-Behtke technique of acid elution is the simplest method for detecting fetal cells in the maternal circulation, the technique obviously cannot be applied to the diagnosis of fetus-to-fetus transfusion, in which multiple gestation characterized by monozygosity and a monochorial placenta is suggestive of the latter complication.

One of the most threatening obstetrical accidents is rupture of the umbilical cord during a precipitous delivery. Often such rupture is caused in part by a short or entangled cord. A short cord may also suggest underlying abnormalities of the fetus, which have contributed to the development of a short cord because of lack of fetal movement.[13] A true obstetrical accident also may result from the application of forceps for traction. Velamentous insertion of the umbilical cord, occurring in approximately 1 percent of all pregnancies, is a complication predisposing to fetal blood loss.[14] Other vascular abnormalities, such as umbilical venous tortuosity and arterial aneurysm or inflammation caused by infection, also may predispose to rupture during normal labor and delivery. Incision of the placenta at the time of cesarean section may produce serious life-threatening fetal hemorrhage.[15] Finally, placenta previa and abruptio placentae are probably the most common causes of blood loss.[16] Especially in smaller infants, iatrogenic blood loss from repeated blood sampling should not be overlooked.

Closed space bleeding in the neonate, usually related to trauma or a hemorrhagic diathesis, may be associated with anemia appearing in the first 24 to 72 hours after birth. Although it may not be associated with early jaundice, it commonly contributes to hyperbilirubinemia later in the first week of life (to be discussed). If there is a large amount of bleeding into a closed space and it is rapid, this complication may not be recognized until the infant shows signs of shock due to blood loss. Although most clinicians would think first of a cephalohematoma, the risk of blood loss to a degree that would cause brain injury or death is unusual in this circumstance because of the confinement of bleeding by periosteal attachments. In contrast, blood loss into the subaponeurotic area of the scalp may be life threatening.[17,18]

Other kinds of closed space bleeding that may contribute to the development of anemia and shock in the newborn include intracranial hemorrhage (typically subarachnoid and subdural in the term infant, as well as periventricular and intraventricular in the premature infant), pulmonary hemorrhage (usually associated with respiratory failure), and gastrointestinal hemorrhage, all of which may be exacerbated by a hemorrhagic diathesis, such as vitamin K deficiency. In particular, breech deliveries have been associated with adrenal, renal, splenic, and hepatic hemorrhages.

Rupture of the liver can be an insidious and immediately life-threatening event. The latter should be suspected after any difficult delivery and probably is underdiagnosed. An infant may appear well for 24 to 48 hours before severe anemia and shock develop. Splenic rupture may present a similar clinical syndrome[19] and is more likely to occur in the presence of splenomegaly, such as that encountered in erythroblastosis fetalis, requiring exchange transfusion. Besides the obvious threat presented by pulmonary hemorrhage and the threat of sudden blood loss, closed space bleeding in the head poses the most direct threat of brain injury. Although periventricular, intraventricular, and parenchymal hemorrhages are generally managed conservatively without surgical intervention (except in the presence of hydrocephalus), subdural parietal hematoma formation or infratentorial posterior fossa bleeding may require neurosurgical procedures in order to prevent injury or death.[2]

HEMOLYSIS

Hemolysis is the other most common cause of anemia presenting at the time of birth or during the first 28 days of life. The causes of hemolysis are summarized in Table 13-5. Although jaundice typically complicates hemolysis during the neonatal period, hemolysis in utero may present with severe anemia and minimal jaundice or jaundice requiring only phototherapy and not exchange transfusion. The clinical syndrome associated with hemolysis is most similar to that observed in association with chronic fetal blood loss, for the blood volume is often normal and the approach to treatment of the anemia per se is also similar. However, because hemolysis often continues in the presence of isoimmune disease, exchange transfusion may be required to remove a large red cell mass subject to continued breakdown or to alleviate hyperbilirubinemia (to be discussed).

Premature infants have a shortened red blood cell life span, which contributes to the physiologic anemia of prematurity.[20] The initial hemoglobin and hematocrit values are lower, and the ultimate nadir between four and eight weeks of age is lower than that in term infants.[21] Transfusion of premature infants (in particular, those with pulmonary disease) is routine in most intensive care

TABLE 13-5   Causes of Hemolytic Process in the Neonatal Period

Immune
  Rh incompatibility
  ABO incompatibility
  Minor blood group incompatibility
  Maternal autoimmune hemolytic anemia
  Drug-induced hemolytic anemia

Infection
  Bacterial sepsis
  Congenital infections
    Syphilis
    Malaria
    Cytomegalovirus
    Rubella
    Toxoplasmosis
    Disseminated herpes

Disseminated intravascular coagulation

Macro- and microangiopathic hemolytic anemias
  Cavernous hemangioma
  Large vessel thrombi
  Renal artery stenosis
  Severe coarctation of aorta

Galactosemia

Prolonged or recurrent acidosis of a metabolic or respiratory nature

Hereditary disorders of the red cell membrane
  Hereditary spherocytosis
  Hereditary elliptocytosis
  Hereditary stomatocytosis
  Other rare membrane disorders

Pyknocytosis

Red cell enzyme deficiency
  Most common are glucose-6-phosphate dehydrogenase deficiency, pyruvate kinase deficiency, 5′ nucleotidase deficiency, and glucose phosphate isomerase deficiency

Alpha thalassemia syndromes

Alpha chain structural abnormalities

Gamma thalassemia syndromes

Gamma chain structural abnormalities

From Nathan DE, Oski FA, eds. Hematology of infancy and childhood. 3rd ed. Philadelphia: WB Saunders, 1987:17.

nurseries. The requirement for transfusion is ultimately based on a clinical judgment that the red cell mass is not adequate for the delivery of oxygen to the tissues. A dependence on supplemental inspired oxygen usually complicates considerations in this regard. Thus, the decision to transfuse premature infants must be individualized, because oxygen consumption as well as cardiovascular and respiratory compensation may vary from infant to infant. Transfusion programs involving "walking donors" and careful screening of blood for cytomegalovirus and other viruses, such as human immunodeficiency virus, can decrease the risk of transfusion in premature infants.[22] Although the administration of erythropoietin to prevent anemia of prematurity is being considered, this strategy requires carefully conducted trials not only to establish efficacy but to ensure safety.

The first important step in the treatment of anemia in the neonate is recognition of the problem. Although pallor is the hallmark of the disease, a variety of conditions can contribute to pallor. Other features may be helpful in differentiating asphyxia with acidosis, acute severe blood loss, chronic severe blood loss, and hemolytic disease in the clinical setting (Table 13-6). Although the need to increase the oxygen carrying capacity is generally recognized, the approach to correcting anemia and the requirement for other supportive measures may vary greatly with the diagnosis. A meticulous diagnostic approach to the anemic newborn is essential in understanding the cause(s) of the pathologic condition and ultimately deciding about diagnosis-specific therapies.[2] However, immediate treatment of anemia in all cases is based on a straightforward generalizable rationale.

The mechanism by which anemia typically threatens the newborn during the transitional period is by compromising the oxygen carrying capacity so that oxygen delivery to the tissues is too low relative to oxygen consumption. If normal cardiorespiratory compensatory responses were not capable of maintaining sufficient oxygen delivery to vital organs relative to tissue utilization, cellular metabolism would be adversely affected, first by becoming more inefficient energetically through utilization of anaerobic metabolism; eventually cells would be irreversibly damaged. Unlike the adult, the neonate is particularly vulnerable to anemia, even when it is chronic, because changes in 2,3 diphosphoglycerate concentration in the cell have less of an effect on the affinity of fetal hemoglobin for oxygen. This is specifically related to the decreased reactivity of 2,3 diphosphoglycerate with the gamma chains of HbF in contrast to the beta chains of HbA. In fact, acute severe anemia or asphyxia accompanied by metabolic acidosis may be associated with a drop in the intracellular pH and, paradoxically, a lowering of the 2,3 diphosphoglycerate levels in red cells. Thus, the neonate is critically dependent on oxygen carrying capacity. Moreover, cellular hypoxia can occur in the presence of a normal P_{O_2} level if the

oxygen content of the blood is low (hypoxemia). The presence of methemoglobins, such as carboxyhemoglobin and methemoglobin, sometimes can confuse the practitioner in this regard.

For example, an infant can be cyanotic and have a normal P_{O_2} level. Moreover, because fetal hemoglobin may not desaturate until P_{O_2} levels less than 40 mm Hg are reached, an infant may appear deceptively pink, though pale, and be at great risk for brain injury because of anemia Cyanosis is recognizable clinically when reduced hemoglobin reaches a level of approximately 3 gm per deciliter. However, the percentage saturation at which this occurs and the oxygen content can vary dramatically, depending on the hemoglobin concentration and the oxygen carrying capacity. Thus, in any infant who is tachypneic, which may be a sign of severe anemia as well as respiratory distress, not only is an arterial blood gas determination indicated, but a hematocrit or hemoglobin concentration should also be obtained. If peripheral perfusion is poor or there are any other signs of intravascular volume depletion, 10 cc per kilogram of packed red cells (hematocrit, 60 to 70 percent) mixed with saline solution or fresh frozen plasma should be infused immediately. Although clinicians almost routinely administer 100 percent oxygen to the depressed neonate at the time of birth and assist ventilation if respiratory efforts appear weak or ineffective, the correction of hypovolemia and anemia is perhaps the most often forgotten yet absolutely essential therapeutic maneuver for effectively resuscitating the neonate and avoiding neonatal brain injury.

BLEEDING DISORDERS

Although the diagnosis and management of inherited and acquired bleeding disorders are beyond the scope of this discussion, as would be an analysis of thrombotic disease in the newborn,[23] the close association of bleeding and thrombosis with hemorrhage and hemolysis warrants some comment. Compared with acquired coagulopathies, inherited coagulopathies are encountered infrequently in the newborn. However, neonates with hereditary bleeding disorders can present with a variety of bleeding problems, some of them life threatening, during the first weeks of life. The differential diagnosis for inherited bleeding disorders as well as their management has been reviewed recently.[24] The hemophilias (deficiencies of factor VIII, IX, or XI) should be seriously considered when the partial thromboplastin time (PTT) is prolonged and the prothrombin time (PT) normal, especially in an infant with a positive family history. The laboratory measurement of specific coagulation factors is essential to the diagnosis. Routinely all infants should be treated prophylactically with vitamin K in order to avoid vitamin K deficiency and

TABLE 13-6   Differential Diagnosis of Pallor in the Newborn

Asphyxia	Acute Severe Blood Loss	Hemolytic Disease
Respiratory findings: retractions, response to oxygen, cyanosis	Decrease in venous and arterial pressure	Hepatosplenomegaly, jaundice
Moribund appearance	Rapid shallow respirations	Positive Coombs' test
Bradycardia	Acyanotic	Anemia
Stable hemoglobin	Tachycardia	
	Drop in hemoglobin	

From Nathan DE, Oski FA, eds. Hematology of infancy and childhood. Vol 1. 3rd ed. Philadelphia: WB Saunders, 1987:37.

hemorrhagic disease of the newborn. In the newborn period coagulopathy should be excluded as a possible cause in any infant with anemia in whom blood loss is suspected clinically.

Thrombocytopenia is one of the most common bleeding diatheses encountered in the newborn.[5,25] In particular, isoimmune thrombocytopenia is probably more common than appreciated. Platelet transfusions (one unit of packed platelets) and treatment with steroids or intravenous nonaggregable gamma globulin can be used to treat active bleeding. If bleeding manifestations are minimal, a more conservative approach of watchful waiting is indicated. In the presence of active bleeding, a platelet transfusion should always be given in a thrombocytopenic neonate. After blood has been drawn for diagnostic tests, fresh frozen plasma should also be administered, since the other most common diagnosis to be considered in the newborn is disseminated intravascular coagulation. The diagnosis is typically difficult to confirm, but can be suspected on the basis of a combination of abnormalities, including prolongation of the PT, PTT, thrombocytopenia, and hypofibrinogenemia. Analysis of factor levels, such as V and VIII, is infrequently performed, unless the bleeding diathesis persists despite nonspecific therapy. Thrombocytopenia and disseminated intravascular coagulation can accompany many different clinical syndromes, such as sepsis and closed space bleeding, and correction of the underlying problem should be the fundamental approach in alleviating any acquired coagulopathy.

A normal hematocrit or hemoglobin value at the time of birth does not exclude severe acute hemorrhage from the differential diagnosis of fetal or neonatal distress. Furthermore, acyanosis does not exclude hypoxemia on the basis of anemia. Hypovolemia or anemia should be considered as a possible cause of apparent respiratory distress or any signs of depression, including metabolic acidosis. Arterial blood gas and hematocrit determinations and an assessment of the intravascular volume should be performed as soon as possible after birth in any depressed or distressed infant. Besides the administration of 100 percent oxygen and assisted ventilation, a 10 cc per kilogram transfusion of packed cells (hematocrit, 60 to 70 percent) mixed with saline solution or fresh frozen plasma always should be given if hypovolemia or anemia cannot be definitively excluded as a cause of the infant's condition. Moreover, in any infant with anemia, coagulopathy should be excluded as a cause. In the presence of active bleeding, a PT, a PTT, the fibrinogen level, and a platelet count should be determined, and a 10 cc per kilogram transfusion of fresh frozen plasma can be given empirically. A platelet transfusion should be given if thrombocytopenia is identified in the bleeding infant.

POLYCYTHEMIA AND THE HYPERVISCOSITY SYNDROME

Ironically, a hematologic condition that represents the opposite extreme of anemia can also threaten the neonate with neonatal brain injury. During the past decade the complications associated with the hyperviscosity syndrome (HVS) in neonates have been the subject of continuing controversy. Several recent reviews of the incidence, signs, and treatment of HVS again have focused attention on the increased morbidity and mortality associated with this disorder.[26-28] HVS is a common disorder, occurring in from 2.9 percent of total births at sea level to 5 percent at 1,612 feet.[29,30] A number of additional variables, for example, cord clamping, intrauterine growth retardation, dysmaturity and postmaturity, macrosomia in infants of diabetic mothers, congenital endocrine disorders (adrenal hyperplasia and thyrotoxicosis), developmental chromosomal abnormalities (trisomies 21, 18, and 13), and Beckwith's syndrome, may be associated with polycythemia or HVS. One problem is that investigators in most studies have had to group these heterogeneous disorders because of their low incidence. Independent of etiology, a recent study revealed that the systemic blood velocity, as measured in the inferior cerebral artery, may be impaired in infants with polycythemia.[31] This study reemphasized the importance of such variables in blood viscosity as red cell deformability and plasma constituents,[32-37] in addition to the hematocrit level in contributing to the signs and symptoms of HVS.

A second problem relates to detecting infants who have HVS without significant polycythemia. Hathaway[26] has emphasized that early signs of HVS (e.g., lethargy, jitteriness, alteration in awareness state, muscular tone, poor feeding) may be too insensitive to be reliable parameters in the clinical assessment. Although the capillary hematocrit level aids in the detection of infants with HVS, a report by Ramamurthy and Brans[38] indicated that the umbilical vein hematocrit level is significantly lower (mean, 63 percent) than the peripheral vein hematocrit level (mean, 71 percent) in infants whose capillary hematocrit levels were 70 percent or greater.

More recently Ramamurthy and Berlanga[39] reported postnatal alterations in the hematocrit level and viscosity in the first 18 hours of life. They found that the peripheral venous hematocrit level was highest at two hours of age and dropped to cord blood levels by 18 hours. The hematocrit level varied similarly in infants considered to be polycythemic (peripheral venous hematocrit level greater than 64 percent), but only a small fraction (38 percent) of the infants with a hematocrit level greater than 64 percent at two hours continued to have a high level beyond 12 hours of age (Fig. 13-1). The viscosity in these infants tended to follow the same pattern of change as the hematocrit level (Fig. 13-2). These investigators also observed that the peripheral venous hematocrit level was better correlated with the cord blood hematocrit than the capillary hematocrit level. However, despite authoritative opinions in the literature, the appropriate screening technique for detecting babies at risk for HVS has not been routinized in practice, and acceptance of such guidelines would depend on further studies of the relationship between clinical signs, hemorheologic changes, and the site used for blood sampling.

Partial exchange transfusion appears to be an effective treatment for HVS in the immediate newborn period,[40] but its efficacy in the prevention of long-term neurologic sequelae remains controversial.[28] Van der Elst et al[41] found no difference at eight months of age between a partially exchanged group and a control group of infants with HVS. Host and Ulrich[42] found 29 of 30 asymptomatic babies with hematocrit levels greater than 65 percent to be normal at two and one-half years of age. On the other hand, Goldberg et al[40] found significant neurologic abnormalities in nonexchanged infants, and Black et al[43] found that 40 percent of asymptomatic infants with HVS who were not exchanged had mild to moderate neurologic sequelae at two-year follow-up.

Blood is a non-newtonian fluid and, thus, does not follow the hydrodynamic laws of simple fluids. Although hematocrit level is the most important variable in determining the viscosity of neonatal blood, the fluidity

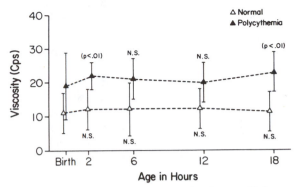

Figure 13-2   The mean +2 SD viscosity values in normal infants was not significantly different at any age. In infants with polycythemia, viscosity rise and fall tend to parallel changes in the hematocrit level. (From Ramamurthy RS, Berlanga M. Postnatal alteration in hematocrit and viscosity in normal and polycythemic infants. J Pediatr 1987; 110:929.)

in the microvasculature is also affected by the aggregation, red cell deformability, and plasma protein concentrations, especially fibrinogen. A number of studies of these variables have been performed in neonates. Linderkamp et al[35] have shown that there is no significant difference in deformability between red cells from fetuses, preterm and term neonates, and adults at any shear stress. They extended those studies recently and demonstrated that the viscoelastic properties as well as the deformability of neonatal red cells deviate only slightly from those of adult red cells.[44] Previous studies have shown that both red cell aggregation and plasma viscosity were very low in preterm infants and increased with increasing gestational age, because of the concomitant increase in the plasma protein concentration.[35,37,45] Reinhart et al[46] and Riopel et al[47] found similarly that the lower viscosity in fetal blood was due to the lower plasma viscosity and could be attributed to a lower plasma protein concentration.

Although polycythemia has been associated with neonatal brain injury, polycythemia also may be considered adaptive. This is a critical point in trying to decide whether polycythemia is the cause of the brain injury or whether it is an epiphenomenon itself, the result of whatever event caused the brain injury. For example, similar hemorheologic disorders have been linked to two readily identifiable groups of infants—those born to mothers who were heavy smokers during pregnancy and those born to mothers with pre-eclampsia.[48] Fetal intrauterine growth retardation, a possible consequence for fetuses in both conditions, has been attributed to chronic fetal hypoxia, which may be a final common pathway for these etiologically distinct clinical entities.

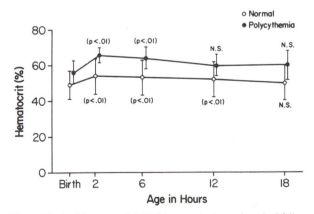

Figure 13-1   The mean +2 SD hematocrit rise and gradual fall are similar in infants with polycythemia and in normal infants up to 12 hours of age. Beyond 12 hours of age, 38 percent of the infants with polycythemia had hematocrit levels greater than 64 percent and the others, values less than 64 percent. (From Ramamurthy RS, Berlanga M. Postnatal alteration in hematocrit and viscosity in normal and polycythemic infants. J Pediatr 1987; 110:929.)

HEAVY MATERNAL SMOKING

Carbon monoxide (CO) is found throughout the environment in varied concentrations as a byproduct of the incomplete combustion of carbonaceous material. Mankind has significantly increased exposure to this toxic gas through the introduction of the internal combustion engine in vehicles and industrial plants and, on an individual basis, through cigarette smoking. In addition, CO is a physiologic gas produced endogenously from the breakdown of heme pigments, as occurs during hemolysis. As protoporphyrin degrades to bilirubin, CO is released from the alpha-methene carbon atom.[49] The causation of intrauterine growth retardation associated with heavy cigarette smoking in pregnancy has not been fully elucidated. However, chronic intrauterine hypoxic stress probably is at least an important contributing factor. Because the affinity of hemoglobin for CO is more than 200 times greater than that for oxygen, inhalation of CO results in disproportionately high carboxyhemoglobin concentrations. Carbon monoxide compromises tissue oxygenation by two mechanisms. First, CO readily displaces oxygen from hemoglobin, thereby decreasing the blood oxygen transport capacity. Second, CO markedly shifts the oxyhemoglobin saturation curve to the left and alters the shape of the curve to a more hyperbolic form.[50] Because CO crosses the placenta and the partial pressure of oxygen in fetal arterial blood is already normally low (20 to 30 mm Hg as compared to a maternal value of 85 mm Hg), developing fetal cells are especially vulnerable to CO-induced hypoxia.[51,52]

Although the nicotine in cigarette smoke may cause placental vasoconstriction,[53] cigarette smokers have a lower incidence of pregnancy-associated hypertension.[54] This suggests that any reduced placental blood flow caused by smoking is unlikely to be related to sustained vasoconstriction. However, hemorheologic effects that reduce peripheral blood flow have been observed in nonpregnant smokers,[55] and such phenomena may contribute to a reduced blood flow in both the fetal and the maternal placental circulations. The importance of these sustained hemorheologic effects, especially when combined with CO induced hypoxia, is suggested by the inability of partial exchange transfusion to alter the prognosis in certain polycythemic infants whose hemorheologic disorder represents a compensatory epiphenomenon, a reaction to chronic oxygen deprivation.[41,42] The link between heavy maternal smoking and intrauterine growth retardation,[56] as well as later behavioral disorders and intellectual impairment, is a legitimate concern.[57,58] Animal studies support the conclusions of clinical observations. Moderate CO exposure has been associated with a decrease in birth weight and an increase in neonatal mortality in rabbits.[59] Prenatal CO exposure differentially affects the postnatal monoamine concentrations and weight of specific brain regions, and

produces a permanent associative deficit restricted to memory impairment in rats.[60,61]

PRE-ECLAMPSIA

Reduced blood flow in both the fetal and the maternal placental circulations may be a contributing factor in the development of pre-eclampsia.[62-64] However, the reduction of intervillus placental blood flow, which has been associated with pre-eclampsia in clinical studies, has been variably described as a cause or an effect of the condition. There is no question that animal experiments have shown that artificially induced uterine ischemia can cause maternal and fetal effects similar to those of pre-eclampsia.[65,66] The occurrence of uteroplacental ischemia with pre-eclampsia may translate to chronic intrauterine fetal hypoxia, indistinguishable clinically from that observed in pregnancies complicated by heavy maternal smoking. Moreover, intrauterine growth retardation and hemorheologic disorders are similar consequences in these two conditions. Preeclamptic women may have elevated hematocrit and fibrinogen levels, increased plasma viscosity, and increased relative blood viscosity as well as reduced erythrocyte deformability.[67-70] Each of these factors not only may reduce placental blood flow and contribute to fetal hypoxia, but may contribute to the maternal pathophysiologic condition, reducing blood flow to organs and causing organ dysfunction. Intravascular coagulation throughout the microcirculation may occur in extreme cases.

HEMORHEOLOGIC PROFILES IN INFANTS BORN TO SMOKING OR PRE-ECLAMPTIC MOTHERS

Hemorheologic disorders have been described in infants born to mothers who were heavy smokers during pregnancy and to those with pre-eclampsia.[48] In particular, HVS has been described in relation to the fetal intrauterine growth retardation associated with these two conditions. Buchan[48] described the hemorheologic profiles in infants born to smoking and nonsmoking mothers and found a significantly decreased birth weight in those born to smoking mothers; they also have elevated hematocrit levels, elevated whole blood viscosity values, and a decreased erythrocyte deformability index. The infants did not differ in terms of gestational age, plasma fibrinogen level, or plasma viscosity. Buchan also reported hemorheologic profiles in infants born to preeclamptic and normotensive mothers. Birth weight was similarly low for the infants of the pre-eclamptic women. Moreover, the hematocrit and whole blood viscosity values were increased, and the erythrocyte deformability index was decreased. The two groups did not differ in terms of gestational age, plasma fibrinogen, or plasma viscosity. Thus, the hemorheologic profiles in infants born to smoking mothers and pre-eclamptic mothers compared with those in the offspring of nonsmoking normotensive mothers were virtually the same. Although the etiology of HVS in these two groups of infants probably differs, the hemorheologic similarities may have common, morbid consequences for the neonates themselves.

POLYCYTHEMIA AND HYPERVISCOSITY AS EPIPHENOMENA

By two weeks after conception, red blood cell production has begun in utero. Although erythropoietin probably affects newborn erythropoiesis throughout most of pregnancy, no erythropiesis activity has been found before the 10th week of gestation in the amniotic fluid. There is general agreement that erythropoietin production is well established in the human fetus during the last trimester of pregnancy. Heavy maternal smoking or other maternal conditions that compromise the delivery of oxygen to fetal tissues, such as pre-eclampsia, may have adverse effects on fetal and neonatal heme catabolism. Heavy smoking potentially has complex effects because of the wide variety of noxious substances present in smoke.

For example, placental vasoconstriction can be caused by nicotine,[53] which also can cause accelerated fetal metabolism.[71] An increased cord blood CO level can cause decreased carbonic anhydrase activity, and possibly chronic fetal hypoxia,[72] because carboxyhemoglobin is unavailable for carrying oxygen, and oxyhemoglobin in the presence of carboxyhemoglobin is less likely to release oxygen to fetal tissues.[50] Either of these effects might lead to increased erythropoietin levels in the fetus and a compensatory polycythemic state. A similar response by the fetus might occur in association with placental vasoconstriction in pre-eclampsia. To date, no clear causal link between the hyperviscosity associated with polycythemia and a poor neurodevelopmental outcome has been proven, although the association has been made a number of times. Moreover, except for the clinical syndrome of hypovolemia related to acute placental overtransfusion perinatally, the use of partial exchange transfusion to correct polycythemia or hyperviscosity has no proven benefit.

When polycythemia is identified, additional variables should be considered by the clinician attempting to understand the cause(s). Information should be sought about the time of cord clamping and the circumstances of the delivery, intrauterine growth retardation, dysmaturity and postmaturity, macrosomia in infants of diabetic mothers, congenital endocrine disorders (adrenal, hyperplasia and thyrotoxicosis), and developmental chromosomal abnormalities (trisomies 21, 18, and

13 and Beckwith's syndrome). If an infant shows signs of acute circulatory overload, such as mild congestive heart failure and respiratory distress, a partial exchange transfusion should be considered to alleviate the effects of probable placental overtransfusion. In a child showing no signs of distress, the role of partial exchange transfusion in preventing neurodevelopmental sequelae remains uncertain. The underlying causes of polycythemia may be the causes of fetal and neonatal brain injury as well. The diagnosis of polycythemia must be considered in the context of postnatal changes in the hematocrit level and differences in the site of sampling. When the peripheral venous hematocrit level is 70 percent or greater in infants younger than 12 hours, the diagnosis of polycythemia should be considered. If the peripheral venous hematocrit level is 64 percent or higher (and in a repeat determination at 12 hours of age), a central hematocrit should be obtained to confirm the diagnosis and partial exchange transfusion should be seriously considered. Any infant with a cord blood hematocrit level of 55 percent or higher should be screened for polycythemia postnatally.

ANEMIA CAUSED BY HEMOLYSIS AND POLYCYTHEMIA LINKED TO HYPERBILIRUBINEMIA

Compared with term infants, infants with polycythemia or hemolysis from any cause produce significantly increased amounts of bilirubin.[73] Under normal conditions, approximately 20 percent of the total bilirubin production in the adult human is derived from sources other than senescent red blood cells and is referred to as "early labeled bilirubin." This type of bilirubin is of both erythropoietic and nonerythropoietic origin. Although there are several sources of erythropoietic early labeled bilirubin, the liver is the major site of nonerythropoietic heme catabolism and is believed to contribute only 10 percent of the total bilirubin production. Under most of the abnormal clinical conditions associated with severe jaundice or hemorheologic disorders, the percentage of total bilirubin production derived from erythroid heme is even greater. Increased bilirubin production is a major factor contributing to all kinds of jaundice in the neonate.

Although classic kernicterus appears to be a syndrome of the past, and yellow staining of the brain is only infrequently seen in premature infants coming to autopsy, the possibility that more subtle bilirubin encephalopathy in premature infants can still occur, contributing to intellectual impairment, motor dysfunction, dyslexia and learning disabilities, and hearing problems, still preoccupies practitioners caring for sick neonates.[74] Several excellent reviews of bilirubin metabolism have been published.[75,76] However, the lack of knowledge about the selective molecular action of bilirubin on brain metabolism, and the lack of agreement about what levels and under what conditions bilirubin really constitutes a risk for neonatal brain injury are less well appreciated.[77,78] All practitioners should be aware of the guidelines provided by the American Academy of Pediatrics, as well as important recommendations in the major pediatric textbooks.[79,80] However, for the purpose of deciding causation in an individual case, the lack of knowledge and the lack of agreement become critical. In fact, most of the experimental work has been in vitro. In such systems the binding of bilirubin to albumin is a critical phenomenon for understanding toxicity.[81] However, its relevance to toxicity in intact animals or humans remains uncertain.[82] Nothing is known with certainty with respect to where bilirubin acts and how it acts. Hypotheses abound in the literature. Overall, the in vitro studies of bilirubin toxicity are inconclusive, and extrapolation to in vivo conditions is uncertain because of confounding uncontrolled factors.

Nonetheless the association between severe hemolysis (Rh disease), hyperbilirubinemia, and kernicterus cannot be ignored.[83] Under such conditions a serum total bilirubin level of 20 mg per deciliter or greater has been empirically associated with an increased risk of neonatal brain injury or death. Thus, "vigintiphobia" has a historical basis, but the extrapolation to other hyperbilirubinemic conditions besides Rh disease is not clear.[84] The standard of care in most communities is that some infants with serum total bilirubin levels greater than 20 mg per deciliter might be managed without exchange transfusion. An infant with the breast milk jaundice syndrome is a typical example. However, despite the assumed benign nature of breast milk jaundice syndrome, some practitioners would recommend exchange transfusion for any infant with a serum total bilirubin level greater than 20 mg per deciliter. Moreover, exchange transfusion might be considered at a lower level if the infant were sick in any way, in particular, if the infant were asphyxiated or infected or had cardiorespiratory or metabolic instability. The many nomograms for guiding the decision making of practitioners with respect to the treatment of hyperbilirubinemia should not be considered irrefutable standards, but rather recommendations for practice that need to be adapted and modified on an individual basis according to the judgment of the clinician. Furthermore, there is no absolute standard level at which phototherapy should be applied, although recommendations have been made.[85] Some investigators have recommended its use in premature infants at very low levels, because kernicterus has been diagnosed in such infants at bilirubin levels between 5 and 8 mg per deciliter. Common sense usually weighs heavily in the decision to start phototherapy in an effort to avoid exchange transfusion, which carries a small but definite risk.

In the future the ability to recognize hemolysis (increased bilirubin production) may help in deciding which infant should be treated, because jaundice associated with hemolysis has represented the most common serious threat.[86] One historical exception to this observation is the clinical experience reported by Silverman et al[87] in 1956 with premature infants treated with sulfoxazole. This tragedy suggested that great caution should be exercised in using any new drug in a neonate. In fact, all drugs considered for use in neonates should be tested for their capacity to displace bilirubin from albumin in order to avoid history's repeating itself. Practically, the prediction of severe jaundice may now be possible by estimating the degree of bilirubin production, combined with an assessment of the ability to handle the load. Such predictive procedures might allow clinicians to make better judgments about which infants should be discharged early, which should be followed more closely over the first week of life, and which require therapy, including home therapy.[88]

Finally, the pathogenesis of kernicterus may be more complex than originally believed. For example, it might result from the combination of anemia and a decreased oxygen carrying capacity with compromised delivery of oxygen to tissues, accumulation of a dyshemoglobin, such as carboxyhemoglobin as a result of massive hemolysis, as well as elevations in the serum bilirubin level, compounded by perinatal asphyxia and cardiorespiratory and metabolic instability. How the factors should be weighted in individual cases cannot be determined with certainty at this time.

There are some particular clinical problems that get practitioners into trouble more often than others. Most of them can be related to the early discharge of infants from the hospital. One example is the breast feeding infant with increased bilirubin production. The source of the increased bilirubin production may be unrecognized hemolytic disease or simply bruising or hematoma formation. The increased bilirubin production combined with a lack of a normal decrease in the enterohepatic circulation may contribute to a very rapid and early rise in the total serum bilirubin level over the first several days of life, which can be missed if the infant is discharged before the time of peak hyperbilirubinemia at approximately 3 to 4 days. The peak may also be later, as is often the case when increased production of bilirubin is a major factor contributing to jaundice. Even a large premature or near-term infant who is breast feeding, and does not have an obvious complication predisposing to increased bilirubin production, may have more difficulty in lowering the bilirubin level and should be followed closely throughout the first two weeks of life. In hemolytic disease, late anemia is a complication that also should not be overlooked once hyperbilirubinemia has been successfully managed. Such anemia may be so severe as to require transfusion by the second to fourth week of life.

In the presence of hemolysis, a total serum bilirubin

level of 20 mg per deciliter or greater has been associated with an increased risk of neonatal brain injury or death. Therefore, exchange transfusion should seriously be considered in any infant under such circumstances. Exchange transfusion should be considered with lower bilirubin levels in any infant who is sick, in particular, if the infant is asphyxiated or infected or has had cardiorespiratory or metabolic instability. The use of drugs capable of displacing bilirubin from albumin in general should be avoided in the newborn. Some displacers, however, are used in doses that do not practically cause a problem (e.g., indomethacin for patent ductus arteriosus closure). New drugs should be used with extreme caution until information about their effect on the binding of bilirubin to albumin is known. The use of Intralipid as a continuous infusion at a rate to prevent essential fatty acid deficiency (0.5 gm per kilogram) is not dangerous, because free fatty acid-albumin ratios are not elevated into the range at which displacement of bilirubin from albumin would be expected. Breast feeding of any infant with a propensity for increased bilirubin production (e.g., bruising, hematoma, prematurity) represents an increased risk for hyperbilirubinemia and warrants close follow-up of the infant throughout the first week and into the second week of life. Early discharge of an infant from the hospital requires that the practitioner arrange for appropriate follow-up to avoid serious hyperbilirubinemia.

REFERENCES

1. Linderkamp O. Placental transfusion: determinants and effects. Clin Perinatol 1982; 9:559.
2. Nathan DE, Oski FA, eds. Hematology of infancy and childhood. 3rd ed. Philadelphia: WB Saunders, 1987:17.
3. Lubin B. Neonatal anaemia secondary to blood loss. Clin Haematolol 1978; 7:19.
4. Glader BE, Platt O. Haemolytic disorders of infancy. Clin Haematol 1978; 7:35.
5. Oski FA, Naiman JL. Hematologic problems of the newborn. Philadelphia: WB Saunders, 1972:54.
6. Diamond LK, Wang WC, et al. Congenital hypoplastic anemia. Adv Pediatr 1976; 22:349.
7. Alter BP, Nathan DG. Red cell aplasia in children. Arch Dis Child 1979; 54:263.
8. Zipursky A, Hull A, et al. Foetal erythrocytes in the maternal circulation. Lancet 1959; 1:451.
9. Kleihauer E, Hildegard B, et al. Demonstration von fetalem hämoglobin in den Erythrocyten eines Blutausstrichs. Klin Wochenschr 1957; 35:637.
10. Benirschke K. Accurate recording of twin placenta. Obstet Gynecol 1961; 18:334.
11. Rausen AR, London RD, et al. Generalized bone changes and thrombocytopenic purpura in association with intra-uterine rubella. Pediatrics 1965; 36:264.
12. Strong SJ, Corney G. The placenta in twin pregnancy. New York: Pergamon Press, 1967.
13. Naeye RL. Umbilical cord length: clinical significance. J Pediatr 1985; 107:278.
14. Kirkman HN, Riley HD Jr. Posthemorrhagic anemia and shock in the newborn. A review. Pediatrics 1959; 24:97.
15. Weiner AS. Diagnosis and treatment of anemia of the newborn caused by occult placental hemorrhage. Am J Obstet Gynecol 1948; 56:717.
16. Novak F. Posthemorrhagic shock in newborns during labor and after delivery. Acta Med Yugosl 1953; 7:280.
17. Robinson RJ, Rossiter MA. Massive subaponeurotic hemorrhage in babies of African origin. Arch Dis Child 1968; 43:684.
18. Packman DJ. Massive hemorrhage in the scalp of the newborn infant. Hemorrhagic caput succedaneum. Pediatrics 1962; 29:907.
19. Erakalis AJ. Abdominal injury related to the trauma of birth. Pediatrics 1967; 39:421.
20. Schulman I. The anemia of prematurity. J Pediatr 1959; 54:633.
21. Melhorn DK, Gross S. Vitamin E dependent anemia in the preterm infant. I. Effects of large doses of medicinal iron. J Pediatr 1971; 79:569.
22. Johnson JD, Malachowski N, Sunshine P, et al. New transfusion program for an intensive care nursery. J Pediatr 1980; 97:806.
23. Barnard DR. Inherited bleeding disorders in the newborn infant. Clin Perinatol 1984; 11:309.
24. Schmidt B, Zipursky A. Thrombotic diseases in newborn infants. Clin Perinatol 1984; 11:461.
25. Andrew M, Kelton J. Neonatal thrombocytopenia. Clin Perinatol 1984; 11:359.
26. Hathaway WE. Neonatal hyperviscosity. Pediatrics 1983; 72:567.
27. Wu PYK. Neonatal hyperviscosity syndrome. West J Med 1985; 142:119.
28. Fischer AF, Sunshine P. The thick blood syndrome. Perinatol Neonat 1984; 8:39.
29. Stevens K, Wirth FH. Incidence of neonatal hyperviscosity at sea level. J Pediatr 1980; 97:118.
30. Wirth FH, Goldberg KE, Lubchenco LO. Neonatal hyperviscosity. I. Incidence. Pediatrics 1979; 63:833.
31. Rosenkrantz TS, Oh W. Cerebral blood flow velocity in infants with polycythemia and hyperviscosity: effects of partial exchange transfusion with Plasmanate. J Pediatr 1982; 101:94.
32. Gross GP, Hathaway WE. Fetal erythrocyte deformability. Pediatr Res 1972; 6:593.
33. Coulombel L, Tchernia G, Feo C, Mohandas N. Echinocytic sensitivity and deformability of human newborn red cells. Biol Neonate 1982; 42:284.
34. Linderkamp O, Wu PYK, Meiselman HJ. Deformability of density separated red blood cells in normal newborn infants and adults. Pediatr Res 1982; 16:964.
35. Linderkamp O, Guntner M, Hiltl W, Vargas VM. Erythrocyte deformability in the fetus, preterm, and term neonate. Pediatr Res 1986; 20:93.
36. Riopel L, Fouron J-C, Bard H. A comparison of blood viscosity between the adult sheep and newborn lamb. The role of plasma and red blood cell type. Pediatr Res 1983; 17:452.
37. Linderkamp O, Versmold HT, Riegel KP, Betke K. Contributions of red cells and plasma to blood viscosity in preterm and full-term infants and adults. Pediatrics 1984; 74:45.
38. Ramamurthy RS, Brans YW. Neonatal polycythemia. I. Criteria for diagnosis and treatment. Pediatrics 1981; 68:168.
39. Ramamurthy RS, Berlanga M. Postnatal alteration in hematocrit and viscosity in normal and polycythemic infants. J Pediatr 1987; 110:929.
40. Goldberg K, Wirth FH, Hathaway WE, et al. Neonatal hyperviscosity. II. Effect of partial plasma exchange transfusion. Pediatrics 1982; 69:419.
41. Van der Elst CW, Moteno CD, Malan AF, et al. The management of polycythaemia in the newborn infant. Early Hum Dev 1980; 4:393.
42. Host A, Ulrich M. Late prognosis in untreated neonatal polycythaemia with minor or no symptoms. Acta Paediatr Scand 1982; 71:629.
43. Black VD, Lubchenco LO, Lackey DW, et al. Developmental and neurologic sequelae of neonatal hyperviscosity syndrome. Pediatrics 1982; 69:426.
44. Linderkamp O, Ozanne P, Wu PYK, Meiselman HJ. Red blood cell aggregation in preterm and term neonates and adults. Pediatr Res 1984; 18:1356.

45. Linderkamp O, Nash GB, Wu PYK, Meiselman HJ. Deformability and intrinsic material properties of neonatal red blood cells. Blood 1986; 67:1244.

46. Reinhart WH, Danoff SF, Usami S, Chien S. Rheologic measurements on small samples with a new capillary viscometer. J Lab Clin Med 1984; 104:921.

47. Riopel L, Fouron JC, Bard H. Blood viscosity during the neonatal period: the role of plasma and red blood cell type. J Pediatr 1982; 100:449.

48. Buchan PC. Fetal intrauterine growth retardation and hyperviscosity. In: Heilman L, Buchan PC, eds. Hemorheological disorders in obstetrics and neonatology. Berlin: FK Schattauer, 1984:7.

49. Sjostrand T. Endogenous formation of carbon monoxide in man under normal and pathological conditions. Scand J Clin Lab Invest 1949; 1:201.

50. Roughton FJW, Darling RC. The effect of carbon monoxide on the oxyhemoglobin dissociation curve. Am J Physiol 1944; 141:17.

51. Longo LD. The biological effects of carbon monoxide on the pregnant woman, fetus, and newborn infant. Am J Obstet Gynecol 1977; 129:69.

52. Longo LD, Ching KS. Placental diffusing capacity for carbon monoxide and oxygen in unanesthetized sheep. J Appl Physiol 1977; 43:885.

53. Suzuki K, Horiguchi T, Comas-Urrutia AC, et al. Pharmacologic effects of nicotine upon the fetus and mother in the rhesus monkey. Am J Obstet Gynecol 1971; 111:1092.

54. Duffus GM, MacGillivray I. The incidence of pre-eclamptic toxaemia in smokers and nonsmokers. Lancet 1968; 1:994.

55. Dintenfass L. Elevation of blood viscosity, aggregation of red cells, haematocrit values and fibrinogen levels with cigarette smokers. Med J Aust 1975; 1:617.

56. Pirani BBK. Smoking during pregnancy. Obstet Gynecol Surv 1978; 33:1.

57. Denson R, Nanson JL, McWatters MA. Hyperkinesis and maternal smoking. Can Psychiatr Assoc J 1975; 20:183.

58. Butler NR, Goldstein GH. Smoking in pregnancy and subsequent child development. Br Med J 1973; 4:573.

59. Astrup P, Olsen HM, Trolle D, Kjeldsen K. Effect of moderate carbon monoxide exposure on fetal development. Lancet 1972; 2:1221.

60. Storm JE, Fechter LD. Prenatal carbon monoxide exposure differentially affects postnatal weight and monoamine concentration of rat brain regions. Toxicol Appl Pharmacol 1985; 81:139.

61. Mactutus CF, Fechter LD. Moderate prenatal carbon monoxide exposure produces persistent, and apparently permanent memory deficits in rats. Teratology 1985; 31:1.

62. McClure Browne JC, Veall N. The maternal placental blood flow in normotensive and hypertensive women. Br J Obstet Gynecol 1953; 60:141.

63. Morris M, Osborn SB, Wright HP. Effective circulation of the uterine wall in late pregnancy measured with ^{24}NaCl. Lancet 1955; 1:323.

64. Prichard JA. Changes in the blood volume during pregnancy and delivery. Anesthesiology 1965; 26:393.

65. Hodari AA. Chronic uterine ischemia and reversible experimental "toxemia of pregnancy." Am J Obstet Gynecol 1967; 97:597.

66. Kumar D. Chronic placental ischemia in relation to toxemias of pregnancy. Am J Obstet Gynecol 1962; 84:1323.

67. Walker J, Turnbull EPN. Haemoglobin and red cells in the human foetus and their relation to the oxygen content of the blood in the vessels of the umbilical cord. Lancet 1953; 2:312.

68. Howie PW. The haemostatic mechanisms of pre-eclampsia. Clin Obstet Gynaecol 1977; 4:595.

69. Matthews JD, Mason TW. Plasma viscosity and pre-eclampsia. Lancet 1974; 3:409.

70. Heilmann L, Mattheck C, Jurz E. Changes in the blood rheology and their influence on the oxygen diffusion in normal and pathological pregnancies. Arch Gynakol 1977; 223:283.

71. Sontag LW, Wallace RF. The effect of cigarette smoking during pregnancy upon the fetal heart rate. Am J Obstet Gynecol 1935; 29:77.

72. Longo LD. Carbon monoxide: effects on oxygenation of the fetus in utero. Science 1976; 194:523.

73. Bartoletti AL, Stevenson DK, Ostrander CR, Johnson JD. Pulmonary excretion of carbon monoxide in the human infant as an index of bilirubin production. I. Effects of gestational and postnatal age and some common neonatal abnormalities. J Pediatr 1979; 94:952.

74. Scheidt PC, Mellits ED, Hardy JB, et al. Toxicity to bilirubin in neonates: infant development during first year in relation to maximum neonatal serum bilirubin concentration. J Pediatr 1977; 91:292.

75. Gartner LM. Disorders of bilirubin metabolism. In: Nathan DG, Oski FA, eds. Hematology of infancy and childhood. 2nd ed. Philadelphia: WB Saunders, 1981:86.

76. Schmid R. Hyperbilirubinemia. In: Stanbury JB, Wyngaarden JB, Frederickson DS, eds. The metabolic basis of inherited disease. 4th ed. New York: McGraw-Hill, 1978:1221.

77. Karp WB. Biochemical alterations in neonatal hyperbilirubinemia and bilirubin encephalopathy. A review. Pediatrics 1979; 64:361.

78. Levine RL. The toxicology of bilirubin. Report of the eighty-fifth Ross conference on pediatric research. Columbus, Ohio: Ross Laboratories, 1983:39.

79. Maisels MJ. Neonatal jaundice. In: Avery GB, ed. Neonatology, pathophysiology and management of the newborn. 2nd ed. Philadelphia: JB Lippincott, 1981:473.

80. Committee on Fetus and Newborn. Home phototherapy. Am Acad Pediatr 1985; 76:136.

81. Cowger ML. Bilirubin encephalopathy. In: Gaull GE, ed. Biology of brain dysfunction. New York: Plenum, 1973:265.

82. Levine RL, Fredericks WR, Rapoport SI. Entry of bilirubin into the brain due to opening of the blood-brain barrier. Pediatrics 1982; 69:255.

83. Mollison PL, Walker W. Controlled trials of treatment of haemolytic disease of the newborn. Lancet 1952; 1:429.

84. Watchko JF, Oski FA. Bilirubin 20 mg/dL = Vigintiphobia (commentary). Pediatrics 1983; 71:660.

85. Maurer HM, Kirkpatrick BV, et al. Phototherapy for hyperbilirubinemia of hemolytic disease of the newborn. Pediatrics 1985; 75:407.

86. Smith DW, Inguillo D, Martin D, et al. Use of noninvasive tests to predict significant jaundice in full-term infants. Pediatrics 1985; 75:278.

87. Silverman WA, Andersen DH, Blanc WA, et al. A difference in mortality rate and incidence of kernicterus among premature infants allotted to two prophylactic antibacterial regimens. Pediatrics 1956; 18:614.

88. Stevenson DK. Home phototherapy: risks versus benefits. Clin Pediatr 1986; 25:300.

14 Nutritional Management

Anjali Malkani, M.D. and John A. Kerner Jr., M.D.

Enteral Feeding
    Gastric Feeding: Intermittent Gavage or Continuous
       Infusion
    Transpyloric Feeding
    Guidelines
Parenteral Feeding
Nutritional Support of the Asphyxiated Infant
    Asphyxia and the Gastrointestinal Tract
Necrotizing Enterocolitis
    Epidemiology
    Clinical Picture
    Management
    Enteral Feeding
       Pathogenesis and Enteral Feeding
       Timing of Enteral Feeding
       Rate and Volume of Enteral Feeds
       Osmolality of Feeds
    Immunologic Considerations
    Ischemia and Hypoxia
    Role of Vitamin E
    Role of Infectious Agents
Conclusion
Recommendations

Optimal nutritional support is critical in the management of the ever increasing number of surviving small premature infants.[1] Although it is important to ensure that the infant receives an adequate caloric intake, the capacity of the very low birth weight infant to digest, absorb, and metabolize enteral nutrients is limited. In addition, these infants often have other major difficulties, such as respiratory distress, cardiovascular instability, hemorrhagic diatheses, and a relatively immature renal system.

To provide proper nutrition to the premature infant, one must have an understanding of the biochemical and physiologic processes that occur during development of the gastrointestinal tract. By 28 weeks of gestation the morphologic development of the gastrointestinal tract in humans is nearly complete, yet as an organ of nutrition the gut is functionally immature. Details of gastrointestinal tract development have been described previously[2-4] and have been summarized recently in tabular form (Table 14–1). Further, complications due to the incomplete development of the gastrointestinal tract in the low birth weight infant have been delineated superbly by Sunshine (Table 14–2).

ENTERAL FEEDING

Gastric Feeding: Intermittent Gavage or Continuous Infusion

Nasogastric feeds may be given continuously or intermittently. Gavage feeds are easy to administer, and it is possible to evaluate the gastric emptying time by checking the gastric residual before each meal. The stomach takes less time to empty with human milk than with formula and when the infant is in the prone or lateral position.[5,6]

Premature infants are predisposed to develop gastroesophageal reflux owing to their incompetent lower esophageal sphincter, small stomach capacity, and delayed gastric emptying. Hence, to prevent this reflux and the subsequent risks of aspiration and apnea, it is necessary to feed these infants small volumes, although more frequently.[7] Also, gastric distention may interfere with respiratory function.[8]

Thus premature infants may benefit from continuous nasogastric feeding. In a study by Toce et al,[9] infants whose birth weight was between 1,000 and 1,249 gm had better weight gain when fed via continuous nasogastric infusion than via gavage feeds. These investigators speculated that this increased weight gain resulted from

Study supported by a grant (RR81) from the General Clinical Research Centers program of the Division of Research Resources, National Institutes of Health, and the Mead Johnson Nutritional Division.

TABLE 14-1   Development of the Human Gastrointestinal Tract

Age (weeks)	Crown-Rump Length (mm)	Stage of Development
2.5	1.5	Gut not distinct from yolk sac
3.5	2.5	Foregut and hindgut present; yolk sac broadly attached at midgut; liver bud present; mesenteries forming
4	5.0	Intestine present as a single tube from mouth to cloaca; esophagus and stomach distinct; liver cords, ducts and gallbladder forming; omental bursa forming; pancreatic buds appear as outpouching of gut
5.6	8.0–12.0	Intestine elongates into a loop and duodenum begins to rotate under superior mesenteric artery; stomach rotates; parotid and submandibular buds appear; cloaca elongates and septum forms to divide cloaca
7	17.0	Circular muscle layer present; duodenum temporarily occluded; intestinal loops herniate into cord; villi begin to develop; pancreatic anlagen fuse
8	23	Villi lined by single layer of cells; small intestine coiling within cord; taste buds appear; microvilli short, thick, and irregularly spaced; lysosomal enzymes detected; cloacal membrane, which sealed the rectum, begins to disappear
9–10	30–40	Auerbach's plexus appears; intestine reenters abdominal cavity; crypts of Lieberkühn develop; active transport of glucose appears aerobically and anaerobically; dipeptidases present; microvilli of enterocytes more regular and glycocalyx present; mitochondria numerous below microvilli
12	56	Parietal cells present in stomach; muscular layers of intestine present; alkaline phosphatase and disaccharidases detectable; active transport of amino acid present; mature taste buds present; enterochromaffin cells appear; pancreatic islet cells appear; bile secretions begin; colonic haustra appear; coelomic extension into umbilical cord obliterated; meconium first detected in ileum
13–14	78–90	Meissner's plexus appears; circular folds appear; peristalsis detected; lysosomes detected ultrastructurally
16	112	Pancreatic lipase and tryptic activity detected; lymphopoiesis present; peptic activity present; swallowing evident—2–7 ml/24 h;
20	160	Peyer's patches present; muscularis mucosae present; mesenteric attachments complete; zymogen granules present and well developed in pancreas (22 weeks); intestine has lost ability to transport glucose anaerobically
24	200	Paneth's cells appear; maltase, sucrase, and alkaline phosphatase very active; ganglion cells detected throughout small and large intestine and in the rectum; amylase activity present in intestine
28	240	Enterokinase activity increases; esophageal glands present; frequency and intensity of duodenal peristaltic contractions increasing
32	270	Lactase activity increases; hydrochloric acid found in stomach
34	290–300	Sucking and swallowing become coordinated; esophageal peristalsis rapid, nonsegmental contraction occurs; small intestinal motility becomes coordinated
36–38	320–350	Maturity of GI tract achieved

Reproduced with permission from Sunshine P. Gastrointestinal. In: Eden RD, Boehm FH, eds. Fetal assessment: physiological, clinical, and medicolegal principles. East Norwalk, Connecticut: Appleton-Century-Crofts, (in press).

improved absorptive capacity. They noted a reduction in stool weight and postulated that continuous feeding resulted in less stimulation of the gastrocolic reflex, with a prolonged transit time allowing for better absorption.

Continuous feeding is not without disadvantages. Nutrients, especially fat, may be lost within the tubing during continuous infusion of breast milk.[10] Preterm formulas with a high mineral content may clot within the tubing.[11] Further, intermittent feeding may be important in the induction of metabolic and endocrine changes that occur in early postnatal life.[12]

Transpyloric Feeding

The advantages of transpyloric feeding are minimal gastric distention, a lower risk of aspiration, and, at least during the first 10 days of life, potentially greater volume tolerance, with less initial weight loss than with nasogastric feeding.[13] Two prospective studies compared continuous nasogastric and transpyloric feeding,[14,15] but only one concluded that there was an advantage to transpyloric feeding during the first two to three weeks

TABLE 14–2   Complications Due to the Incomplete Development of the Gastrointestinal Tract in the Low Birth Weight Infant

Incomplete development of motility
  Poor coordination of sucking and swallowing
  Aberrant esophageal motility
  Biphasic esophageal peristalsis
  Decreased or absent lower esophageal sphincter pressure
  Delayed gastric emptying time
  Poorly coordinated motility of the small and large intestine
    Stasis
    Dilation
    Impaired blood supply
    Functional obstruction

Delayed ability to regenerate new epithelial cells
  Decreased rates of proliferation
  Decreased cellular migration rates
  Shallow crypts
  Shortened villi
  Decreased mitotic indices

Inadequate host resistance factors
  Decreased gastric acidity
  Decreased concentrations of immunoglobulins in lamina
    propria and intestinal secretions
  Impaired humoral and cellular response to infection

Inadequate digestion of nutrients
  Decreased digestion of protein
    Decreased activity of enterokinase
    Trypsin activity low prior to 28 weeks' gestation
    Decreased concentration of gastric hydrochloric acid and
      pepsinogen
  Decreased digestion of carbohydrates
  Decreased hydrolysis of lactose
  Decreased ability to transport glucose actively
  Decreased activity of pancreatic amylase
  Decreased digestion of lipids
    Decreased production and reabsorption of bile acids
    Decreased activity of pancreatic lipase

Increased incidence of other problems that may indirectly lead
  to poor gastrointestinal function
  Hyaline membrane disease
  Intraventricular hemorrhage
  Patent ductus arteriosus
  Hypoxemic ischemic states

Reproduced with permission from Sunshine P. Gastrointestinal. In: Eden RD, Boehm FH, eds. Fetal assessment: physiological, clinical, and medicolegal principles. East Norwalk, Connecticut: Appleton-Century-Crofts, (in press).

of life.[14] Roy et al[16] compared every-two-hour bolus nasogastric feeds with nasojejunal feeds in healthy-by-birth weight infants and found no difference in growth or weight gain in the two groups. Since the stomach was bypassed in the nasojejunal group and fat digestion starts in the stomach, more fat malabsorption occurred in the nasojejunally fed babies. The fat malabsorption may be minimized by duodenal placement.[14]

Further, in two studies transpyloric feeding was not recommended in infants requiring either ventilatory support via a face mask or nasopharyngeal suctioning,[17,18] owing to the risk of dislodgment and subsequent aspiration.[17,18]

Polyvinyl chloride tubes were used initially because they are relatively stiff and easily positioned. However, if left in the duodenum for several days, they harden and may perforate the intestine.[19] Silastic tubes are now commonly used, but they are more flexible and, hence, difficult to position. They are usually weighted at the tip and placed with the help of gravity. Being more flexible, they can curl back into the stomach. Perforation with the Silastic tubes has been reported.[20]

A change in the microbial flora of the upper intestine of infants fed via transpyloric feeds has been reported. The upper intestine of the normal infant is sterile or contains sparse gram-positive flora. However, Dellagrammaticus et al[21] have shown that the presence of a tube facilitates colonization with a "fecal type" of flora in which *S. faecalis* and gram-negative bacteria predominate.[21] Theoretically a heavy resident flora in the upper intestine could lead to poorer assimilation of feeds. Conflicting data exist in regard to the relationship of necrotizing enterocolitis to transpyloric feeds.[17,22] As we shall see, it is likely not the *route* of feeding that was responsible for the necrotizing enterocolitis in the foregoing studies but rather the increased osmolality of the formula used. In controlled studies necrotizing enterocolitis was proven not to be more frequent during transpyloric feeds than in nasogastric feeds.[14,17,23]

Guidelines

The European Society of Paediatric Gastroenterology and Nutrition has recently issued guidelines for feeding the preterm infant:[15]

"Enteral feeding should be introduced as soon as it is safe to do so.

1. Intermittent gastric tube feeding seems more physiological than transpyloric feeding and whenever possible should be preferred.
2. When there are feeding difficulties such as regurgitation, poor gastric emptying or gastric distension, continuous gastric feeding or even transpyloric feeding may be necessary, as they are useful alternatives either to reduced oral feeding or total parenteral nutrition.
3. The success of any feeding technique is at least partly the result of the skill of the staff of the unit in following their own practised routines.
4. Nursery routines should encourage the mother to play an active role in feeding. This will help her to become confident in the care of her baby."

PARENTERAL FEEDING

Because sick and premature newborns often are not fed enterally, the alternative is parenteral nutrition. In a recent review by Moyer-Mileur and Chan,[24] parenteral feeding in very low birth weight infants requiring assisted ventilation for more than six days led to a decrease in the percentage of weight loss from birth weight and a decrease in the amount of time required for recovery of birth weight than in those fed enterally or by a combination of enteral and parenteral feeding. Furthermore, a delay in enteral feeding increased the tolerance to subsequent enteral feeding in these infants. Tolerance was defined as an absence of residuals, abdominal distention, or guaiac-positive, reducing substance-positive stools.[24] Another recent retrospective study presented conflicting data regarding the benefits and risks of parenteral nutrition.[25]

Limited data exist relating to the potential benefit of parenteral nutrition in the treatment of preterm infants. A controlled study of peripheral total parenteral nutrition (TPN) composed of casein hydrolysate, dextrose, and soybean emulsion in 40 premature infants with the respiratory distress syndrome showed that TPN neither favorably altered the clinical course of the syndrome nor worsened an infant's pulmonary status.[26] Among the infants weighing less than 1,500 gm those who received TPN had a greater incidence of survival when compared with a control group (71 versus 37 percent).

Yu and co-workers[27] carried out a controlled trial of TPN in 34 preterm infants with birth weights less than 1,200 gm. Infants in the TPN group had a greater mean daily weight gain in the second week of life and regained birth weight sooner than did the control infants. Four in the milk-fed control group developed necrotizing enterocolitis, whereas none did in the TPN group.

The results of a study conducted by our group of 40 infants who weighed less than 1,500 gm at birth were in agreement with the two aforementioned controlled studies.[28] We found no increased risk in using peripheral parenteral nutrition as compared with conventional feeding techniques, and we also found comparable growth in the two groups.

Recently 59 infants weighing less than 1,500 gm were randomly assigned either to a parenteral nutrition regimen via a central catheter or to a transpyloric feeding regimen (mother's milk or SMA Gold Cap [Wyeth Laboratories]) via a Silastic nasoduodenal tube.[29] The authors postulated that some of the problems of enteral feeding in very low birth weight infants might be overcome if enteral nutrients were delivered beyond the pylorus.[30] The parenteral nutrition group had a higher incidence of bacterial sepsis. Conjugated hyperbilirubinemia occurred only in the parenteral nutrition group. In spite of the observations that 34 percent of the infants (10 of 29) in the transpyloric group failed to establish full enteral feeding patterns by the end of the first week of life, and therefore had achieved lower protein-energy intake than the parenteral nutrition group, no beneficial effect on growth or mortality was found in the parenteral nutrition group.

The authors concluded that "Parenteral nutrition does not confer any appreciable benefit and because of greater complexity and higher risk of complications should be reserved for those infants in whom enteral nutrition is impossible."[29] My colleagues and I agree with the comment of Zlotkin and co-workers:[31] "Had peripheral-vein feeding been used rather than central venous alimentation, or had nasogastric gavage feeding been used in preference to transpyloric feeding, the morbidity and mortality would have declined and the results comparing TPN with enteral feeds would have been quite different."

A classic study that remains a model for nutritional support in the very low birth weight infant was performed by Cashore and associates.[32] They described 23 infants who weighed less than 1,500 gm in whom peripheral parenteral nutrition was begun on day two of life to *supplement* enteral feedings, thus allowing for adequate nutrition while avoiding overtaxing the immature gastrointestinal tract. These infants regained their birth weight by the age of eight to 12 days and achieved growth rates that approximated intrauterine rates of growth. Interestingly, infants weighing less than 1,000 gm were still not taking all their nutrients enterally by 25 days of age.

A recent survey of 269 neonatal intensive care units showed that TPN was used exclusively during the first week of life in 80 percent of the infants weighing 1,000 gm or less at birth.[33] The others received a combination of parenteral and enteral feedings in the first week. As a general rule we, like Adamkin,[34] begin parenteral nutrition by 72 hours of age in neonates with a birth weight less than 1,000 gm in whom respiratory disease and intestinal hypomotility limit the safety of feedings in the first one to two weeks of life. In addition, premature infants, especially those who have the respiratory distress syndrome and are incapable of taking full oral feeds, often receive parenteral nutrition because of their extremely limited substrate reserve, very rapid growth rate, and perceived susceptibility to irreversible brain damage secondary to malnutrition.[31]

In some nurseries umbilical arterial catheters are used for infusing parenteral nutrition. Few studies have been carried out to define safety of this practice. Yu et al[27] studied 34 infants with birth weight less than 1,200 gm and randomly assigned them to TPN via umbilical artery catheters or enteral feeds. The TPN group had better nitrogen balance, weight gain, less necrotizing enterocolitis, and unchanged mortality than the enterally fed group. No data on catheter-related complications were presented, although bacterial or fungal septicemia did not occur in either group during the study period.

Higgs and co-workers[35] described a controlled trial of TPN versus formula feeding by continuous nasogastric drip. The study included 86 infants weighing 500 to 1,500 gm. The TPN, including glucose, amino acids, and fat emulsion, was administered by an umbilical artery catheter for the first two weeks of life. There was no difference in neonatal morbidity or mortality between the two groups. Specifically, there was no difference in the incidence of septicemia, although four of the 43 TPN babies had "catheter problems," described in the text only as "blockage" of the catheter.

Hall and Rhodes[36] delivered TPN to 80 infants by umbilical artery lines and to nine infants by indwelling umbilical venous catheters; all 89 were "high risk" infants who were unable to tolerate enteral feedings. Results were compared with those in 23 infants with tunneled jugular catheters inserted for chronic medical or surgical problems that prevented use of the gastrointestinal tract. All infants studied ranged in weight from under 1,000 to over 2,500 gm. As in the study by Higgs et al,[35] Hall and Rhodes[36] found that morbidity, mortality, and the common complications, such as infection and thrombosis, were similar in both groups.

Hall and Rhodes[36] concluded that TPN delivered by indwelling umbilical catheters presents no greater risk than infusion through tunneled jugular catheters. However, careful analysis of their data raises questions about their conclusions. According to the authors, "Six deaths may have been catheter-related." Five of those deaths occurred in the *umbilical artery catheter* group; death resulted from the thrombosis of the aorta in one patient, candidal septicemia in two, streptococcal septicemia in one, and enterococcal septicemia in one. One death occurred in the jugular venous catheter group, with right atrial thrombosis—superior vena cava syndrome and *Staphylococcus epidermidis* on blood culture.

Merritt[37] cautions against the use of umbilical arterial catheters for TPN because this practice is associated with a high incidence of arterial thrombosis. Dr. Arnold Coran,[38] a pediatric surgeon, strongly recommends that parenteral nutrition not be given through either umbilical arteries or umbilical veins. Parenteral nutrition through the umbilical vein causes phlebitis, which may lead to venous thrombosis and portal hypertension. Coran is especially concerned about infusing parenteral nutrition solutions into an umbilical artery line, since this practice can lead to thrombosis of the aorta or iliac vessels. Furthermore, *severe damage* can occur to an artery *without being recognized*. There may even be thrombosis of the aorta without recognition. Only over an extensive period of time will the side effects of umbilical artery catheter use (such as inappropriate growth of one limb[38]) be known. Even 12.5 percent dextrose infused through an umbilical artery line has increased osmolality that is clearly shown to cause thrombophlebitis.[38] Although the first three studies described earlier claimed that there were no short-term complications, they did not address the problem of long-term complications.

Coran[38] states that if parenteral nutrition is required and peripheral veins are not usable or if peripheral vein delivery is inadequate to provide necessary calories, he would consider percutaneous subclavian vein catheterization, which he can perform successfully even in a 900 gm infant.

Like Coran and Merritt, we are reluctant to use umbilical catheters for the parenteral infusion of nutrients. We attempt to provide needed calories by peripheral vein. If more calories are needed or if parenteral nutrition must be provided for longer than two weeks, a central venous line is placed.[39]

In a recent study by Sadig, complications associated with the Broviac catheter (a central venous line) were compared in very low birth weight infants and in older infants (n = 48). Sixty-nine percent of the catheter-associated infections occurred in very low birth weight infants and only 20 percent in infants weighing more than 1,500 gm. Seventy-eight percent (14 of 18) of these infections were successfully treated with antibiotics without catheter removal. The incidence of thrombosis was also higher in very low birth weight infants.

NUTRITIONAL SUPPORT OF THE ASPHYXIATED INFANT

In an asphyxiated infant, in addition to the complications due to incomplete development of the gastrointestinal tract, there is a superimposed insult to the gut from the asphyxia itself.

Most centers do not enterally feed an asphyxiated infant for the first five days to two weeks. This practice is based on animal data relating to cellular proliferation and migration. The intestinal mucosa of newborn and suckling rats has a very slow rate of cellular proliferation and migration compared with that in adult animals.[41] Although the turnover of intestinal epithelium in the adult jejunum is 48 to 72 hours, the duration in the 10-day-old animal is at least twice that long and in the two-to three-day-old animal it may be even longer.[42] In a study by Sunshine and colleagues[43] in the adult animal, labeled cells reached the tips of the villi within 48 hours. During the same period of time the labeled cells had migrated only one-eighth to one-fourth the length of the villi in the suckling animal. There are indications that the same slower rate of turnover of intestinal epithelium exists in the newborn human.[44]

Asphyxia per se may cause significant injury to the gastrointestinal tract. Further, asphyxia may predispose an infant to necrotizing enterocolitis.

Asphyxia and the Gastrointestinal Tract

Asphyxia may cause varying degrees of injury to the premature infant's gastrointestinal tract. During acute episodes of shock or hypoxemia the "vital structures," which include the heart, brain, and adrenal glands, are preferentially perfused. Perfusion of the "nonvital" organs, including the skin, muscle, lungs, kidney, and gastrointestinal tract, is decreased significantly. With limited periods of hypoxia the newborn has some autoregulatory capabilities of maintaining blood flow to the intestine. When bleeding occurs, it is usually superficial, involving only the mucosa. However, if ischemia is maintained for a period of time, perforation and significant hemorrhage may occur.[45]

Coupled with asphyxia, feeding in the premature infant poses a significant risk of the development of neonatal necrotizing enterocolitis.

NECROTIZING ENTEROCOLITIS

Necrotizing enterocolitis is a well described and extensively investigated affliction of the high risk newborn. The etiology of this multifactorial disorder remains elusive, and currently there is no universally accepted theory of pathogenesis.[46,47]

Epidemiology

The incidence varies widely, some centers reporting rare isolated cases while others report an incidence of 3 to 5 percent of all neonatal admissions.[48,49] Among patients in whom necrotizing enterocolitis develops, the average birth weight is 1,400 to 1,500 gm and the mean gestational age is 30 to 32 weeks.[50] In one study by Stoll and co-workers,[51] the overall incidence was 3 per 1,000 live births, but increased to 66 per 1,000 live births in infants weighing less than 1,500 gm. Similarly, the mortality was zero in infants weighing more than 2,500 gm but increased to 40 percent in infants weighing less than 1,500 gm. The age at diagnosis ranged from two to 44 days and was inversely related to the gestational age. All babies of less than 35 weeks' gestational age were diagnosed by one week of age. Stoll et al believed that there may be two populations who develop necrotizing enterocolitis—an early population consisting of term and preterm infants, and a later group of solely preterm babies who are smaller and sicker, who presumably sustain continuing insults to the gastrointestinal tract and who therefore are at continued risk of developing the disease. These babies must be closely monitored for the possible development of necrotizing enterocolitis later in the hospital course.[51] It is important to appreciate that approximately 10 percent of all cases of necrotizing enterocolitis occur in full-term neonates.[46]

There are two distinct patterns of necrotizing enterocolitis: endemic and epidemic.[52] Superimposed on an endemic incidence, epidemics (referring to cases clustered in location and time) may be observed. No seasonal pattern of occurrence of these epidemics has been demonstrated. Patient characteristics appear to differ during epidemics: infants are more mature, with fewer antece-

dent neonatal illnesses, acquire necrotizing enterocolitis later, and have been fed for a longer period of time than those who develop necrotizing enterocolitis during nonepidemic times.

Clinical Picture

Necrotizing enterocolitis may assume a broad spectrum of clinical severity. Some infants have little in the way of signs and symptoms with a benign course, and others have fulminating disease characterized by extensive gangrene, perforation, shock, and death.

The diagnosis is suspected when two or more typical gastrointestinal signs and symptoms occur simultaneously with nonspecific signs.[50] The initial signs and symptoms in 123 consecutive patients are presented in Table 14–3, as noted by Kliegman and Walsh[53] in a nine-year study. Not all patients have every symptom, and the signs vary chronologically in their appearance, depending on the severity of the illness (Table 14–4).

TABLE 14–3 Initial Signs and Symptoms of Necrotizing Enterocolitis

Signs	Percentage of Patients*
Abdominal distention	73
Bloody stool	28
Apnea, bradycardia	26
Abdominal tenderness	21
Retained gastric contents	18
Guaiac-positive stool	17
"Septic appearance"	12
Shock	11
Bilious emesis	11
Acidosis	10
Lethargy	9
Diarrhea	6
Cellulitis of abdominal wall	6
Right lower quadrant mass	2

* Total exceeds 100 percent, as many patients had more than one sign.
Reproduced with permission from Walsh MC, Kliegman RM. Necrotizing enterocolitis: treatment based on staging criteria. Pediatr Clin North Am 1986; 3:181.

TABLE 14–4 Unusual Manifestations of Necrotizing Enterocolitis

10% occur in term infants

10–12% occur in infants who have never been fed

10–15% will not have pneumatosis intestinalis

10–15% will have no blood in stools

10–15% will develop intestinal strictures

Reproduced with permission from Sunshine P. Gastrointestinal. In: Eden RD, Boehm FH, eds. Fetal assessment: physiological, clinical and medicolegal principles. East Norwalk, Connecticut: Appleton-Century-Crofts, (in press).

Because the initial symptoms of necrotizing enterocolitis are nonspecific and the findings on physical examination may be deceptively benign, radiographic findings are used to support the diagnosis. Radiographic examination of the abdomen may show nonspecific findings of distention, ileus, and ascites. The two diagnostic radiologic signs are pneumatosis intestinalis (intramural intestinal gas) and intrahepatic portal venous gas. One of these is essential to confirm the diagnosis. More severe disease results in perforation and pneumoperitoneum. However, pneumatosis intestinalis may be subtle and fleeting. It typically is first seen in the ileocecal area but may be seen anywhere from the stomach to the rectum. Two patterns are described: a curvilinear intramural radiolucency probably representing subserosal gas, and a cystic form assuming a foamy or bubbly appearance, probably representing submucosal gas. Gas mixed with stool in the bowel, however, can be difficult to distinguish from pneumatosis intestinalis.[54] Pneumatosis also may be present in other clinical situations—intestinal gangrene secondary to vascular occlusion, Hirschsprung's disease with enterocolitis, obstruction at the site of bowel atresia, pyloric stenosis, and meconium ileus.

Investigators have developed screening tests for necrotizing enterocolitis, such as breath hydrogen analysis and urinalysis for D-lactate (produced by enteric flora when the infant is fed excess carbohydrate),[55-57] but these tests have not become routine in clinical monitoring up to the present.

Management

There is no universal acceptance of a unifying theory regarding the pathogenesis of necrotizing enterocolitis. Numerous controlled studies have been performed in order to delineate the neonate at risk. Stoll et al[51] determined that affected infants were similar to controls and identified no risk factors. Kliegman et al[59] failed to delineate any important risk factor. They therefore concluded that perinatal problems that precede necrotizing enterocolitis are equally common in all high risk infants. Figure 14-1 demonstrates the persistence of considerable confusion surrounding predisposing phenomena and factors of etiologic importance.

A unifying theory must explain the development of necrotizing enterocolitis in the enterally fed or fasted high risk neonate and in the healthy term newborn.[50] It seems likely that necrotizing enterocolitis represents the final response of the immature gastrointestinal tract to one or more unrelated stresses. Because there are many stressful factors, there may be a wide range in the severity of bowel injury and therefore a continuous spectrum of clinical disease. Perhaps in the mildly affected infant the

RISK FACTOR FOR NEC	REFERENCE						
	78	101	51	87	29	76	17
APGAR 1		S					S
APGAR 5	S						S
UMBILICAL ARTERIAL CATH					S		S
UMBILICAL VENOUS CATH					S		S
EXCHANGE TRANSFUSION		S					
NO RDS			S				
ENTERIC FEEDING					S	S	
PROM	S	S					
PDA	S						
HYPEROSMOLAR FEEDS	S	S					
RECURRENT APNEA		S					
PLACENTAL ABRUPTION				S			
SHOCK		S					
GAVAGE FEEDING	S						
HYPERALIMENTATION	S						
10% DEXTROSE	S						
MARRIED MOTHERS							
MATERNAL ANTIBIOTICS	S						
MATERNAL ANESTHESIA	S						
NO GENTAMICIN	S						

Figure 14-1   Purported risk factors for necrotizing enterocolitis (summary of seven controlled studies). S, parameter significantly more common in patients with necrotizing enterocolitis. □, parameter not significant. ■, parameter not investigated. (Reproduced with permission from Barnard J, Greene H, Cotton R. Necrotizing enterocolitis. In: Kretchmer N, Minkowski A, eds. Nutritional adaptation of the gastrointestinal tract of the newborn. Nestle nutrition. Vol 3. New York: Raven Press, 1983:115. Copyright 1983, Raven Press.)

stresses are not so injurious, and in the severely affected infant multiple stresses act synergistically to produce more severe damage (Fig. 14–2).[50]

Enteral Feeding

Since necrotizing enterocolitis can manifest within a wide range of severity along a continuum of various stages of bowel disease, the true nature or clinical course that the disease will follow usually is not known until 48 hours after onset.

Bell and associates[58] proposed important clinical staging criteria for necrotizing enterocolitis that allowed accurate comparisons of patients with disease of similar severity. Kliegman and associates[59] modified Bell's staging criteria to include systemic intestinal and radiogra-

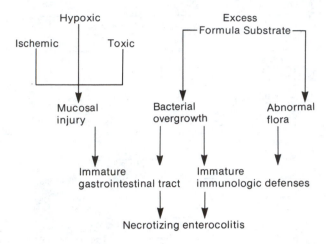

Figure 14–2 Proposed schema by which multiple factors combine to initiate necrotizing enterocolitis. (Modified from Walsh MC, Kliegman R, Fanaroff A. Necrotizing enterocolitis: a practitioner's perspective. Pediatr Rev 1988; 9:220. Copyright 1988, American Academy of Pediatrics.)

phic signs and suggested treatment regimens based on the stages (Table 14–5).

In addition to the recommendations in Table 14–5, a large bore, double lumen nasogastric tube also should be placed to decompress the stomach. The length of time the bowel is allowed to "rest" depends on the progression or lack of progression of the disease and the philosophy of the institution. Parenteral nutrition is recommended in patients with documented necrotizing enterocolitis during the period of intestinal recovery. When prolonged parenteral feedings are required, a central venous line may need to be placed. Parenteral nutrition allows for a slow return to enteral feeding; it is common for this transition to take one to three weeks to reestablish full enteral feedings. Infants requiring surgical resection of the bowel have a more protracted course, especially with extensive resection, and may develop the "short bowel syndrome." The specific details of such management are described elsewhere.[60]

Pathogenesis and Enteral Feeding

Conflicting opinions exist regarding the relationship of enteral feeding practices and the development of necrotizing enterocolitis. It is important to bear in mind that 5 to 10 percent of the patients who develop necrotizing enterocolitis have never been fed.[46] Controlled studies comparing feeding techniques in infants with and without necrotizing enterocolitis consistently fail to support feeding as an important precursor, although controversy persists.

There are numerous ways by which feedings might contribute to the pathogenesis or progression of necrotizing enterocolitis:

1. Direct mucosal injury by hypertonic feeds.
2. Alteration intestinal flora.
3. Structural of immaturity of the premature infant's intestine.
4. Absence of breast milk's immunologically protective effect in formula-fed infants.
5. The effect of early or large volume feedings on an alimentary tract compromised by adverse perinatal events.[43]

Timing of Enteral Feeding

There is a definite trend to delay enteral feeding in the sick premature infant. In a recent survey of 269 neonatal intensive care units Churella et al[33] (described previously), most (80 percent) gave parenteral feedings during the first week of life to infants weighing less than 1,000 gm at birth. None started enteral feeding alone, and 20 percent used a combination of enteral and parenteral feeding. Sixty-nine percent of the infants weighing between 1,001 and 2,399 gm received a combination of parenteral and enteral feeds.

The first enteral feeding was begun at a mean of seven days after birth in infants with birth weights less than 1,000 gm, five days after birth in those with a birth weight of 1,001 to 1,500 gm, and three days after birth in infants weighing more than 1,500 gm.[33]

In a prospective study by Eyal et al[61] the delaying of feedings in very low birth weight infants (less than 1,500 gm) from two to three days to two to three weeks decreased the incidence of necrotizing enterocolitis from 18 to 3 percent. It is interesting that in patients (3 percent) who developed necrotizing enterocolitis after a delayed onset of enteral feeding, the time of onset of the first symptoms ranged from 23 to 60 days, compared with 7 to 23 days in infants fed enterally within the first week of life. Hence, infants in whom enteral feeding is delayed must be observed for a longer period of time to detect the development of necrotizing enterocolitis.

Brown and Sweet[48] believed that necrotizing enterocolitis was virtually eliminated from their nursery with the initiation of an extremely cautious feeding protocol, which fostered late initiation of enteral feeding, slow advancement to reach full feeds after two weeks following the onset of feeds, and prompt discontinuation of feeds when untoward signs suggesting hypoxia, hypoperfusion, or gastrointestinal dysfunction developed (i.e., distention, guaiac-positive stools, or apnea).

On the other hand, Ostertag et al[63] in a prospective study of 34 low birth weight infants (less than 1,500 gm) who were fed on day one or day seven did not show any significant increase in the incidence of necrotizing enterocolitis: 29 percent of those enterally fed on day one compared with 35 percent fed enterally on day seven developed necrotizing enterocolitis. There were no differences in the perinatal risk factors in both groups. In another study by Unger and co-workers,[64] delayed initiation of enteral feeding was associated with a decreased

TABLE 14–5   Modified Bell's Staging Criteria for Necrotizing Enterocolitis (NEC)

Stage	Systemic Signs	Intestinal Signs	Radiologic Signs	Treatment
IA—Suspected NEC	Temperature instability, apnea, bradycardia, lethargy	Elevated pregavage residuals, mild abdominal distention, emesis, guaiac-positive stool	Normal or intestinal dilation, mild ileus	NPO, antibiotics 3 days pending culture
IB—Suspected NEC	Same as above	Bright red blood from rectum	Same as above	Same as above
IIA—Definite NEC Mildly ill	Same as above	Same as above, *plus* absent bowel sounds, +/− abdominal tenderness	Intestinal dilation, ileus, pneumatosis intestinalis	NPO, antibiotics for 7–10 days if exam is normal in 24–48 hours
IIB—Definite NEC Moderately ill	Same as above, *plus* mild metabolic acidosis, mild thrombocytopenia	Same as above, *plus* absent bowel sounds, definite abdominal tenderness, +/− abdominal cellulitis or right lower quadrant mass	Same as IIA, *plus* portal vein gas, +/− ascites	NPO, antibiotics for 14 days NaHCO₃ for acidosis
IIIA—Advanced NEC Severely ill, bowel intact	Same as IIB, *plus* hypotension, bradycardia, severe apnea, combined respiratory and metabolic acidosis, disseminated intravascular coagulation, neutropenia	Same as above, *plus* signs of generalized peritonitis, marked tenderness, and distention of abdomen	Same as IIB, *plus* definite ascites	Same as above, *plus* 200+ ml/kg fluids, inotropic agents, ventilation therapy, paracentesis
IIIB—Advanced NEC Severely ill perforated	Same as IIIA	Same as IIIA	Same as IIB, *plus* pneumoperitoneum	Same as above, *plus* surgical intervention

Reproduced with permission from Walsh MC, Kliegman RM. Necrotizing enterocolitis: treatment based on staging criteria. Pediatr Clin North Am 1986; 3:187.

incidence of necrotizing enterocolitis only among male infants with birth weights less than 775 gm; hence their study did not support the elective withholding of enteral feeding in other groups of low birth weight infants.

Rate and Volume of Enteral Feeds

Aggressive feeding practices were found to be associated with necrotizing enterocolitis by Krousop.[62] In his case material, infants who developed necrotizing enterocolitis received an average of 43 ml per kilogram during the initial day of enteral feeding and 72 ml per kilogram during the second day.

Book and associates,[65] in a small prospective study comparing fast and slow feeding rates (an increase of 20 ml per day versus 10 ml per day) designed to attain complete enteral feedings at seven and 14 days, respectively, did not find any difference in the incidence of necrotizing enterocolitis. Goldman,[66] however, in a retrospective uncontrolled study found an increased incidence of necrotizing enterocolitis when feedings were advanced by large volumes--more than 40 to 60 ml per kilogram per day. He also found a higher incidence of disease more than in infants receiving volumes greater than 150 ml per kilogram per day. Anderson et al[67] noted

an increased incidence of necrotizing enterocolitis among low birth weight infants fed aggressively—advanced at a rate exceeding 20 ml per kilogram per day.

The mechanism by which excessive feeding predisposes to necrotizing enterocolitis is uncertain. There may be relative mucosal ischemia as a result of an imbalance between mucosal blood flow and oxygen extraction due to an excessive load.[50] Alternatively the already low concentration of lactase in preterm infants may be overwhelmed by the excessive lactose load. The excess lactose is then fermented by the microflora, resulting in hydrogen production, initiating necrotizing enterocolitis.[50] Reducing substances are also a byproduct of this bacterial fermentation. Book and co-workers[68] found that 75 percent of the infants who developed necrotizing enterocolitis had 3 to 4 + reducing substances in the stools one to four days prior to clinical manifestations of disease.

In a recent review, Walsh and co-workers[50] recommended starting enteral feeds at 1 ml every one to two hours and advancing feeds slowly, no more than 20 ml per kilogram per day. They successfully feed 1 kg infants who require ventilatory support. However, the infant is monitored continuously for intolerance— increased residuals, distention, guaiac-positive stools, or reducing substances in the stools.

Sweet[69] recommended with-holding feeds if there are residuals in the stomach prior to feeding. If residue persists, the bowel is rested for five to seven days. If abdominal distention develops during feeding appropriate cultures and radiographs are obtained. Even if studies are inconclusive, he does not feed the infant for one to two weeks. In his conservative approach, infants who develop sudden episodes of apnea, pallor, bradycardia, or poor skin perfusion are not fed for one week or more. With this approach his group has had only one episode of necrotizing enterocolitis in five years among 89 infants weighing less than 1,000 gm and 211 weighing between 1,000 and 2,500 gm.

Osmolality of Feeds

Both animal studies and clinical data have implicated hypertonic feeds in causing mucosal injury. DeLemos et al[70] produced enterocolitis in goats fed a hypertonic formula. Book et al[71] found that feeding infants weighing less than 1,200 gm an elemental formula containing 650 mosm per liter resulted in an 87 percent incidence of necrotizing enterocolitis, in comparison with 25 percent of neonates fed a standard cow's formula (359 mosm per liter). Willis et al[72] noted a higher frequency of necrotizing enterocolitis among infants fed undiluted calcium lactate than among those whose feeds were unsupplemented or supplemented with diluted calcium lactate. The American Academy of Pediatrics[73] has recommended that infant feedings have an osmolarity of less than 400 mosm per liter (osmolality approximately 450 mosm per kilogram of water).

Hypertonic formulas may be the result of added oral medications. In an excellent review by White and Harkavy, the osmolalities of five oral preparations were studied—theophylline, calcium glubionate, digoxin, phenobarbital, and dexamethasone. The osmolalities of all five were greater than 3,000 and hence should be given undiluted orally with extreme caution. When mixed with formula, theophylline, calcium glubionate, and digoxin had acceptable osmolalities (less than 400), but dexamethasone and phenobarbital elixirs still had osmolalities of approximately 1,000 when 3.8 and 1 cc, respectively, were mixed with 15 cc of formula.[74] Ernst et al[75] showed that 1 ml of MVI Pediatric added to 30 ml of a standard formula increased the osmolality from 375 to 744 mosm per kilogram of water. If an intravenous line is required for other reasons, the intravenous route of drug administration may be preferred over the oral route.

Immunologic Considerations

The newborn protects its mucosa by the formation of secretory IgA (SIgA). SIgA inhibits bacterial adherence to mucosal cells in addition to preventing other toxins and antigenic material from binding to the epithelial cells, but in term infants SIgA is not demonstrable in intestinal fluids until one week of age, and adult values are not reached until one month of age.[76] However, nature has its way of protecting the newborn. SIgA-producing plasma cells in the maternal gut are antigenically stimulated and migrate to the breast where specific antibodies are secreted into the colostrum. Thus, the breast-fed newborn receives some passive protection against the bacteria he is most likely to harbor (i.e., his mother's).

In the non–breast-fed premature infant, whose intestine is already immature, there is no protection against bacteria when microbial colonization occurs. Hence, maternal milk has importance in protecting the newborn. Barlow's work in rats substantiates the importance of breast milk in preventing necrotizing enterocolitis.[77] She consistently produced a disease similar to necrotizing enterocolitis by producing a hypoxic insult in rats fed artificial formula. All breast-fed asphyxiated rats were protected from disease. She concluded that breast milk induced protective enteric immunity for newborn rats, and similarly it may protect premature infants. However, necrotizing enterocolitis has been reported in neonates fed fresh human milk.[78]

Most nurseries tend to feed premature infants pooled frozen milk. Kliegman et al[79] found that there was no difference in the incidence of necrotizing enterocolitis among these infants and those fed commercial formula. The reasons for this, despite the theoretical advantages of breast milk, could include the adverse affects of storage on the viability and functional integrity of the cellular components of milk, in addition to the possibility of contamination. In a recent study by Stevenson et al[80] there was no difference in the intestinal flora of preterm hospitalized infants fed stored frozen breast milk and a proprietary formula. However, all the infants fed breast milk had been treated with parenteral doses of antibiotics.

Ischemia and Hypoxia

Ischemia with subsequent damage to the intestinal mucosa has been hypothesized in the pathogenesis of necrotizing enterocolitis. Investigators developed an ischemic model of necrotizing enterocolitis in piglets and postulated a "diving reflex." This is a well-documented reflex in marine animals when there is arterial constriction in the vascular beds of the skin, kidney, and gastrointestinal tract in an attempt to preserve cardiac and cerebral blood flow during prolonged diving. Premature infants may respond in a similar manner to repeated episodes of gut ischemia. Factors implicated in the "ischemia–hypoxia" pathogenesis of necrotizing enterocolitis include prenatal asphyxia, hypotension, hypothermia, umbilical vessel catheterization, patent ductus arteriosus, polycythemia, and exchange transfusion. Nonetheless necrotizing enterocolitis does not develop in the majority of infants with these risk factors,[49,51] and necrotizing enterocolitis has been reported in premature infants with no risk factors.[81]

Umbilical vessel catheterization has been widely implicated in the pathogenesis of mucosal ischemia; 80 percent of the infants with umbilical artery catheters have been found to have distinct arterial thrombosis.[82] Plasticizer levels in tissues of neonates with necrotizing enterocolitis were found to be significantly higher than in those without catheters.[83] A significant increase in the portal venous pressure was noted in newborn piglets undergoing exchange transfusion via umbilical venous catheter. The investigator concluded that alterations in mucosal vascular pressures produced ischemia secondary to vascular congestion and hemorrhage.[84]

Role of Vitamin E

Premature infants weighing less than 1,500 gm maintained at high serum levels of vitamin E for prophylaxis of retinopathy of prematurity have been found to have a higher incidence of necrotizing enterocolitis.

Johnson et al[85] found that premature infants weighing less than 1,500 gm who received prophylactic vitamin E had a higher incidence of necrotizing enterocolitis and sepsis if maintained at pharmacologic levels (more than 3.0 mg per deciliter) for more than one week. Therefore, they recommend that serum vitamin E levels be kept between 1.0 and 3.0 mg per deciliter. In a recent study by Kerner et al[86] high serum vitamin E levels (more than 3.5 mg per deciliter) were found in premature infants weighing less than 1,500 gm who received the recommended dosage of MVI Pediatric; thus they recommend weekly serum vitamin E level determinations in infants weighing 1 to 3 kg. Further, infants with elevated vitamin E levels or those weighing less than 1 kg should receive 1 ml per day of MVI concentrate, with supplemental vitamin B_{12} and folic acid (instead of MVI Pediatric) to avoid elevations in the serum vitamin E level and the increased risk of necrotizing enterocolitis.[86]

The most likely reason for the increased incidence of necrotizing enterocolitis is that pharmacologic serum vitamin E levels result in a decrease in oxygen-dependent intracellular killing capacity, which leads to an increased susceptibility to infection in preterm infants.

Role of Infectious Agents

Many consider necrotizing enterocolitis to be an infectious disease because many infants are colonized with a resistant and invasive organism. These organisms are capable of producing hydrogen gas, which leads to pneumatosis.

The organisms most commonly encountered have been *E. coli*, *Klebsiella*, and *Clostridium*, and more recently *Staphylococcus epidermidis* has been implicated in a number of patients.[45] The premature infant has decreased resistance, and coupled with the inability to mount an appropriate immune response, these infections can be overwhelming.

The prophylactic oral use of aminoglycosides was initially hailed as a means of either preventing necrotizing enterocolitis altogether or preventing perforation if the disease had already developed. Prospective studies have demonstrated that oral doses of gentamicin do not prevent intestinal perforation or alter the course of the disease. Further, oral doses of aminoglycosides can be absorbed across the damaged intestine and increase serum levels, possibly leading to drug toxicity.[50] In addition, Neu and co-workers[87] showed that in animals who had been asphyxiated, the use of gentamicin significantly decreased jejunal lactase levels.

CONCLUSION

Because approximately 95 percent of the patients with necrotizing enterocolitis have been fed, many nurseries have attempted to prevent the disease by delaying enteral feedings. In the excellent controlled study by Yu et al[27] there was a documented reduction of necrotizing enterocolitis in patients randomized to receive TPN and receive nothing enterally. Yet Walsh et al[50] pointed out that the lower incidence of necrotizing enterocolitis was confined to that study period. Once those assigned to receive TPN were fed, necrotizing enterocolitis subsequently was observed. It appeared that prolonging enteral feedings. In the excellent controlled study by Yu et al[63] showed that providing dilute enteral calories early (starting on day 1 of life) did not adversely affect the incidence of necrotizing enterocolitis in comparison with a group given TPN until day 7 of life. The same investigators also showed that there was no protection against necrotizing enterocolitis in a group of premature infants weighing under 1,500 gm who were given nothing by mouth for two weeks.[88] Book et al,[65] in a small prospective study, compared fast and slow feeding rates designed to attain complete enteral nutrition at seven and 14 days, respectively. No difference in the incidence of necrotizing enterocolitis was found, yet large daily increases in feeds or large absolute daily volumes may contribute to the development of necrotizing enterocolitis.[66,67]

Further, Eyal et al[61] performed a two-year study of the influence of feeding practices on the incidence of necrotizing enterocolitis. During the first year neonates were fed expressed breast milk on days 2 to 5 of life and were advanced at increments of 10 to 20 ml per kilogram per day. In the second year infants were first fed at two to three weeks of age. The incidence of necrotizing enterocolitis was 18 percent in the first year and 3 percent in the second year. In addition, in patients exposed to any risk factors that may lead to poor bowel perfusion, Brown and Sweet[89] have employed a regimen of prolonged periods of bowel rest to allow for recovery of the intestinal mucosa, while supplying all nutrients by the parenteral route. After a variable period of time (five to 10 days), rigorous attention is paid to a slow progressive feeding regimen for these patients, with careful examination of gastric residual and reducing substances in the stool. By strict adherence to this regimen, they have shown a marked reduction and almost elimination of necrotizing enterocolitis in their institution.

The downside of prolonged periods of bowel rest is that bowel maturation may be delayed. There is evidence that enteral feeding may be the critical element that triggers postnatal gut maturation through release of gut peptide hormones.[90] Recent research in our laboratory confirms that intestinal development is arrested when animals receive TPN with no enteral nutrients, but that resumption of intestinal maturation occurs on reintroduction of intraluminal nutrients.[91]

RECOMMENDATIONS

Several preventive measures can be proposed for at-risk infants. At-risk infants are those who are suspected of having had an intrauterine or neonatal episode of asphyxia or shock leading to poor bowel perfusion.

Late Introduction of Feedings.   At-risk infants should receive nothing enterally for the first one to two weeks of life; they receive TPN. Enteral feedings are then initiated slowly, but at the first sign of abdominal distention, increasing gastric residuals, regurgitation, or guaiac-positive or Clinitest-positive stools, enteral feedings are stopped and are not reintroduced for several days to weeks.

Slow Advancement of Feedings.   At the end of one to two weeks, or if feedings are to be initiated earlier than already stated (e.g., in tiny newborns on ventilators), one should begin with 1 ml every one to two hours and advance slowly to increase the total feeding by no more than 20 ml per kilogram per day.

Low Osmolality Feedings.   The infant should be fed human milk or a premature formula that is isotonic. High osmolality feeds may result in reduced mesenteric perfusion. One must avoid the addition of oral doses of medicines or vitamins with high osmolality in any high risk infant.

Human Milk.   Although early studies suggested that human milk would protect necrotizing enterocolitis, the disease has been described even in infants receiving fresh human milk. However, the immune protection from fresh human milk is thought by many to be very important to the preterm infant. Since human milk may not meet calcium, phosphorus, caloric, and protein needs of low birth weight infants, it can be supplemented with Enfamil Human Milk Fortifier. In our laboratory

we have shown that such supplementation has no adverse effects on key anti-infective factors in human milk.[92]

Route of Feeding.   Intermittent gavage tube feeding appears to be more physiologic than transpyloric feeding and whenever possible is preferred. If the patient has regurgitation, poor gastric emptying or gastric distention, continuous nasogastric feeding or even transpyloric feeding may be required.[13]

Observe for Early Signs of Necrotizing Enterocolitis.   Carefully monitor all high risk infants for early signs of necrotizing enterocolitis. These signs may occur up to 60 days of life in infants whose first feeding is delayed beyond the first week of life. If the diagnosis of necrotizing enterocolitis is suspected, feedings are stopped, and the infant receives no enteral nutrition for several days to two weeks, depending on the severity of symptoms.

REFERENCES

1. Committee on Nutrition. Nutritional needs of low-birthweight infants. Pediatrics 1985; 75:976.
2. Grand RJ, Watkins JB, Torti FM. Development of the human gastrointestinal tract. Gastroenterology 1976; 70:790.
3. Lebenthal E, Lee PC. Interactions of determinants in the ontogeny of the gastrointestinal tract: a unified concept. Pediatr Res 1983; 17:19.
4. Milla PJ. Development of intestinal structure and function. In: Tanner MS, Stocks RJ, eds. Neonatal gastroenterology—contemporary issues. Newcastle upon Tyne: Intercept, 1984:10.
5. Cavell B. Gastric emptying in preterm infants. Acta Paediatr Scand 1979; 68:725.
6. Yu VYH. Effect of body position on gastric emptying in the neonate. Arch Dis Child 1975; 50:500.
7. Herbst JJ, Minton SD, Book LS. Gastroesophageal reflux causing respiratory distress and apnea in newborn infants. J Pediatr 1979; 95:763.
8. Pitcher-Wilmott R, Shutack JG, Fox WW. Decreased lung volume after nasogastric feeding of neonates recovering from respiratory distress. J Pediatr 1979; 96:914.
9. Toce SS, Keenan WJ, Homan SM. Enteral feeding in very-low-birth-weight infants—a comparison of two nasogastric methods. Am J Dis Child 1987; 141:439.
10. Narayanan I, Singh B, Harvey D. Fat loss during feeding of human milk. Arch Dis Child 1984; 59:475.
11. Moyer L, Chan GM. Clotted feeding tubes with transpyloric feeding of premature infant formula. J Pediatr Gastroenterol Nutr 1982; 1:55.
12. Lucas A, Bloom SR, Aynsley-Green A. Metabolic and endocrine events at the time of the first feed of human milk in preterm and term infants. Arch Dis Child 1978; 53:731.
13. Bremer HJ, Brooke OG, Orzalesi M, et al. Nutrition and feeding of preterm infants. Oxford, Blackwell Scientific, 1987:197.
14. Van Caillie M, Powell GK. Nasoduodenal versus nasogastric feeding in the very low birth weight infant. Pediatrics 1975; 56:1065.
15. Whitfield MF. Poor weight gain of the low birth weight infant fed nasojejunally. Arch Dis Child 1982; 57:597.
16. Roy RN, Pollnitz RP, Hamilton JR, et al. Impaired assimilation of nasojejunal feeds in healthy low-birth-weight infants. J Pediatr 1977; 90:431.
17. Beddis I, McKenzie S. Transpyloric feeding in the very low birthweight (1,500 gm and below) infant. Arch Dis Child 1979; 54:213.

18. Whittfield MF. Transpyloric feeding in infants undergoing intensive care. Arch Dis Child 1980, 55:571.

19. Hayhurst EG, Wyman M. Morbidity associated with prolonged use of polyvinyl feeding tubes. Am J Dis Child 1975; 129:72.

20. Rodriguez JP, Guero J, Frias EG, Omenaca F. Duodenorenal perforation in a neonate by a tube of silicone rubber during transpyloric feeding. J Pediatr 1978; 92:113.

21. Dellagrammaticus HD, Duerden BI, Milner RDG. Upper intestinal bacterial flora during transpyloric feeding. Arch Dis Child 1983; 58:115.

22. Vazquez C, Arroyos A, Valls A. Necrotizing enterocolitis: increased incidence in infants receiving nasoduodenal feeding. Arch Dis Child 1980; 55:826.

23. Pereira GR, Lemons JA. Controlled study of transpyloric and intermittent gavage feeding in the small preterm infant. Pediatrics 1981; 67:68.

24. Moyer-Mileur L, Chan GM. Nutritional support of very-low-birth-weight infants requiring prolonged assisted ventilation. Am J Dis Child 1986; 140:929.

25. Unger A, Goetzman BW, Chan C, et al. Nutritional practices and outcome of extremely premature infants. Am J Dis Child 1986; 140:1027.

26. Gunn T, Reaman G, Outerbridge EW. Peripheral total parenteral nutrition for premature infants with the respiratory distress syndrome: a controlled study. J Pediatr 1978; 92:608.

27. Yu VYH, James B, Hendry P, et al. Total parenteral nutrition in very low birthweight infants: a controlled trial. Arch Dis Child 1979; 54:653.

28. Kerner JA, Hattner JAT, Trautman MS, et al. Postnatal somatic growth in very low birth weight infants on peripheral parenteral nutrition. J Pediatr Perinat Nutr (in press).

29. Glass EJ, Hune R, Lang MA, et al. Parenteral nutrition compared with transpyloric feeding. Arch Dis Child 1984; 59:131.

30. Dryburgh E. Transpyloric feeding in 49 infants undergoing intensive care. Arch Dis Child 1980; 55:879.

31. Zlotkin SH, Stallings VA, Pencharz PB. Total parenteral nutrition in children. Pediatr Clin North Am 1985; 32:381.

32. Cashore WJ, Sedaghatian MR, Usher RH. Nutritional supplements with intravenously administered lipid, protein hydrolysate, and glucose in small premature infants. Pediatrics 1975; 56:8.

33. Churella HR, Bachhuber BS, MacLean WC. Survey: methods of feeding low-birth-weight infants. Pediatrics 1985; 76:243.

34. Adamkin DA. Nutrition in very low birth weight infants. Clin Perinatol 1986; 13:419.

35. Higgs SC, Malan AF, Heese H DeV, et al. A comparison of oral feeding and total parenteral nutrition in infants of very low birthweight. S Afr Med J 1974; 48:2169.

36. Hall RT, Rhodes PG. Total parenteral alimentation via indwelling umbilical catheters in the newborn period. Arch Dis Child 1976; 51:929.

37. Merritt RJ. Neonatal nutritional support. Clin Consult Nutr Support 1981; 1:10.

38. Coran AG. Parenteral nutritional support of the neonate (a group telephone workshop). Tele Session Corporation, New York, August 17, 1981.

39. Kerner JA. The use of umbilical catheters for parenteral nutrition. In: Kerner JA, ed. Manual of pediatric parenteral nutrition. New York: John Wiley 1983:303.

40. Sadig HF. Broviac catheterization in low birth weight infants: incidence and treatment of associated complications. Crit Care Med 1987; 15:47.

41. Koldovsky O, Sunshine P, Kretchmer N. Cellular migration of intestinal epithelia in suckling and weaned rats. Nature 1966; 212:1389.

42. Herbst JJ, Sunshine P. Postnatal development of the small intestine of the rat. Pediatr Res 1969; 3:27.

43. Sunshine P, Herbst JJ, Koldovsky O, Kretchmer N. Adaptation of the gastrointestinal tract to extrauterine life. Ann NY Acad Sci 1971; 176:16.

44. Herbst JJ, Sunshine P, Kretchmer N. Intestinal malabsorption in infancy and childhood. Adv Pediatr 1969; 16:11.

45. Sunshine P. Gastrointestinal. In: Eden RD, Boehm FH, eds. Fetal assessment: physiological, clinical and medicolegal principles. East Norwalk, Connecticut: Appleton-Century-Crofts, (in press).

46. Kliegman RM, Fanaroff AN. Necrotizing enterocolitis. N Engl J Med 1984; 310:1093.

47. Kosloske AM. Pathogenesis and prevention of necrotizing enterocolitis: a hypothesis based on personal observation and a review of the literature. Pediatrics 1984; 74:1086.

48. Brown E, Sweet AY. Preventing necrotizing enterocolitis in neonates. JAMA 1978; 240:2452.

49. Frantz ID, L'Heureux P, Engel RR, Hunt CE. Necrotizing enterocolitis. J Pediatr 1975; 56:259.

50. Walsh MC, Kliegman R, Fanaroff A. Necrotizing enterocolitis: a practitioner's perspective. Pediatr Rev 1988; 9:219.

51. Stoll B, Kanto W, Glass R, et al. Epidemiology of necrotizing enterocolitis: a case control study. J Pediatr 1980; 96:447.

52. Moonijian AS, Peckham G, Fox W. Necrotizing enterocolitis: endemic vs epidemic. Pediatr Res 1978; 12:530.

53. Walsh MC, Kliegman RM. Necrotizing enterocolitis: treatment based on staging criteria. Pediatr Clin North Am 1986; 33:179.

54. Mata AG, Rosenpart RM. Intraobserver variability in the radiographic diagnosis of necrotizing enterocolitis. Pediatrics, 1980; 66:68.

55. Kirschner B, Lahr C, Lahr D. Detection of increased breath hydrogen in infants with necrotizing enterocolitis. Gastroenterology 1980; 72:A57/1080.

56. Stevenson DK, Shahin SM, Ostrander CR, et al. Breath hydrogen in preterm infants: correlation with changes in bacterial colonization of the gastrointestinal tract. J Pediatr 1982; 101:607.

57. Garcia J, Smith FR, Cucinelli SA. Urinary D-lactate in infants with necrotizing enterocolitis. J Pediatr 1984; 104:268.

58. Bell MJ, Ternberg TJ, Feigin RD, et al. Neonatal necrotizing enterocolitis: therapeutic decisions based upon clinical staging. Ann Surg 1978; 197:1.

59. Kliegman RM, Hack M, Jones P, Fanaroff AA. Epidemiologic study of necrotizing enterocolitis among low-birth-weight infants: absence of identifiable risk factors. J Pediatr 1982; 100:440.

60. Kerner JA Jr, Hartman GE, Sunshine P. The medical and surgical management of infants with the short bowel syndrome. J Perinatol 1985; 5:517.

61. Eyal F, Sagi E, Avital A. Necrotizing enterocolitis in the very low birthweight infant: expressed breast milk feeding compared with parenteral feeding. Arch Dis Child 1982; 57:274.

62. Krousop RW. The influences of feeding practices. In: Brown EG, Sweet AY, eds. Necrotizing enterocolitis. New York: Grune & Stratton, 1980:570.

63. Ostertag SG, LaGamma EF, Reisen CE, Ferrentino RL. Early enteral feeding does not affect the incidence of necrotizing enterocolitis. Pediatrics 1986; 77:275.

64. Unger A, Goetzman BW, Chan C, et al. Nutritional practices and outcome of extremely premature infants. Am J Dis Child 1986, 140:1027.

65. Book LS, Herbst JJ, Jung AL. Comparison of fast-and-slow-feeding rate schedules to the development of necrotizing enterocolitis. J Pediatr 1976; 89:463.

66. Goldman HI. Feeding and necrotizing enterocolitis. Am J Dis Child 1980; 134:553.

67. Anderson DM, Rome ES, Kleigman RM. Relationship of endemic necrotizing enterocolitis to alimentation. Pediatr Res 1985; 19:331A.

68. Book LS, Herbst JJ, Jung AL. Carbohydrate malabsorption in necrotizing enterocolitis. Pediatrics 1976; 57:201.

69. Sweet AY. Necrotizing enterocolitis: feeding the neonate weighing less than 1500 grams—nutrition and beyond. In: Sunshine P, ed. Report of the 79th Ross conference on pediatric research. Columbus, Ohio: 1980.

70. DeLemos RA, Rogers JH, McLaughlin GW. Experimental production of necrotizing enterocolitis in newborn goats. Pediatr Res 1974; 8:380.

71. Book LS, Herbst JJ, Atherton SO, Jung AL. Necrotizing enterocolitis in low-birth-weight infants fed an elemental formula. J Pediatr 1975; 87:602.

72. Willis DM, Chabot J, Radde IC, Chance GW. Unsuspected hyperosmolality of oral solutions contributing to necrotizing

enterocolitis in very-low-birth weight infants. Pediatrics 1977; 60:535.

73. American Academy of Pediatrics Committee on Nutrition. Commentary on breast feeding and infant formulas including proposed standards for formulas. Pediatrics 1976; 57:278.

74. White KC, Harkavy KZ. Hypertonic formula resulting from added oral medications. Am J Dis Child 1982; 136:931.

75. Ernst JA, Williams JM, Glick MR. Osmolality of substance used in the intensive care nursery. Pediatrics 1983; 72:347.

76. Barnard J, Greene H, Cotton R. Necrotizing enterocolitis. In: Kretchmer N, Minkowski A, eds. Nutritional adaptation of the gastrointestinal tract of the newborn. Nestle nutrition. Vol. 3. New York: Raven Press, 1983:103.

77. Barlow B, Santulli TV, Heird WC, Pitt J, Blanc WA, Schullinger JN. An experimental study of acute neonatal necrotizing enterocolitis—The importance of breast milk. J Pediatr Surg 1974; 9:587.

feeding. Lancet 1977; 2:507.

79. Kliegman RM, Pittard WB, Fanaroff AA. Necrotizing enterocolitis in neonates fed human milk. J Pediatr 1979; 95:450.

80. Stevenson DK, Yang C, Kerner JA, Yeager AS. Intestinal flora in the second week of life in hospitalized preterm infants fed stored frozen breast milk or a proprietary formula. Clin Pediatr 1985; 24:338.

81. Kliegman RM, Fanaroff AA. Neonatal necrotizing enterocolitis: a nine-year experience: epidemiology and uncommon observations. Am J Dis Child 1981; 135:603.

82. Lehmiller DH, Kanto WF. Relationship of mesenteric thromboembolism, oral feeding and necrotizing enterocolitis. J Pediatr 1978; 92:96.

83. Hillman LS, Goodwin SL, Sherman WR. Identification and measurement of plasticiser in neonatal tissues after umbilical catheters and blood products. N Eng J Med 1975; 292:381.

84. Touloukian RJ, Kadaw A, Spencer RP. The gastrointestinal complications of umbilical venous exchange transfusion: a clinical and experimental study. Pediatrics 1973; 51:36.

85. Johnson L, Bowen FW, Abbasi S, et al. Relationship of prolonged pharmacologic serum levels of vitamin E to incidence of sepsis and necrotizing enterocolitis in infants with birth weight 1500 grams or less. Pediatrics 1985; 75:619.

86. Kerner JA, Poole RL, Sunshine P, Stevenson DK. High serum vitamin E levels in premature infants receiving MVI-Pediatric. J Pediatr Perinatal Nutr 1987; 1:75.

87. Neu J, Masi M, Stevenson DK, et al. Effects of asphyxia and oral gentamicin on intestinal lactase in the suckling rat. Pediatr Pharmacol 1981; 1:215.

88. LaGamma E, Ostertag S, Birnbaum H. Failure of delayed oral feedings to prevent necrotizing enterocolitis. Am J Dis Child 1985; 139:385.

89. Brown E, Sweet A. Neonatal necrotizing enterocolitis. Pediatr Clin North Am 1982; 29:114.

90. Aynsley-Green A. Metabolic and endocrine interrelation in the human fetus and neonate. Am J Clin Nutr 1985; 41:399.

91. Feng JJ, Kwong LK, Kerner JA, et al. Resumption of intestinal maturation upon reintroduction of intraluminal nutrients: functional and biochemical correlations. Clin Res 1987; 35:228A.

92. Kerner JA Jr, Yang C, Stevenson DK. Effects of nutritional supplements on anti-infective factors in human milk. Gastroenterology 1988 94:A223.

ASSESSING THE CAUSES OF PERMANENT NEUROLOGIC DISABILITY AND THE RISKS OF PRACTICE

15 Electroencephalography in the Assessment of the Premature and Full–Term Infant

Barry R. Tharp, M.D.

Technical Aspects of Electroencephalography
Maturation of the Electroencephalogram in
  Normal Newborns
The Abnormal Electroencephalogram
  Use of the Electroencephalogram in Assessment
    of the Severity and Progression of
    Neonatal Encephalopathy
  The Iatrogenically Paralyzed Infant
  The Value of Electroencephalography in Identifying
    Specific Neurologic Disorders
Videoelectroencephalographic Monitoring in the
  Intensive Care Nursery

The electroencephalogram (EEG) has been used in the clinical evaluation of neonates for over two decades. Early studies, particularly in France and the United States, were devoted to the assessment of brain function in healthy full-term infants. Subsequent publications presented the spectrum of abnormalities in the EEGs of term infants, and ultimately, the prognostic value of the neonatal EEG vis-a-vis the risk of neurologic sequelae.[1] With advances in neonatal intensive care and the accompanying reduction in the age at which premature infants are viable, EEG assessment of premature infants has become a routine in a small number of neonatal intensive care units.[2] It was found that specific EEG patterns characterized each gestational age, and that a skilled pediatric electroencephalographer could determine the conceptional age of a healthy infant to within two weeks. This maturational progression of the EEG background acitivity occurs in healthy infants whether they are growing in utero or are in the intensive care nursing isolette. Neurologic syndromes in the premature infant therefore are associated not only with abnormal patterns similar to those in term infants, but with a permanent or transient disruption in the expected maturational sequence of EEG background patterns when serial recordings are obtained during the neonatal period.

Continuous EEG recording, accompanied by video surveillance, recently has been introduced into a few nurseries. this technique not only is an excellent way to monitor the integrity of cerebral function in critically iss or iatrogenically paralyzed newborns but has resulted in a major adjustment in our thinking about neonatal seizures.[3,4] Many types of aberrant behavior, heretofore considered seizures, have been shown to be unassociated with EEG ryhthms considered to be diagnostic of seizures. The exact origin and nature of this nonseizure behavior are unclear, but it is though to represent brain stem release phenomena that are not amenable to anticonvulsants (see Chapter 11).

The goal in this chapter is to acquaint the reader with the fundamentals of neonatal EEG, including a brief discussion of the maturational features of the premature infant's cerebral electrical activity and the abnormal patterns seen in sick neonates, with particular emphasis on patterns that are correlated with specific neurologic disorders, the use of the EEG in the timing of the brain insult, and its prognostic value. Additionally, I will describe the importance of long-term continuous monitoring of newborns, not only in predicting the outcome and detecting seizures but also in assessing the impact of postnatal events, both acute and chronic, on cerebral function.

TECHNICAL ASPECTS OF ELECTROENCEPHALOGRAPHY

Electroencephalography is a noninvasive procedure that can be performed in the clinical neurophysiology laboratory or, more commonly when neonates are involved, at the infant's bedside. Electrodes usually are applied with paste or occasionally with collodion if a prolonged recording is anticipated. The site of attachment of each electrode is determined by an international measurement system; approximately nine to 22 electrodes are applied, the number depending on the size of the infant's head, the presence of scapl intravenous infusions, the age of the infant, the purpose of the study, and the preference of the particular laboratory. The various technical parameters of the actual recording are discussed elsewhere and are not reiterated here.[5] A routine EEG usually records 45 to 60 minutes of cerebral electrical activity on paper.

For a study to be considered adequate, the EEG should be recorded during all stages of sleep (active [REM] sleep onset, transitional sleep, quiet [non-REM] sleep, and postquiet sleep active sleep) and wakefulness. Sleep states are less well developed in premature infants. Early periods of active sleep, with eye movements, small body movements, and continuous EEG background activity, can be seen in some healthy infants at 28 to 30 weeks' conceptional age (see section on EEG maturation). By 32 to 34 weeks' conceptional age most normal infants have easily identifiable sleep states. The first stage of sleep in infants is usually active (REM) sleep, which may last up to 40 minutes in healthy infants or even longer in sick infants. EEG abnormalities may not be obvious in active sleep and appear only during the following quiet sleep stage; therefore it is imperative that the technologist continue the recording until both major sleep states have been monitored.

If longer recording is to be accomplished, the data can be stored on magnetic tape, including miniaturized cassettes or video cassette tape, with or without an accompanying video picture of the infant.[4, 6, 7] Extreme compression of EEG data on paper (several hours on a single page) is accomplished by using a variety of small devices that display a limited number of channels of EEG.[8] Most recording systems also can store other important physiologic variables, e.g., mean arterial blood pressure, heart rate and electrocardiographic findings, PCO_2 and PO_2 values, and intracranial pressure.[4]

It should be emphasized that neonatal EEG recording requires the services of a skilled EEG technologist who not only is well versed in the technical aspects of EEG but has an intimate knowledge of infant behavior and perinatal neuropathologic conditions. He or she must also interact well with nursery personnel and parents and feel comfortable with very ill and often clinically fragile newborns. The technologist must keep a well-annotated record of every infant, chronicling particularly the infant's behavior during the recording (to assist in sleep staging) as well as pertinent clinical information, such as drugs received, conceptional age, and recent changes in blood gas levels. EEG background rhythms may be significantly but transiently disturbed by the emergency administration of many drugs and by abrupt drops in the PO_2 level and blood pressure. The absence of this information at the time of the interpretation could lead to an exaggeration of the severity of the infant's encephalopathy and a misstatement of the long-term prognosis.

The majority of newborn EEGs are obtained as isolated studies, which are usually interpreted "off line." In many laboratories a single recording is obtained, often at the time of discharge—a time when the infant may have clinically recovered from the neurologic problem that prompted the EEG in the first place. As is discussed in a later section, the EEG also may show significant improvement by that time and the most useful information for prognostic purposes may be lost (i.e., the very abnormal patterns present during the acute phase of the encephalopathy). The timing of the EEG therefore is critical.

The initial tracing should be taken when the infant is most critically ill, including the first 24 hours of life. Early recordings may be helpful not only in predicting the long-term outcome, but also in selecting infants at high risk for seizures who will require serial EEGs over the next week or, if available, continuous monitoring. EEGs also should be done when there are changes in the neurologic status, when seizures are suspected, in all infants who are iatrogenically paralyzed,[9] and as a follow-up in infants receiving antiepileptic drugs for clinical seizures, because subclinical (clinically silent) seizures may persist in an infant whose neurologic function is depressed by the encephalopathy and an antiepileptic drug, particularly phenobarbital.

Long-term monitoring of cerebral function has only recently been introduced into neonatal intensive care units.[4] At the moment two approaches are being used for continuous recording:

1. In our laboratory and others, the EEG is recorded on magnetic or video tape with or without an accompanying video image of the infant, and both tapes are synchronized by a time code generator so that a second by second analysis of EEG changes and infant's behavior is possible.[3,4] These systems also accept input from other physiologic monitoring equipment, such as those recording transcutaneous gas levels, blood pressure, electrocardiographic changes, and intracranial pressure.

2. In Europe and in a few laboratories in the United States, small recording units are available for recording the EEG and other physiologic variables on paper for long periods of time, i.e., several hours of data compressed on a few inches of paper printout. These units have been used particularly to identify and quantify neonatal seizures.[8]

Before ending these introductory remarks, I should like to emphasize one last point, which may appear obvious but often is overlooked by physicians ordering EEGs. The accuracy of EEG interpretation is entirely dependent on the skill and experience of the physician reviewing the record. At present, there are few electro-encephalographers with extensive experience in this area. Physicians who want to read neonatal EEGs require additional training even if they are well versed in pediatric electroencephalography. The literature is replete with publications about neonatal EEGs that are of dubious value because of questionable interpretation of the tracings. Neonatal EEG interpretation is also complicated by the fact that it is not a test that is well standardized or amenable to computer interpretation, as is the electrocardiogram, for example. In the newborn, as we will see in the next section, there are rapid maturational changes in EEG patterns that occur over a period of weeks, and each laboratory must have its own set of norms for each gestational age. Additionally norms must be established for each state (active, quiet, and transitional sleep and wakefulness) at each conceptional age. Laboratories must accumulate enough records to gather this normative data and to adequately train their technologists. Once this level of expertise has been reached, neonatal EEGs must be done on a regular basis to maintain the laboratory's proficiency. A laboratory carrying out electroencephalography in one or two newborns each month probably will never develop the experience necessary to interpret newborn records beyond a very rudimentary level.

MATURATION OF THE ELECTROENCEPHALOGRAM IN NORMAL NEWBORNS

The rate of brain maturation in the premature infant is rapid, striking changes in brain size and complexity taking place over the last three months of a full-term pregnancy. One has only to look at reviews of brain development [10] to be impressed by the striking differences at a gross level between the relatively smooth cortical surface with its simple sulcal pattern in the 26- to 28-week conceptional age infant, and the complex cortical gyral pattern present a mere 12 to 14 weeks later in the full-term newborn. Complex and rapid histologic and biochemical changes accompany these morphologic changes.

It therefore is not surprising that similarly dramatic electrophysiologic changes are also taking place in this group of infants. A variety of EEG patterns appear and disappear over the last trimester and during the first year of life. Maturational changes occur most rapidly from 25 weeks' gestational age to approximately one month after term and occur at about the same rate whether the infant is in utero or in the intensive care nursery. This means that the EEG of a 12-week-old infant born at 28 weeks'

gestational age will be virtually identical to that of a two-day-old infant born at 40 weeks gestational age, assuming that the premature infant had a benign postnatal course. Over the first few months after term, infantile EEG and behavioral patterns disappear and more "adult" EEG patterns appear. This loss of infantile EEG patterns occurs at a well-established rate so that deviations from normal can be appreciated at these early ages and suggest the presence of acquired or congenital pathologic disorders.

Sleep states can be identified in all healthy premature infants (Figs. 15–1, 15–2). Active sleep (REM sleep) is the first clearly recognizable behavioral state to appear at 28 to 30 weeks' conceptional age and is characterized by rapid eye movements, continuous background EEG activity, frequent small body and limb movements, irregular respirations, and an increased incidence of apnea (as compared with quiet sleep). Quiet sleep is well characterized by 31 to 34 weeks conceptional age and is associated with regular respirations, discontinuous EEG background activity, a paucity of motor activity and eye movements, and infrequent apnea. The concordance between behavior and EEG background activity increases as term approaches; e.g., frequent body movements and eye movements become more associated with the continuous portion of the EEG (active sleep) than they were in small prematures, in whom certain aspects of active sleep behavior may spill over into discontinuous portions of the EEG (a background EEG pattern more typically seen in older prematures during quiet sleep). Each of these sleep states, as well as wakefulness, is associated with characteristic EEG activity at each conceptional age. Therefore, in order to properly interpret a neonatal EEG, the reader must be familiar with a large number of age- and state-related patterns and the significance of deviations from this normal activity in sick infants.

To illustrate the rapid changes in brain electrical activity, three common patterns can be chosen (Fig. 15–3). Delta brushes are an easily recognized transient consisting of a short run of fast activity (beta) superimposed on a slow wave (delta) (small arrow, Fig. 15–3). The frequency of these transients (number per minute) is highest at 31 to 32 weeks' conceptional age in active sleep.[12] They gradually disappear over the next two months, initially in active sleep and wakefulness and finally in quiet sleep. A few are present in quiet sleep at term and for a few weeks after term. The location of the maximal number of brushes (frontal, temporal, parietal, occipital lobe) also depends on the sleep state as well as on the conceptional age. Temporal theta bursts (large arrow, Fig. 15–3) are most abundant at 29 to 31 weeks' conceptional age and diminish rapidly over the next two months, being absent at term. Frontal sharp waves (underlined, Fig. 15–3), on the other hand, appear at about 33 to 35 weeks and increase in abundance to term, at which they are of maximal frequency in transitional

C♀   CA31–32W ACTIVE SLEEP

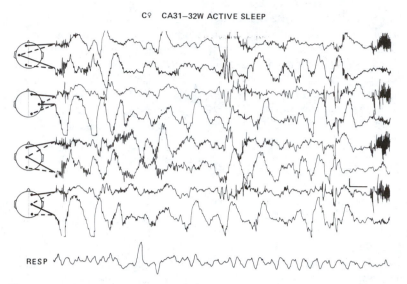

RESP

Figure 15–1   Normal EEG during active (REM) sleep in a premature infant of 31 to 32 weeks' conceptual age. Continuous EEG background, irregular respirations, and frequent muscle artifact due to movement (electromyographic artifact at right of 20 second EEG sample). Calibration (in this illustration and in Figures 15–2 and 15–3): one second, 50 microvolts.

C♀   CA31–32W QUIET SLEEP

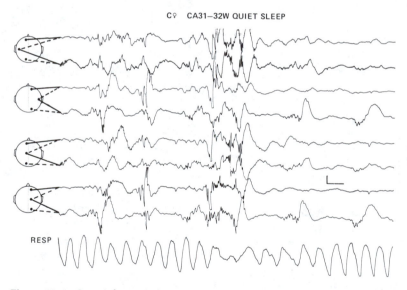

RESP

Figure 15–2   Same infant as in Figure 15–1 during quiet (non-REM) sleep. Background more discontinuous. Marked attenuation of background EEG activity (except for slow waves in occipital regions) during last seven to eight seconds of sample. Respirations deeper and more regular.

sleep (between active sleep and quiet sleep). They gradually disappear over the next four weeks.[11]

When the experienced pediatric electroencephalographer takes all these EEG features into consideration, he or she can determine a healthy infant's conceptional age (from earliest prematurity approximating 25 weeks to a few weeks after term) with an error of one to two weeks, solely on the basis of EEG patterns and background activity. The rate of maturational change slows after term, and EEG changes occur over periods of months rather than weekly as in the premature. Sleep

spindles, for example, appear in some infants as young as two weeks after term but are delayed in other normal infants until two months.[13]

Most healthy newborns pass almost immediately into active sleep when falling asleep (as do adults with narcolepsy). The switch to adult behavior—quiet sleep onset—occurs three to nine weeks after term, although occasional normal infants may have an initial period of active sleep beyond these limits.

Many pathologic conditions slow the rate of maturation of the brain. For example, infants with Down

NORMAL PATTERNS

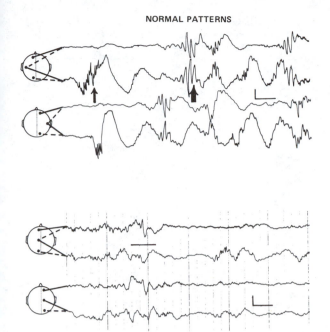

Figure 15–3 Samples of normal EEG patterns in premature infants: delta brush (small arrow), temporal theta burst (large arrow), frontal sharp wave (underlined).

syndrome usually have normal EEGs, but the rate of maturation is slowed, with the tracé alternant pattern (discontinuous pattern in quiet sleep in term infants) disappearing at a later age and concomitant with a delay in the appearance of rolandic sleep spindles.[13]

This brief discussion of EEG maturation has been presented in order to emphasize several points:

1. Maturation is rapid enough in the preterm infant to allow the experienced electroencephalographer to estimate the conceptional age.
2. These rapid EEG fluctuations inject a significant degree of complexity into the interpretation of the EEG in infants, particularly those under three months of post-term age.
3. The brain matures in an extrauterine environment at approximately the same rate as it does in utero, provided there are no major insults to the brain during the neonatal course.
4. This maturation can be impaired transiently or permanently by a variety of primary (e.g., intracranial hemorrhage) or secondary (e.g., hypoxia and hypoglycemia) disorders that occur frequently in the high risk newborn.

ABNORMAL ELECTROENCEPHALOGRAM

It is beyond the scope of this chapter to discuss the spectrum of EEG abnormalities that occur in the new-

born. Readers interested in a more detailed description of these patterns can refer to several recent publications on the subject.[5, 14, 15] In most laboratories EEG abnormalities are graded as mild, moderate, or marked. Unfortunately there is no standardized classification of EEG abnormalities, and each laboratory has developed its own criteria. This leads to some difficulty in comparing EEG results from laboratory to laboratory, particularly in regard to abnormalities graded as mild and moderate. There is much better agreement, particularly among laboratories performing large numbers of neonatal EEGs, about what is considered a marked EEG abnormality. We use the terminology and criteria from our laboratory in the following discussion (see references 5 and 16 for details of our classification system).

The EEG most commonly is used to grade the severity and progression of diffuse encephalopathies—hypoxic ischemic encephalopathy being responsible for the largest number of referrals to our laboratory. Additionally it is of value in identifying specific neurologic syndromes (Table 15–1). In this chapter I discuss the areas listed in Table 15–1 except for neonatal seizures, which are the topic of Chapter 11.

Use of the Electroencephalogram in Assessment of the Severity and Progression of Neonatal Encephalopathy.

In the majority of cases, abnormal EEG patterns in newborns are etiologically nonspecific. Suppression burst patterns, generalized voltage depression, and dysmature backgrounds can accompany a range of disorders, from hypoxic-ischemic encephalopathy and infection to congenital malformation and inherited metabolic disorders. The timing and persistence of the EEG abnormality and the clinical state of the child at the time of the recording are helpful in arriving at a more specific etiologic diagnosis and predicting the long-term outcome.[5,17]

TABLE 15–1   Value of the Electroencephalogram in the Assessment of the At-Risk Newborn

1. Determines the severity of the encephalopathy
2. Follows the progression of the encephalopathy and the impact of acquired postnatal events on brain function
3. Contributes to the formulation of long-term neurologic prognoses
4. Identifies and quantitates seizures and the response to therapy
5. Assesses cerebral function in the iatrogenically paralyzed infant
6. Identifies specific pathologic entities:
   a. Herpes encephalitis
   b. Metabolic disorders, e.g., aminoacidopathies and organic acidurias
   c. Deep white matter lesions, e.g., periventricular leukomalacia
   d. Cerebral infarctions and other lateralized abnormalities
   e. Certain congenital malformations of brain
   f. Chronic neurologic syndrome associated with bronchopulmonary dysplasia

The EEG usually is the most sensitive method for determining the presence of an encephalopathy. In many instances, findings in the neurologic examination appear normal, particularly in the small premature infant, or the examination cannot be performed (iatrogenically paralyzed infant), yet the EEG is abnormal. In a study from our laboratory, serial EEGs and neurologic examinations were performed in 62 premature infants (less than 1,200 gm birth weight) in the neonatal period.* The EEG was a more efficient predictor of outcome than the neurologic examination (90 versus 82 percent). More important, the sensitivity (the number of correctly diagnosed positives [infants with sequelae or who died] compared with the total number of positive) was 72 percent for the EEG versus 39 percent for the neurologic examination.

The grading of the EEG from mild to marked reflects the severity of the encephalopathy and in the case of a marked abnormality is predictive of poor outcome. A single markedly abnormal EEG in a term or premature infant is usually indicative of a severe and permanent encephalopathy.[14, 16, 18, 19] One must be cautious, however, in making such a prognostic statement in certain circumstances, such as when an infant has received large amounts of central nervous system–active medication prior to the EEG, which may lead to a transient deterioration of background rhythms. This is noted particularly with the benzodiazepam class of drugs. If an EEG is obtained immediately after acute deterioration of oxygenation, the background may transiently worsen. EEGs obtained during the first 48 hours of life may also have somewhat less value as predictors of long-term outcome than tracings obtained at an older age.[19] A suppression burst background appearing within the first 24 hours of life, for example, occasionally may be associated with a normal outcome, whereas in older infants it almost always connotes a severe irreversible encephalopathy.

In a recent unpublished study from our laboratory the predictive value of the EEG in the first 48 hours of life was evaluated in 86 full-term and 27 premature infants.† Preliminary results are shown in Table 15–2. The EEG was more predictive of the long-term outcome (determined by examination after two years of age) in term infants than in prematures, particularly when recorded in the second 24 hours of life. We attributed the difference between term and premature infants to the difference in the time of onset of neurologic syndromes at different gestational ages; e.g., hypoxic-ischemic encephalopathy in term infants is usually worse shortly after delivery, with subsequent improvement, whereas the onset of intraventricular hemorrhage or periventricular leukomalacia in premature infants occurs several days or more following delivery. The EEG in the

---

*Tharp B, Scher M, Clancy R. Study to be published in Neuropediatrics.
†Weinstein S, Monyer H, Tharp B.

TABLE 15–2   Predictive Value of the Electroencephalogram in the First 48 Hours of Life and the Outcome

Premature Infants

EEG	Outcome			
	Normal	Suspect	Abnormal	Dead
Normal to mild abnormality	23	10	7	15
Moderate abnormality	9	8	4	4
Marked abnormality	3	6	7	8

Term Infants

EEG	Outcome			
	Normal	Suspect	Abnormal	Dead
Normal to mild abnormality	20	0	1	9
Moderate abnormality	11	2	2	12
Marked abnormality	6 (4, 2)*	1 (1, 0)*	12 (8, 4)*	10 (3, 7)*

* Day 1 and day 2 EEGs.

first few hours of life also may be influenced by maternal anesthesia and drug ingestion, although usually only to a mild degree.

The later onset of neurologic disorders in premature infants led to the proposal that serial EEGs, i.e., on a weekly or every other week basis, might be a better method of following high risk infants.[2] In the study of 62 premature infants with birth weights less than 1,200 gms already mentioned, EEGs were obtained shortly after birth and at one- to three-week intervals until death or discharge from the nursery.‡ Neurologic follow-up was carried out at two and three years of age. We found that serial recordings added further information beyond that obtained with a single random EEG and provided interesting insights into the timing of the neurologic insult (Table 15–3).

TABLE 15–3   Electroencephalogram Versus Outcome

EEG	Outcome			
	Normal	Suspect	Abnormal	Died
1. Normal, mild, moderate abnormality X 1	35	6	2	3
2. Moderate abnormality > 2, marked abnormality	1	1	10	4

---

‡ Tharp B, Scher M, Clancy R. Unpublished observations.

All the infants with at least one markedly abnormal EEG had neurologic sequelae or died. At least one moderately abnormal EEG was recorded in 21 infants (excluding the four infants with markedly abnormal tracings); five infants were normal at follow-up, and 16 had neurologic sequelae (mental retardation and static motor syndromes), were suspect (developmental delay, subtle neurologic abnormalities), or died. However, when we considered infants with two or more moderately abnormal tracings at at least weekly intervals, an abnormal outcome was even more likely. Of 12 infants in the latter category, one was normal at follow-up, one was suspect, eight had neurologic sequelae, and two died in the neonatal period.

On the other hand, 37 infants had normal or mildly abnormal EEGs during the neonatal period: 31 were normal at follow-up, three were suspect, two were abnormal, and one died. Two of the latter three infants (abnormal and dead) had acquired neurologic syndromes that occurred after the last EEG was recorded. Therefore, serial normal neonatal EEGs were recorded in a single infant with neurologic sequelae. This infant had a benign clinical neonatal course as well. At three years of age he was found to have an IQ of 129 and spastic paraparesis, suggesting a congenital syndrome rather than an acquired perinatal disorder.

The timing of central nervous system damage was suggested by the trend of the EEG abnormalities. Figure 15–4 illustrates the serial EEGs in four infants with major sequelae. Deterioration of cerebral electrical activity appeared to occur at the onset of the encephalopathy, which was thought to be responsible for the child's chronic neurologic sequelae. In patient 8, intraventricular hemorrhage and a small intraparenchymal hemorrhage were detected by ultrasonography in the first week of life, yet the EEG (and the findings on the neurologic examination) remained normal until progressive hydrocephalus appeared. We believe that the combination of neurologic insults was responsible for the severe neurologic sequelae, and that the deterioration of the EEG reflects the point at which irreversible brain injury occurred. Patient 45 had chronic lung disease but remained neurologically normal until acute deterioration occurred at conceptional age 41 weeks as a result of pneumonia and severe hypoxia.

In some infants with perinatal asphyxia, the onset of the neurologic syndrome occurs at the time of delivery or earlier. For example, in subject 65 with clinical evidence of perinatal asphyxia (Apgar scores of 0/0/2), it is probable that the encephalopathy occurred at the time of delivery. The EEG obtained on day 2, however, was only moderately abnormal and contained positive rolandic sharp waves, an EEG pattern that is highly correlated with periventricular leukomalacia.

It usually takes several days or longer for positive rolandic sharp waves to appear in isolated cases of periventricular leukomalacia, suggesting that this infant's initial hypoxic ischemic event may have occurred several

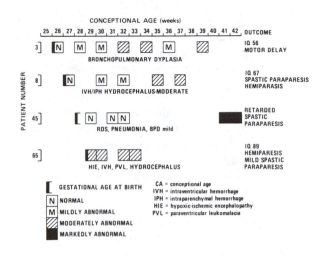

Figure 15–4   EEG results in four premature infants with neurologic sequelae. Presumed cause of encephalopathy noted under EEG results; neurologic findings at three-year examination listed at the right (see text for more details). (From Tharp B. The electroencephalographic aspects of ischemic-hypoxic encephalopathy and intraventricular hemorrhage. In: Yabuuch H, Watanabe K, Okada S, eds. Neonatal brain and behavior. Nagoya, Japan: University of Nagoya Press, 1987:71.)

days prior to delivery and that there were additional problems at birth accounting for the low Apgar scores.

We believe therefore that if they persist unchanged for several weeks, certain EEG patterns may reflect an already established encephalopathy, whereas others, particularly if they improve or are replaced by other types of abnormalities over the ensuing days or weeks, reflect a more dynamic, and therefore acute, process.

A particularly interesting result of this prospective study concerned the evolution of EEG abnormalities in infants with bronchopulmonary dysplasia. Patient 3 in Figure 15–4 illustrates the characteristic pattern of EEG deterioration that occurred in infants with bronchopulmonary dysplasia and neurologic sequelae. Bronchopulmonary dysplasia ocurred in 17 infants; four were left with sequelae and five died. A common EEG abnormality in the latter infants was a dysmature background, i.e., a background that was more typical of a conceptional age at least two weeks younger than the true conceptional age. When this dysmaturity persisted on serial records, a poor outcome ensued. Typically EEGs recorded in the first few weeks of life were normal. At 32 to 35 weeks the normal maturation of EEG background activity slowed, and by 37 to 40 weeks the EEG resembled that of an infant at least two to three weeks younger. Of the nine infants with persistently dysmature EEGs, two were suspect, three were abnormal at follow-up, and four died. The neonatal EEGs of eight infants with bronchopulmonary dysplasia were normal or contained other nonspecific abnormalities; four were normal, two were suspect, and one each were abnormal and died.

Neuropathologic examination of infants who die following bronchopulmonary dysplasia shows the spectrum of changes typical of hypoxic ischemic encephalopathy, including diffuse neuronal loss, periventricular

In some instances more subtle pathologic changes are seen, including a maturational arrest of neuronal growth, which we speculate might be the substrate of the arrest of electrophysiologic maturation we recorded with serial EEGs.[21]

Two neurologic syndromes have been described with bronchopulmonary dysplasia, one progressive and fatal and the second nonprogressive.[22-24] Intraventricular hemorrhage, pulmonary air leaks, and a prolonged hospital stay (suggesting more severe lung disease) have been associated with neurologic sequelae in infants with bronchopulmonary dysplasia.[23, 24] In our series intraventricular hemorrhage was relatively uncommon in infants with bronchopulmonary dysplasia, occurring in only one of the nine infants who died or suffered neurologic sequelae.

It is our impression that the encephalopathy is caused by chronic severe hypoxemia, exacerbated by episodes of more acute hypoxia and hypotension due to pneumothorax and perhaps complicated by nutritional and other metabolic factors.

Lombroso,[14] who originally described the clinical significance of dysmature, EEG background activity in a large series of patients with a variety of neurologic disturbances, reported results similar to ours. In his latest series, infants with transiently dysmature EEG background activity usually had good outcomes (26 of 32 infants), whereas persistent dysmaturity was followed by neurologic sequelae in 32 of 46 infants. His series did not specifically identify infants with bronchopulmonary dysplasia.

Persistently moderately abnormal EEGs in term infants with hypoxic-ischemic encephalopathy are also associated with poor neurologic outcomes.[1, 14, 25] The EEG is usually most disturbed immediately following the initial asphyxic insult at birth. There is gradual improvement in the EEG background even though permanent neuronal damage may have occurred. The cause of this apparent "normalization" is unknown. The initial EEG therefore should be recorded as close as possible to the peak of symptomatic neurologic impairment if an accurate prognostic statement is to be made. A mildly abnormal EEG obtained three weeks following a severe asphyxic event could lead to a falsely optimistic prognosis. A significantly abnormal EEG several weeks following an asphyxic event, however, is indicative of severe encephalopathy.[1, 25]

The Iatrogenically Paralyzed Infant

We and others have shown the value of routine EEGs in infants treated with neuromuscular blocking drugs.[9, 26, 27] The EEG is the only means of assessing the integrity of cerebral function in paralyzed infants, the majority of whom are in a high risk category because of compromised cardiopulmonary function. Many have had difficult deliveries and perinatal hypoxia, which predisposes them to intraventricular hemorrhage, hypoxic-ischemic encephalopathy, and periventricular leukomalacia. Seizures are also abundant in this group and can be identified in most instances only by the EEG. In our study of 40 paralyzed infants, seizures occurred in 16; eight infants had seizures only during the period of paralysis, which would have been missed if an EEG had not been performed.[9] We now recommend more continuous EEG monitoring of paralyzed newborns, particularly if they were asphyxiated at birth, have deterioration of the cardiopulmonary status during paralysis, demonstrate rhythmic fluctuations in vital signs and oxygenation (which may reflect the autonomic perturbations that occasionally accompany seizures[9, 27]), and if the initial EEG is moderately or markedly abnormal. Ideally all paralyzed infants should undergo continuous EEG surveillance.[4]

The Value of Electroencephalography in Identifying Specific Neurologic Disorders.

Although the majority of EEG abnormalities are nonspecific, a few patterns are highly correlated with specific neurologic disorders (Table 15-1). The EEG pattern per se may not be pathognomonic, but in association with a particular clinical course is suggestive of a specific disorder. The infant with a congenital malformation of the brain often has a markedly abnormal EEG yet may have relatively normal results on neurologic examination, mild or no dysmorphic features, and a history suggesting mild perinatal asphyxia (particularly when fetal monitoring is considered).[28] In the more severe forms of brain malformation, e.g., holoprosencephaly, a markedly abnormal and at times characteristic EEG pattern appears,[5] whereas in less severe anomalies the EEG abnormalities are less specific. Occasionally in an infant with a central nervous system malformation, an EEG is performed solely because of neonatal seizures. The marked disparity between the gross EEG abnormalities, the relatively normal-appearing infant, and the benign neonatal course should suggest the diagnosis and lead to neuroradiologic and genetic investigation.

Infants with congenital inborn errors of metabolism may develop markedly abnormal EEG patterns after beginning protein feeding. The history is usually that of an unremarkable pregnancy and perinatal period, followed by the gradual appearance of lethargy, vomiting, and seizures. A suppression burst or other markedly abnormal pattern in the EEG of an infant with this history suggests a metabolic problem. The EEG abnormalities are nonspecific, but occasional patterns such as that seen in maple syrup urine disease may suggest a specific disorder (unpublished personal observations).[29]

We recently described an EEG discharge, the positive rolandic sharp wave, in infants with deep white matter infarcts (periventricular leukomalacia in the premature) or necrosis (meningitis or metabolic disorders in term infants).[16,30] Positive rolandic sharp waves usually appear during the precystic stage of periventricular leukomalacia, commonly between the second and fourth weeks of life, when cranial ultrasound examination shows echodense periventricular lesions. These characteristic sharp waves appear several days or more after the onset of periventricular leukomalacia and therefore when present in the first few days of life suggest a prenatal onset, a not uncommon occurrence.[31,32] Several reports have suggested that prenatal events are often responsible for this disorder, which occurs in 5 to 10 percent of premature infants studied with serial head ultrasonography.[31-35]

Additionally, the presence of positive rolandic sharp waves in an infant with echodense lesions on ultrasonography should provoke a repeat scan in four to seven days and serially thereafter until the scan normalizes or cystic lesions appear. It is now well established that cystic lesions, particularly if they are extensive or located in the posterior periventricular region, are associated with major neurologic sequelae.[36,37] In our experience the presence of positive rolandic sharp waves on the EEG of an infant with periventricular leukomalacia suggests an extensive lesion and a poor long-term outcome.[30]

Persistent lateralized EEG abnormalities, particularly attenuation of background rhythms over one hemisphere, usually are associated with focal disease, i.e., hemorrhage and infarction.[38] The computed tomographic (CT) scan may be normal in the first few days after an acute cerebral infarction, whereas the EEG shows significant hemispheric electrical disturbance. In such a clinical setting a repeat CT scan in one week is warranted.[39] Focal seizures are also common in infants with perinatal cerebral infarctions.[40] If serial EEGs reveal that seizures are arising from one hemisphere, a CT scan is warranted.

Pathognomonic EEG patterns are seen in herpes encephalitis and are associated with a poor neurologic outcome.[41] There is usually no difficulty in ultimately arriving at the proper diagnosis in this infection, but often it is overlooked for days and treatment is delayed, particularly in infants presenting with focal seizures and a history of perinatal asphyxia.

VIDEO ELECTROENCEPHALOGRAPHIC MONITORING IN THE INTENSIVE CARE NURSERY

The newborn infant is subjected to a variety of stresses following delivery, particularly if delivery is premature. In order to assess the impact of postnatal events on cerebral function and determine their role in the development of a static encephalopathy, frequent intermittent or continuous EEG recording is necessary.*

Until recently continuous monitoring of the EEG was undertaken primarily to detect seizures in high risk infants and those receiving neuromuscular blocking drugs.[27,42] In the last few years several centers have initiated studies of the value of continuous monitoring in asphyxiated infants without seizures.[4,6,8] Two of these groups are using the interburst interval as an index of cerebral function in preterm infants.[4,6] As discussed earlier in this chapter, the EEG background normally is discontinuous in premature infants, with periods of continuous background lasting seconds to minutes, interrupted by low-voltage EEG activity or flat periods of variable duration (see Fig. 15–2). The length of these interburst intervals in normal infants is correlated with the conceptional age, longer intervals occurring in the younger premature infants. Normative data are now being collected in our laboratory in infants at different conceptional ages and are to be used as standard values for future studies of the use of the EEG in identifying infants with cerebral dysfunction. When an infant's brain is compromised, the interburst interval lengthens and exceeds the norms for conceptional age. This may become permanent and is classified as a suppression burst pattern. Transient increases in interburst interval occur when reversible disturbances of brain function occur, as from hypoxia or reduction of the cerebral blood flow.[4] Research presently being conducted in our laboratory concerns the impact of perturbations of gas exchange, cerebral blood flow, blood pressure, and caretaker manipulation on cerebral electrical activity (as quantified by the overall assessment of background rhythms using spectral analysis techniques and, more specifically, continuous measurement of interburst interval). Continuous EEG monitoring will be available to all infants undergoing extracorporeal membrane oxygenation therapy in order to determine the impact of changes in blood gas levels, perfusion pressures, and intrinsic events such as cerebral hemorrhages on brain integrity. It is anticipated that these measurements ultimately will be adapted to on-line computer surveillance of cerebral integrity. In the future continuous EEG monitoring should join transcutaneous gas monitors, arterial blood pressure measurements, electrocardiography, and heart rate recording as routine intensive care procedure.

The EEG is an excellent noninvasive technique for assessing the integrity of cerebral function in high-risk newborns. Serial recordings or continuous EEG monitoring usually identifies infants with significant encephalopathies who are likely to have neurologic sequelae and may provide critical information about the timing of the insult(s) responsible for the neurologic deficits seen at long-term follow-up. The EEG also may contain specific

---

* See reference 4 for a comprehensive review of video electroencephalographic recording in newborns.

patterns that are highly correlated with certain pathologic entities or may provoke further neurodiagnostic studies, such as CT scanning or metabolic evaluation. Neonatal intensive care units should have access to high-quality EEG facilities if comprehensive neurologic assessment is to be offered to high risk newborns and if the parents of these infants are to be provided with an accurate statement about the long-term outcomes of their infants. The EEG also provides valuable data to the neonatologist who is struggling with complex treatment issues of continuing support or invasive procedures in critically ill infants.

REFERENCES

1. Monod N, Pajot N, Quidasci S. The neonatal EEG: statistical studies and prognostic value in full-term and preterm babies. Electroencephalogr Clin Neurophysiol 1972; 32:529.
2. Tharp B, Cukier F, Monod N. The prognostic value of the electroencephalogram in premature infants. Electroencephalogr Clin Neurophysiol 1981; 51:219.
3. Mizrahi E, Kellaway P. Characterization and classification of neonatal seizures. Neurology 1987; 37:1837.
4. Tharp B. Intensive video/EEG monitoring of neonates. In: Gumnit RJ, ed. Advances in Neurology. New York: Raven Press, 1987:107.
5. Tharp B. Neonatal and pediatric electroencephalography. In: Aminoff M, ed. Electrodiagnosis in clinical neurology. New York: Churchill Livingstone, 1986:77.
6. Connell J, Oozeer R, Dubowitz V. Continuous 4-channel EEG monitoring: a guide to interpretation, with normal values, in preterm infants. Neuropediatrics 1987; 18:138.
7. Shewmon A, Krentler K. Off-line montage reformatting. Electroencephalogr Clin Neurophysiol 1984; 57:591.
8. Hellstrom-Westas L, Rosen I, Swenningsen N. Silent seizures in sick infants in early life. Acta Paediatr Scand 1985; 74:741.
9. Tharp B, Laboyrie P. The incidence of EEG abnormalities and outcome of infants paralyzed with neuromuscular blocking agents. Crit Care Med 1983; 11:926.
10. Holmes G. Morphological and physiological maturation of the brain in the neonate and young child. J Clin Neurophysiol 1986; 3:209.
11. Ellingson R, Peters J. Development of EEG and daytime sleep patterns in normal full-term infants during the first 3 months of life: longitudinal observations. Electroencephalogr Clin Neurophysiol 1980; 49:112.
12. Watanabe K, Iwase K. Spindle-like fast rhythms in the EEGs of low birth weight infants. Dev Med Child Neurol 1972; 14:373.
13. Ellingson R, Peters J. Development of EEG and daytime sleep patterns in trisomy-21 infants during first year of life: longitudinal observations. Electroencephalogr Clin Neurophysiol 1980; 50:457.
14. Lombroso C. Neonatal polygraphy in full-term and premature infants: a review of normal and abnormal findings. J Clin Neurophysiol 1985; 2:105.
15. Coen R, Tharp B. Neonatal electroencephalography. Adv Perinatal Med 1985; 4:278.
16. Clancy R, Tharp B, Enzmann D. EEG in premature infants with intraventricular hemorrhage. Neurology 1984; 34:583.
17. Tharp B. The electroencephalographic aspects of ischmic hypoxic encephalopathy and intraventricular hemorrhage. In: Yabuuchi H, Watanabe K, Okada S, eds. Neonatal brain and behavior. Nagoya, Japan: University of Nagoya Press, 1987:71.
18. Holmes G, Rowe J, Hafford J, et al. Prognostic value of the EEG in neonatal asphyxia. Electroencephalogr Clin Neurophysiol 1982; 53:60.
19. Pezzani C, Radvanyi-Bouvet M, Relier J, Monod N. Neonatal electroencephalography during the first twenty-four hours of life in full-term newborn infants. Neuropediatrics 1986; 17:11.
20. Brand M, Bignami A. The effects of chronic hypoxia on the neonatal and infantile brain. Brain 1969; 92:233.
21. Takashima S, Becker L, et al. Retardation of neuronal maturation in premature infants compared with term infants of the same postconceptional age. Pediatrics 1982; 69:33.
22. Ellison P, Farina M. Progressive central nervous system deterioration: a complication of advanced chronic lung disease of prematurity. Ann Neurol 1980; 8:43.
23. Lifschitz M, Seilheimer D, Wilson G, et al. Neurodevelopmental status of low birth weight infants with bronchopulmonary dysplasia requiring prolonged oxygen supplementation. J Perinatol 1987; 7:127.
24. Campbell L, McAlister W, Volpe J. Neurological aspects of bronchopulmonary dysplasia. Clin Pediatr 1988; 27:7.
25. Watanabe K, Miyazaki S, Hara K, Hakamada S. Behavioral state cycle, background EEGs and prognosis of newborns with perinatal hypoxia. Electroencephalogr Clin Neurophysiol 1980; 49:618.
26. Staudt F, Roth J, Engel R. The usefulness of electroencephalography in curarized newborns. Electroencephalogr Clin Neurophysiol 1981; 51:205.
27. Goldberg R, Goldman S, Ramsay R, Feller R. Detection of seizure activity in the paralyzed neonate using continuous monitoring. Pediatrics 1982; 69:583.
28. Garite T, Linzey E, Freeman R, et al. Fetal heart rate patterns and fetal distress in fetuses with congenital anamolies. Obstet Gynecol 1979; 53:716.
29. Vidailhet M, Brocard O, Weber N. Aspects electro-cliniques des leucinoses. Rev Electroencephalogr Neurophysiol Clin 1978; 8:61.
30. Novotny E, Tharp B, Coen R, et al. Positive rolandic sharp waves in the EEG of the premature infant. Neurology 1987; 37:1481.
31. Bejar R, Vigliocco G, Solana C, et al. Prenatal white matter necrosis in multiple gestations. Ann Neurol 1987; 22:424.
32. Roland E, Norman M, Hill A. Antenatal periventricular white matter infarction. Ann Neurol 1987; 22:423.
33. Leviton A, Gilles F, Neff R, Yaney P. Multivariate analysis of risk of perinatal telencephalic leukoencephalopathy. Am J Epidemiol 1976; 104:621.
34. Gilles F, Leviton A, Kerr C. Endotoxin leukoencephalopathy in the telencephalon of the newborn kitten. J Neurol Sci 1976; 27:183.
35. Calvert S, Hoskins E, Fong K, Forsyth S. Etiological factors associated with the development of periventricular leukomalacia. Acta Paediatr Scand 1987; 76:254.
36. DeVries L, Dubowitz L, Dubowitz V, et al. Predictive value of cranial ultrasound in the newborn baby: a reappraisal. Lancet 1985; 2:137.
37. Guzzetta F, Shackleford G, Volpe S, et al. Periventricular intraparenchymal echodensities in the premature infant: critical determinant of neurologic outcome. Pediatrics 1986; 78:995.
38. Scher M, Tharp B, Sylvestri L. Significance of focal abnormalities in neonatal electroencephalograms: radiological correlation and outcome. Ann Neurol 1982; 12:217.
39. Mannino F, Trauner D. Stroke in neonates. J Pediatr 1983; 102:605.
40. Levy S, Abroms I, Marshall P, Rosquete E. Seizures and cerebral infarction in the full-term newborn. Ann Neurol 1985; 17:366.
41. Mizrahi E, Tharp B. A characteristic EEG pattern in neonatal herpes simplex encephalitis. Neurology 1982; 32:1215.
42. Coen R, McCutchen C, Wermer O, et al. Continuous monitoring of the electroencephalogram following perinatal asphyxia. J Pediatr 1982; 100:628.

16

New Noninvasive Technologies to Evaluate Brain Function

William D. Rhine, M.D., Ricardo R. González-Méndez, Ph.D., and
David K. Stevenson, M.D.

Cerebral Blood Flow Measurement
   Positron Emission Tomography
   Technical Considerations
   Single Photon Emission Computed Tomography
   Other Noninvasive Technologies to Measure
      Cerebral Blood Flow
Cerebral Metabolism and Biochemistry
   Nuclear Magnetic Resonance Spectroscopy
   Theory
   Neonatal Studies
   Related Studies
   Technical Considerations
   Positron Emission Tomographic Scanning
Measurement of Cerebral Oxygenation
Recommendations

Noninvasive technologies are available to assess brain function as well as structure. As with their imaging counterparts described elsewhere in this book, the techniques to evaluate function have depended on the extension to biologic applications of well-established techniques in chemistry and physics. The first applications of noninvasive methods in neonates were developed to measure cerebral blood flow. The impetus to study cerebral blood flow came in large part from the desire to understand the relationship between cerebral blood flow and intraventricular hemorrhage, which occurs in approximately 40 percent of premature infants with birth weights less than 1,500 gm. Further understanding of cerebral blood flow and metabolism becomes important with the development of extracorporeal membrane oxygenation, a treatment that is used in babies whose internal carotid arteries are permanently ligated to permit prolonged cardiopulmonary bypass. Recently the use of nuclear magnetic resonance (NMR) spectroscopy to study human subjects has enabled physicians to start investigating a wider range of cerebral functions noninvasively. The other noninvasive technology applied to human neonates to date has been near infrared light absorption studies to measure cerebral oxygenation status.

CEREBRAL BLOOD FLOW MEASUREMENT

Neonatologists have long sought the means to measure cerebral blood flow in newborns. Understanding cerebral blood flow provides a cornerstone in understanding the neuropathologic conditions common to neonates, especially premature infants: intraventricular hemorrhage, periventricular leukomalacia, and porencephalic cysts. Kety and Schmidt[1] first measured cerebral blood flow in adults in the 1940s on the basis of inhaled nitrous oxide uptake by the brain. Later studies applied this technique to children.[2] However, because this invasive method required repeated jugular venous sampling, it had limited applicability to neonates. The same measurements later were made noninvasively by positron emission tomography (PET). Other techniques using plethysmography, both venous occlusion and electrical impedance, have since been developed to measure the cerebral blood flow in neonates. Finally, cerebral blood flow also can be determined by Doppler flow ultrasound studies and in the future may be measurable by NMR imaging techniques (see Chapter 17).

Positron Emission Tomography

PET starts with the introduction of a positron emitting isotope, e.g. ^{11}C, ^{15}O, or ^{133}Xe, by either injection or inhalation. When a positron emitted from the isotrope strikes a nearby electron, two gamma-rays are released at 180 degrees to each other. A concentric scintillation detector then measures simultaneous gamma-rays and calculates isotope concentrations for a specified location within the detection field. Computed calculations similar to those of conventional x-ray computed tomographic (CT) scanning are used to reconstruct two-dimensional images of the isotope accumulation. The earliest studies described the use of PET to measure the cerebral blood flow in adults and animals.

Lou et al[3] first used PET to measure cerebral blood flow in neonates in 1977. Eight newborns, most with respiratory distress, underwent PET studies using ^{133}Xe injected intra-arterially. Cerebral blood flow values ranged from 17 to 55 ml per 100 gm per minute, and the cerebral blood flow was shown to vary with the systemic blood pressure. A larger population of 19 newborns had a mean cerebral blood flow of 40 ml per 100 gm per minute, compared with an average of 64 in adults.[4] The variance of cerebral blood flow with systemic blood pressure in all weight groups suggested that cerebral blood flow may not be well autoregulated in distressed newborns. Another study by the same group showed that the cerebral blood flow decreased with bicarbonate infusion;[5] this could have significant implications in neonatal resuscitation, in which bicarbonate is frequently administered.

Ment et al[6] described PET studies in 16 babies with birth weights less than 1,250 gm using inhalation of [133]Xe. They were able to distinguish the cerebral blood flow of each brain hemisphere. In four of five patients with asymmetrical intraventricular hemorrhages, the side with the highest cerebral blood flow had the worse bleed. Younkin et al[7] used eight scintillation detectors simultaneously to measure the cerebral blood flow within specific regions of the neonatal brain. A more recent comparison of ^{133}Xe inhalation PET and Doppler flow measurement of the cerebral blood flow showed a correlation of PET values with Doppler mean flow velocity, with the end diastolic flow velocity, and, less well, with the pulsatility index.[8]

Volpe et al[9] injected [15]O in water as a positron emitting isotope in newborns and correlated the cerebral blood flow measurements with available neuropathologic findings. On the basis of adult baboon studies, they calculated that [15]O PET estimated the cerebral blood flow within 5 percent of the values obtained by direct invasive measurement. [15]O has the advantage of depending on the blood-brain barrier partition coefficient of water, versus that of xenon, which is not a biologically abundant or important compound. The blood-brain partition coefficient of water has been shown to change less than 5 percent in rats after hypoxic ischemic injury. In this first study cerebral blood flow measurements were lower than those estimated by previous xenon studies.[9] However, this was due in part to a more sick patient population and in part to a technical artifact known as partial voluming. In one infant with hypoxic ischemic encephalopathy, PET with [15]O during a seizure showed an increased flow to the hemisphere with the seizure focus (80 versus 57 ml per 100 gm per minute).[10] In asphyxiated newborns [15]O PET

has shown a decrease (25 to 50 percent reduction) in parasagittal flow compared with flow in the sylvian cortex (Fig. 16–1).[11] This provides evidence that the area with the most impaired flow is the cerebrovascular area at greatest risk for intraventricular hemorrhage.

Technical Considerations

Positron emission tomography requires transport and stabilization of the newborn to the scintillation detector and adequate sedation for the duration of cerebral blood flow measurement. With the use of short-lived radioactive isotopes, radiation exposure can be reduced to less than that of a chest x-ray exposure. However, most of these isotopes require a nearby cyclotron for preparation. The spatial resolution of PET is limited to 2 to 3 cm for ^{133}Xe and 1 to 1.5 cm for [15]O. PET is not very effective in evaluating posterior cerebral circulation and cannot distinguish extracerebral flow.[12] [15]O PET requires frequent blood sampling, e.g., every five seconds, to correct for its rapid radioactive decay; this technology therefore by definition is invasive.

Single Photon Emission Computed Tomography

A newly developed technology related to PET scanning is single photon emission computed tomography (SPECT). SPECT utilizes inhaled or injected radioactive tracers such as iodine or xenon that emit single photons that are detected by several detectors surrounding the patient. These tracers are attached to compounds that can pass through the blood-brain barrier, e.g., I[123] iodoamphetamine. The data obtained are processed using computed tomographic techniques and images then can be constructed in any plane. Resolution of SPECT images is now approaching 3 to 5 mm. Besides determining cerebral blood flow, SPECT can be used to study other aspects of cerebral metabolism once radioactive labeling can be added to specific markers of metabolism. SPECT has been used to study cerebral changes associated with Alzheimer's disease, schizophrenia, and aphasia in adults.[13-16] SPECT has yet to be used to study neonates, probably because higher resolution equipment is only now becoming available. SPECT has the advantage over PET in that SPECT does not require a cyclotron to produce labeled compounds of interest.

Other Noninvasive Technologies to Measure Cerebral Blood Flow

Venous occlusion plethysmography (VOP) is used to estimate cerebral blood flow on the basis of expansion of the relatively mobile neonatal skull after occlusion of

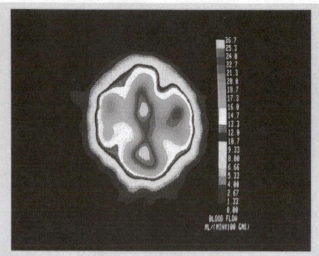

Patient 9

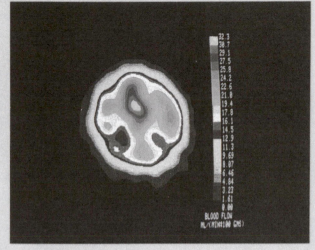

Patient 16

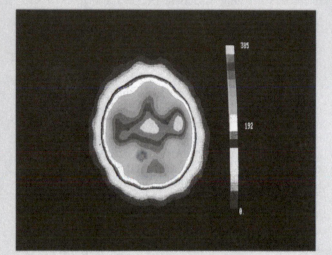

Patient 13

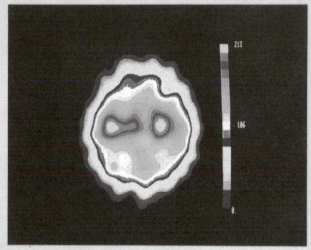

Patient 14

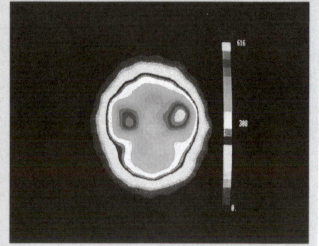

Patient 17

Figure 16–1   Positron emission tomographic measurements of regional cerebral blood flow in five infants with clinically overt hypoxic ischemic encephalopathy. Actual values of cerebral blood flow were obtained for patients 9 and 16. (From Volpe JJ, et al. Positron emission tomography in the asphyxiated newborn. Ann Neurol 1985; 17:287.)

the jugular veins.[17-19] Skull expansion is measured by a strain gauge encircling the skull. VOP provides only an estimate of the total cranial flow because it cannot distinguish between extracerebral and intracerebral blood flow. Furthermore, cranial venous return outside the jugular veins via the vertebral veins is not accounted for and may increase significantly with jugular occlusion. Partial occlusion of the carotid arteries during venous occlusion would lead to erroneously low estimates of the cerebral blood flow. Finally, the hazards of handling sick newborns and possibly increasing intracranial pressure, albeit transiently, have limited clinical acceptability of VOP.

Electrical impedance plethysmography has been used for many years to measure flow in organs, including the brain.[20] Use of this technique to measure cerebral blood flow, known as rheoencephalography, has been modified for application in neonates.[21] This technique requires placement of four small electrodes over the scalp. Constant current, usually 100 Hz, is applied through two electrodes while voltage changes are measured in the other two, thereby allowing calculations of changes in impedance over time. Changes in impedance have been shown to correlate with cerebrovascular resistance and flow. These changes have to be corrected for changes caused by respiration and movement. Mochalova[22] used rheoencephalography in 37 "healthy" newborns to estimate the cerebral blood flow, with mean values of 36 ml per 100 gm per minute on the first day of life and 41 ml per 100 gm per minute on the fourth to fifth day. Induction of hypercapnia by inhalation of carbon dioxide–rich gas caused variable changes in cerebral blood flow but seemed to increase the flow in offspring of mothers with late toxemia. Weindling et al[23] have shown changes in impedance with the onset of pneumothorax, during an exchange transfusion, and even during feedings. Electrical impedance plethysmography can be carried out at the bedside and has not demonstrated any adverse side effects, such as heating from the electrical current. It does not distinguish intracerebral from extracerebral flow, nor can it compare flow between hemispheres.

CEREBRAL METABOLISM AND BIOCHEMISTRY

Nuclear Magnetic Resonance Spectroscopy

In recent years magnetic resonance imaging (MRI) has become accepted as a clinical tool (see Chapter 17). Magnetic resonance spectroscopy (MRS) has shown that many important biochemical processes can be monitored in vivo. In some cases there have been observations of changes in molecular processes in pathologic states. Although most studies have used animal models, some studies involving human neonates have been carried out. Therefore, MRS has shown the potential for becoming a useful clinical tool to observe molecular biochemistry in a dynamic way.

Theory

The following is an elementary description of MRS in vivo. For a more detailed description the reader should refer to references 24 to 26.

A nucleus with a magnetic moment can absorb energy at a specific frequency when placed in a strong magnetic field. The energy used for in vivo MRS, at existing magnetic field strengths (1.5 to 2.3 telsa), lies in the radiofrequency range. This energy is very small, roughly 10^{10} times less than that used for x-ray examination. What makes this technique useful is that one can observe slightly different resonance frequencies for nuclei of the same type, depending on the surrounding atoms, therefore obtaining very useful chemical species information. For example, one can observe a separate signal for each of the three phosphorous nuclei of ATP, since each nucleus is slightly different from the others from an electronic standpoint. Usually a reference signal is selected (e.g., phosphocreatine [PCr] in the ^{31}P spectra of brain, heart, and muscle), and the "chemical shift," the difference between the signal of interest and the reference signal, is determined. Since the chemical shift in terms of frequency is dependent on the magnetic field strength surrounding the sample, the chemical shift is expressed in terms of parts per million. This allows for comparison of chemical shifts obtained in different MRS instruments.

The area (intensity) of an MRS peak, but not the height, is directly proportional to the concentration of nuclei contributing to the peak. If the concentration of nuclei contributing to resonance (e.g., N-acetylaspartate in the ^{1}H spectra of the brain) is known, it can be used to calculate the concentration of other resonances in the spectrum. A set of important NMR parameters are the relaxation times T_1 (spin-lattice) and T_2 (spin-spin). They affect the signal intensities and widths of MRS measurements. When a sample has absorbed, there are radiationless processes by which the energy dissipates and the nuclei return to the unperturbed state. Since there is no emission of energy in MRS, all the energy is dissipated as heat (to be discussed).

Because of the specific properties of each nucleus and their varying natural abundances, different nuclear species have different sensitivities. Table 16–1 illustrates this fact. It is easily seen why proton MRI has developed so rapidly. With the water ^{1}H concentration of 110 M in human tissues, with the highest sensitivity and 100 percent natural abundance, one can see that this will translate into some extremely high signal-to-noise ratios. However, given the highly specific biochemical information that can be obtained from other nuclei, it is well worth the effort to pursue that knowledge.

It should be noted that nuclei with spins larger than ½ undergo a much faster type of relaxation, and therefore have much broader lines, but that signal averaging can occur much faster, making up for their lower sensitivity. Most aspects of biologic MRS and MRI have been reviewed recently.[26-28]

The nucleus most studied by in vivo MRS to date is ^{31}P. Because of the ability to detect molecules such as ATP, PCr, and inorganic phosphate (P_i), phosphorous MRS can be used to study cerebral energy metabolism. Furthermore, the signal of the P_i has proven extremely useful for the noninvasive study of pH. It has been

TABLE 16-1   Properties of Biologically Relevant Visible Nuclei

Nucleus	Natural Abundance	Relative Sensitivity
^{1}H	99.98	100.00
^{13}C	1.11	1.59
^{14}N	99.60	0.04
^{15}N	0.37	0.10
^{19}F	100.00	83.30
^{23}Na	100.00	9.25
^{31}P	100.00	6.63
^{39}K	93.10	0.01

From James TL. Nuclear magnetic resonance in biochemistry: principles and applications. New York: Academic Press, 1975.

shown that the chemical shift of the P_i, when referenced to another signal such as PCr, correlates extremely well with intracellular pH (pH_i).[29] This method has been shown to correlate well with classic methods for measuring the pH_i.[30-31] Although the absolute pH can be determined only to ± 0.1 pH unit, changes in pH of 0.05 unit can be detected in vivo. Among the parameters determined from ^{31}P MRS, the parameter most often reported is the PCr/P_i ratio, an index of the sufficiency of oxygen and of oxidative phosphorylation.[32,33] The ATP level also has been used as an index to determine the sufficiency of overall cellular energy metabolism.

Neonatal Studies*

Cady et al[35] first reported the application of MRS to investigate human brain energy metabolism in 1983, claiming that the PCr/P_i ratio was low (0.2 to 1.0) in neonates (37, 39, and 40 weeks gestational age) studied 42, 44, and 50 hours after severe birth asphyxia. Each was studied more than once, two of them several times—up to 26 days of life in one case. Thus, the few serial data relating to these babies may provide some preliminary information about intrasubject variability, but interpretation remains limited. Moreover, these data are uninterpretable biologically, because no physiologic data are presented. The PCr/P_i ratios in four other infants are presented; none of the children was normal, although one (infant 7) is believed by the authors to have had a normal brain (PCr/P_i ratio, 1.7). The diagnosis of questionable congenital muscular dystrophy is consistent with having a normal brain, but the information provided in the report is insufficient to exclude congenital muscular dystrophy associated with cerebral nervous system abnormalities (e.g., the Fukuyama type).

Furthermore, the requirement for mechanical ventilation is less common in congenital muscular dystrophy, and its use for infant 7, as well as the child's immaturity (33 weeks' gestational age) and "germinal layer hemorrhage," places the subject at high risk for also having brain injury and neurodevelopmental problems. Although infant 7 weighed 1,620 gm at birth, even a small subependymal intraventricular hemorrhage may be associated with an increased risk of impaired development, as has been suggested in a recent review of the correlation of echoencephalographic findings and neurodevelopmental outcome in infants with birth weights of 1,000 gm or less.[36] Thus, the article by Cady et al[35] stands as a landmark of the application of MRS to study the human brain, but it can go no further than to record the fact that the ^{31}P MRS spectrum of the neonatal brain can be determined and to suggest what might be possible in terms of future applications.

In 1984 Hope et al[37] reported a small controlled study comparing the ratios of phosphorous metabolites and pH in six normal and 10 asphyxiated infants (Fig. 16-2). That asphyxiated and normal infants could be differentiated on the basis of changes in PCr and P_i builds on the earlier anecdotal experience. However, the study represents nothing more than an expanded version of the original survey.[35] Interpretation is again limited because the control group is small, presumably represents a collection of chronologically older prematurely born infants and term infants (16 hours to 97 days of age), and assumes that term gestation–equivalent age ensures comparability with term gestation infants. Despite the reasonable nature of the assumption, no data have been presented to support it. Moreover, anyone who has cared for very low birth weight infants (even those who may appear perfectly normal by neurobehavioral examination) must doubt this assumption prima facie, because of the poor extrauterine growth commonly evidenced by such infants when they are compared at a postconceptual age of "term" with infants born at full gestation. The authors express appropriate perplexity about the fact that the mean PCr/P_i ratio of the asphyxiated infants was normal on the first day of life and later was not; lack of clinical data makes it impossible to evaluate the physiologic significance of the nadir PCr/P_i ratio, which occurred over a wide range of times (16 hours to nine days). For example, the role of post-asphyxial cerebral edema, typically peaking over the first several days of life, remains obscure. Although this article concludes that the low PCr/P_i ratios may portend death or serious injury, the design of the study does not test this hypothesis, and thus its findings should not serve as the basis for any prognostication.

In 1986 a survey of infants with increased cerebral echodensities found a positive correlation of PCr/P_i with gestational plus postnatal age, and an association between a low PCr/P_i ratio and gross neurologic outcome among infants with increased cerebral echodensities.[38]

---

* Most of this section is derived from González-Méndez R, Stevenson DK, Jardetzky O. NMR in biology and medicine: spectroscopy in vivo. Magn Reson Med Biol (in press).

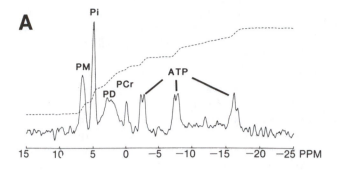

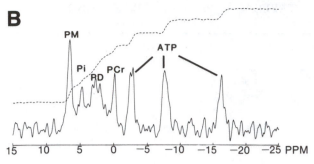

Figure 16-2 ^{31}P NMR spectrum recorded from *A*, normal full-term infant 16 hours old and *B*, full-term infant 48 hours old following severe birth asphyxia. The x-axis is chemical shift in parts per million and the y-axis is signal intensity. ATP = adenosine triphosphate (from right to left, β, α, and γ); PCr = phosphocreatine; PD = phosphodiester and phospholipids; Pi = inorganic orthophosphate; PM = phosphomonoester, mainly phosphoethanolamine. The interrupted line is the integral of the spectrum. (From Hope PI, Reynolds. Investigation of cerebral energy metabolism in newborn infants by phosphorous nuclear magnetic resonance spectroscopy. Clin Perinatol 1985; 12:261. Data from Hope PL, Costello AM de L, Cady EB, et al. Cerebral energy with phosphorous NMR spectroscopy in normal and birth-asphyxiated infants. Lancet 1984; 2:366.)

Interpretations of the presentation is difficult for several reasons:

1. The subjects with increased cerebral echodensities represented a fraction (less than half) of a group of infants whose lesions were not characterized or graded with respect to severity; they were heterogeneous developmentally and diagnostically; they were exclusive of other infants with similar cerebral echodensities based on temporal considerations.
2. Although the measurement of energy metabolism may be assumed to be the physiologic "bottom line," it is notable that no attempt was made to analyze for possible confounding variables (e.g., maternal high risk factors); however, the sample size was probably too small to make possible a meaningful analysis in this regard.
3. Besides death and autopsy findings, neurodevelopmental data were completely lacking. Prima facie, the follow-up was inadequate, as it was apparently less than three years in all infants and less than one year in some.

Within the United States, the researchers at Children's Hospital in Philadelphia have reported the most experience with the use of NMR spectroscopy to study neonates.[39-40] In their initial study of six asphyxiated newborns, they also showed falls in the intracellular pH level in the brain, with an average nadir of 7.1 ±0.1 (SD). However, the nadir for the PCr/P_i ratio was 1.3, significantly higher than that reported in England. This may be explained by differences in the severity of the asphyxia and/or population variability.

From a critical perspective most clinical studies, such as those just briefly discussed, have not been adequately designed, and the data have been too scanty to decide whether PCr/P_i or some other MRS measure of cellular well-being will be a predictor of neurodevelopmental outcome among human neonates, or of tissue

injury. The authors deserve credit for their pioneering work and promise in this regard.[35,37-39, 40] However, if MRS is destined to have a role eventually in clinical practice, this future will not be fulfilled unless appropriate attention is given to sample size (relative to the sort of effect that is being looked for and the differences that would be clinically important). In statistical language, failure to consider sample size makes type II errors* more likely and leads to a tendency to overestimate true differences when they occur. Moreover, when study design is considered, it should be remembered that repeated measurements over time may increase the risk of type I errors.[†41,42] The preceding comments assume the use of procedures to "blind" the investigators (as much as this is possible) to the independent variables, so that the dependent outcomes could not possibly bear even the unconscious systematic influence of the researchers. As clinical interventions are tested (e.g., mannitol), the additional required ingredient of randomization must complete the design of good clinical investigation. In summary, the positive and negative predictive accuracies of the PCr/P_i ratio for neurodevelopmental outcome in human neonates have yet to be defined, and the usefulness of MRS as a clinical monitoring technique has yet to be estalished.

Related Studies

An early use of NMR spectroscopy in humans studied ^{31}P energetics in muscle as a marker for myopathies.[43] The ability to study other organs depended on technical improvements that provided an adequate bore of the magnet. A recent report of metabolic disease

---

* A false acceptance of the null hypothesis; that is, an acceptance of the null hypothesis when in fact an alternative hypothesis is true.
† A false rejection of the null hypothesis; that is, a rejection of the null hypothesis when in fact it is true.

recognizable by NMR spectroscopy outside the neonatal period was that of a 15-year-old girl with mitochondrial encephalomyopathy.[44] [31]P spectra were abnormal in both brain and muscle, which correlated with histochemical and electron microscopic studies of a muscle biopsy specimen. As more centers develop the ability to perform NMR spectroscopy, we would anticipate more studies of brain cellular metabolism in children and adults.

Numerous studies have used NMR spectroscopy to study brain physiology in animals. Most have examined ^{31}P spectra to evaluate energy metabolism and intracellular pH. Studies in newborn animals have evaluated normal development as well as pathologic states, including cerebral ischemia, hypoxia, hypotension, brain edema, seizures, hypercarbia, hypothermic cardiac arrest, bilirubin injury, and hypoglycemia (Fig. 16–3).[45-60] Species studied included rats, gerbils, rabbits, lambs, monkeys, and dogs.[51, 53-59] High resolution ^{1}H spectroscopy to evaluate metabolites such as lactate has been used in animal brains, sometimes in conjunction with ^{31}P NMR spectroscopy (Fig. 16–4).[48,60,61] [31]P spectroscopy also has been used to study phototoxicity of a hematoporphyrin derivative in the cat brain.[62] This might be applicable to human neonates with hyperbilirubinemia when treatment with metalloporphyrins becomes available.[63] ^{19}F NMR spectroscopy has been used to study the effects and kinetics of anesthetics in animal brains.[64] In this study the authors demonstrate several of the pitfalls of MRS in vivo that can lead to erroneous conclusions, and the way to avoid such pitfalls is demonstrated. ^{15}N NMR spectroscopy potentially can be used to evaluate protein synthesis in various organs, including the brain, using labeled amino acids as precursors of protein synthesis. ^{13}C-labeled compounds have been used to study liver biochemistry.

Technical Considerations

NMR spectroscopy has only begun to be applied clinically to the field of neonatology, mainly as a research tool. Broader use will depend on increased understanding of potential applications, based on the types of animal research in this field already described. There are important technical considerations that will also limit the spread of this new technology. NMR magnets are expensive; at the high field strengths needed for spectroscopy, with a bore large enough to study humans, an MRI/MRS instrument with its associated facilities costs over $2 million. These strong magnets have fringe fields that require special siting and physical shielding from metal objects; therefore they require an abundance of associated space. Even with shielding, these magnets cannot be used in close proximity to most ferrous objects, which would be drawn into the magnet at great risk to the patient. Furthermore, NMR equipment requires a special radiofrequency shielded room to prevent interference by external radiofrequency sources.

For the sick newborn, this applies to the incubator providing warmth, intravenous lines and pumps, ventilator support, and cardiopulmonary monitoring. The latter can be accomplished with nonferrous electrocardiographic leads. All necessary monitoring equipment must be optically coupled to the patient in order to prevent interference with the NMR spectrum, and to prevent the radiofrequency from producing damage to the monitoring unit. Babies also have to be screened for the presence of loose metallic objects such as identification bands and snaps on clothes. Appropriate sedation or restraints must be used, because NMR spectroscopic studies take 60 minutes or more, during which time the baby must be still.

Because of the need to shield them from radiofrequency and metallic objects, most NMR facilities are at a distance from the intensive care nursery, frequently in another building. Therefore, the nursery has to provide adequate transport for the baby, who has to be stable enough for transport. Supplies for full resuscitation have

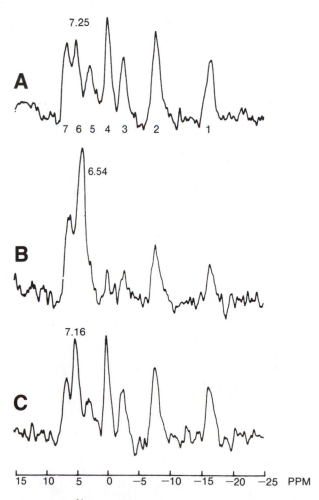

Figure 16–3 ^{31}P spectra (148 scans at two-second intervals) during and after cerebral ischemia. *A*, Control; *B*, after clipping carotid arteries and reduction of mean arterial blood pressure to 15 mm Hg; *C*, 3½ hours after reperfusion of brain. Estimated intracellular pH values are indicated beside inorganic phosphate resonance. (From Delpy DT, et al. Noninvasive investigation of cerebral ischemia by phosphorous nuclear magnetic resonance. Pediatrics 1982; 70:310.)

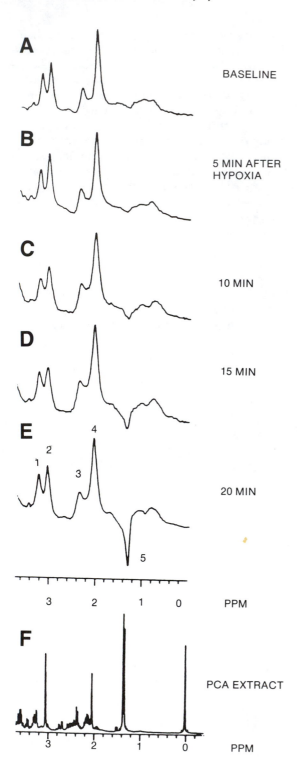

EEG

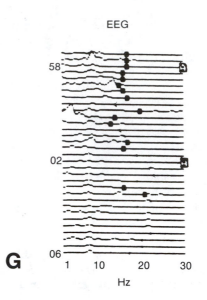

G

BASELINE

5 MIN AFTER
HYPOXIA

10 MIN

15 MIN

20 MIN

PPM

PCA EXTRACT

PPM

Figure 16-4 ^{1}H NMR spectra of a hypoxic rat brain. *A*, In vivo NMR spectrum of a normal rat brain. *B*, five minutes after initiation of hypoxia; *C*, 10 minutes after; *D*, 15 minutes after; *E*, 20 minutes after. *F*, Quantitative in vitro NMR spectrum of the extracted brain metabolites. *G*, Electroencephalographic recording of the brain during hypoxia showing decreased brain activity at the end of the experiment. Signal assignments are as follows: 1, choline/phosphoryl choline; 2, creatine/creatine phosphate; 3, glutamate; 4, *N*-acetylaspartate; 5, lactate. (From Chang L -H, et al. Comparison of concentration determinations in ischemic and hypoxic rat brains by in vivo and in vitro ^{1}H NMR spectroscopy. Magn Reson Med 1987; 4:575.

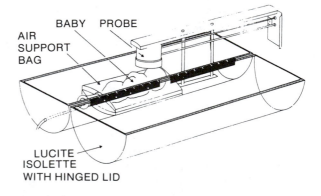

Figure 16-5 Isolette designed for use in the magnet. The baby is swaddled in an infant blanket placed on a heated mattress, and positioned with the temporo parietal region under a 4 cm diameter radiofrequency surface coil. The isolette allows continuous visual observation. In addition, heart rate, respiratory rate, transcutaneous oxygen, and electroencephalogram can be monitored. If necessary, no mechanical ventilation can be continued during measurements. (From Younkin DP, et al. Unique aspects of human cerebral metabolism evaluated with phosphorus nuclear magnetic resonance spectroscopy. Ann Neurol 1984; 16:581.)

to be available at the NMR facility. With careful planning, NMR facilities for both imaging and spectroscopy have been built in close proximity to an intensive care nursery (Fig. 16–5).[40] The development of self-shielded superconductive magnet technology can lead to the removal of many siting constraints. Because of the smaller size that babies have, small bore research magnets (30 to 40 cm clear bore) have been available to study neonates for almost six years. Currently one can obtain a high field (2 to 4.7 telsa), self-shielded magnet (5 gauss line of fringe field at less than 6 feet) with a 40 to 50 cm bore that can perform both imaging and spectroscopy. Owing to the small size of the bore, only infants can be examined. Because of the small fringe field, the need for shielding from ferrous objects would be minimal. Owing to its small size, such a magnet could be sited in a standard-size hospital room, requiring only radiofrequency shielding and access for cryogens. Such a "neonatal" MR unit would be significantly cheaper and could be sited within the nursery, or next door to it, thereby obviating the need for transport of the babies. This unit would be fully dedicated to the nursery. Also the exponential growth of computer technology to handle larger databases more quickly will allow use of more rapid and higher resolution MRS.

Finally, in regard to the issue of safety, no ill side effects are known to be caused by MRS. However, because all the energy absorbed is dissipated as heat, there may be some risk of burns from overheating. To prevent such burns, the Food and Drug Administration has instituted guidelines for the specific absorption rate of radiofrequency. One should use caution in carrying out spectroscopy because these specific absorption rates are based on studies done in adults, and the models used by most manufacturers to calculate specific absorption rates are relatively crude.

Positron Emission Tomographic Scanning

PET can also be used to study cerebral metabolism as well as blood flow. PET using ^{18}F-deoxyglucose has been used to measure cerebral metabolic rates in adults. [11]C can be used to measure other aspects of cerebral physiology such as glucose metabolism; however, this has not yet been described in newborns. PET metabolic studies are still not generally available to newborns owing to the high dose of radiation involved.

MEASUREMENT OF CEREBRAL OXYGENATION

Brazy et al[65] recently have described a noninvasive optical method to measure cerebral oxygenation, named near infrared oxygen sufficiency scope or NIROS-SCOPE. NIROS-SCOPE measures skin absorption of

three or four near infrared lasers at fixed frequencies, which correlate with quantities of hemoglobin, both deoxygenated and oxygenated, and cytochrome aa3. Cytochrome aa3 is a primary enzyme involved in oxidative phosphorylation in mitochondria. Measurement of near infrared absorption, along with calculations of total blood volume, provides an index of cerebral oxygenation status (Fig. 16–6). Recovery of cytochrome aa3 to baseline values is slower if there has been underlying or prolonged hypoxia, or even after recurrent episodes of hypoxia. In one patient with a patent ductus arteriosus, there were decreases in cytochrome aa3 levels not detected by transcutaneous measurement of the PO_2; this suggested the presence of more significant "cerebral steal" by the ductus than had been appreciated previously.

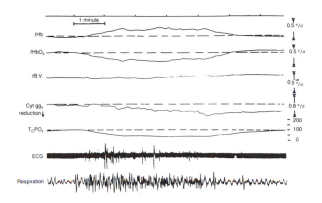

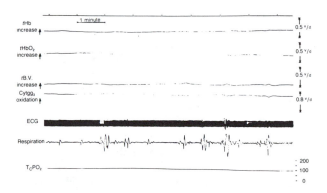

Figure 16-6 Tracing from baby A (top), characteristic of stable monitoring period. Slight fluctuations of deoxygenated hemoglobin (tHb), oxygenated hemoglobin (tHbO₂), tissue blood volume (tBV), and cytochrome aa3 occur with deep respirations; otherwise little change is noted over several minutes. Tracing from baby B (bottom) during five-minute spontaneous episode of decreased oxygenation. Oxygenated hemoglobin (tHbO₂), cytochrome aa3, and transcutaneous PO₂ all decrease together with the increase in deoxygenated hemoglobin (tHb). Recovery of hemoglobin oxygenation is followed rapidly by a return in transcutaneous PO₂ to its baseline value; however, aa3 remained reduced and did not return to its baseline value for six additional minutes. tBV = tissue blood volume. The instrument is calibrated in units of "variation in density" (v/d) where one v/d equals order of magnitude change in signal received. (From Brazy JE, et al. Noninvasive monitoring of cerebral oxygenation in preterm infants: preliminary observations. Pediatrics 1985; 75:217.)

NIROS-SCOPE is a technology that is readily applicable within the intensive care nursery. The equipment used can be brought to the bedside and the baby need only be restrained enough to prevent major head movements. The lasers used are not hazardous to the skin; however, bilirubin eye masks must be used to prevent exposure to the eyes. Further studies and more widespread availability of NIROS-SCOPE will help increase our understanding of cerbral oxygenation and its relationship to neuropathologic conditions in newborns.

RECOMMENDATIONS

Many technologies are now available to assess different aspects of brain function noninvasively. Several methods described here have been fundamental to the understanding of cerebral blood flow and its importance in the premature and sick newborn. The most accurate of these, PET, has several technical limitations that have limited its routine clinical use in measuring cerebral blood flow. However, PET potentially can be used to measure other aspects of cerebral metabolism. The increasingly widespread availability of Doppler equipment and the ease of its bedside use have led to its being the most common means to evaluate cerebral blood flow. The increased resolution and availability of SPECT may lead to its use more often in the study of neonatal cerebral metabolism. As the role of the cerebral blood flow in normal and pathologic neurodevelopment is better understood, the practice of routinely monitoring cerebral blood flow by one of these technologies will increase.

NMR spectroscopy has already been used to study cerebral energy metabolism and molecular biochemistry in normal and asphyxiated neonates. We anticipate that it will be used increasingly to study many aspects of cellular physiology within the brain. PET may have similar applicability. Finally, near infrared absorption studies have recently shed more light on important aspects of cerebral oxygenation. Improved ability to assess brain function with these technologies should improve the recognition, prevention, and treatment of brain injury in neonates.

REFERENCES

1. Kety SS, Schmidt CF. The determination of cerebral blood flow in man by the use of nitrous oxide in low concentration. Am J Physiol 1945; 143:53.
2. Kennedy C, Sokoloff L. An adaptation of the nitrous oxide method to the study of the cerebral circulation in children: normal values for cerebral blood flow and cerebral metabolic rate in childhood. J Clin Invest 1957; 36:1130.
3. Lou HC, Lassen NA, Friis-Hansen B. Low cerebral blood flow in hypotensive perinatal distress. Acta Neurol Scand 1977; 56:343.
4. Lou HC, Lassen NA, Friis-Hansen B. Impaired autoregulation of cerebral blood flow in the distressed newborn infant. J Pediatr 1979; 94:118.
5. Lou HC, Lassen NA, Friis-Hansen B. Decreased cerebral blood flow after administration of sodium bicarbonate in the distressed newborn infant. Acta Neurol Scand 1978; 57:239.
6. Ment LR, Ehrenkranz RA, Lange RC, et al. Alterations in cerebral blood flow in preterm infants with intraventricular hemorrhage. Pediatrics 1981; 68:763.
7. Younkin DP, Reivich M, Obrist W, Delivoria-Papadopolous M. Noninvasive method of estimating human regional cerebral blood flow. J Cereb Blood Flow Metab 1982; 2:415.
8. Greisen G, Johansen K, Ellison PH, et al. Cerebral blood flow in the newborn infant: comparison of Doppler ultrasound and ^{133}xenon clearance. J Pediatr 1984; 104:411.
9. Volpe JJ, Herscovitch P, Perlman JM, Raichle ME. Positron emission tomography in the newborn: extensive impairment of regional cerebral blood flow with intraventricular hemorrhage and hemorrhagic intracerebral involvement. Pediatrics 1983; 72:589.
10. Perlman JM, Herscovitch P, Kreusser KL, et al. Positron emission tomography in the newborn: effect of seizure on regional cerebral blood flow in an asphyxiated infant. Neurology 1985; 35:244.
11. Volpe JJ, Herscovitch P, Perlman JM, et al. Positron emission tomography in the asphyxiated term newborn: parasagittal impairment of cerebral blood flow. Ann Neurol 1985; 17:287.
12. Kirsch JR, Traystman RJ, Rogers MC. Cerebral blood flow measurements in infants and children. Pediatrics 1985; 75:887.
13. Andreasen NC. Brain imaging: applications in psychiatry. Science 1988; 239:1381.
14. Hellman RS, Collier BD. MRI and SPECT I-123 iodoamphetamine imaging of a patient with progressive dementia. Adv Funct Neuroimag 1988; 1:18.
15. Van Heertum RL, O'Connell RA. The evaluation of psychiatric disease with IMP cerebral SPECT imaging. Adv Funct Neuroimag 1988; 1:4.
16. Tikofsky RS. SPECT brain studies: potential role of cognitive challenge in language and learning disorders. Adv Funct Neuroimag 1988; 1:12.
17. Cross KW, Dear PRF, Warner RM, Watling GB. An attempt to measure cerebral blood flow in the newborn infant. J Physiol 1976; 260:42.
18. Cooke RWI, Rolfe P, Howat P. A technique for the non-invasive estimation of cerebral blood flow in the newborn infant. J Med Eng Technol 1977; 1:263.
19. Cooke RWI, Rolfe P. Cerebral blood flow measurement using venous occlusion plethysmography in the newborn human infant. In: Rolfe P, ed. Non-invasive physiological measurements. New York: Academic Press, 1979:175.
20. Gedes LA, Hoff HE, Hull CW, Millar HD. Rheoencephalography. Cardiovasc Res Cent Bull 1964; 2:112.
21. Murdoch N, Murray P, Rolfe P, Weindling AM. Computer modelling of cerebral electrical impedance in the newborn baby for comparison with in vivo measurements. Proc 5th Nordic Meeting Med Biol Eng 1981; 2:418.
22. Mochalova LD, Khodov DA, Zhukova TP. Cerebral circulation control in healthy full-term neonates. Acta Paediatr Scand [Suppl] 1983; 311:20.
23. Weindling AM, Rolfe P, Tarassenko L, Costeloe K. Cerebral haemodynamics in newborn babies studied by electrical impedance. Acta Paediatr Scand [Suppl] 1983; 311:14.
24. Gadian DG. Nuclear magnetic resonance and its applications to living systems. Oxford: Clarendon Press, 1982.
25. James TL, Margulis AR, eds. Biomedical magnetic resonance. San Francisco: UCSF Radiology Research and Education Foundation, 1984.
26. Jardetzky O, Roberts GCK. NMR in molecular biology. New York: Academic Press, 1981.
27. James TL. Nuclear magnetic resonance in biochemistry: principles and applications. New York: Academic Press, 1975.
28. Rabenstein DL, Guo W. Nuclear magnetic resonance spectroscopy. Anal Chem 1988; 60:1R.
29. Moon RB, Richards JH. Determination of intracellular pH by ^{31}P magnetic resonance. J Biol Chem 1973; 248:7276.
30. González-Méndez R, Hahn GM, Wade-Jardetzky NJ, Jardetzky O. Comparison of intracellular pH measurements by ^{31}P NMR and weak acid partitioning in Chinese hamster ovary fibroblasts. Mag Reson Med 1988; 6:373.

31. Petroff OAC, Pritchard JW, Behar KL, et al. Cerebral intracellular pH by ^{31}P nuclear magnetic resonance spectroscopy. Neurology 1985; 35:781.

32. Gyulai L, Roth Z, Leigh JS Jr., Chance B. Bioenergetic studies of mitochondrial oxidative phosphorylation using ^{31}phosphorus NMR. J Biol Chem 1985; 260:3947.

33. Chance B, Leigh JS Jr., Clarck BH, et al. Control of oxidation metabolism and oxygen delivery in human skeletal muscle: a steady state analysis of the work/energy cost transfer function. Proc Natl Acad Sci USA 1985; 82:8384.

34. González-Méndez R, Stevenson DK, Jardetzky O. NMR in biology and medicine: spectroscopy in vivo. Magn Reson Med Biol (in press).

35. Cady EB, Costello AMdeL, Dawson MJ, et al. Non-invasive investigation of cerebral metabolism in newborn infants by phosphorous nuclear magnetic resonance spectroscopy. Lancet 1983; 1:1059.

36. Salomon WL, Benitz WE, Enzmann DR, Bravo RH, et al. Correlation of echoencephalographic findings and neurodevelopmental outcome: intracranial hemorrhage and ventriculomegaly in infants of birth weights 1,000 gm or less. J Clin Monit 1987; 3:178.

37. Hope PL, Costello AMdeL, Cady EB, et al. Cerebral energy metabolism studied with phosphorous NMR spectroscopy in normal and birth-asphyxiated infants. Lancet 1984; 2:366.

38. Hamilton PR, Cady EB, Wyatt JS, et al. Impaired energy metabolism in brains of newborn infants with increased cerebral echodensities. Lancet 1986; 1:1242.

39. Chance B, Younkin DP, Warnell R, et al. ^{31}P NMR of cortical oxidative metabolism in neonates. Pediatr Res 1983; 17:307A.

40. Younkin DP, Delivoria-Papadopoulos M, Leonard JC, et al. Unique aspects of human cerebral metabolism evaluated with phosphorous nuclear magnetic resonance spectroscopy. Ann Neurol 1984; 16:581.

41. Brown BW Jr., Hollander M. Statistics: a biomedical approach. New York: John Wiley, 1977:373.

42. Pocock SJ, Hughes MD, Lee RJ. Statistical problems in the reporting of clinical trials: a survey of three medical journals. N Engl J Med 1987; 317:426.

43. Radda GK, Bore PJ, Rajagopalan B. Clinical aspects on ^{31}P nuclear magnetic resonance spectroscopy. Br Med Bull 1984; 40:155.

44. Hayes DJ, Hilton-Jones D, Arnold DL, et al. A mitochondrial encephalopathy. A combined ^{31}P magnetic resonance and biochemical investigation. J Neurol Sci 1985; 71:105.

45. Tofts P, Wray S. Changes in brain phosphorous metabolites during the post-natal development of the rat. J Physiol 1985; 359:417.

46. Delpy DT, Gordon RE, Hope PL, et al. Noninvasive investigation of cerebral ischemia by phosphorous nuclear magnetic resonance. Pediatrics 1982; 70:310.

47. Thulborn KR, duBoulay GH, Duchen LW, Radda G. A ^{31}P nuclear magnetic resonance in vivo study of cerebral ischemia in the gerbil. J Cereb Blood Flow Metab 1982; 2:299.

48. Hope PL, Cady EB, Chu A, et al. Brain metabolism and intracellular pH during ischaemia and hypoxia: an in vivo ^{31}P and ^{1}H nuclear magnetic resonance study in the lamb. J Neurochem 1987; 49:75.

49. González-Méndez R, McNeill A, Gregory GA, et al. Effects of hypoxic hypoxia on cerebral phosphate metabolism and pH in the anesthetized infant rabbit. J Cereb Blood Flow Metab 1985; 5:512.

50. Young RS, Briggs RW, Yagel SK, Gorman I. ^{31}P nuclear magnetic resonance study of the effect of hypoxemia on neonatal status epilepticus. Pediatr Res 1986; 20:581.

51. Cowan BE, Young RS, Briggs RW, et al. The effect of hypotension on brain energy state during prolonged neonatal seizure. Pediatr Res 1987; 21:357.

52. Bartowski HM, Pitts LH, Nishimura M, et al. NMR imaging and spectroscopy of experimental brain edema. J Trauma 1985; 25:192.

53. Bederson JB, Bartowski HM, Moon K, et al. Nuclear magnetic resonance imaging and spectroscopy in experimental brain edema in a rat model. J Neurosurg 1986; 64:795.

54. Petroff OA, Prichard JW, Behar KL, et al. In vivo phosphorous nuclear magnetic resonance spectroscopy in status epilepticus. Ann Neurol 1984; 16:169.

55. Young RS, Osbakken MD, Briggs RW, et al. ^{31}P NMR study of cerebral metabolism during prolonged seizures in the neonatal dog. Ann Neurol 1985; 18:14.

56. Young RS, Cowan B, Briggs RW. Brain metabolism after electroshock seizure in the neonatal dog: a [^{31}P] NMR study. Brain Res Bull 1987; 18:261.

57. Litt L, González-Méndez R, Severinghaus JW, et al. Cerebral intracellular changes during supercarbia: an in vivo ^{31}P nuclear magnetic resonance study in rats. J Cereb Blood Flow Metab 1985; 5:537.

58. Stocker F, Herschkowitz N, Bossi E, et al. Cerebral metabolic studies in situ by ^{31}P nuclear magnetic resonance after hypothermic circulatory arrest. Pediatr Res 1986; 20:867.

59. Ahlfors CE, Bennett SH, Shoemaker CT, et al. Changes in the auditory brainstem response associated with intravenous infusion of unconjugated bilirubin into infant rhesus monkeys. Pediatr Res 1986; 20:511.

60. Behar KL, den Hollander JA, Petroff OA, et al. Effect of hypoglycemic encephalopathy upon amino acids, high-energy phosphates, and pH$_i$ in the rat brain in vivo: detection by sequential ^{1}H and ^{31}P NMR spectroscopy. J Neurochem 1985; 44:1045.

61. Chang L-H, Pereira BM, Weinstein PR, et al. Comparison of lactate concentration determinations in ischemic and hypoxic rat brains by in vivo and in vitro ^{1}H NMR spectroscopy. Magn Reson Med 1987; 4:575.

62. Chopp M, Helpern JA, Frinak S, et al. In vivo ^{31}P NMR or photoactivated hematoporphyrin derivative in cat brain. Med Phys 1985; 12:256.

63. Kappas A, Drummond GS, Manola T, et al. Sn-protoporphyrin use in the management of hyperbilirubinemia in term newborns with direct Coombs-positive ABO incompatibility. Pediatrics 1988; 81:485.

64. Litt L, González-Méndez R, James TL, et al. An in vivo study of halothane uptake and elimination in the rate brain with fluorine nuclear magnetic resonance spectroscopy. Anesthesiology 1987; 67:161.

65. Brazy JE, Lewis DV, Mitnick MH, vander Vliet J. Noninvasive monitoring of cerebral oxygenation in preterm infants: preliminary observations. Pediatrics 1985; 75:217.

17

Imaging of Hypoxic-Ischemic Cerebral Damage

Dieter R. Enzmann, M.D.

Hypoxic-Ischemic Injury
  Subependymal-Intraventricular Hemorrhage
    Ultrasound Scanning
    Computed Tomographic Scanning
    Sequelae
  Extracorporeal Membrane Oxygenation
    Other Intracranial Hemorrhages
  Periventricular Leukomalacia
    Imaging: Ultrasound, Computed Tomography,
      and Magnetic Resonance Imaging
    Benign Cysts
  Focal Infarction
    Ultrasound
    Computed Tomography
  Diffuse Hypoxic-Ischemic Injury
    Imaging with Ultrasound and Computed
      Tomography
  Hypoglycemia

Imaging of the brain has become important in premature infants in assessing potential hypoxic-ischemic damage. Computed tomography (CT) was the first imaging method widely used to investigate the neonatal brain. It was CT's accurate depiction of intracranial hemorrhage that led to greater interest in and understanding of the central nervous system complications of prematurity.[1] The accuracy of CT was confirmed by neuropathologic correlation.[2,3] Shortly after CT raised the awareness level of investigators in regard to intracranial hemorrhage, real-time ultrasound scans began to prove their value in detecting and delineating subependymal-intraventricular hemorrhage.[4,5] CT–neuropathologic–ultrasound correlation showed good agreement, ultrasound being highly sensitive to most forms of subependymal-intraventricular hemorrhage.[2] Because of ultrasound's portability, low risk, ease of performance, and accuracy, its use increased rapidly so that it has become the dominant imaging test for the diagnosis of subependymal-intraventricular hemorrhage in the premature newborn. The recent introduction of magnetic resonance (MR) imaging has opened up other opportunities, which promise to yield new information about hypoxic-ischemic brain damage.

Current practice is such that for the diagnosis of subependymal-intraventricular hemorrhage, the ultrasound scan is the initial study of choice. Often it provides all the information necessary for diagnosis and follow-up. The ultrasound scan does have the disadvantage of not visualizing the entire brain. Because the anterior fontanelle serves as an acoustic window to the brain, ultrasound is less sensitive to abnormalities either very close to the internal table of the skull (i.e., over the convexities) or at some distance from the transducer (i.e., low in the brain and in the posterior fossa). In the face of an unusual or confusing ultrasound scan or when the clinical history is highly suggestive of central nervous system disease but the ultrasound scan is negative, a CT or MR scan is indicated to visualize the brain more completely.

For long-term follow-up the ultrasound scan becomes less useful as the anterior fontanelle (which is necessary for its performance) closes. That leaves CT and MR for use in assessing the long-term sequelae of a hypoxic-ischemic insult, and a MR scan is superior to CT.[6-8] The MR scan is equivalent to or more sensitive than CT in depicting morphologic and structural abnormalities in the brain.[8] The MR scan also more accurately shows abnormalities of and delays in the pattern of myelination.[7] Some disease entities, such as periventricular leukomalacia in their less severe end stages are undetectable by CT but are well seen by MR.[6] For long-term follow-up, therefore, the MR scan is likely to become the examination of choice. Even in the acute stage this technique may supplant CT, although the latter still has the advantage of allowing better physical access to the neonate with life support systems and making possible very rapid scans (i.e., two or three seconds).

These imaging tests, in addition to delineating hypoxic-ischemic brain damage, also show central nervous system abnormalities of other disorders. All three types of studies are capable of detecting such abnormalities, which can range from congenital malformations to congenital infections. More acute processes, such as meningoencephalitides, also can be detected. The findings in these disease entities are usually different enough from the hypoxic-ischemic spectrum that they can be diagnosed with confidence.

HYPOXIC-ISCHEMIC INJURY

The findings in hypoxic-ischemic brain damage include a broad spectrum of abnormalities. The two broad categories are hemorrhage and infarction; subependymal-intraventricular hemorrhage being the most common. Isolated intraparenchymal hemorrhage without a subependymal-intraventricular hemorrhagic component is much less common, although such hemorrhages do occur in a new group of premature infants—those treated by extracorporeal membrane oxygenation.

The other major pathologic entity is cerebral infarction, which can present in several ways. Infarction may occur in a watershed distribution and manifest as periventricular leukomalacia. The infarction, however, can be similar to that seen in adult patients and assume a more typical segmental vascular distribution. Finally, the insult can be so extensive as to cause global ischemia, resulting in diffuse infarction of the entire brain. Spanning these two broad categories of hemorrhage and infarction is the hemorrhagic form of periventricular leukomalacia. This has been termed periventricular hemorrhagic infarction, but it is not clear at this time whether this entity should be classified differently from nonhemorrhagic periventricular leukomalacia.

Subependymal-Intraventricular Hemorrhage

Subependymal-intraventricular hemorrhage has been one of the most common complications reported in the central nervous system in premature infants. Its specific etiology is still debated, although it appears to be related to fluctuations in cerebral blood flow and perfusion pressures. Since the neonatal brain does not exhibit autoregulation, changes in the systemic blood pressure are transmitted directly to the brain, and vessels in the subependymal germinal matrix appear to be particularly vulnerable to rupture under such conditions. With the availability of imaging tests—ultrasound and CT—it has become apparent that the incidence of this complication, although initially high, has been decreasing, with more recent reports showing an incidence of approxi-

mately 30 percent in infants weighing less than 1,500 gm.[9,10] Not only has the incidence decreased, but the severity of subependymal-intraventricular hemorrhage also appears to have decreased, although grading systems differ and have not been standardized.[9,10] It is also apparent that with this decreased incidence and severity of subependymal-intraventricular hemorrhage there has also been a decrease in mortality and morbidity.[10]

This chapter uses the combined term subependymal-intraventricular hemorrhage because although there is close correlation between CT and ultrasound scans with neuropathologic findings in terms of hemorrhage size, it is not always possible by these imaging studies to distinguish the subependymal from the intraventricular component.[2,9] It is therefore more accurate to combine the terms. These two hemorrhagic components do not carry any different prognosis or imply any different pathogenesis. Serial ultrasound scans often can tease out the intraventricular component of subependymal-intraventricular hemorrhage over time by virtue of its clot retraction within the ventricle. At times a part of the hemorrhage disappears rapidly, indicating that this portion was intraventricular and was cleared rapidly from the ventricular system. The subependymal component evolves more slowly. Therefore, although serial ultrasound scans may delineate an intraventricular component, on any single scan the subependymal component cannot be definitively distinguished from the intraventricular component. Hence, the term subependymal-intraventricular hemorrhage.

Various grading methods have been used to assess the size of subependymal-intraventricular hemorrhage in the hope of using such a grading system as a prognostic measure of the outcome.[11] The earliest grading scale developed by Papile et al[12] was too simple and grouped pathologic findings that in subsequent studies have been shown to be better evaluated separately.[9,13] At present the following three pathologic findings probably should be considered and graded separately: subependymal-intraventricular hemorrhage, intraparenchymal hemorrhage, and periventricular leukomalacia. Although commonly associated, these manifestations of hypoxic-ischemic damage, at least from an imaging point of view, appear to be related to outcome. The lesser grades of subependymal-intraventricular hemorrhage are associated with lower mortality and a lower incidence of hydrocephalus than higher grades. The incremental finding of intraparenchymal hemorrhage seems to result in a higher mortality and an increased incidence of hydrocephalus no matter what the grade of the underlying subependymal-intraventricular hemorrhage.[9] It is clear that subependymal-intraventricular hemorrhage alone does not explain all the neurologic sequelae in these infants. In fact it is imaging evidence of parenchymal damage, infarction, and porencephaly that most consistently correlates with subsequent neurologic deficits.

Ultrasound Scanning

The natural history of subependymal-intraventricular hemorrhage has been well delineated by ultrasound (Figs. 17–1, 17–2).[14] The hallmark on the ultrasound scan is an area of increased echogenicity in a subependymal and intraventricular location, most often near the head of the caudate nucleus. This increased echogenicity is usually well marginated and may be unilateral or bilateral. When small, it is usually limited to a very focal region in the lateral ventricle near the caudate nucleus. With increasing size the hyperechoic region may conform to the shape of the lateral ventricle and, if extensive enough, may produce a cast of it. With larger hemorrhages the lateral ventricle is enlarged and distorted, forming a more rounded, expanded area filled with echogenic hemorrhage. When extensive, the subependymal-intraventricular hemorrhage can form a cast of the entire lateral ventricle, inlcuding the temporal and occipital horns. Although the most common site of hemorrhage is near the head of the caudate nucleus, subependymal-intraventricular hemorrhage may occur anywhere in the subependymal germinal matrix of the lateral ventricle. Therefore, at times the hemorrhage may be localized posteriorly near the atrium and in unusual situations in the temporal horn (Fig. 17–3). No one side shows a greater predisposition for the development of subependymal-intraventricular hemorrhage.[9]

A hemorrhage may be quite small and limited to the choroid plexus, in which case it is not a subependymal-intraventricular hemorrhage but a choroid plexus hemorrhage, which has a benign natural history.[15] An important diagnostic criterion for distinguishing hemorrhage from choroid plexus is extension of the hyperechoic mass into the frontal horn where choroid plexus is not found, i.e., anterior to the foramen of Monro.

The onset of subependymal-intraventricular hemorrhage usually occurs in the first seven days of life, day 3 being the most commonly reported.[9] Subependymal-intraventricular hemorrhage appears to be a single event within a 24-hour period in most neonates. In some neonates it shows progression over a 48-hour period. (Fig. 17–4). This means that a unilateral hemorrhage may become a bilateral hemorrhage, or the grade of a unilateral hemorrhage may increase over this time. Documentation of subependymal-intraventricular hemorrhage progression over 48 hours carries a poor prognosis and a mortality rate of approximately 50 percent (Fig. 17–4).[9] A few neonates show late onset of subependymal-intraventricular hemorrhage occurring between three weeks and three months of age. Such late onset hemorrhages are usually of low grade, are clinically silent, and result in few sequelae.[9,16]

Subependymal-intraventricular hemorrhage progresses through characteristic ultrasound stages as it evolves toward resolution. In the acute stage the hemorrhage is homogeneously hyperechoic. In the one to three week posthemorrhage interval the appearance of the hemorrhage changes, losing echogenicity in its central portion while retaining an echogenic rim (see Figs. 17–1, 17–2). The hemorrhage therefore begins to assume the shape of a hyperechoic rim around a hypoechoic center.[14] After this stage further resolution is seen as a progressive decrease in the diameter of the hyperechoic ring. Resolution takes place over four to six weeks, large hemorrhages taking somewhat longer to resolve (see Figs. 17–1, 17–2). Patients with a significant intraventricular component to the subependymal-intraventricular hemorrhage can show increased echogenicity of the ventricular walls that contained intraventricular blood. These findings, suggestive of ependymitis, resolve slowly.

An intraparenchymal hemorrhagic component of subependymal-intraventricular hemorrhage is identified on the ultrasound scan when the hyperechoic region extends beyond the ventricular wall and subependymal region into the deep white matter of the centrum semiovale (Figs. 17–5, 17–6). An intraparenchymal hemorrhagic component is usually identifiable as an area of hyperechogenicity beyond the confines of even a dilated ventricular system.[14] The intraparenchymal hemorrhagic component evolves in a similar fashion to that of subependymal-intraventricular hemorrhage, with loss of central echogenicity. With the loss of central echogenicity the hemorrhage appears to retract, leaving an anechoic region between the irregular clot and the remaining brain parenchyma. As this retraction continues, depending on the size of the intraparenchymal hemorrhage, the hemorrhagic tissue may fragment and collapse into the ventricular system, leaving a large area of porencephaly, i.e., an anechoic appendage to the ventricle (Fig. 17–6).[14,17–19] This area of porencephaly does not decrease in size and in fact may increase in size over time.

Computed Tomographic Scanning

Acute subependymal-intraventricular hemorrhage appears as an area of increased density on the CT scan (Fig. 17–7). This increased density typically is seen in or adjacent to the lateral ventricle near the head of the caudate nucleus. The size varies from a small focal lesion in the ventricular wall to a hemorrhage of increased density forming a cast on the entire lateral ventricle, which may be either normal in size or dilated. A free flowing ventricular hemorrhagic component may be visualized in the occipital horns where it settles in a supine position. As the subependymal-intraventricular hemorrhage evolves, however, it becomes less apparent on the CT scan because it decreases in density. This occurs at approximately two weeks when the hemorrhage may be difficult to detect on a CT scan, since it has a density similar to that of adjacent brain tissue. At this time it is possible for the CT scan to be falsely negative, whereas

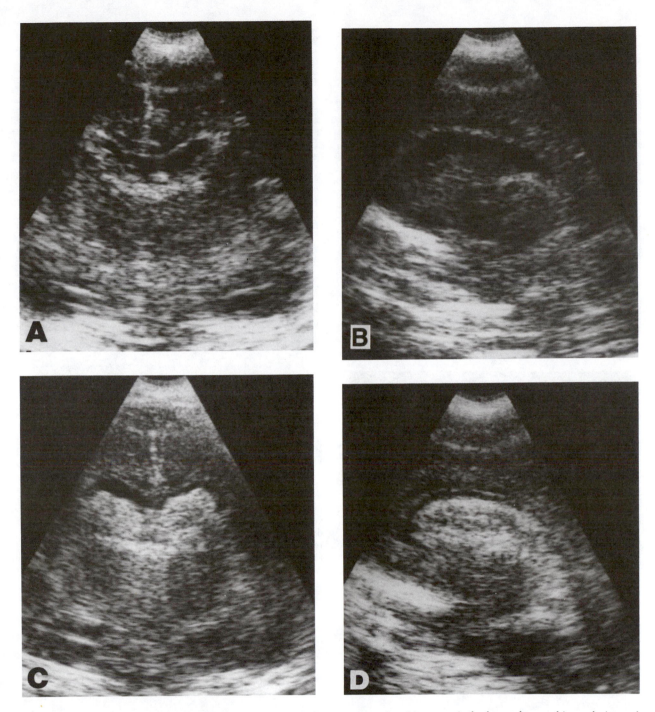

Figure 17-1 This series of ultrasound scans shows the development of subependymal-intraventricular hemorrhage and its evolution and resolution. On day 1 of life, the coronal (*A*) and sagittal (*B*) scans show a normal ventricular system except for mild asymmetry. On the following day bilateral subependymal-intraventricular hemorrhage is seen in the coronal (*C*) and sagittal (*D*) views. *Figure continues.*

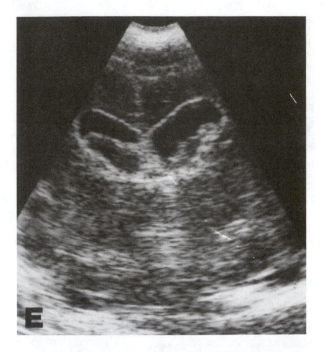

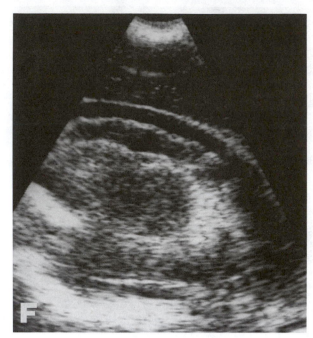

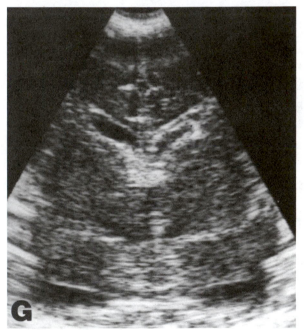

Figure 17–1 (Continued)   In our grading system this would represent grade IV disease without intraparenchymal hemorrhage. A scan at two weeks of life shows evolution of subependymal-intraventricular hemorrhage into the typical pattern of a hyperechoic rim around a hypoechoic center seen in both coronal (*E*) and sagittal (*F*) views. The ventricular system remains enlarged comparable to the findings on day 2, but the intraventricular component of the hemorrhage has retracted. At four weeks of life the coronal scan (*G*) shows a decrease in ventricular size and a small residual subependymal-intraventricular hemorrhage in the left lateral ventricle; it still has a hyperechoic rim and hypoechoic center pattern. *Figure continues.*

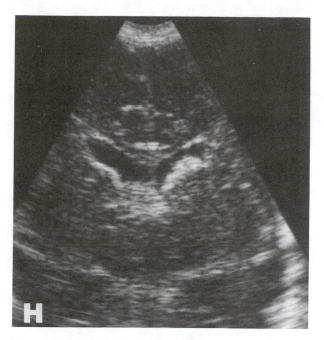

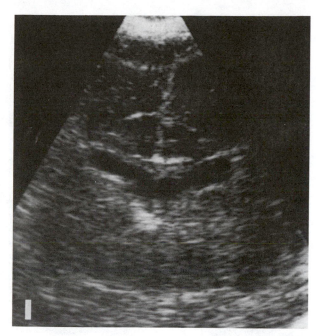

Figure 17–1 (Continued)   The ultrasound scan at eight weeks of life shows no significant change in the ventricular size, but the hemorrhage in the left lateral ventricle is now echogenic. This does not indicate rehemorrhaging but simply a decrease in the size of the hypoechoic center, leaving only the collapsed hyperechoic rim (*H*). At 10 weeks the coronal ultrasound scan shows no evidence of subependymal-intraventricular hemorrhage but persistent mild enlargement of the ventricular system (*I*). In this neonate severe bilateral subependymal-intraventricular hemorrhage resulted in only minimal structural sequelae and mild ventricular enlargement.

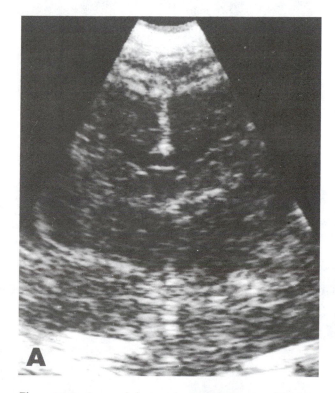

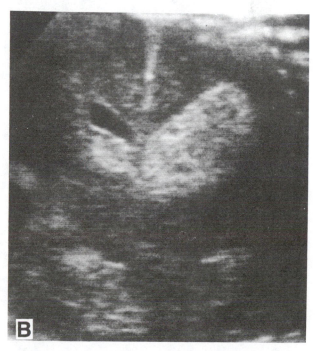

Figure 17–2   A coronal ultrasound scan on the first day of life shows a normal ventricular system with no evidence of hemorrhage on the coronal (*A*) and sagittal (*D*) images. On day 4 of life subependymal-intraventricular hemorrhage is detected bilaterally; it is greater on the left where it causes expansion of the left lateral ventricle. The hemorrhage is homogeneously echogenic on both the coronal (*B*) and sagittal (*E*) scans. In our grading systems this would be a grade IV hemorrhage without intraparenchymal hemorrhage. *Figure continues.*

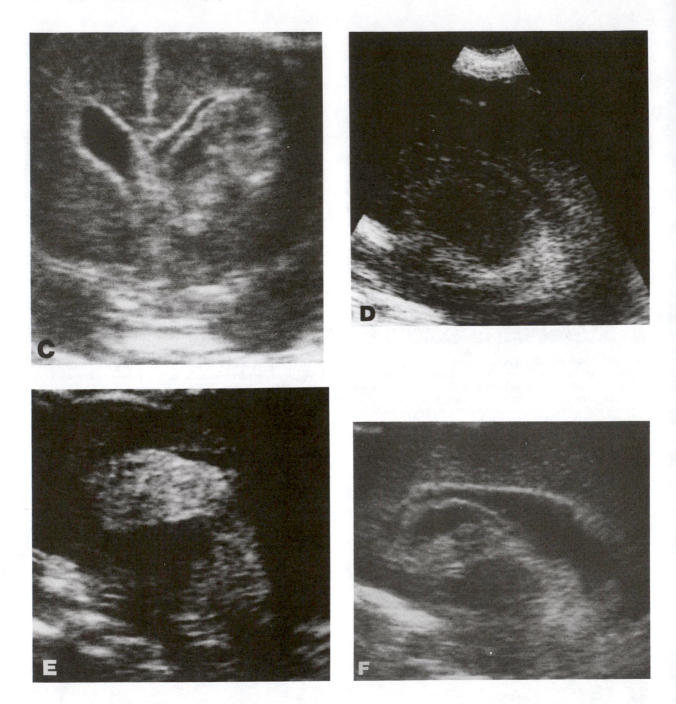

Figure 17-2 (Continued)   On day 18 of life the hemorrhage has evolved to the typical intermediate stage characterized by central hypoecho-genicity surrounded by a rim of hyperechogenicity (C, F). In the interval the ventricular system has dilated (C). This sequence of scans therefore shows the onset of subependymal-intraventricular hemorrhage in the first week of life, the typical evolution from the homogeneous echogenic state to the typical hypoechoic center–hyperechoic ring stage, and the complication of moderate hydrocephalus. (A, B, and C, from Baker LL, Stevenson DK, Enzmann DR. End-stage periventricular leukomalacia: MR evaluation. Radiology, 1988; 168:812.)

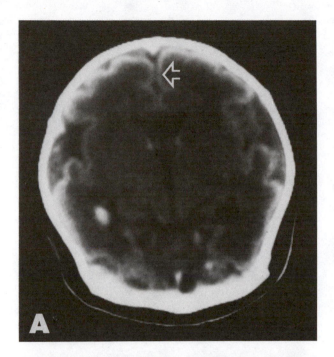

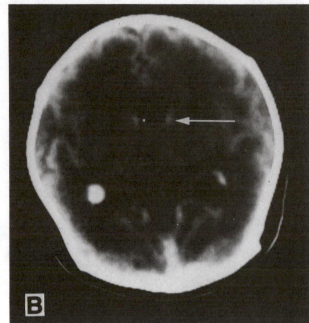

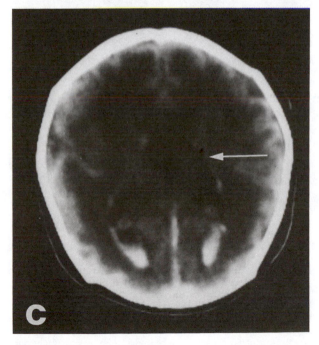

Figure 17-3 These three images from a CT scan show a small subependymal-intraventricular hemorrhage in the right temporal horn (A, B) and a smaller, more subtle subependymal-intraventricular hemorrhage in the left atrium (B). An intraventricular component of the hemorrhage is seen to layer in both occipital horns (C). These peripherally located subependymal-intraventricular hemorrhages can be difficult to detect by ultrasound. The CT scan shows the normal differentiation between the thin cortical ribbon of gray matter (open arrow, A) and underlying unmyelinated white matter. The subtle increase in density along the ventricular wall (long arrows) represents the normal slightly increased density of the subependymal germinal matrix (B, C).

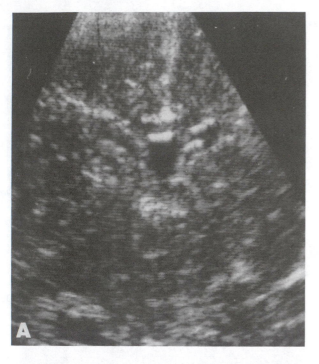

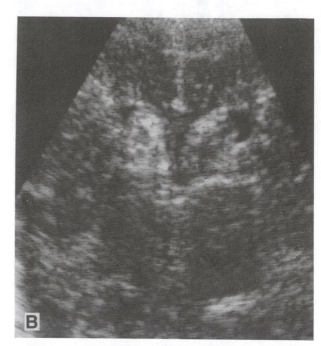

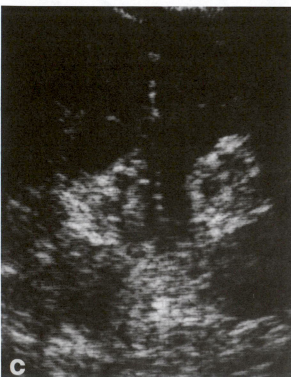

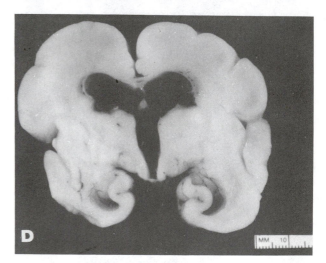

Figure 17–4   The serial coronal ultrasound scans show evidence of progressive subependymal-intraventricular hemorrhage. The initial scan shows a normal ventricular system (*A*). On the following day bilateral hemorrhaging is noted, as is minimal ventricular dilation (*B*). On the following day the hemorrhage has increased in severity bilaterally, indicating further progression over 48 hours, as has the ventricular enlargement (*C*). Progressive subependymal-intraventricular hemorrhage such as this carries a poor prognosis. The gross pathologic specimen confirms the bilateral grade IV hemorrhage without intraparenchymal hemorrhage (*D*). (*A* and *B*, from Baker LL, Stevenson DK, Enzmann DR. End-stage periventricular leukomalacia: MR evaluation. Radiology 1988; 168:813.)

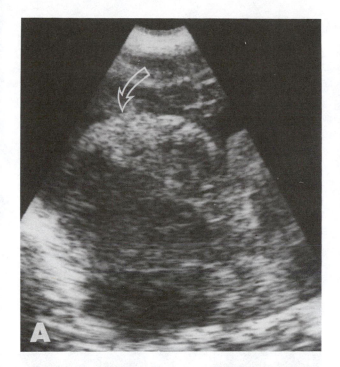

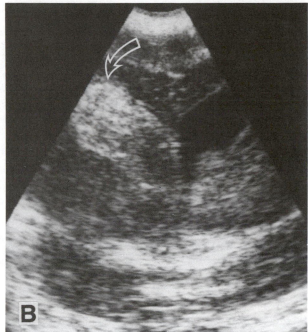

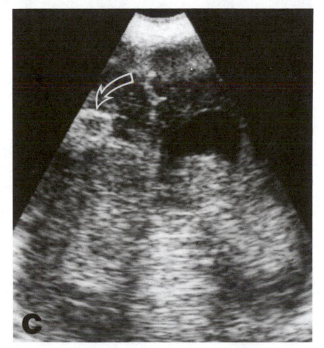

Figure 17–5   These three coronal ultrasound scans (anterior to posterior) show subependymal-intraventricular hemorrhage on the right side with an extension into the adjacent centrum semiovale representing an intraparenchymal hemorrhagic component. The latter component is denoted by curved arrows (*A, B, C*). The subependymal-intraventricular hemorrhagic component occupies most of the dilated right lateral ventricle. The left ventricle shows marked enlargement.

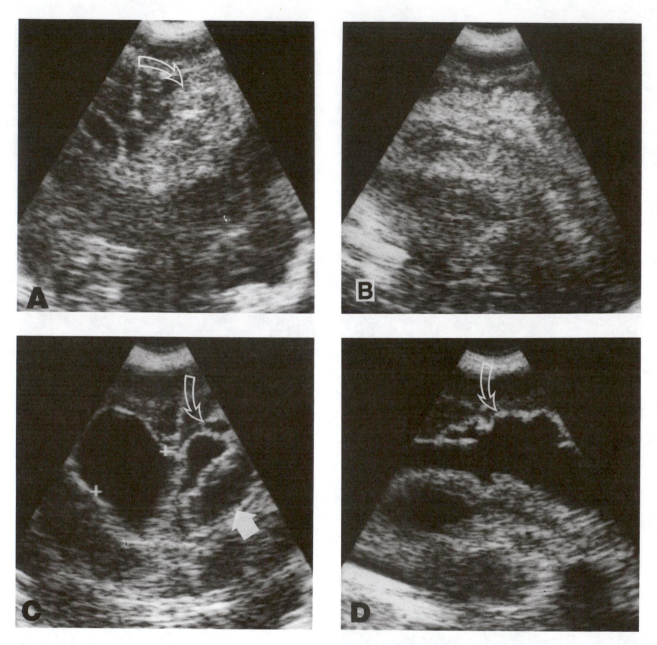

Figure 17-6   The initial ultrasound scan in the coronal view shows an extensive subependymal-intraventricular hemorrhage in the left lateral ventricle, with extension of this hemorrhage into the centrum semiovale causing an intraparenchymal hemorrhage (open arrow, *A*). The sagittal ultrasound scan shows diffuse increased echogenicity in the centrum semiovale above the lateral ventricle, which is compressed and not visualized. An ultrasound scan performed two weeks later shows interval development of marked hydrocephalus as shown by enlargement of the right lateral ventricle and also the left lateral ventricle. The subependymal-intraventricular hemorrhage has undergone the typical evolution, resulting in the appearance of a hyperechoic rim around a hypoechoic center (straight arrow, *C*). An anechoic region above the lateral ventricle shows the development of porencephaly (open arrow, *C, D*). This area of porencephaly is better visualized on the concomitant sagittal scan (arrow, *D*) where the anechoic region is seen to communicate with the body of the left lateral ventricle. This anechoic region of porencephaly develops when the hemorrhagic contents of the intraparenchymal hemorrhage collapse into the lateral ventricle.

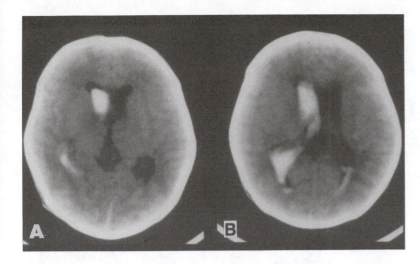

Figure 17-7   This pair of CT scans show the typical findings in subependymal-intraventricular hemorrhage. The increased density representing the hemorrhage is seen conforming to the ventricular system in the typical pericaudate location on the right. Some layering of free flowing "blood" is noted in both occipital horns.

on the ultrasound scan the hemorrhage is easily detectable. At this stage the ultrasound scan shows the typical appearance of a hyperechoic rim around a hypoechoic center. Once this stage has been reached, the subependymal-intraventricular hemorrhage will be difficult to detect directly on a CT scan.

The use of MR imaging in following the natural history of subependymal-intraventricular hemorrhage has only limited documentation, in part because of the logistics involved in using this technology. Cerebral hemorrhage, however, typically shows high signal intensity on T1 weighted images (Fig. 17-8).[8] These images show brain as an intermediate shade of gray, cerebrospinal fluid as a dark shade of gray or black, and hemorrhage as a very bright area, i.e., high signal intensity.[8] T2 weighted MR images are not as useful for detecting subependymal-intraventricular hemorrhage. Signal intensity changes of evolving cerebral hemorrhage can be complicated on the MR images, and all the changes are not yet fully understood. Despite these signal changes, detection of hemorrhage is accurate, more so than with CT scanning after the acute stage.

Sequelae

One of the sequelae of subependymal-intraventricular hemorrhage is ventricular enlargement (see Fig. 17-2). This enlargement may be mild, especially with the lower grades of hemorrhage. The enlargement may be asymmetrical and relatively static. The term *ventricular enlargement* is used in patients in whom this enlargement is of a mild degree, develops slowly, and remains stable. Some patients, however, develop what can rightfully be called hydrocephalus in which ventricular enlargement

progresses relatively rapidly, causing ventricular enlargement of a moderate to severe degree.[20] Hydrocephalus is unusual with the mild form of subependymal-intraventricular hemorrhage but is more common with the higher grades.[9] The time course of hydrocephalus development is variable, but the most severe forms show a rapid increase in ventricular size to a maximum in approximately three weeks.[9]

The natural history of hydrocephalus seems to show some regression even without therapeutic intervention. The milder forms of hydrocephalus may show regression to normal ventricular size, whereas the severe forms may show improvement but rarely a return to normal (see Figs. 17-1, 17-2).[9] Ultrasound can be used to monitor the effect of serial lumbar punctures if that treatment modality is used. When this procedure is performed, intermittent decreases in ventricular size can be documented, but usually the ventricle expands to its pretreatment size after 24 to 48 hours. Over a longer time the hydrocephalus seems to recede. The presence of hydrocephalus does not appear to be directly related to the prognosis.[13] Porencephaly results from an intraparenchymal hemorrhage of significant size. The porencephalic cyst is located at the site of hemorrhage and represents a cerebrospinal fluid space extending into brain parenchyma but in direct communication with the ventricular system.[14,17-19] As the severity of subependymal-intraventricular hemorrhage has decreased, so have such sequelae.

Extracorporeal Membrane Oxygenation

This treatment modality represents a more aggressive approach in premature infants who need temporary

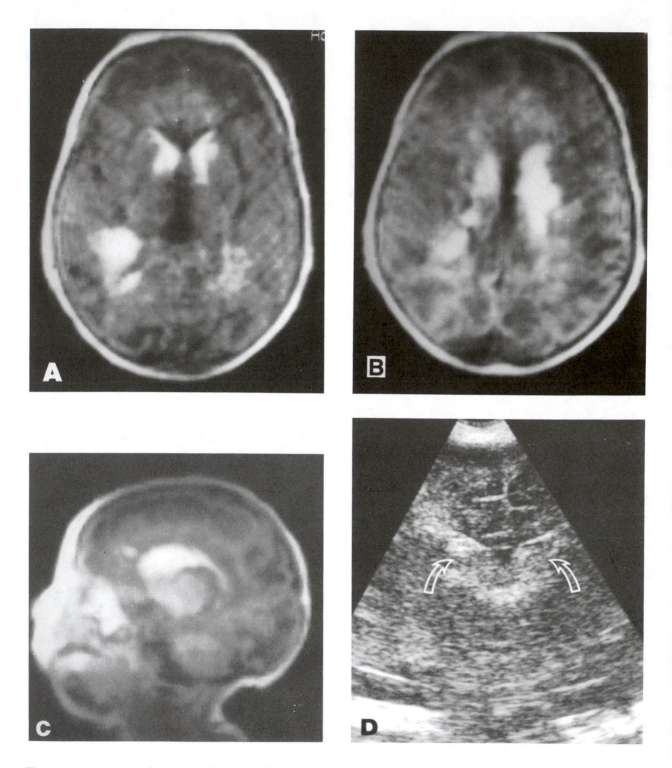

Figure 17-8   Concurrent ultrasound and MR scans of subependymal-intraventricular hemorrhage. The axial T1 weighted scans show the hemorrhage to be of high signal intensity (bright) and in the typical pericaudate location (*A*), extending along the body of the lateral ventricle and into the right temporal horn (*A, B*). The sagittal T1 weighted scan shows the typical configuration of subependymal-intraventricular hemorrhage in the wall of the lateral ventricle (left side, *C*). The ultrasound shows bilateral subependymal-intraventricular hemorrhage at the level of the caudate nuclei (arrows, *D*).

cardiorespiratory support. An important feature of this treatment is anticoagulation with heparin to prevent clotting in the pump oxygenator. Therefore, in addition to the usual risk of intracranial hemorrhage, further risk is introduced by the anticoagulation. Intracranial imaging studies, primarily ultrasound, are important in assessing the candidacy of an infant for this treatment, since the presence of intracranial hemorrhage is a contraindication.

In addition, once the infant is given extracorporeal membrane oxygenation, daily ultrasound scans are used to detect the appearance of any intracranial hemorrhage. While these infants are receiving extracorporeal membrane oxygenation they can develop the garden variety of subependymal-intraventricular hemorrhage, but they seem to have an increased susceptibility to intraparenchymal hemorrhage without a concomitant subependymal-intraventricular hemorrhage (Fig. 17–9).[20] Intraparenchymal hemorrhage without subependymal-intraventricular hemorrhage is unusual in the premature infant who is not receiving extracorporeal membrane oxygenation. Since the intraparenchymal hemorrhage can occur anywhere in the brain, the ultrasound scan requires careful scrutiny in areas other than the expected sites of subependymal-intraventricular hemorrhage. The ultrasound scan does carry some possibility of missing the intraparenchymal hemorrhage because of its limited view of the intracranial space. Infants receiving extracorporeal membrane oxygenation are also at increased risk for focal infarction.[20]

Other Intracranial Hemorrhages

Other hemorrhages occur in premature infants, but they are often related to a traumatic delivery. Subdural hemorrhages occur but differ from the usual subdural hematomas seen in adults. In the neonate subdural hematomas often occur around the tentorium near the straight sinus. They are more common around the falx and tentorium than over the convexities. Subdural and epidural hematomas, however, do occur under skull fractures, which may be related to traumatic delivery. Subarachnoid hemorrhages are relatively uncommon on imaging tests. They may be related to a traumatic delivery or to a diffuse hypoxic-ischemic insult. The ultrasound scan is insensitive to subarachnoid hemorrhage, as is the MR scan. The CT scan provides the best opportunity for the diagnosis of subarachnoid hemorrhage, showing increased density in cisternal spaces, which are normally of low density. A subarachnoid hemorrhage must be significant for it to be detectable by CT. In most instances subdural hematomas and subarachnoid hemorrhages resolve without specific treatment.

Periventricular Leukomalacia

Periventricular leukomalacia is an important manifestation of hypoxic-ischemic central nervous system disease in the premature infant. Its presence should be noted and graded separately from subependymal-intraventricular hemorrhage. This entity is responsible for significant morbidity involving visual, auditory, and motor dysfunction. The major sequelae of periventricular leukomalacia is spastic diplegia because of its involvement of the corticospinal tracts, especially those to the lower extremities. Fibers of the optic radiations may also be affected, causing visual deficits.[21]

The incidence of periventricular leukomalacia depends on the diagnostic test used to detect it. In autopsy series the incidence has been reported to be as high as 22 percent, but lower incidences have been reported in ultrasound series (5 to 7 percent).[21-23] Its incidence depends on birth weight. Different imaging tests have varying sensitivities to this pathologic process, and the sensitivity changes with the different stages of periventricular leukomalacia (see later).

Periventricular leukomalacia is essentially a watershed infarction, occurring in the periventricular region at the junction of the ventriculopedal and ventriculofugal vessels, which penetrate into deep white matter. Damage is caused by decreased blood flow in these watershed zones. These zones characteristically involve the superolateral border of the periventricular white matter, the areas where the major abnormalities are seen on imaging tests. The region most commonly afflicted is the periventricular white matter adjacent to the trigone of the lateral ventricles. These infarctions progress through characteristic pathologic stages, which correlate well with the ultrasound findings (see later). They vary in size and can be unilateral or bilateral. In addition, they can have a hemorrhagic component, which may be small in the form of petechial hemorrhages or massive as evidenced by gross hemorrhage.

Imaging: Ultrasound, Computed Tomography, and Magnetic Resonance Imaging

Evidence of periventricular leukomalacia is often detected on the ultrasound scan in the first week of life. The major finding is a diffuse, somewhat ill-defined area of increased echogenicity in the periventricular region (Fig. 17–10).[24-28] This most often occurs along the superolateral edge of the lateral ventricle and the superolateral posterior border of the trigone of the lateral ventricle. The findings are often bilateral, although they may be asymmetrical. This hyperechogenicity should be visualized in both coronal and sagittal views, since mild degrees of hyperechogenicity, especially in the periatrial

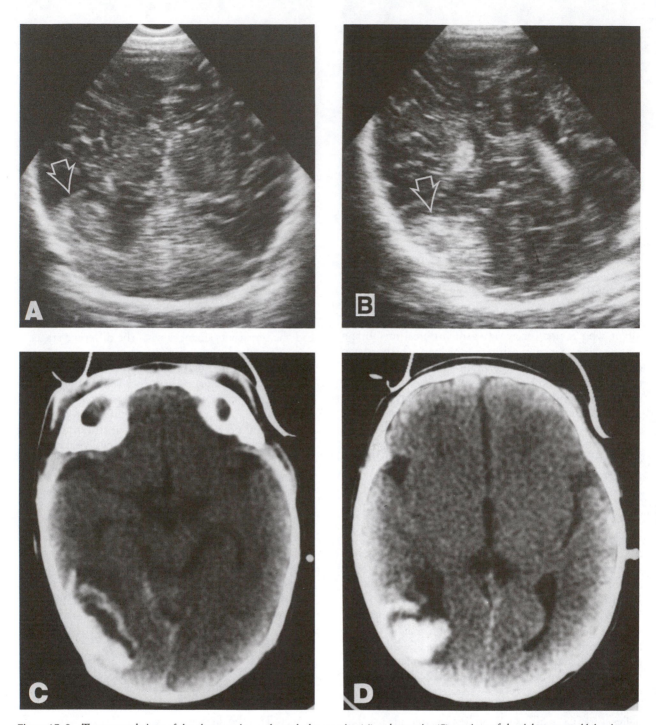

Figure 17-9   Two coronal views of the ultrasound scan through the anterior (*A*) and posterior (*B*) portions of the right temporal lobe show an area of increased echogenicity representing an intraparenchymal hemorrhage (open arrows, *A*, *B*). On the CT scan the intraparenchymal hemorrhage is an inhomogeneous area of increased density in the mid and posterior right temporal lobe (*C, D*). The low density in the hemorrhage suggests some segregation of red cells from plasma. These findings are typical of the intraparenchymal hemorrhages seen in neonates given extracorporeal membrane oxygenation.

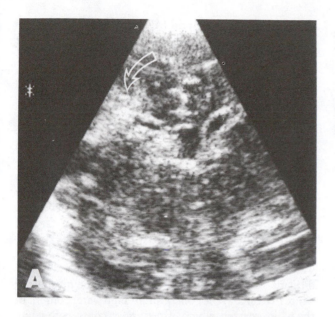

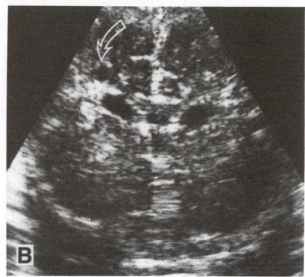

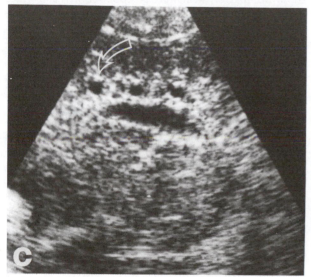

Figure 17-10   The initial coronal ultrasound scan on day 4 of life showed two distinct lesions. One area of increased echogenicity in the right frontal horn represents subependymal-intraventricular hemorrhage. Geographically separate from this lesion is another area of increased echogenicity in the periventricular white matter adjacent to the right lateral ventricle (curved arrow, *A*). This represents the early stage of periventricular leukomalacia. Coronal (*B*) and sagittal (*C*) ultrasound scans performed at six weeks of life show transition from the echogenic periventricular leukomalacia stage (*A*) to the "cystic" stage (*C*). In this patient the cysts are small, well circumscribed, and limited to the immediate periventricular region (arrows, *B, C*). This transition from echogenic to cystic appearance is typical of periventricular leukomalacia. The small subependymal-intraventricular hemorrhage has resolved.

region, can be seen normally in the sagittal view.[29] The pathologic correlate of this stage is primarily vascular congestion with some degree of petechial hemorrhage and very early coagulative necrosis.[30] The findings are striking in that the lesion, although relatively extensive, is associated with a minimal mass effect. Often there is no subependymal-intraventricular hemorrhage component. This periventricular leukomalacia echogenic lesion usually is easily distinguishable from the intraparenchymal hemorrhagic component of subependymal-intraventricular hemorrhage; the latter usually has a significant mass effect and the intraparenchymal hemorrhagic component often shows contiguity with the subependymal-intraventricular hemorrhage.

Over a period of two to three weeks this hyperechoic region begins to show changes, the most characteristic of which is the formation of anechoic areas, i.e., "cystic" changes. These cysts initially are small, but as they become more numerous, they begin to coalesce into larger cystic lesions (see Figs. 17–10, 17–11). This later stage is therefore characterized by an inhomogeneous area of echogenicity, which has a multicystic appearance.[24-28] Again, despite the formation of cysts, the mass effect remains minimal or absent. In very mild forms of periventricular leukomalacia a single cyst may be visualized, although most often in this late stage it is characterized by a multicystic appearance. The pathologic correlate of this stage is cyst formation within areas of coagulative necrosis.[30] The cysts are the end stage after the liquefied necrotic tissue is cleared by macrophages. These cysts do not persist but eventually collapse and coalesce, resulting in a ex vacuo phenomenon in the adjacent lateral ventricle, which enlarges. In the end stage only glial scars remain as evidence of this watershed infarction.[30]

Periventricular leukomalacia may be hemorrhagic or nonhemorrhagic.[31] There is some debate whether the hemorrhagic form represents a different type of lesion. A new term, periventricular hemorrhagic infarction, has been suggested (Fig. 17–12). These two forms of periventricular leukomalacia cannot be distinguished by ultrasound, since both are equally echogenic. CT scanning discriminates between these two entities, because the CT scan detects the high density of hemorrhage in the periventricular region in the hemorrhagic form (see Fig. 17–12). On the CT scan this can be distinguished from subependymal-intraventricular hemorrhage, since hemorrhagic periventricular leukomalacia (or periventricular hemorrhagic infarction) often only shows as a high density in the periventricular region without high density within the ventricular system that would indicate subependymal-intraventricular hemorrhage. If they are associated, the area of periventricular leukomalacia is often geographically separate from the subependymal-intraventricular hemorrhage (see Fig. 17–10).

Ultrasound, CT, and MR imaging are sensitive in the detection of periventricular leukomalacia at different stages of the disease. In the acute stage when the ultrasound scan shows a highly echogenic lesion, the CT scan may be negative or at best may show very subtle low density in the periventricular region. This is indeed a subtle change because in a premature infant this periventricular white matter is normally of low density because of its high water content. The MR scan on T1 weighted images can show periventricular areas of low signal intensity indicative of necrosis. Although documentation is sparse at this time, there is a suggestion that MR imaging may detect periventricular leukomalacia even when the ultrasound scan is negative or equivocal. The pattern of abnormality on MR imaging may have a "cystic" appearance without cysts being obvious by ultrasound. On a T2 weighted MR image these early abnormalities are more difficult to detect because of the lack of myelinated white matter and the concomitant high water content of the white matter, which affords poor contrast in white matter to highlight the infarction. If in the acute stage periventricular leukomalacia is hemorrhagic, this characteristic of the lesion can be detected by CT because of the high density caused by hemorrhage and the hemorrhagic component should be detectable by MR imaging as easily as it is by CT on T1 and T2 weighted images.[8]

The subacute cystic stage of periventricular leukomalacia is readily detected by ultrasound, and the transition from a hyperechoic to a cystic lesion is the sine qua non of the ultrasound diagnosis.[24-28] The cystic stage may or may not be detected by CT, depending on its severity (see Fig. 17–11). If the cysts are large enough, narrow, low density lesions in a periventricular distribution may be detected, but this can be difficult because they may not be easily separable from the ventricles themselves or from the adjacent low density white matter (see Fig. 17–11). Only severe forms of this subacute stage of periventricular leukomalacia are detected by CT. These cysts are detectable on T1 weighted images as multiple round low signal abnormalities in a periventricular distribution. In this late stage they are also more readily detectable on T2 weighted images because the cysts often have a dark rim. This low signal rim results from a magnetic susceptibility effect caused by the deposition of hemosiderin. The presence of this rim is consistent with the necrosis and petechial hemorrhage seen in the acute stages of this type of infarction.[30]

The end stage of periventricular leukomalacia, the glial scar, is also not directly detected by CT unless it is very large. The CT scan may show indirect evidence of previous periventricular leukomalacia by virtue of ventricular enlargement and evidence of loss of white matter, i.e., cortical gyri adjacent to the trigone. Ultrasound

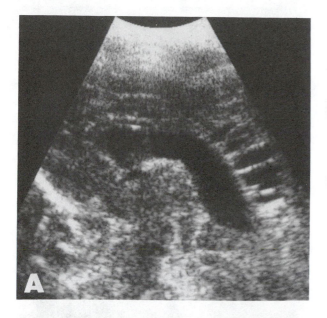

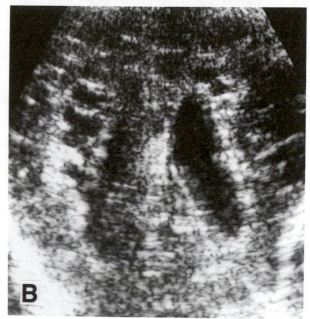

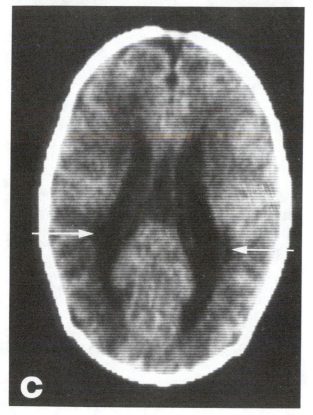

Figure 17–11   In this patient with severe bilateral periventricular leukomalacia the ultrasound findings (*A*, *B*) are compared with the CT scan findings (*C*). The ultrasound scans performed during the sixth week of life show prominent large cyst formation in the peri-atrial white matter. This is a typical location for periventricular leukomalacia on the sagittal scan (*A*) and coronal scan (*B*). Findings on the noncontrast CT scan are somewhat more subtle, but linear low density abnormalities are seen in the immediate periventricular region (arrows, *C*). These are the CT equivalent of the cystic stage of periventricular leukomalacia. (*C*, from Enzmann D, Murphy-Irwin K, Stevenson D, et al. The natural history of subependymal dural matrix hemorrhage. Am J Perinatol 1985; 2:130.)

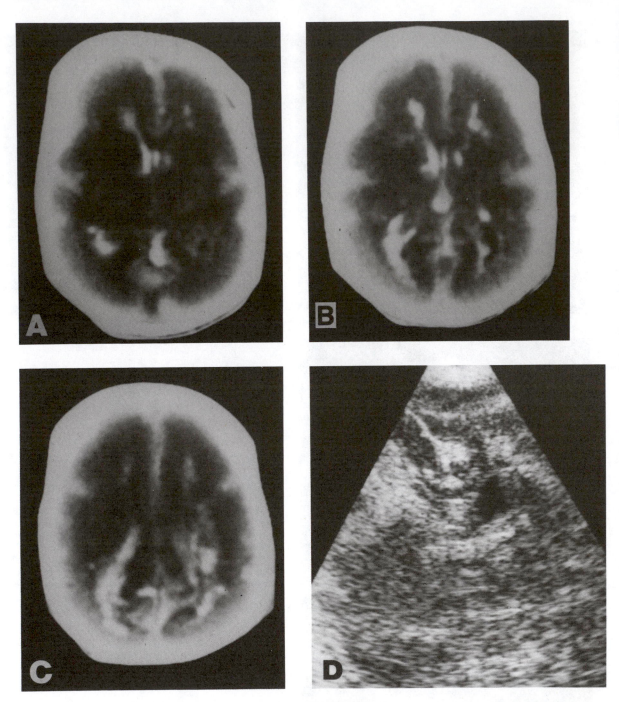

Figure 17-12   The CT scan in a patient with the hemorrhagic form of periventricular leukomalacia (or PVHI) shows diffuse, multifocal increased density in the periventricular white matter (*A, B, C*). In this patient it is extensive and nearly symmetrical. Coronal ultrasound views at this time show ill-defined increased echogenicity in the white matter of the centrum semiovale superolateral to the ventricular system (*D, E*). *Figure continues*.

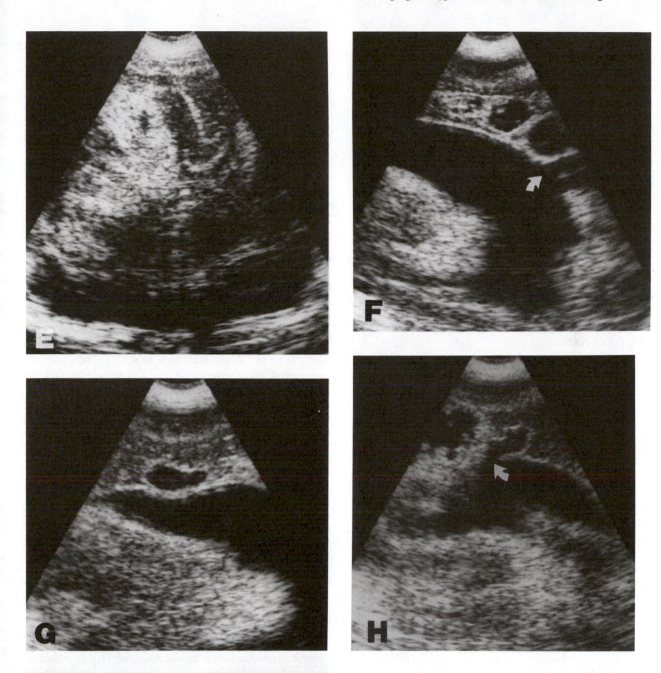

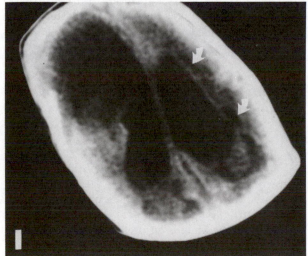

Figure 17–12 (Continued)   The areas of hemorrhagic periventricular leukomalacia are extensive and irregular. An ultrasound scan performed three weeks later shows the expected multicystic appearance of the periventricular white matter (see Fig. 17-4). Some areas of cavitation within the area of hemorrhagic periventricular leukomalacia communicate with the ventricular system (arrows, *F, H*); this will result in focal ventricular dilation or porencephaly. A CT scan performed at this time shows marked ventricular enlargement in the interval and prominent low density areas within the periventricular white matter (*I*). A large low density region in the right frontal area causes a mass effect on the enlarged ventricle (*I*). Many of the periventricular cysts are subtle (curved arrows, *I*). A mass effect from these cysts was also evident on the ultrasound scan (*G*). The hemorrhagic form of periventricular leukomalacia cannot be distinguished from the nonhemorrhagic form by ultrasound.

is not appropriate for use in this late stage because the anterior fontanelle is closed and no other acoustic window is available. The best examination for detecting this late stage of periventricular leukomalacia appears to be the MR scan, specifically the T2 weighted sequence of such a study (Fig. 17–13). MR imaging allows direct detection of the glial scar, which is seen as an area with an abnormal high signal on the T2 weighted images in the periventricular region, typically the trigone.[6] This area of abnormal signal characteristically abuts the ventricular wall and often has a flame shaped appearance extending into the subcortical white matter.[6] The indirect evidence for periventricular leukomalacia, consisting of ventricular enlargement and loss of white matter, also is well visualized on the MR scan. A pulse sequence on MR that is sensitive to myelination, such as a T1 weighted or inversion recovery scan, can show in addition to glial scarring, a delay or lack of myelination in white matter.

Benign Cysts

One should be aware that small periventricular cysts may be found in the first week of life that are similar to the subacute stage of periventricular leukomalacia normally seen later.[32] These cysts are in a different location, usually adjacent to the frontal horn near the caudate nucleii (Fig. 17–14). They do not change over the first few weeks of life and are believed to be benign. They do not have an abnormal echogenicity, and they have thin walls. Although the onset of periventricular leukomalacia may occur in utero and the cystic stage may therefore be present in neonates in the first week of life, this unusual. One should at least be aware of this entity so as not to automatically attach prognostic significance to the presence of cysts. Although our experience is limited, these small cysts may remain stable for several weeks and then slowly involute. Their exact nature is not known, but current evidence suggests that no serious consequences are associated with such cysts.

Focal Infarction

Cerebral infarction similar to that seen in adult patients is seen in neonates.[33] It is a somewhat uncommon manifestation of hypoxic-ischemic disease compared with subependymal-intraventricular hemorrhage and periventricular leukomalacia. Focal infarcts appear to be most common in neonates given extracorporeal membrane oxygenation.[20]

Ultrasound

Focal infarcts have a vascular distribution and have characteristic locations in the brain. They typically have a "wedge" shape. On ultrasound scans a focal infarct presents as a wedge shaped area of moderately increased echogenicity in a vascular distribution, usually in the middle cerebral artery distribution. The abnormal echogenicity involves both gray and white matter.[33] The mass effect is a function of the size and age of the infarct; with acute and larger infarcts some ventricular compression or midline shift can be detected. In the later stages of the infarct the parenchymal echogenicity decreases and atrophic changes appear, i.e., compensatory sulcal and ventricular enlargement. When sulci dilate, they appear more echogenic.

Computed Tomography

Infarcts on the CT scan are similar to those seen in adult patients.[33] In the very acute stage the CT scan may show no abnormality in the infarcted zone. Within two to three days, however, the infarction develops an abnormal low density in a vascular distribution involving both gray and white matter. The wedge shape may be somewhat less obvious on the CT scan, which is in the axial projection, compared with the ultrasound scan, which is in a coronal projection. As the infarct evolves, the low density increases and a mass effect may be detected, depending on the size of the infarct. There is a short period at approximately two weeks when there may be some increase in the density of the infarct, but this usually is not enough to obscure its delineation. In the very late stages of the infarction the low density becomes more prominent and the borders of the infarct are more sharply marginated. At this stage adjacent atrophic changes become evident as ventricular dilation occurs with dilation of adjacent cortical sulci.[33]

Diffuse Hypoxic-Ischemic Injury

Damage to the central nervous system due to diffuse hypoxic-ischemic insult can vary from neuronal dropout caused by hypoxia to a severe form consisting of global cerebral edema and infarction. The latter process is caused by extended periods of asphyxia or cardiorespiratory arrest.

Imaging with Ultrasound and Computed Tomography

A severe global hypoxic-ischemic insult results in diffuse cerebral edema in the acute stage. On the ultrasound scan the major finding is a lack of visualization of the ventricualr system (Fig. 17–15). There is no midline shift because the brain is diffusely swollen. The paren-

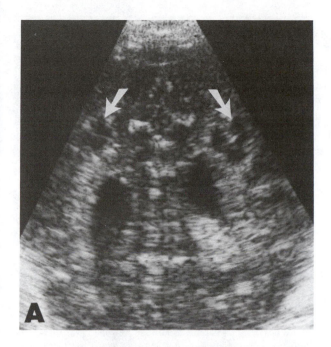

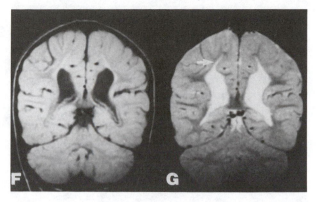

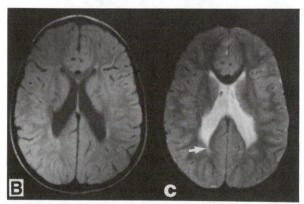

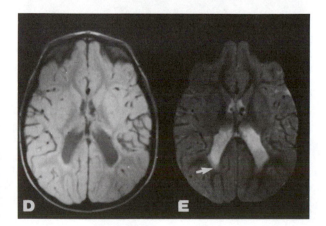

Figure 17–13   A coronal ultrasound scan shows the cystic stage of periventricular leukomalacia in the superolateral region of the atria. Small cysts are identified (arrows, *A*) within a larger area of increased echogenicity in this periventricular location. This child's MR scan at the age of four years shows abnormal high signal intensity on the first (*B, D*) and second (arrows, *C, E*) echoes of a T2 weighted sequence. This abnormal high signal is seen on the first echo images (*B, D*) adjacent to the lateral ventricles, which are of low signal intensity. On the second echo images (*C, E*) this abnormal high signal intensity seems to cap the ventricle and extend into the white matter of the centrum semiovale. A coronal T2 weighted scan shows this increased signal intensity on the first (*F*) and second (arrow, *G*) images. Note that the abnormal signal intensity is immediately adjacent to the ventricle on both axial (arrows, *C, E*) and coronal (arrow, *G*) views. This is characteristic of periventricular leukomalacia and differentiates it from the normal area of delayed myelination located in this region.

chyma may show inhomogeneous echogenicity, but because of the symmetry of findings this may be difficult to detect. The diencephalon may exhibit a relatively increased echogenicity (see Fig. 17–15). Diagnosis by ultrasound is complicated because normal neonates may show a very small ventricular system, which could have an appearance similar to that in a neonate with diffuse cerebral edema. An important finding is the diminution of vascular pulsation as detected in real time as the scan is being performed.

The CT scan in this early stage shows a diffuse symmetrical low density of the entire cerebrum with sparing of the diencephalon (Fig. 17–16). There is a lack of distinction between gray and white matter. The ventricular system is either slitlike or barely identifiable. Normal cisternal structures such as the quadrigeminal cistern are compressed. The low density in the cerebrum is symmetrical and contrasts with the relatively normal density of the cerebellum and diencephalon.

As this injury evolves, it often follows a final common pathway to multicystic encephalomalacia. Other

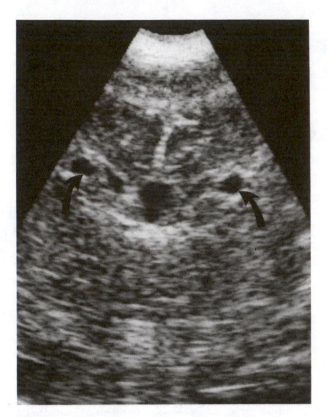

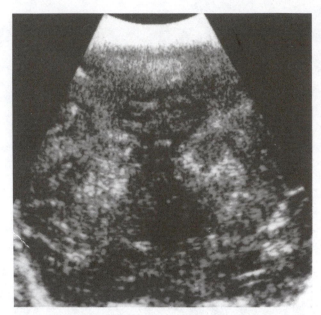

Figure 17-15 This coronal ultrasound scan shows the findings of diffuse cerebral edema. The ventricular system is not identifiable. There is increased diffuse symmetrical echogenicity in the region of the diencephalon. Although the lack of visualization of ventricular system can be normal, this degree of abnormal echogenicity in the parenchyma is not normal. When the examination is performed, it is important to assess the pulsatility of the intracerebral vessels; it would be decreased with diffuse edema.

Figure 17-14 This coronal ultrasound scan shows the typical appearance of benign periventricular cysts that could be mistaken for periventricular leukomalacia. These cysts can be identified in the first week of life and remain unchanged for several weeks. In this patient the cysts are bilaterally symmetrical (arrows) and situated lateral to the frontal horns, lower than where cysts of periventricular leukomalacia would be expected.

what increased density. These findings represent the end stage of multicystic encephalomalacia in which, in essence, most neural tissue in the cerebral hemispheres has been destroyed and replaced by cystic degeneration. Pathologically such a brain is described by the descriptive term *status marmoratus*.

Hypoglycemia

Isolated neonatal hypoglycemia is unusual but can occur with maternal diabetes mellitus or toxemia. The manifestations of hypoglycemia are similar to those of hypoxia, since the relative lack of glucose inhibits the normal utilization of oxygen. A wide spectrum of structural changes therefore may occur, ranging from neuronal dropout, which has no correlate on imaging studies, to diffuse cortical infarction. With diffuse cortical infarction the CT scan may show an abnormal density in the cerebral cortex, usually bilaterally symmetrically. With the intravenous use of a contrast medium, an abnormal increase in the pattern of cortical gyral enhancement is seen.[35] Hemorrhage is not part of the spectrum of hypoglycemia.[36] In the endstage, atrophic changes are the residua of neuronal dropout and frank infarction. This is manifested as ventricular enlargement and dilation of cortical sulci.[36]

severe brain injuries also may follow this final common pathway, i.e., diffuse meningoencephalitis. On the ultrasound scan the earliest evidence of cystic encephalomalacia is the appearance of small scattered anechoic regions in the cerebral hemispheres.[28] This occurs two to three weeks after the insult.[34] The small anechoic regions coalesce to form larger cysts. The cysts are better seen as discrete entities on the ultrasound scan compared with the CT scan. On the CT scan one can visualize the development of the cysts as areas that have a progressively lower density crisscrossed by apparent septations (Fig. 17–16).[28] The cysts develop symmetrically throughout the cerebral hemispheres.

During this process some symmetrical ventricular enlargement occurs, but it is not massive (Fig. 17–16).[28] In fact, given the amount of tissue destruction, ventriculomegaly is modest. In addition, characteristically a symmetrical band of relatively normal density remains between the frontal and parietal lobes (see Fig. 17–16).[28] The diencephalon is relatively spared compared with the cerebral cortex, giving it a normal density or a some-

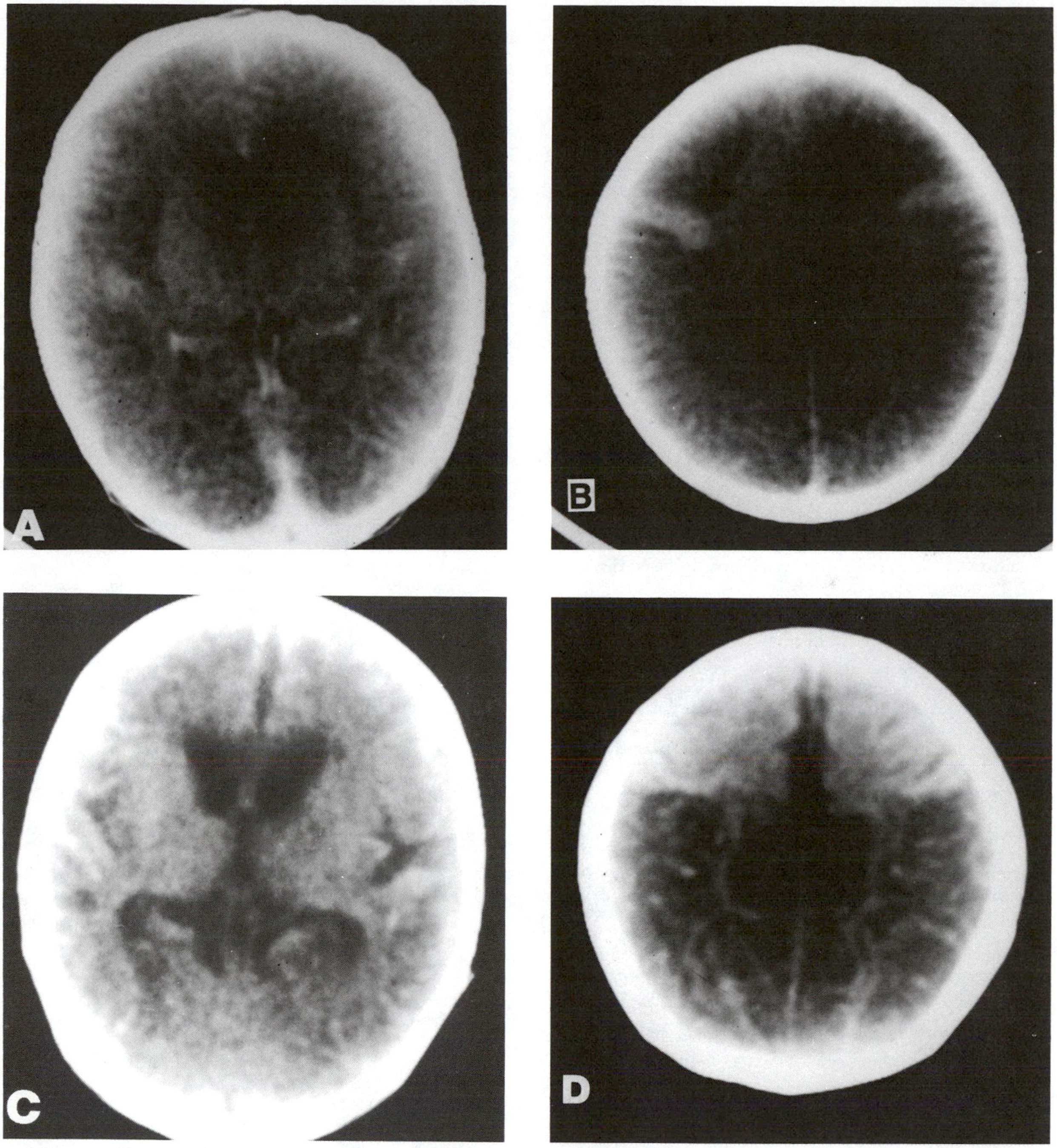

Figure 17-16   The CT scans obtained a few days after a global hypoxic-ischemic insult to the brain show diffuse abnormal signal intensity of the entire cerebrum (*A, B*), with relative sparing of the basal ganglia (diencephalon) and a thin ribbon of tissue between the frontal and parietal lobes (*B*). A subtle compressed gyral pattern is still evident. A CT scan obtained two weeks later shows interval enlargement of the ventricles and sylvian fissures; the enlargement is indicative of atrophic changes resulting from tissue loss. The temporoparietal and high parietal regions are developing the typical "septated" appearance of multicystic encephalomalacia. The signal density of the diencephalon has remained within normal limits.

REFERENCES

1. Rumack CM, McDonal MM, O'Meara OP, et al. CT detection and course of intracranial hemorrhage in premature infants. AJR 1978; 131:493.
2. Babcock DS, Bove KE, Han BK. Intracranial hemorrhage in premature infants: sonographic-pathologic correlation. AJNR 1982; 3:309.
3. Ludwig B, Becker K, Rutter G, Bohl J, Brand M. Postmortem CT and autopsy in perinatal intracranial hemorrhage. AJNR 1983; 4:27.
4. Grant ED, Borts F, Schellinger D, et al. Real-time ultrasonography of neonatal intraventricular hemorrhage and comparison with computed tomography. Radiology 1981; 139:687.
5. Silverboard G, Horder MH, Ahmann PA, et al. Reliability of ultrasound in diagnosis of intracerebral hemorrhage and posthemorrhagic hydrocephalus: comparison with computed tomography. Pediatrics 1980; 66:507.
6. Baker LL, Stevenson DK, Enzmann DR. End-stage periventricular leukomalacia: MR evaluation. Radiology 1988; 168:809.
7. Johnson MA, Pennock JM, Bydder GM, et al. Serial MR imaging in neonatal cerebral injury. AJNR 1987; 8:83.
8. McArdle CB, Richardson CJ, Hayden CK, et al. Abnormalities of the neonatal brain: MR imaging. Part I. Intracranial hemorrhage. Radiology 1987; 163:387.
9. Enzmann D, Murphy-Irwin K, Stevenson D, et al. The natural history of subependymal germinal matrix hemorrhage. Am J Perinatol 1983; 2:123.
10. Shinnar S, Molteni RA, Gammon K, et al. Intraventricular hemorrhage in the premature infant. N Engl J Med 1982; 306:1464.
11. Shankaran S, Slovis TL, Bedard MP, Poland RL. Sonographic classification of intracranial hemorrhage. A prognostic indicator of mortality, morbidity, and short-term neurologic outcome. J Pediatr 1982; 100:469.
12. Papile LA, Burstein J, Burstein R, Koffler H. Incidence and evolution of subependymal and intraventricular hemorrhage: a study of infants with birth weights less than 1500 g. J Pediatr 1978; 92:529.
13. Salomon WL, Benitz WE, Enzmann DR, et al. Correlation of echoencephalographic findings and neurodevelopmental outcome: intracranial hemorrhage and ventriculomegaly in infants of birth weight 1,000 grams or less. J Clin Monit 1987; 3:178.
14. Bowerman RA, Donn SM, Silver TM, Jaffe MH. Natural history of neonatal periventricular-intraventricular hemorrhage and its complications: sonographic observations. AJNR 1984; 5:527.
15. Reeder JD, Kaude JV, Setzer ES. Choroid plexus hemorrhage in premature neonates: recognition by sonography. AJNR 1982; 3:619.
16. Hecht ST, Filly RA, Callen PW, Wilson-Davis SL. Intracranial hemorrhage: late onset in the preterm neonate. Radiology 1983; 149:697.
17. Fleischer AC, Hutchison AA, Bundy AL, et al. Serial sonography of posthemorrhagic ventricular dilatation and porencephaly after intracranial hemorrhage in the preterm neonate. AJNR 1983; 4:971.
18. Grant EG, Kerner M, Schellinger D, et al. Evolution of porencephalic cysts from intraparenchymal hemorrhage in neonates: sonographic evidence. AJNR 1982; 3:47.
19. Smith WL, McGuiness G, Cavanaugh D, Courtney S. Ultrasound screening of premature infants: longitudinal follow-up of intracranial hemorrhage. Radiology 1983; 147:445.
20. Eelkema EA, Bowen A'Delbert, Latchow RE. Cranial ultrasound in infants treated with extracorporeal membrane oxygenation (ECMO). AJNR, in press.
21. Chow PP, Horgan JG, Taylor KJW. Neonatal periventricular leukomalacia: real-time sonographic diagnosis with CT correlation. AJNR 1985; 6:383.
22. Bejar R, Coen RW, Merrit TA, et al. Focal necrosis of the white matter (periventricular leukomalacia): sonographic, pathologic, and electroencephalographic features. AJNR 1986; 7:1073.
23. Shuman RM, Selednik LJ. Periventricular leukomalacia, a one-year autopsy study. Arch Neurol 1980; 37:231.
24. Bowerman RA, Donn SM, DiPietro MA, et al. Periventricular leukomalacia in the pre-term newborn infant: sonographic and clinical features. Radiology 1984; 151:382.
25. Grant EG, Schellinger D. Sonography of neonatal periventricular leukomalacia: recent experience with a 7.5-MHz Scanner. AJNR 1985; 6:781.
26. Grant EG, Schellinger D, Smith Y, Uscinski RH. Periventricular leukomalacia in combination with intraventricular hemorrhage: sonographic features and sequelae. AJNR 1986; 7:443.
27. Schellinger D, Grant EG, Richardson JD. Cystic periventricular leukomalacia: sonographic and CT findings. AJNR 1984; 5:439.
28. Schellinger D, Grant EG, Richardson JD. Neonatal leukencephalopathy: a common form of cerebral ischemia. Radiographics 1985; 5:221.
29. Grant EG, Schellinger D, Richardson JD, et al. Echogenic periventricular halo: normal sonographic finding or neonatal cerebral hemorrhage. AJNR 1983; 4:43.
30. Fawer CL, Calame A, Perentes E, Anderegg A. Periventricular leukomalacia: a correlation study between real-time ultrasound and autopsy findings. Periventricular leukomalacia in the neonate. Neuroradiology 1985; 27:292.
31. Hill A, Melson GL, Clark HB, Volpe JJ. Hemorrhagic periventricular leukomalacia: diagnosis by real time ultrasound and correlation with autopsy findings. Pediatrics 1982; 69:282.
32. Keller MS, DiPietro MA, Teele RL, et al. Periventricular cavitations in the first week of life. AJNR 1987; 8:291.
33. Hill A, Martin DJ, Daneman MB, Titz CR. Focal ischemic cerebral injury in the newborn: diagnosis by ultrasound and correlation with computed tomographic scan. Pediatrics 1983; 71:790.
34. Slovis TL, Shankaran S, Bedard MP, Poland RL. Intracranial hemorrhage in the hypoxic-ischemic infant: ultrasound demonstration of unusual complications. Radiology 1984; 151:163.
35. Kaiser MC, Pettersson H, Harwood-Nash DC, et al. Computed tomography of the brain in severe hypoglycaemia. J Comput Tomogr 1981; 5:757.
36. Hirabayashi S, Kitahara T, Hishida T. Computed tomography in perinatal hypoxic and hypoglycemic encephalopathy with emphasis on follow-up studies. J Comput Tomogr 1980; 4:451.

18 Etiology and Timing of Static Encephalopathies of Childhood (Cerebral Palsy)

Steven L. Weinstein, M.D. and Barry R. Tharp, M.D.

Historical Overview
Cerebral Palsy
  Definition
  Clinical Phenotypes
    Quadriplegia
    Spastic Diplegia
    Hemiplegia
    Athetosis-Choreoathetosis
    Dystonia
    Ataxia
  Mental Retardation and Seizures
  Trends in the Prevalence of Cerebral Palsy
Brain Morphology in Cerebral Palsy
  Pathologic Findings
  Radiologic Findings
Time of Injury
  Postnatal and Familial Cerebral Palsy
  Perinatal Risk
  Prepregnancy and Pregnancy Risks
    Optimality of Pregnancy
    Maternal Age
    Reproductive History
    Socioeconomic Status
    Race
    Maternal Neurologic Disorder
    Gestational Age
    Growth Retardation
    Head Circumference
    Malformations
    Congenital Infection
    Placental Abnormality
    Umbilical Cord Length
    Presentation
    Twins

Neonatal Depression and Asphyxia
  Meconium
  Fetal Monitoring
  Apgar Scores
Neonatal Neurologic Status
  Term Infants
    Clinical Examination
    Seizures
    Birth Trauma
    Stroke
  Premature Infants
    Clinical Examination
    Periventricular Hemorrhage and Leukomalacia
  Antecedents of Central Nervous System
    Hemorrhage and Periventricular Leukomalacia
    Pregnancy
    Labor and Delivery
    Perinatal Asphyxia
    Neonatal Period
Summary

Encephalopathies that are apparent at birth or in the first few months after delivery are usually categorized as "cerebral palsy." The afflicted child often becomes a burden to the family and society and has significant caretaking needs as well as medical and educational expenses. Physicians caring for the mother and the newborn infant are often held culpable for the subsequent motor and intellectual handicaps because of the commonly held view that most injuries are sustained immediately before or during the birth process. Parents also seek reassurance that subsequent pregnancies will not produce a similarly impaired offspring. This chapter points out that most cases of so-called cerebral palsy have no connection with perinatal asphyxia and that those caused by perinatal events may be identifiable in the immediate postnatal period. Each case of this syndrome therefore should be approached as a unique diagnostic problem rather than being lumped under the rubric of cerebral palsy.

HISTORICAL OVERVIEW

Crippling neurologic disabilities are described in writings and paintings from ancient civilizations. Courville's monograph displays artwork of the ancient Egyptians of an individual with the posture of spastic diplegia, a posture similar to Raphael's illustration of the Biblical description of a cripple "lame from [his] mother's womb" (Acts 3:21) begging alms at the gate of the temple.[1]

Little,[2] credited with the early clinical descriptions of cerebral palsy, attributed the disorder to "premature birth, difficult labours, mechanical injuries during parturition to head and neck, where life had been saved" although recognizing that "the great majority of apparently stillborn infants, whose lives are saved by the attendant accoucheur, recover unharmed from such conditions."

Freud[3] took issue with the origins of the syndrome, stating that "difficult birth and premature birth can certainly not be considered the etiology of the case wherever it may occur. It may be just an accidental combination of etiologic factors; a child conditioned by intrauterine fate to develop cerebral palsy could have been born prematurely or could have undergone difficult birth. ... difficult birth and premature birth are not always accidental happenings, but may frequently be results of a deeper cause, or its expressions, without being the actual etiological factor. Thus it may well be possible that the same pathogenic factors that rendered intrauterine development abnormal also extended their influence to parturition; abnormal birth is then the final result of abnormal pregnancy." Freud also had the insight to note a case report in which an infant at "9 months then developed convulsions after an intestinal catarrh, and from then on had symptoms of severe general rigidity ... with impairment of mental development." When the child died at the age of $3\frac{1}{2}$ years, the autopsy showed "bilateral porencephaly...deep microgyric orifice and atypical gyri, and changes ... [that] indicated with certainty a fetal origin of the disease." Freud expressed frustration in differentiating some forms of cerebral palsy from familial neurologic syndromes because of the ambiguity of the clinical manifestations. Finally, in reviewing the pathology literature, he concluded that "the initial lesion of infantile cerebral paralysis consists of vascular disturbances in a large number of cases: hemorrhage, embolism, or thrombosis of the same nature and effect as in the adult brain."[3]

Almost 100 years later the issues raised by Little and Freud remain unresolved in spite of growing medical sophistication: When does the insult occur, what is the role of labor and how is it influenced by an abnormal fetus, how do postnatal influences affect the child, can familial disorders be discriminated, and what is the role of the cerebrovascular system in the pathogenesis of the cerebral disease? This chapter addresses some of these questions.

CEREBRAL PALSY

The clinical syndrome called cerebral palsy has been utilized as a marker for cerebral damage during early brain maturation. The disorder, however, should not be considered as synonymous with perinatal injury but rather as a nonspecific motor abnormality secondary to any central nervous system insult. The syndrome is identifiable by physical examination, but its expression may change as the child matures.

Definition

Cerebral palsy is defined by the Little Club to be "a disorder of movement and posture due to a defect or lesion of the immature brain."[4] Bax et al[4] excluded motor disorders of short duration, degenerative illnesses, and isolated mental deficiency. Children with cerebral palsy who also have congenital anomalies (except obvious malformations of the brain) and postnatally acquired brain injury during the first years of life are usually included in pathologic and epidemiologic series.

The spectrum of neurologic syndromes typically classified as cerebral palsy can be diagnosed during the first year of life, but more mildly impaired infants may not be identified until school entry.[5,6] The majority of children in the National Collaborative Perinatal Project (NCPP) with cerebral palsy at seven years were at least suspected of having a brain abnormality prior to discharge from the nursery.[7] At four months 64 percent and at one year 60 percent of the children destined to have cerebral palsy were considered at least neurologically suspect; conversely, 40 percent of the children had not yet been diagnosed.[5,8] False positive findings were a significant problem in that 52 percent of the children considered to have cerebral palsy at one year "outgrew" the disorder.[5,9] Recent follow-up studies in premature infants also demonstrated the need for waiting until school age to make the final diagnosis, for the grade of motor and cognitive handicap was reclassified between one year and three to five years of age in 22 to 37 percent of the cases.[10,11]

Clinical Phenotypes

Heterogeneity of the clinical syndromes is the rule. Children are subcategorized according to the pattern of involvement: tone either increased or decreased; associated adventitious movements including choreoathetosis, dystonia or ataxia, and varying combinations; limbs involved; degree of functional impairment; and associated neurologic abnormalities.[12] Rigid categorization fails owing to the lack of interobserver agreement regarding both the type and the severity of the handicap as well as the changing character of the deficits over time.[13] Nonetheless there is a need for these categories when designing interventions for subsequent care as well as stratagems for improving our understanding of the underlying pathophysiology.

Spastic syndromes account for 51 to 87 percent of the cases, with a variable frequency of the pattern of limb involvement.[9,14-19] The most common syndromes considered under the term cerebral palsy include the following:

Quadriplegia

In this spastic syndrome there is relatively equal impairment of the upper and lower extremities. The children are usually multiply handicapped with severe motor involvement, profound mental retardation, epilepsy, and microcephaly.[17-19] Early death is not unusual.[9]

Spastic Diplegia

Spasticity is noted in all the extremities, but the legs are disproportionately impaired. This syndrome is commonly seen in low birth weight survivors.[17,18] The motor disability is severely handicapping in only 11 to 20 percent of the cases, and mental retardation when present is not so profound as in quadriplegics.[17,18,20]

Hemiplegia

This frequently seen syndrome is usually the most common of the postnatally acquired phenotypes.[9,14,18,21] The motor handicaps are the least likely to be disabling, and intelligence in most instances is normal to dull normal. Seizures may occur.[17,18,22]

Athetosis-Choreoathetosis

This rare disorder is dominated by involuntary motor activity with poorly coordinated, exaggerated movements, often considered the hallmark of kernicterus. The movement disorder is relatively nonincapacitating and is infrequently associated with mental retardation or seizures.[17,18,23]

Dystonia

This uncommon entity is characterized by abnormal shifts of tone, spastic signs, retention of primitive reflexes, and the assumption of dystonic postures. The disorder correlates primarily with perinatal "asphyxia" and less frequently with kernicterus. The motor difficulties are usually incapacitating, and cognitive abilities are significantly impaired in the majority of instances. Seizures are a frequent concomitant and early death is not unusual.[17,18,23,24]

Ataxia

In rare cases ataxia predominates. It may be difficult to distinguish from spastic diplegia as well as the familial cerebellar disorders. The ataxia occasionally may be incapacitating and can be associated with mental retardation.[17,18]

We use the terms *motor syndrome* and *static encephalopathy* interchangeably with cerebral palsy throughout most of the chapter in order to emphasize the nonspecific etiology of these disorders. We use the term cerebral palsy when we are citing the studies of others who clearly identified their study group as having cerebral palsy.

Mental Retardation and Seizures

A common pathogenesis in cerebral palsy and profound mental retardation is suggested by their coexistence in some patients. For example, Nelson et al[25] found that 90 of the 189 infants in the NCPP with moderate to severe cerebral palsy were also severely retarded. An underlying etiology could be established for 40: postnatal neurologic catastrophes (13), gross malformations of the central nervous system (13), and neonatal infections, metabolic disorders, and chromosomal aberrations (14). The remaining 50 infants had no identifiable disorder, but neonatal neurologic signs such as intracranial hemorrhage (no radiologic confirmation) and seizures (no electroencephalographic confirmation) were the best independent discriminators of these 50 infants from normal controls.

Isolated profound mental retardation is rarely a consequence of a perinatal event.[26] McQueen et al[27] found a high frequency of chromosomal and other dysmorphic syndromes in the majority of infants with profound retardation. Mild retardation, without associated motor impairment, is also poorly correlated with perinatal events and is more dependent on socioeconomic status and maternal education.[26,28] Sameroff et al[28] demonstrated that a multifactorial measure of family functioning was the best predictor of cognitive abilities.

Finally, epilepsy occurs in approximately 25 to 30 percent of the children with static encephalopathies classified as cerebral palsy.[17,29-31] When the children with cerebral palsy were removed from a cohort of epileptics, the remaining population did not have an increased incidence of delivery complications.[29,32]

Trends in the Prevalence of Cerebral Palsy

A recent review by Paneth et al[33] cited a prevalence for cerebral palsy of 1.4 to 2.9 per 1,000 live births. Since 1949, population-based surveys have demonstrated no consistent trends of change across geographic locations.[33] Table 18–1 presents recent data on prevalence by birth weight. Term infants (2,500 gm or more) show no statistically significant difference between the time periods.[34,35] Low birth weight babies show no consistent change, with incidences in neonatal survivors decreasing,[34] increasing,[16,36,37] or remaining unchanged.[35] Comparisons of these data are complicated by changes in population demographics and differing ages of assessment.[37] Furthermore, accounting for postneonatal deaths is necessary if we are to determine an accurate incidence of cerebral palsy; as many as 53 percent of neurologically impaired children died within the first year of life and an additional 11 percent of one-year-old children with cerebral palsy died by age seven years.[7,9]

Correct interpretation of prevalence data is crucial because there are societal concerns that neonatal intensive care is increasing the number of children with cerebral palsy. This presumed increase may be a consequence of the "continuum of reproductive wastage," a theory that states that a falling mortality leads to the salvaging of increased numbers of damaged children.[38,39] The increase could also be iatrogenic owing to inexperience with new technologic methods. Alternatively the incidence, when expressed in terms of live births, may only appear to increase but in reality the incidence per neonatal survivor is decreasing. If there is no concomitant decrease in the incidence per survivor, as mortality falls, there will be more children with cerebral palsy, which will cause the incidence per number of live births (denominator unchanged) to increase.[36]

The recent prevalence data relating to cerebral palsy suggest that no major changes are occurring and that the overall number of normal children being saved far exceeds those that eventually will be identified with static motor syndromes.[34,40]

BRAIN MORPHOLOGY IN CEREBRAL PALSY

Morphologic studies of the central nervous system provide a basis for understanding the clinical features of cerebral palsy and clues to the pathogenesis of brain injury. Autopsy observations cannot be extrapolated to all children with cerebral palsy for the series are biased toward the more severely afflicted individuals whose brain lesions may be different from those of surviving infants.[41] Radiologic imaging, which allows us to study living children, is limited by the relatively gross nature of the identifiable disease. All pathologic and radiologic studies to date have not been done on random selections of children with cerebral palsy nor have they been performed with controls and the examiners blinded to the categories under study.

TABLE 18–1   Trends in the Prevalence of Cerebral Palsy

Study	Year	Birth Weight (gm)	Incidence*	Year	Incidence*
Western Australia[34]	1968–1971	<1,500	44.34 (14.4)	1979–1981	37.7 (26.9)
		1,500–2,499	11.2 (10.5)		10.3 (10.0)
		>2,500	1.7 (1.7)		1.6 (1.6)
Rochester, USA[35]	1950–1958	<2,500	12.0	1968–1976	12.0
		>2,501	1.8		1.1
United Kingdom[16,36]	1974–1977	<1,500	25.6 (12.0)	1979–1981	77.6 (42.1)
		1,501–2,500	9.2 (8.8)		
		>2,500	1.1 (1.5)		
Melbourne, Australia[37]	1966–1970	500–1,500	26	1980–1982	110

* Calculated incidence rate per 1,000 neonatal survivors (incidence per 1,000 live births).

Pathologic Findings

The heterogeneity of disorders classified as cerebral palsy is apparent when one examines three of the largest recent autopsy series. Gross et al[42] reported neuropathologic findings in the brains of 891 children with mental retardation and neurologic disorders that became clinically evident during the first three years of life. Christensen et al[43] described 69 brains collected from the University Clinic of Pediatrics in Copenhagen from 1948 to 1964, and Malamud et al[44] detailed the pathologic findings in 68 brains examined between 1955 and 1960 obtained from a chronic care state facility; entry criteria for the latter study excluded tumors and metabolic, neurocutaneous, and chromosomal disorders.

Spasticity was evident in 45 percent (N = 401) of the infants in the series reported by Gross et al;[47] defined causes in this subgroup included metabolic disorders (10 percent; e.g., cretinism, leukodystrophies, lipidoses, mucopolysaccharidoses, phenylketonuria, and infantile neuroaxonal dystrophy) and cerebral malformations (32 percent). The causes are similar to those in the two other series, in which pathologic diagnoses included gliomas (4 percent),[43] metabolic disorders (13 percent),[43] and cerebral malformations, including microdysplasias (23 to 35 percent).[43,44] Significantly, the cerebral malformations were found to coexist with encephaloclastic changes, suggesting a superimposed hypoxic-ischemic event.

It is almost impossible to time the onset of encephaloclastic lesions after the child matures. Insults occurring early in brain development interfere with the formation of normal architecture; however, once a structure has been formed, the gross pathologic changes are nonspecific.[45] In some instances the response to injury may help in timing the lesions. For example, microscopy of encephaloclastic lesions prior to the 20th week of gestation shows a reactive monocytosis as the major cellular response producing a smooth-walled cyst, whereas later injuries produce an astrocytic reaction whether in utero or after birth.[46] If the brain is examined in the immediate newborn period, better definition of timing may be possible since acute ischemic injury has a characteristic progression of maturation consisting of staining pallor, neuronal necrosis, cellular response, and vascular changes.[46]

Radiologic Findings

Modern neuroimaging is now used to examine less severely affected individuals, but to date no large series of randomly selected children with cerebral palsy have been reported. Cranial computed tomography (CT) finds a higher frequency of abnormalities in postnatally acquired cases than in encephalopathies presumably acquired prior to or at the time of birth. This suggests different mechanisms of injury.[47,48] Overall, 54 to 92 percent of the scans in children with motor syndromes demonstrate lesions, with a higher incidence of abnormalities in children with hemiplegia. No sizable study using magnetic resonance imaging has been published.

Children with spastic quadriplegia have abnormalities in 75 to 85 percent of the scans; central atrophy with ventricular enlargement being the most common abnormality.[47-49] Other findings include irregular ventricular walls, low density periventricular white matter, infarcts, porencephalic cysts, and malformations.[47-49] Spastic diplegic children have abnormal studies in 41 to 74 percent of scans.[47,48,50] The greater the degree of gait impairment, the higher the probability of an abnormality on the CT scan.[50] Central atrophy involving the lateral ventricular walls is most common, although frontal horn involvement is noted primarily in nonambulatory individuals.[50] Paraplegic infants appear to have a greater involvement of areas anterior to the trigone, with loss of tissue from the posterior aspects of the centrum semiovale.[47]

Scans in hemiplegic patients are abnormal in 73 to 92 percent on the cases, unilateral atrophy or a porencephalic cyst being the most frequent finding.[22,47-49,51] Cortical and subcortical disease is associated with a higher incidence of seizures and mental retardation than are lesions more confined to the periventricular and basal ganglia areas.[22,51]

Children with choreoathetosis have abnormal scans with minor degrees of atrophy or ventricular enlargement, often without basal ganglia abnormalities.[45]

TIME OF INJURY

An accurate determination of the time of brain injury is difficult in the majority of infants. Epidemiologic studies often arbitrarily note central nervous system injury as having occurred prenatally or perinatally, depending on the presence of a complication at delivery. Estimates of the percentage of cases with onsets at these times include: prenatally 18 to 50 percent, perinatally 29 to 46 percent, postnatally 6 to 15 percent, and mixed or unknown compromising the remainder.[14,15,52] It is reported that a greater number of term infants with cerebral palsy sustained injury antenatally as compared with preterm infants, who had a higher incidence of perinatal injury.[14,52] As is to be discussed, this method of the assignment of the central nervous system insult to a particular stage of brain development probably overestimates the incidence of perinatal injury. We will now review epidemiologic features that presumably predisposes infants to cerebral injury in each of these time periods.

Postnatal and Familial Cerebral Palsy

Brain injury in the postnatal period usually follows a discrete event, such as trauma, anoxia, an infectious disease, and stroke. Stanley and Blair[21] found that some children may be predisposed to "postnatally acquired" cerebral palsy as evidenced by a higher incidence of immediate postnatal problems than in control subjects (i.e., neonatal seizures, irritability, drowsiness, poor feeding, and increased admissions to an intensive care nursery). This is suggestive of a chronic neurologic disorder that began prenatally or perinatally and is manifested at an older age as "near miss" sudden infant death syndrome,[53,54] "brain damage" from seizures,[55,56] and pertussis vaccine "reaction."[56] An underlying neurologic impairment due to a cerebral malformation or an inborn error of metabolism (e.g., mitochondrial and fatty acid oxidation defects, aminoacidopathies, organic acidopathies, and leukodystrophies) may also present as an acute encephalopathy in the first year of life.

Familial neurologic syndromes may be responsible for an additional small percentage of cases of cerebral palsy. These syndromes inlcude enzyme deficiencies, neurocutaneous syndromes, and familial ataxias and spastic diplegias (e.g., olivopontocerebellar degeneration and Charcot-Marie-Tooth disease). Taking the genetic issue one step further, complications of pregnancy such as toxemia may also be inherited.[57] Additionally, apparent genetic influences in reality may be a reflection of intrauterine environment; e.g., mothers who have low birth weight infants are at higher risk for subsequent low birth weight infants,[58] perhaps because of uterine abnormalities, maternal illnesses including poor nutritional status, cigarette smoking, alcohol and drug abuse, and other toxin exposure.

Perinatal Risk

The current thinking is that an infant who has had an asphyxial episode during parturition manifests changes in the level of consciousness and tone in the immediate postdelivery period. It is also thought that the extent and duration of the abnormal neurologic signs are directly proportional to the degree and duration of the alterations of brain metabolism. If the signs are present without known asphyxia, one has to presume that the hypoxic-ischemic event occurred prior to delivery or that one is dealing with a nonasphyxial disorder.

The contribution of known complications at birth in the overall population with cerebral palsy is relatively small. The NCPP prospectively enrolled infants between 1959 and 1966, and although dated by improvements in neonatal intensive care, the results are probably relevant for term infants given their stable incidences of cerebral palsy (see Table 18–1). Late obstetrical complications occurred in approximately 63 percent of the term pregnancies (more than 2,500 gm), and if associated with low Apgar scores the mortality was increased but usually not the risk of cerebral palsy.[29,59] The combination of a complicated delivery and signs suggesting hypoxic-ischemic encephalopathy in the infant (decreased activity beyond the first day, feeding difficulties including poor

suck, seizures, prolonged incubator care, respiratory difficulties) was associated with an increased risk of cerebral palsy. The degree of encephalopathy (number of abnormal signs and their persistence) further improved the ability to predict cerebral palsy. Nonetheless, the combination of a complicated delivery and a five minute Apgar score of 5 or less was found in only 13 percent of the cerebral palsy population.[29] In a separate analysis infants with at least one of the aforementioned signs of hypoxic-ischemic encephalopathy (exclusive of Apgar scores) accounted for 32 percent of the cerebral palsy population.[59] Conversely 68 percent of the children with cerebral palsy had neither a low Apgar score nor abnormal signs. The risk of cerebral palsy was not increased in children born following late obstetrical complications with low Apgar scores in the absence of these signs of hypoxic-ischemic encephalopathy.[59]

A case control project in Western Australia involving infants of all gestational ages supports this finding. Infants with cerebral palsy born during the period 1975 to 1980 were matched with control subjects for birth weight, race, sex, plurality, and year of birth.[60] Birth asphyxia was defined as "abnormalities" in fetal heart rate detected by either continuous electronic monitoring or intermittent auscultation, the presence of meconium, a one minute Apgar score less than 7, or a delay of two minutes or longer in the onset of spontaneous respirations. Signs considered to be suggestive of hypoxic-ischemic encephalopathy included alterations of consciousness (jitteriness, irritability, lethargy), hypotonia, poor suck, and seizures. Presumed birth asphyxia was present in more than 60 percent of the infants weighing less than 1,500 gm and occurred with equal frequency in infants with cerebral palsy and in those without. The odds ratio of the risk of cerebral palsy following birth asphyxia for infants weighing 1,501 to 2,500 gm was 2.38 and for infants weighing more than 2,500 gm, 3.50. Overall in only 14 percent of the cerebral palsy population could the disorder be attributed to birth asphyxia, and only those with signs of hypoxic-ischemic encephalopathy demonstrated an increased risk.[60]

Suboptimal obstetrical care as defined by Niswander et al[61] did not appear to "cause" cerebral palsy in the majority of children, meaning that changes in the management of pregnancy may have a negligible impact on the incidence of cerebral palsy. A case control methodology was utilized to blindly grade the complexity of pregnancy and to assess the impact of suboptimal antenatal and intrapartum care on the incidence of cerebral palsy. All cases in which the management was questioned, as well as a sampling of cases with good management, were reviewed by a third obstetrician. Suboptimal prenatal care increased the incidences of fetal "asphyxial" death and neonatal seizures in term infants (not electroencephalographically confirmed) whereas suboptimal intrapartum management was associated with a higher frequency of neonatal depression and neonatal seizures.

Neither group had a higher incidence of cerebral palsy at 18 months.[61]

The apparent minimal contribution of labor and delivery to the cerebral palsy population and the relatively low association with poor obstetrical care suggests either that the majority of children with static encephalopathies are damaged prenatally or that the present measures of assessing fetal distress and neonatal asphyxia are inadequate.

Prepregnancy and Pregnancy Risks

Optimality of Pregnancy

Prechtl[62] introduced the concept of obstetrical "optimality" in an attempt to demonstrate a relationship between prenatal and perinatal events and the neonatal examination. Optimality was defined by 42 items that increased the probability of the birth of a normal child. When this scoring method was applied retrospectively to a group of children with spastic diplegia and hemiplegia and dyskinetic cerebral palsy, a higher incidence of abnormal pregnancies (lower optimality scores) was found than in normal infants.[63-65]

Maternal Age

The mean age of mothers of children with cerebral palsy is not significantly different from that of controls.[66] An interaction of risk and maternal age is suggested by the presence of a U shaped incidence curve for spastic diplegia, teenage and mid-30s mothers having more afflicted children.[20] Parity, when simultaneously considered, is more strongly associated with a risk of cerebral palsy than maternal age.[20]

Reproductive History

A poor maternal reproductive history has been suggested as a risk factor in cerebral palsy,[38] especially spastic diplegia.[67] Infants with spastic diplegia tend to be somewhat growth retarded (see later discussion of growth retardation).[68] When infants with cerebral palsy are matched to controls for birth weight and gestational age, there is no difference in the reproductive histories of the mothers. However, mothers with growth retarded infants, with or without cerebral palsy, have worse reproductive histories.[68]

Socioeconomic Status

Socioeconomic status as an independent variable does not significantly alter the incidence of cerebral palsy.[17,20,69]

Race

Race does not influence the incidence of cerebral palsy in full-grown infants.[20,62] In the NCPP, nonwhite race was associated with a higher incidence of low birth weight infants. The incidence of cerebral palsy in nonwhite low birth weight infants, however, was lower than that in comparable-weight white children.[30,58,66]

Maternal Neurologic Disorder

Maternal epilepsy (seizure within the five years prior to delivery) was associated with a statistically increased incidence of mixed cerebral palsy with mental retardation and microcephaly in the NCPP.[69] A hereditary encephalopathy was suggested in some cases by the increased incidence of associated maternal mental retardation compared with controls. Evidence against a genetic disorder was the lack of other anomalies, including cleft lip, cleft palate, and cardiac defects in the affected children.[69] Adverse intrauterine influences in an epileptic mother could also affect the fetus in the following ways: a direct toxic effect of anticonvulsants on brain development or blood flow (although no statistical difference between therapy or no-therapy groups was observed in the NCPP),[69] an increased frequency of obstetrical complications,[69] a maternal systemic disorder causing seizures but also involving the placenta (e.g., an increased incidence of placental sickling in black epileptics),[69] and a predisposition to fetal distress during labor.[70-72] Whatever the mechanism, maternal epilepsy contributed only minimally to the number of cases of cerebral palsy in the NCPP study.[69]

Gestational Age

The majority of infants (64 to 69 percent) with cerebral palsy have a birth weight of 2,500 gm or more.[16,17,30,33,34,40] The risk of cerebral palsy, however, is much greater in the premature infant (see Table 18–1.) This implies that the gestational age of a cerebral palsy population should be matched to that of the control group when assessing any risk factor for cerebral palsy. An apparently significant contribution to the incidence of cerebral palsy may merely reflect a factor's relationship to premature birth.[58]

Growth Retardation

The relationship of birth weight and gestational age to cerebral palsy is complex and is confused by the lack of distinction in the literature between symmetrical (all growth parameters) and asymmetrical (normal head size) smallness.[73] Different mechanisms of cerebral injury probably exist in these two groups of growth-retarded infants. Symmetrical retardation usually has its origins early in pregnancy and is often secondary to intrinsic fetal abnormalities, i.e., "genetic" influences (maternal size, chromosome or dysmorphic syndromes (2 to 20 percent) or exposure to abnormal maternal or environmental influences.[73] Asymmetrical growth retardation can reflect those factors but commonly is a consequence of uteroplacental insufficiency.[73]

In the NCPP the preterm infants with cerebral palsy were not overtly growth retarded but were clustered between the 10th and 50th percentiles for race-specific weight norms. The premature babies had a higher risk of developing cerebral palsy than growth-retarded term infants of the same birth weight. Term infants with cerebral palsy did not show this subtle growth retardation, but small-for-gestational-age infants (birth weights less than the 5th percentile of normal) were overrepresented.[30] The dysmature infant (absence of vernix, desquamating skin, and perhaps meconium staining) was usually born after term and did not have an increased risk of cerebral palsy.[74] Overall only 0.7 percent of the term infants with birth weights from 1,501 to 2,500 gm had cerebral palsy (as compared with an incidence of 0.3 percent in appropriate-for-gestational-age term infants).[30]

Growth-retarded infants had a higher incidence of spastic cerebral palsy syndromes in English and Australian populations, whereas Swedish infants (especially terms) with decreased birth weight–length ratios had higher incidences of spastic diplegia and dyskinetic cerebral palsy.[20,64,65,75,76]

The majority of infants with growth retardation, excluding those with malformations and "birth asphyxia," are normal.[77,78]

Head Circumference

Head circumference reflects brain growth. Abnormal sizes may be associated with an increased risk of subsequent cerebral palsy. The NCPP found that after correcting for gestational age, sex, and race, the relative risk of cerebral palsy was increased if the head size deviated above or below the mean (five to nine times the risk if 2 standard deviations from the mean and 21 to 26 times if 3 standard deviations). Infants with congenital infections and dysmorphic syndromes were not excluded.[7] Growth-retarded infants, including prematures, with a head circumference 3 standard deviations below the mean did not have an increased probability of an abnormal outcome (excluding infants with congenital malformations) unless there was superimposed birth asphyxia.[78] A disproportionately small head for body size was not associated with an increased risk of an

abnormal neurologic outcome if infants at the extremes of the population (less than the 10th percentile and more than the 90th percentile) and those asphyxiated (one and five minute Apgar scores less than 7) were excluded.[79] A large head circumference is caused by a multitude of well-defined neurologic syndromes, which must be excluded before discussing the risk of cerebral palsy in infants with isolated macrocrania.[80,81]

Malformations

The presence of cerebral anomalies suggests an intrauterine onset of neurologic impairment. Major malformations of the central nervous system usually are excluded from studies addressing the causes of cerebral palsy, although it must be recalled that many malformations are visible only at the microscopic level.

New imaging techniques, such as magnetic resonance imaging, will almost certainly increase our ability to identify brain maldevelopment and categorize more accurately a significant subgroup of infants with static encephalopathy. Geneticists are describing new syndromes at an ever increasing rate, and it is becoming apparent that many children with presumed asphyxic encephalopathies have instead a genetic syndrome.

Brain malformations were noted in 23 to 35 percent of the autopsies of children with cerebral palsy, although certain acquired lesions, such as porencephaly, hydranencephaly, and micropolygyria, were included in this category.[42-44] Small dysplastic lesions are of uncertain significance. They are thought to appear late in brain maturation and theoretically could develop postnatally in the small premature infant.[82] Studies of living children with cerebral palsy have demonstrated central nervous system malformations in 3 to 17 percent of the cases.[47,52,83]

Dysmorphic features and major non–central nervous system congenital anomalies have been found in an increased incidence in children with cerebral palsy, although studies of older children are less reliable because the examiner cannot be blind to the child's underlying neurologic status. The incidence of non–central nervous system malformations in children with cerebral palsy in the NCPP was 22 percent (29 percent if the birth weight was less than 2,000 gm) compared with 6.8 percent in the non–cerebral palsy population.[84] These anomalies included abnormalities of the vertebrae, eye (excluding cataracts), and musculoskeletal system, micrognathia, and unilateral undescended testes.[84] Others report an equally high incidence of three to four times that in control populations.[85,86] Arima (reported by Stanley[87]) found an incidence that was double that expected in the non–cerebral palsy population. The most common features were face anomalies (saddle nose, low set ears, high arched palate), abnormal dermatoglyphics, and skin abnormalities.

Dental anomalies and abnormal dermatoglyphics were found more frequently in two nonblinded studies of children with nonspecific neurologic abnormalities and children with cerebral palsy.[88,89] A blinded study of neurologically impaired children also demonstrated a higher incidence of enamel hypoplasia and abnormal dermatoglyphics than that in control subjects. Antenatal "timing" of injury in at least 59 percent of the children was suggested by using both measures.[90]

The relationship of non–central nervous system anomalies to cerebral palsy is a matter of conjecture. It is possible that both are markers of a single shared insult to the fetus (e.g., there is a higher incidence of microdysplasia and white matter gliosis in a variety of non–central nervous system malformations[91,92] and that the non–central nervous system malformation predisposes to perinatal asphyxia. The latter mechanism is suggested by the simultaneous occurrence of encephaloclastic changes and brain anomalies at autopsy.[43] Additionally 14 of 40 (35 percent) of the asphyxiated newborns with cerebral palsy in the NCPP also had non–central nervous system anomalies.[84] The predisposition to asphyxia in the malformed infant could be based on a higher incidence of low birth weight,[73] antepartum hemorrhage,[85] breech presentation,[84,93] short umbilical cord,[94] and fetal distress.[95]

Congenital Infection

Intrauterine infections of the fetal-placental unit increase the probability of death and the incidence of encephalopathy. The asymptomatically infected newborn with a static encephalopathy must be identified in the immediate postnatal period before the infant is exposed to the organism during the first year of life if the relationship between infection and later cerebral palsy is to be recognized. Infections of concern include rubella, cytomegalovirus, toxoplasmosis, herpes simplex, syphilis, and human immunodeficiency virus.

Placental Abnormality

Placental infarcts (larger than 3 cm) are associated with an increased incidence of fetal and neonatal death but not cerebral palsy.[29,96] The infarcts may be caused by underlying disorders that themselves contribute to the morbidity. Maternal factors include hypertension, increased hematocrit, malnutrition, working throughout pregnancy in an upright position, as well as the presence of twins.[96] Placental growth retardation (in the absence of large infarcts or fetal malformations) also increases the risk of death and approaches statistical significance vis-à-vis late moderate to severe motor impairment.[25,96]

Placenta previa and abruption significantly increase the risk of infant death, but only placenta previa is associated with higher risks of cerebral palsy.[29,96] Underlying predisposing problems should be considered; e.g., both placental disorders may be "caused" by cigarette smoking, and abruption may be secondary to hypertension, chorioamnionitis, placenta previa and circumvallate placenta, maternal malnutrition, and placental infarcts.[96]

Chorioamnionitis is an important risk factor in early death and cerebral palsy, triggering premature delivery and increasing the risk of neonatal infection.[58,96] Neonates in the NCPP suspected of having sepsis or meningitis had higher incidences of cerebral palsy.[66] Of the children with cerebral palsy, 37 percent received antibiotics in the neonatal period (as compared with 10 percent in the non–cerebral palsy survivors), but only 13 percent of the infants destined to have cerebral palsy had positive cultures. The high incidence of antibiotic use in the infants with cerebral palsy in spite of negative cultures could be explained by inadequate culturing techniques, prophylactic use of antibiotics following chorioamnionitis or premature rupture of membranes, or an increased incidence of respiratory distress of the newborn. Possibly, too, the antibiotics in some way caused an encephalopathy, or the infant had a noninfectious encephalopathy that clinically resembled sepsis.[66]

Umbilical Cord

Neurologic outcome is related to the length of the umbilical cord, which in turn is dependent in part on gestational age, amniotic fluid volume, and fetal activity.[94,96] Short cords are associated with abruptio placentae, cord compression, and abnormal labor as well as congenital malformations in the fetus. Shorter cords when studied by univariate analysis are associated with greater degrees of hypotonia in infants of less than 34 weeks' gestation and with cerebral palsy, mental retardation, and seizures, but this relationship disappears with multivariate analysis.[29,96]

Presentation

Breech presentation (in contrast with breech delivery) is associated with an increased risk of cerebral palsy in term infants.[84] Abnormal fetal presentation can be secondary to a variety of causes, including an aberrantly shaped uterus (uterine and placental abnormalities), less fetal constraint (prematurity, growth retardation, polyhydramnios), excessive fetal constraint (twins, oligohydramnios), and intrinsic fetal anomalies.[94] In reference to the latter point, it should be noted that one-third of the children in the NCPP with cerebral palsy who presented in the breech presentation had non–central nervous system malformations.[84]

Twins

Twins account for 5 to 10 percent of cerebral palsy populations.[97-100] Genetic factors theoretically would produce similar phenotypes of encephalopathy in both monozygotic twins. Environmental influences could affect either one or both twins and possibly produce differing phenotypes of neurologic impairment. The observed incidence of cerebral palsy in same-sex twins is higher than in opposite-sex infants. Interpretation of these data is limited by incomplete zygosity information,[20,97-100] unrecognized first trimester twin loss, and an elevated fetal and perinatal mortality rate among twins.[98,99] Explanations for the greater morbidity in twins could include genetic factors, fetal demise associated with multicystic encephalomalacia in the survivor,[101,102] an increased incidence of prematurity compared with unaffected twin pairs,[98,99] growth retardation,[98-100] and an increased incidence of delivery complications.[98,99]

The influence of birth order on the clinical picture suggests that different mechanisms may create cerebral injury in twins. When the first born infant has cerebral palsy, the twins are likely to have been premature, in the vertex presentation, and delivered without incident. The involved twin usually has spastic diplegia on follow-up. The second born twin who has cerebral palsy is a product of a more mature twin pair than the former group. It is also more likely to have been a product of a complicated delivery and to have spastic quadriparesis or athetosis.[99]

NEONATAL DEPRESSION AND ASPHYXIA

Meconium

In utero meconium passage is suggestive of fetal asphyxia and is associated with a higher infant mortality. If other signs of possible fetal asphyxia are present (i.e., abnormal fetal heart rate pattern or acidosis), there is an increased probability of neonatal depression.[103-105] Although meconium may appear to increase the incidence of cerebral palsy, multivariate analysis demonstrated that it is the neonatal depression that is predictive of subsequent cerebral palsy.[25]

The time of appearance of meconium and the presence of staining suggest the time of onset of the fetal distress. The in utero stress can be considered acute when meconium passage occurs after the appearance of clear amniotic fluid, whereas staining of the placenta and infant suggests that the stress (which may be minor and merely superimposed on a more chronic depressed state) occurred several hours or more prior to delivery.[103,106,107] As a matter of fact, infants dying of meconium aspiration and those with meconium staining do indeed appear to have a higher incidence of chronic abnormalities, e.g.,

erythroblastosis fetalis, congenital heart lesions, chorioamnionitis, and abnormal muscularization of the small intra-acinar arteries.[108,109] It would seem, therefore, that meconium passage per se has no relationship to cerebral palsy.

Fetal Monitoring

One criticism of the older epidemiologic studies of cerebral palsy is that the introduction of continuous electronic fetal heart rate monitoring has revolutionized care and produced better babies. The premise for monitoring is that certain "abnormal" fetal heart rate patterns identify the fetus in distress and obstetrical interventions can be performed prior to central nervous system injury. The many patterns suggesting fetal distress are beyond the scope of this chapter; however, it is important to note that they lack specificity in the identification of asphyxia.

The question remains whether fetal heart rate monitoring has altered the incidence of cerebral palsy. A recent critical methodologic review of seven clinical trials found that universal monitoring had not significantly altered the perinatal mortality, frequency of Apgar scores less than 7, and neonatal intensive care unit admissions.[110] A subsequent study in Denver addressed the issue of selective versus universal continuous fetal heart rate monitoring. Selective monitoring (on alternate months) of high risk mothers (37 percent of the total obstetrical population) and universal monitoring (79 percent of the population) were compared. There was no decrease in the incidence of intrapartum stillbirths, low Apgar scores, admissions to the intensive care nursery, or the need for respiratory support when universal monitoring was employed. The authors concluded that continuous monitoring of low risk mothers was unproductive.[111] The Dublin prospective randomized trial of electronic monitoring noted that the cohort followed by intermittent auscultation, compared with the group continuously monitored, did have a higher incidence of seizures (not confirmed by electroencephalography) and abnormal neurologic signs during early infancy but no increase in cerebral palsy at one year.[112] The Western Australia registry did not find a change in cerebral palsy incidences despite increased electronic monitoring.[60]

We do not mean to imply that fetal distress causing significant neurologic morbidity cannot be noted in infants by monitoring heart tones. In the NCPP fetal bradycardia on intermittent auscultation was a significant but small risk factor for cerebral palsy.[66] Severe bradycardia (less than 60 beats per minute) was found in 1 percent of the total NCPP population, but only 6 percent of the children with cerebral palsy had this as an antecedent risk factor.

Assessment of fetal pH, the "gold standard" of the biophysical tests, also has less predictive value than originally suggested.[113] Sykes et al[114] prospectively sampled umbilical cord pH in 1,210 consecutive deliveries of all gestational ages. Severe acidosis (pH less than 7.11 and a base deficit greater than 12 mmol per liter) was associated with only 27 percent and 14 percent of infants having Apgar scores less than 7 at one and five minutes, respectively. Conversely, depression (Apgar score of 3 or less at one minute) was associated with this acidosis in only 29 percent of the instances. The former discrepancy may be explained by an asphyxia of such short duration that postnatal depression was not produced. Low Apgar scores in the presence of normal fetal blood gas levels suggest that the neonatal depression was not caused by late intrapartum asphyxia.

Apgar Scores

The assessment of the impact of delivery on the fetal central nervous system includes the time until first breath or cry, the need for resuscitation, and the Apgar score. The latter instrument is the most commonly used and serves as the measure of outcome in most biophysical studies during delivery. Apgar's method of newborn assessment at one minute was meant to be used as "a basis of discussion and comparison of the results of obstetric practices, types of maternal pain relief and the effects of resuscitation."[115] She subsequently noted that the score is useful but that it has "its limitations. It is no substitute for a careful physical exam or serial observations over the first few hours of life. Nor will it predict neonatal death or survival in individual infants."[116] Drage and Berendes[117] in an early analysis of the NCPP data noted that the "value of the one-minute score in identification of the newborn in need of resuscitation is supplemented by the five-minute score's stronger association with neonatal mortality and infant morbidity. The categorization is crude .... The condition reflected by the low score may accentuate an existing pathologic condition, or the low score in itself may reflect the damaging event." Despite early concerns, the scoring system has become almost synonymous with neonatal asphyxia and the standard by which all obstetrical practices are judged. The American Academy of Pediatrics expressed in 1986 its own reservations about the abuse of the scores when used in this manner.[118]

There was a significant inverse relationship between the Apgar score and an abnormal infant outcome.[117,119] In a cohort of infants weighing more than 2,500 gm who had five minute scores of 3 or less, but 10 minute scores of 4 or more, the mortality was 7.7 percent and the incidence of cerebral palsy, 0.9 percent. If the low score persisted until 20 minutes, these incidences were 59.0 and 57.1 percent, respectively.[119] However, only 15 percent of the children with cerebral palsy had a five minute Apgar score of 3 or less.[119]

Peters[120] utilized the time of establishment of spontaneous respirations at birth as a measure of depression and found that apnea for three minutes in a term infant was associated with a cerebral palsy incidence of only 9.14 per 1,000 neonatal survivors. Other investigators found similar results; prolonged depression or protracted apnea at birth was associated with high mortality, yet only 7 to 26 percent of the survivors had cerebral palsy.[121-125]

The Apgar score may be less useful in the premature infant because of the confounding variable of gestational age. Catlin et al[126] studied 73 infants with gestational ages of 22 to 42 weeks who were products of uncomplicated pregnancies and without evidence of perinatal ischemia (no labor complications, normal fetal heart rate on monitoring, and normal cord blood gas levels). A significant inverse relationship was found between the gestational age and the Apgar score. For example, infants of less than 30 weeks' gestational age usually had one minute scores between 4 and 6. An additional problem in interpreting the Apgar score in the premature infant was that 14 of the 22 smallest infants were intubated prophylactically.[120] Finally, the presence of a low Apgar score in this population should not automatically be interpreted as normal. Acidotic premature babies, unlike term infants, almost always have depressed Apgar scores.[127,128]

NEONATAL NEUROLOGIC STATUS

Term Infants

Clinical Examination

Neurologic abnormalities following presumed birth asphyxia are rarely restricted to a single sign.[124,129,130] Multisystem dysfunction is frequently present as well.[131] The mildest manifestation of encephalopathy is hyperexcitability with increased flexor tone, stimulus hypersensitivity, jitteriness, hyperreflexia, and seizures.[124,130] These signs usually resolve within two weeks but may progress within the first day to decreasing consciousness, hypotonia, hyporeflexia, and increasing seizures.[132,133] The infant may stabilize at this depressed level or progress into coma, characterized by flaccidity with episodic decerebrate posturing and poor brainstem function.[124,129,130] If the child recovers, a period of extensor hypertonus and brainstem dysfunction (abnormal swallowing, sucking, eye movements) may occur.[124,129] Rarely extensor hypertonia (without the brainstem signs) and joint contractures can be present at birth and suggest an earlier insult. Acute hypoxic-ischemic encephalopathy resulting from birth asphyxia may be superimposed on these chronic findings.[129] The timing of the asphyxial event on the basis of the clinical symptoms alone is therefore difficult, for although these signs evolve over time, the range of rate of change is wide and may not follow a given sequence.

The degree of neonatal encephalopathy following presumed birth asphyxia (as determined by clinical and electroencephalographic criteria) is directly related to the subsequent neurologic outcome (see Chapter 15). The incidences of handicap range from 17 to 53 percent, depending on the exclusion criteria, age at follow-up, and definition of outcome measures.[122,124,129-134] A cohort of children surviving the first year and considered to have had definite or suspect central nervous system abnormalities in the nursery, regardless of etiology or presumed time of onset (11 percent of the total NCPP population), accounted for 57 percent of the children with subsequent cerebral palsy; conversely, 43 percent of the cerebral palsy population were apparently normal in the neonatal period.[7]

Seizures

Neonatal seizures have been cited as a measure of the optimality of pregnancy and the adequacy of obstetrical management.[61,112,135-138] The demonstration that the severity of neonatal depression in the delivery room was predictive of outcome in most seizing infants suggests that the seizures closely reflect antenatal and intrapartum events.[139] Also the assumption that seizures have their onset solely after delivery is only partially correct, for in utero seizures have been reported and may be unrecognized.[139,140] (A further discussion of neonatal seizures may be found in Chapter 11.)

Birth Trauma

Birth trauma was a major cause of perinatal abnormalities during the early 20th century but is less common today.[141] Subdural hemorrhage is seen more frequently in the term infant and is often accompanied by other evidence of traumatic delivery, e.g., facial paresis.[142-144] Subarachnoid, intraventricular, or parenchymal hemorrhage may occur independently or with the subdural bleeding. The mortality and morbidity following intracranial bleeding in the term infant are not well defined owing to the small size of the series, ascertainment of the worst cases, and the young age at follow-up.[145] These hemorrhages have been found in stillborn infants and with intrauterine central nervous system imaging, suggesting that birth trauma is not the only etiology.[146-148] Predisposing factors include maternal trauma, coagulopathy, primiparity, and difficult deliveries.[145]

Birth asphyxia may lead to the urgent delivery of a depressed hypotonic infant who in turn will be more vulnerable to obstetrical trauma. Midforceps delivery illustrates this complex relationship between birth trauma and cerebral palsy. The NCPP found that children delivered by midforceps extraction and infants with peripheral nerve injuries (no mention of method of delivery) had a higher incidence of cerebral palsy.[25] Subsequently Dierker et al[149] retrospectively studied infants delivered with midforceps and compared them with a group delivered by cesarean section, matching for indications for surgery or forceps delivery, fetal heart rate abnormalities, birth weight, gestational age, sex, race, and time of birth. The developmental outcome was the same at two years, suggesting that the complexity of labor rather than the method of delivery predisposed to the neurologic morbidity.

Stroke

Ischemic injury usually occurs in term infants as a large vessel stroke and in the premature infant as periventricular leukomalacia. Neonatal strokes are relatively infrequent and series are small and often anecdotal so that assessment of risk factors is difficult. Many different patterns of damage are seen, often associated with more global anoxic cerebral involvement. Patterns of ischemic lesions include telencephalic white matter (including periventricular leukomalacia), diencephalic infarcts, brainstem necrosis, cerebral infarcts in a major vessel distribution, and areas of widespread damage with multicystic encephalomalacia. As we have emphasized, these lesions cannot be attributed solely to intrapartum or postnatal events because each has been described in still births or has been seen by ultrasound imaging prior to or immediately after birth.[92,101,102,150-156]

Premature Infants

Clinical Examination

The neurologic examination of the asphyxiated premature infant has not been adequately detailed, in part owing to the confounding variables of gestational age, concomitant systemic illness, and the use of sedative and paralytic drugs for pulmonary care. Additionally there are superimposed postnatal events, such as intracranial hemorrhage with shock, acidosis, renal failure, necrotizing enterocolitis, and pulmonary disease, making it difficult to determine the signs attributable to perinatal asphyxia and those due to acquired lesions.[157-159]

The persistence of neurologic abnormalities in premature babies (less than 34 weeks' gestational age) at a conceptual age of approximately 40 weeks increases the risk of cerebral palsy. Infants with normal findings on examination at that age are usually normal at one year; those with only hypotonia may be normal in about two-thirds of the cases, and babies demonstrating other tone changes, asymmetries, poor orientation and excessive irritability, tremors, and startles tend to do poorly, with overt motor abnormalities and developmental delay.[160]

Periventricular Hemorrhage and Leukomalacia

Early studies of the etiology of cerebral injury in the premature infant were biased because they included primarily autopsy material. The introduction of bedside imaging of the central nervous system has made possible better definition of the frequency and timing of hemorrhagic and ischemic lesions. It is well known that two common neurologic syndromes occurring almost exclusively in premature infants are followed by a relatively high incidence of static encephalopathy—subependymal-intraventricular hemorrhage and periventricular leukomalacia. The overall incidence of these disorders is dependent on gestational age; for the very low birth weight infant the incidence of subependymal-intraventricular hemorrhage approximates 46 to 60 percent and periventricular leukolmalacia, 2 to 26 percent.[161-169] Concurrent hemorrhage is frequently seen with periventricular leukomalacia. Ultrasound studies underestimate the frequency of periventricular leukomalacia owing to technical limitations of the equipment (small lesions may be missed) and scanning at inappropriate times. Periventricular leukomalacia appears to be an acquired lesion, which may disappear during the first few weeks to months of life, and scanning may be performed too early or too late.[170,171] In some series outborn infants have been included, which may increase the incidence of subependymal-intraventricular hemorrhage and periventricular leukomalacia.

The severity of the intraventricular hemorrhage, as measured by the extent of ventricular engorgement with blood, is relatively poorly correlated with outcome unless intraparenchymal hemorrhage is present.[164,165,172,173] The severity of the accompanying hypoxic-ischemic encephalopathy is more predictive of the risk of later neurologic sequelae.[173] Periventricular leukomalacia, on the other hand, is often followed by a static encephalopathy, the severity of which is determined by the location and size of the ischemic or hemorrhagic periventricular lesion.[165-169,172,174]

Antecedents of Central Nervous System Hemorrhage and Periventricular Leukomalacia

Identification of antecedent events in subependymal-intraventricular hemorrhage has been difficult because of incomplete case ascertainment. Older studies have relied on clinical data or CT scanning to identify hemorrhage, whereas more recent studies have used the more sensitive bedside ultrasound. Future analyses should consider creating cohorts based on the time of the hemorrhage, early (less than 12 hours) bleeding reflecting intrapartum events and later bleeding, the consequences of neonatal care,[175] and on closely (less than two weeks) matched controls.[176]

The identification of risk factors in periventricular leukomalacia is complicated because the characteristic periventricular hyperechoic signals are not seen for one day or more after a postulated insult. Therefore it is difficult to distinguish physiologic activity or caretaker intervention that may have preceded the onset of the periventricular leukomalacia from a case that was a consequence of encephalopathy.

Pregnancy

Prematurity is the most significant risk factor in subependymal-intraventricular hemorrhage and periventricular leukomalacia, most lesions occurring in infants of less than 32 weeks' gestations.[177] Studies of pregnancy risk factors for subependymal-intraventricular hemorrhage and periventricular leukomalacia that match control infants for gestational age demonstrate no consistent antecedents. Antepartum hemorrhage is associated in the very low birth weight infant with intracranial hemorrhage and periventricular leukomalacia, but the results are not consistently replicated.[171,177-181] Infants have normal birth weights for conceptual age.[177,179-182] Both lesions, however, occur in utero, as shown in autopsies of stillborns, by fetal ultrasound, and by the presence of cystic lesions in the first day of life.[154-156,183-186]

Labor and Delivery

Significant controversy exists whether labor or the method of delivery increases the risk of central nervous system hemorrhage or white matter infarction. Most studies that compare age matched controls find no difference in the incidence of subependymal-intraventricular hemorrhage or periventricular leukomalacia when the results with cesarean section are compared to those with vaginal deliveries.[177-182,187] These incidences are independent of fetal presentation. Once labor has begun, intervention with cesarean section may not alter the incidence of hemorrhage.[180,188,189] There is the suggestion that surgical delivery prior to the onset of labor may decrease the overall mortality.[189]

Perinatal Asphyxia

Fetal heart rate monitoring data demonstrate no consistent increase in the frequency of abnormal patterns preceding subependymal-intraventricular hemorrhage.[178,181,187] The Apgar score also does not identify infants at increased risk for hemorrhage compared with age-matched controls.[178-180] The relationship between the Apgar score and the risk of periventricular leukomalacia is uncertain, most series being small and uncontrolled for gestational age and birth weight. It would be safe to state that a substantial percentage of infants are not depressed at birth.[161,165,166,168,174,179,183,190]

Neonatal Period

Neonatal factors consistently associated with subependymal-intraventricular hemorrhage are the respiratory distress syndrome and ventilatory intervention, although there is contamination of the analyses in many studies by inadequate matching with controls of identical gestational ages. Perhaps reflecting the severity of the pulmonary disease, abnormal arterial blood gas levels, increased amounts of bicarbonate infusion, fluctuating cerebral blood flow velocities, coagulopathy, and other features appear to be related to subependymal-intraventricular hemorrhage and have been suggested as causal factors. Reviews of these features are available elsewhere and are beyond the scope of this discussion.[191] Neonatal factors inconclusively suggested as increasing risk of ischemic lesions (periventricular leukomalacia) include ventilator support, patent ductus arteriosus, pneumothorax, septicemia, apnea, and seizures.

SUMMARY

Static motor encephalopathies included under the term "cerebral palsy" have diverse origins and clinical expressions. Care needs to be exercised when assigning an etiology to these syndromes and, in particular, attributing the neurological deficit to perinatal events. Disorders with a well established relationship to abnormal development need to be excluded (e.g., brain anomalies, genetic and dysmorphic syndromes, congenital infection, inborn errors of metabolism, and postnatally acquired anoxic, infectious, and traumatic lesions).

A prenatal origin of the encephalopathy is suggested by the presence of medical complications of pregnancy, abnormal placental pathology, and non–central nervous system malformations. These factors cannot be assumed to be causative because they may simply reflect a more remote in utero insult or genetic abnormality which is responsible for the entire constellation of findings. These prenatal abnormalities may ill prepare the infant for delivery and result in what appears to be a perinatal asphyxic encephalopathy.

The attributable risk of labor and delivery to the incidence of static encephalopathy is approximately 15 percent. The presence of meconium, fetal heart rate abnormalities, fetal acidosis, and neonatal depression (low Apgar scores) are not definitive evidence of brain injury during parturition. Infants with major central nervous system malformations, for example, may have all these signs at delivery. It is worth emphasizing that the Apgar score is a nonspecific description of neonatal behavior, and although related to infant outcome, may be depressed from a multitude of causes other than birth asphyxia. Without clinical evidence of a significant encephalopathy in the neonatal period it is unlikely that a low Apgar score is of etiologic significance following a complication of delivery.

The contribution of neonatal intensive care to neurologic sequelae is difficult to assess. Premature infants constitute the majority of babies within this group and it is still only speculative as to whether their care adds to the higher incidence of motor abnormalities. Central nervous system hemorrhagic or ischemic lesions such as periventricular leukomalacia and stroke are markers of increased risk for adverse outcome in term and premature infants. However, identifying the event which caused the cerebral lesion or even determining the exact time of onset of the bleed or infarction is difficult. The vascular lesion which is thought to be responsible for these lesions may begin to develop prenatally and the full-blown hemorrhage or infarct appears as a result of postnatal events. If we are to fully understand these syndromes the analysis of variables must extend back into the infant's intrauterine life.

Crothers and Paine[192] stated that the term cerebral palsy "does not designate a disease in the usual medical sense. It is, however, a useful administrative term, which covers individuals who are handicapped by motor disorders." To this we add that the encephalopathies considered to be responsible for cerebral palsy represent a diverse group of entities, only a portion of which are related to events that took place at the time of birth.

REFERENCES

1. Courville CB. Cerebral palsy. Los Angeles: San Lucas Press, 1954.
2. Little WJ. On the influence of abnormal parturition, difficult labours, premature birth, and asphyxia neonatorum, on the mental and physical condition of the child, especially in relation to deformities. Trans Obstet Soc London 1861; 3:293.
3. Freud S (translated by Russin LA). Infantile cerebral paralysis (1897). Miami: University of Miami Press, 1968.
4. Bax MCO. Terminology and classification of cerebral palsy. Dev Med Child Neurol 1964; 6:295.
5. Nelson KB, Ellenberg JH. Children who "outgrew" cerebral palsy. Pediatrics 1982; 69:529.
6. Stanley FJ. Using cerebral palsy data in the evaluation of neonatal intensive care: a warning. Dev Med Child Neurol 1982; 24:93.
7. Nelson KB, Ellenberg JH. Neonatal signs as predictors of cerebral palsy. Pediatrics 1979; 64:225.
8. Ellenberg JH, Nelson KB. Early recognition of infants at high risk for cerebral palsy: examination at age four months. Dev Med Child Neurol 1981; 23:705.
9. Nelson KB, Ellenberg JH. The epidemiology of cerebral palsy. Adv Neurol 1978; 19:421.
10. Ross G, Lipper EG, Auld PAM. Consistency and change in the development of premature infants weighing less than 1501 grams at birth. Pediatrics 1985; 76:885.
11. Kitchen W, Ford G, Orgill A, et al. Outcome in infants of birth weight 500 to 999 g: a continuing regional study of 5-year-old survivors. J Pediatr 1987; 111:761.

12. Ingram TTS. A historical review of the definition and classification of the cerebral palsies. Clin Dev Med 1984; 87:1.

13. Blair E, Stanley F. Interobserver agreement in the classification of cerebral palsy. Dev Med Child Neurol 1985; 27:615.

14. Holm VA. The causes of cerebral palsy: a contemporary perspective. JAMA 1982; 247:1473.

15. O'Reilly DE, Walentynowicz JE. Etiological factors in cerebral palsy: an historical review. Dev Med Child Neurol 1981; 23:633.

16. Pharoah POD, Cooke T, Rosenbloom I, Cooke RWI. Trends in birth prevalence of cerebral palsy. Arch Dis Child 1987; 62:379.

17. Lagergren J. Children with motor handicaps: epidemiological, medical and socio-paediatric aspects of motor handicapped children in a Swedish country. Acta Paediatr Scand 1981; Suppl 289.

18. Hagberg B, Hagberg G, Olow I. The changing panorama of cerebral palsy in Sweden 1954–1970. II. Analysis of the various syndromes. Acta Paediatr Scand 1975; 64:193.

19. Evans P, Elliott M, Alberman E, Evans S. Prevalence and disabilities in 4 to 8 year olds with cerebral palsy. Arch Dis Child 1985; 60:940.

20. Atkinson S, Stanley FJ. Spastic diplegia among children of low and normal birth weight. Dev Med Child Neurol 1983; 25:693.

21. Stanley F, Blair E. Postnatal risk factors in the cerebral palsies. Clin Dev Med 1984; 87:135.

22. Cohen ME, Duffner PK. Prognostic indicators in hemiparetic cerebral palsy. Ann Neurol 1981; 9:353.

23. Kyllerman M, Bager B, Bensch J, et al. Dyskinetic cerebral palsy. I. Clinical categories, associated neurological abnormalities and incidences. Acta Paediatr Scand 1982; 71:543.

24. Kyllerman M. Dyskinetic cerebral palsy. II. Pathogenetic risk factors and intra-uterine growth. Acta Paediatr Scand 1982; 71:551.

25. Nelson KB, Broman SH. Perinatal risk factors in children with serious motor and mental handicaps. Ann Neurol 1977; 2:371.

26. Broman SH. Prenatal anoxia and cognitive development in early childhood. In: Field TM, ed. Infants born at risk: behavior and development. New York: SP Medical and Scientific Books, 1979:29.

27. McQueen PC, Spence MW, Winsor EJT, et al. Causal origins of major mental handicap in the Canadian maritime provinces. Dev Med Child Neurol 1986; 28:697.

28. Sameroff AJ, Seifer R, Barocas R, et al. Intelligence quotient scores of 4-year-old children: social-environmental risk factors. Pediatrics 1987; 79:343.

29. Nelson KB, Ellenberg JH. Obstetric complications as risk factors for cerebral palsy or seizure disorders. JAMA 1984; 251:1843.

30. Ellenberg JH, Nelson KB. Birth weight and gestational age in children with cerebral palsy or seizure disorder. Am J Dis Child 1979; 133:1044.

31. Drillien CM. Studies in mental handicaps. II. Some obstetric factors of possible aetiological significance. Arch Dis Child 1968;43:283.

32. Nelson KB, Ellenberg JH. Antecedents of seizure disorders in early childhood. Am J Dis Child 1986; 140:1053.

33. Paneth N, Kiely J. The frequency of cerebral palsy: a review of population studies in industrialized nations since 1950. Clin Dev Med 1984; 87:46.

34. Stanley FJ, Watson L. The cerebral palsies in Western Australia: trends, 1968 to 1981. Am J Obstet Gynecol 1988; 158:89.

35. Kudrjavcez T, Schoenberg BS, Kurland LT, Groover RV. Cerebral palsy—trends in incidence and changes in concurrent neonatal mortality: Rochester, MN, 1950–1976. Neurology 1983; 33:1433.

36. Powell TG, Pharoah POD, Cooke RWI. Survival and morbidity in a geographically defined population of low birthweight infants. Lancet 1986; 1:539.

37. Kitchen WH, Rickards A, Ryan MM, et al. Improved outcome to two years of very low-birthweight infants: fact or artifact? Dev Med Child Neurol 1986; 28:579.

38. Lilienfeld AM, Parkhurst E. A study of the association of the factors of pregnancy and parturition with the development of cerebral palsy. Am J Hyg 1951; 53:262.

39. Kitchen WH, Rickards AL, Ryan MM, et al. A longitudinal study of very low-birthweight infants. II. Results of controlled trial of intensive care and incidence of handicaps. Dev Med Child Neurol 1979; 21:582.

40. Hagberg B, Hagberg G, Olow I. Gains and hazards of intensive neonatal care: an analysis from Swedish cerebral palsy epidemiology. Dev Med Child Neurol 1982; 24:13.

41. Gilles FH. Neuropathologic indicators of abnormal development. In: Freeman JM, ed. Prenatal and perinatal factors associated with brain disorders. NIH publication 85-1149. Washington, DC: Department of Health and Human Services, 1985:53.

42. Gross H, Jellinger K, Kaltenback E, Rett A. Infantile cerebral disorders: clinical-neuropathological correlations to elucidate the aetiological factors. J Neurol Sci 1968; 7:551.

43. Christensen E, Melchior J. Cerebral palsy: a clinical and neuropathological study. Clin Dev Med 1967; 25:1.

44. Malamud N, Itabashi HH, Castor J, Messinger HB. An etiologic and diagnostic study of cerebral palsy. J Pediatr 1964; 65:270.

45. Volpe JJ. Neurology of the newborn. Philadelphia: WB Saunders, 1987.

46. Rorke LB. Pathology of perinatal brain injury. New York: Raven Press, 1982.

47. Pedersen H, Taudorf K, Melchior JC. Computed tomography in spastic cerebral palsy. Neuroradiology 1982; 23:275.

48. Koch B, Braillier D, Eng G, Binder H. Computerized tomography in cerebral-palsied children. Dev Med Child Neurol 1980; 22:595.

49. Kulakowski S, Larroche JC. Cranial computerized tomography in cerebral palsy. An attempt at anatomo-clinical and radiological correlations. Neuropediatrics 1980; 11:339.

50. Kanda T, Suzuki J, Yamori Y, Fukase H. CT findings of spastic diplegia with special reference to grade of motor disturbance. Brain Dev 1982; 4:239.

51. Kotlarek F, Rodewig R, Brull D, Zeumer H. Computed tomographic findings in congenital hemiparesis in childhood and their relation to etiology and prognosis. Neuropaediatrics 1981; 12:101.

52. Hagberg B, Hagberg G. Prenatal and perinatal risk factors in a survey of 681 Swedish cases. Clin Dev Med 1984; 87:116.

53. Naeye RL, Ladis B, Drage JS. Sudden infant death syndrome: a prospective study. Am J Dis Child 1976; 130:1207.

54. Steinschneider A, Weinstein SL, Diamond E. The sudden infant death syndrome and apnea/obstruction during neonatal sleep and feeding. Pediatrics 1982; 70:858.

55. Palm L, Blennow G, Brun A. Infantile spasms and neuronal heterotopias: a report on six cases. Acta Paediatr Scand 1986; 75:855.

56. Bellman MH, Ross EM, Miller DL. Infantile spasms and pertussis immunization. Lancet 1983; 1:1031.

57. Chesley LC, Cooper DW. Genetics of hypertension in pregnancy: possible single gene control of pre-eclampsia and eclampsia in the descendants of eclamptic women. Br J Obstet Gynaecol 1986; 93:898.

58. Nelson KB, Ellenberg JH. Predictors of low and very low birth weight and the relation of these to cerebral palsy. JAMA 1985; 254:1473.

59. Nelson KB, Ellenberg JH. The asymptomatic newborn and risk of cerebral palsy. Am J Dis Child 1987; 141:1333.

60. Blair E, Stanley FJ. Intrapartum asphyxia: a rare cause of cerebral palsy. J Pediatr 1988; 112:515.

61. Niswander K, Henson G, Elbourne D, et al. Adverse outcome of pregnancy and the quality of obstetric care. Lancet 1984; 2:827.

62. Prechtl HFR. Neurological findings in new born infants after pre- and paranatal complications. In: Jonxis JHP, Visser HKA, Troelstra JA, eds. Aspects of praematurity and dysmaturity. Springfield, IL: Charles C Thomas, 1968:303.

63. Michaelis R, Rooschuz B, Dopfer R. Prenatal origin of congenital spastic hemiparesis. Early Hum Dev 1980; 4:243.

64. Veelken N, Hagberg B, Hagberg F, Olow I. Diplegic cerebral palsy in Swedish term and preterm children: differences in reduced optimality, relations to neurology and pathogenetic factors. Neuropediatrics 1983; 14:20.

65. Kyllerman M. Reduced optimality in pre- and perinatal condi-

tions in dyskinetic cerebral palsy-distribution and comparison to controls. Neuropediatrics 1983; 14:29.

66. Nelson KB, Ellenberg JH. Antecedents of cerebral palsy. I. Univariate analysis of risks. Am J Dis Child 1985; 139:1031.

67. Drillien CM, Ingram TTS, Russell EM. Comparative aetiological studies of congenital diplegia in Scotland. Arch Dis Child 1962; 37:282.

68. Spiers PS, Davis N. Spastic diplegia and the significance of mothers' previous reproductive loss. Dev Med Child Neurol 1982; 24:20.

69. Nelson KB, Ellenberg JH. Maternal seizure disorder, outcome of pregnancy, and neurologic abnormalities in the children. Neurology 1982; 32:1247.

70. Hiilesmaa VK, Bardy A, Teramo K. Obstetric outcome in women with epilepsy. Am J Obstet Gynecol 1985; 152:499.

71. Fedrick J. Epilepsy and pregnancy: a report from the Oxford record linkage study. Br Med J 1973; 2:442.

72. Yerby M, Koepsell T, Daling J. Pregnancy complications and outcomes in a cohort of women with epilepsy. Epilepsia 1985; 26:631.

73. Brar HS, Rutherford SE. Classification of intrauterine growth retardation. Semin Perinatol 1988; 12:2.

74. Ting RY, Wang MH, Scott TFM. The dysmature infant: associated factors and outcome at 7 years of age. J Pediatr 1977; 90:943.

75. Pharoah POD, Cooke T, Rosenbloom L, Cooke RWI. Effects of birth weight, gestational age, and maternal obstetric history on birth prevalence of cerebral palsy. Arch Dis Child 1987; 62:1035.

76. Stanley FJ. Spastic cerebral palsy: changes in birthweight and gestational age. Early Hum Dev 1981; 5:167.

77. Tenovuo A, Kero P, Korvenranta H, et al. Developmental outcome of 519 small for gestational age children at the age of two years. Neuropediatrics 1988; 19:41.

78. Commey JOO, Fitzhardinge PM. Handicap in the preterm small-for-gestational age infant. J Pediatr 1979; 94:779.

79. Brennan TL, Funk SG, Frothingham TE. Disproportionate intra-uterine head growth and developmental outcome. Dev Med Child Neurol 1985; 27:746.

80. Cochrane DD, Myles ST, Nimrod C, et al. Intrauterine hydrocephalus and ventriculomegaly: associated abnormalities and fetal outcome. Can J Neurol Sci 1985; 12:51.

81. Babcock DS, Han BK, Dine MS. Sonographic findings in infants with macrocrania. AJNR 1988; 9:307.

82. Barth PG. Disorders of neuronal migration. Can J Neurol Sci 1987; 14:1.

83. Rantakallio P, Von Wendt L. A prospective comparative study of the aetiology of cerebral palsy and epilepsy in a one-year birth cohort for Northern Finland. Acta Paediatr Scand 1986; 75:586.

84. Nelson KB, Ellenberg JH. Antecedents of cerebral palsy: multivariate analysis of risk. N Engl J Med 1986; 315:81.

85. Illingworth RS. Why blame the obstetrician? A review. Br Med J 1979; 1:797.

86. Eastman NJ, Kohl SG, Maisel JE, Kavaler F. The obstetrical background of 753 cases of cerebral palsy. Obstet Gynecol Surv 1962; 17:459.

87. Stanley F. Prenatal risk factors in the cerebral palsies. Clin Dev Med 1984; 87:87.

88. Cohen HJ, Diner, H. The significance of developmental dental enamel defects in neurological disorders. Pediatrics 1970; 46:737.

89. Martin JK, Thompson MW, Castaldi CR. A study of the clinical history, tooth enamel and dermal patterns in 175 cases of cerebral palsy. Guy's Hosp Res 1960; 109:139.

90. Jaffe M, Attias D, Dar H, et al. The etiology of brain damage in children: unusual dermatoglyphics and enamel hypoplasia as markers of fetal and perinatal insult. In: Harel S, Anatasiow NJ eds. The at-risk infant: psycho/socio/medical aspects. Baltimore: Brookes Publishing, 1985:227.

91. Veith G, Wicke R. Cerebrale Differenzierungsstörungen bei Epilepsie. In: Meencke JH, Janz D, eds. Neuropathological findings in primary generalized epilepsy: a study of eight cases. Epilepsia 1984; 25:8.

92. Leviton A, Gilles FH. Acquired perinatal leukoencephalopathy. Ann Neurol 1984; 16:1.

93. Braun FHT, Jones KL, Smith DW. Breech presentation as an indicator of fetal abnormality. J Pediatr 1975; 86:419.

94. Miller ME, Higginbottom M, Smith DW. Short umbilical cord: its origin and relevance. Pediatrics 1981; 67:618.

95. Garite TJ, Linzey EM, Freeman RK, Dorchester W. Fetal heart rate patterns and fetal distress in fetuses with congenital anomalies. Obstet Gynecol 1979; 53:716.

96. Naeye RL, Tafari N. Risk factors in pregnancy and diseases of the fetus and newborn. Baltimore: Williams & Wilkins, 1983.

97. Illingworth RS, Woods GE. The incidence of twins in cerebral palsy and mental retardation. Arch Dis Child 1960; 35:333.

98. Russell EM. Cerebral palsied twins. Arch Dis Child 1961; 36:328.

99. Griffiths M. Cerebral palsy in multiple pregnancies. Dev Med Child Neurol 1967; 9:713.

100. Hagberg G, Hagberg B, Olow I. The changing panorama of cerebral palsy in Sweden 1954–1970. III. The importance of foetal deprivation of supply. Acta Paediatr Scand 1976; 65:403.

101. Smith JF, Rodeck C. Multiple cyctic and focal encephalomalacia in infancy and childhood with brainstem damage. J Neurol Sci 1975; 25:377.

102. Yoshioka H, Kadomoto Y, Mino M, et al. Multicystic encephalomalacia in liveborn twin with a stillborn macerated co-twin. J Pediatr 1979; 95:798.

103. Miller FC, Sacks DA, Yeh SY, et al. Significance of meconium during labor. Am J Obstet Gynecol 1975; 122:573.

104. Starks GC. Correlation of meconium-stained amniotic fluid, early intrapartum fetal pH, and Apgar scores as predictors of perinatal outcome. Obstet Gynecol 1980; 56:604.

105. Meis PJ, Hobel CJ, Ureda JR. Late meconium passage in labor—a sign of fetal distress? Obstet Gynecol 1982; 59:332.

106. Miller PW, Coen RW, Benirschke K. Dating the time interval from meconium to birth. Obstet Gynecol 1985; 66:459.

107. Desmond MM, Lindley JE, Moore J, Brown CA. Meconium staining of newborn infants. J Pediatr 1956; 49:540.

108. Fujikura T, Klionsky B. The significance of meconium staining. Am J Obstet Gynecol 1975; 121:45.

109. Murphy JD, Vawter GF, Reid LM. Pulmonary vascular disease in fatal meconium aspiration. J Pediatr 1984; 104:758.

110. Thacker SB. The efficacy of intrapartum electronic monitoring. Am J Obstet Gynecol 1987; 156:24.

111. Leveno KJ, Cunningham FG, Nelson S, et al. A prospective comparison of selective and universal electronic fetal monitoring in 34,995 pregnancies. N Engl J Med 1986; 315:615.

112. MacDonald D, Grant A, Sheridan-Pereira M, et al. The Dublin randomized controlled trial of intrapartum fetal heart rate monitoring. Am J Obstet Gynecol 1985; 152:524.

113. Clark SL, Paul RH. Intrapartum fetal surveillance: the role of fetal scalp blood sampling. Am J Obstet Gynecol 1985; 153:717.

114. Sykes GS, Molloy PM, Johnson P, et al. Do Apgar scores indicate asphyxia? Lancet 1982; 1:494.

115. Apgar V. A proposal for a new method of evaluation of the newborn infant. Curr Res Anesth Analg 1953; 32:260.

116. Apgar V, James LS. Further observations on the newborn scoring system. Am J Dis Child 1962; 104:419.

117. Drage JS, Berendes H. Apgar scores and outcome of the newborn. Pediatr Clin North Am 1966; 13:635.

118. American Academy of Pediatrics: Committee of Fetus and Newborn. Use and abuse of the Apgar score. Pediatrics 1986; 78:1148.

119. Nelson KB, Ellenberg JH. Apgar scores as predictors of chronic neurologic disability. Pediatrics 1981; 68:36.

120. Peters TJ, Golding J, Lawrence CJ, et al. Delayed onset of regular respiration and subsequent development. Early Hum Dev 1984; 9:225.

121. Steiner H, Neligan G. Perinatal cardiac arrest: quality of the survivors. Arch Dis Child 1975; 50:696.

122. Scott H. Outcome of very severe birth asphyxia. Arch Dis Child 1976; 51:712.

123. Thomson AJ, Searle M, Russell G. Quality of survival after severe birth asphyxia. Arch Dis Child 1977; 52:620.

124. DeSouza SW, Richards B. Neurological sequelae in newborn babies after perinatal asphyxia. Arch Dis Child 1978; 53:564.

125. Ergander U, Eriksson M, Zetterstrom R. Severe neonatal ashphyxia: incidence and prediction of outcome in the Stockholm area. Acta Paediatr Scand 1983; 72:321.

126. Catlin EA, Carpenter MW, Brann BS, et al. The Apgar score revisited: influence of gestational age. J Pediatr 1986; 109:865.

127. Goldenberg RL, Huddleston JF, Nelson KG. Apgar scores and umbilical arterial pH in perterm newborn infants. Am J Obstet Gynecol 1984; 149:651.

128. Tejani N, Verma UL. Neonatal depression and birth asphyxia in the low birthweight neonate. Am J Perinatol 1988; 2:85.

129. Brown JK, Purvis RJ, Forfar JO, Cockburn F. Neurological aspects of perinatal asphyxia. Dev Med Child Neurol 1974; 16:567.

130. Sarnat HB, Sarnat MS. Neonatal encephalopathy following fetal distress: a clinical and electroencephalographic study. Arch Neurol 1976; 33:696.

131. Sexson WR, Sexson SB, Rawson JE, Brann AW. The multisystem involvement of the asphyxiated newborn. Pediatr Res 1976; 10:432.

132. Robertson C, Finer N. Term infants with hypoxic-ischemic encephalopathy: outcome at 3.5 years. Dev Med Child Neurol 1985; 27:473.

133. Ishikawa T, Ogawa Y, Kanayama M, Wada Y. Long-term prognosis of asphyxiated full-term neonates with CNS complications. Brain Dev 1987; 9:48.

134. Mulligan JC, Painter MJ, O'Donoghue PA, et al. Neonatal asphyxia. II. Neonatal mortality and long-term sequelae. J Pediatr 1980; 96:903.

135. Spellacy WN, Miller S. Neonatal seizures: an obstetrician's concern. J Perinatol 1986; 6:157.

136. Derham RJ, Matthews TG, Clarke TA. Early seizures indicate quality of perinatal care. Arch Dis Child 1985; 60:809.

137. Keegan KA, Waffarn F, Quilligan EJ. Obstetric characteristics and fetal heart rate patterns of infants who convulse during the newborn period. Am J Obstet Gynecol 1985; 153:732.

138. Minchom P, Niswander K, Chalmers I, et al. Antecedents and outcome of very early seizures in infants born at or after term. Br J Obstet Gynaecol 1987; 94:431.

139. Mellits ED, Holden KR, Freeman JM. Neonatal seizures. II. A multivariate analysis of factors associated with outcome. Pediatrics 1982; 70:177.

140. Clarke M, Gill J, Noronha M, McKinley I. Early infantile epileptic encephalopathy with suppression burst: Ohtahara Syndrome. Dev Med Child Neurol 1987; 29:520.

141. Schwartz P. Birth injuries of the newborn: morphology, pathogenesis, clinical pathology and prevention. New York: Hafner Publishing, 1961.

142. Towbin A. Central nervous system damage in the human fetus and newborn infant. Mechanical and hypoxic injury incurred in the fetal-neonatal period. Am J Dis Child 1970; 119:529.

143. Welch K, Strand R. Traumatic parturitional intracranial hemorrhage. Dev Med Child Neurol 1986; 28:156.

144. Hayashi T, Hashimoto T, Fukuda A, et al. Neonatal subdural hematoma secondary to birth injury: clinical analysis of 48 survivors. Childs Nerv Syst 1987; 3:23.

145. Pierre-Kahn A, Renier D, Sainte-Rose C, Hirsh JF. Acute intracranial hematomas in term neonate. Childs Nerv Syst 1986; 2:191.

146. Fedrick J, Butler NR. Certain causes of neonatal death. V. Cerebral birth trauma. Biol Neonate 1971; 18:321.

147. Mateos F, Esteban J, Ramos JT, et al. Fetal subdural hematoma: diagnosis in utero: case report. Pediatr Neurosci 1987; 13:125.

148. Gunn TR, Mok PM, Becroft DMO. Subdural hemorrhage in utero. Pediatrics 1985; 76:605.

149. Dierker LJ Jr, Rosen MG, Thompson K, Lynn P. Midforceps deliveries: long-term outcome of infants. Am J Obstet Gynecol 1986; 154:764.

150. Parisi JE, Collins GH, Kim RC, Crosley CJ. Prenatal symmetrical thalamic degeneration with flexion spasticity at birth. Ann Neurol 1983; 13:94.

151. Dambska M, Laure-Kamionowska M, Liebhart M. Brainstem lesions in the course of chronic fetal asphyxia. Clin Neuropathol 1987; 6:110.

152. Barmada MA, Moossy J, Shuman RM. Cerebral infarcts with arterial occlusion in neonates. Ann Neurol 1979; 6:495.

153. Ong BY, Ellison PH, Browning C. Intrauterine stroke in the neonate. Arch Neurol 1983; 40:55.

154. Skullerud K, Skjaeraasen J. Clinicopathological study of germinal matrix hemorrhage, pontosubicular necrosis, and periventricular leukomalacia in stillborn. Childs Nerv Syst 1988; 4:88.

155. Sims ME, Turkel SB, Halterman G, Paul RH. Brain injury and intrauterine death. Am J Obstet Gynecol 1985; 151:721.

156. Szymonowicz W, Yu VYH. Outcome of intrauterine periventricular haemorrhage and leukomalcia. Aust Paediatr J 1985; 21:261.

157. Harrison VC, Heese HV, Klein M. Intracranial haemorrhage associated with hyaline membrane disease. Arch Dis Child 1968; 43:116.

158. Deonna T, Payot M, Probst A, Prod'hom LS. Neonatal intracranial hemorrhage in preterm infants. Pediatrics 1975; 56:1056.

159. Lazzara A, Ahmann P, Dykes F, et al. Clinical predictability of intraventricular hemorrhage in preterm infants. Pediatrics 1980; 65:30.

160. Dubowitz LMS, Dubowitz V, Palmer PG, et al. Correlation of neurologic assessment in the preterm newborn infant with outcome at 1 year. J Pediatr 1984; 105:452.

161. Sinha SK, Davies JM, Sims DG, Chiswick ML. Relation between periventricular haemorrhage and ischaemic brain lesions diagnosed by ultrasound in very pre-term infants. Lancet 1985; 2:1154.

162. Trounce JQ, Shaw DE, Levene MI, Rutter N. Clinical risk factors and periventricular leucomalacia. Arch Dis Child 1988; 63:17.

163. Szymonowicz W, Yu VYH. Periventricular hemorrhage and leukomalacia in extremely low birthweight infants. Aust Paediatr J 1986; 22:207.

164. Szymonowicz W, Yu VYH, Bajuk B, Astbury J. Neurodevelopmental outcome of periventricular haemorrhage and leukomalacia in infants 1250 g or less at birth. Early Hum Dev 1986; 14:1.

165. Guzzetta F, Shackelford GD, Volpe S, et al. Periventricular intraparenchymal echodensities in the premature newborn: critical determinant of neurological outcome. Pediatrics 1986; 78:995.

166. Weindling AM, Rochefort MJ, Calvert SA, et al. Development of cerebral palsy after ultrasonographic detection of periventricular cysts in the newborn. Dev Med Child Neurol 1985; 27:800.

167. Fawer CL, Diebold P, Calame A. Periventricular leucomalacia and neurodevelopmental outcome in preterm infants. Arch Dis Child 1987; 62:30.

168. Calvert SA, Hoskins EM, Fong KW, Forsyth SC. Periventricular leukomalacia: ultrasonic diagnosis and neurological outcome. Acta Paediatr Scand 1986; 75:489.

169. Smith YF. Incidence and outcome: periventricular leukomalacia. In: Grant EG, ed. Neurosonography of the pre-term neonate. New York:Springer-Verlag, 1986:91.

170. Trounce JQ, Fagan D, Levene MI. Intraventricular haemorrhage and periventricular leucomalacia: ultrasound and autopsy correlation. Arch Dis Child 1986; 61:1203.

171. Szymonowicz W, Schafler K, Cussen LJ, Yu VYH. Ultrasound and necropsy study of periventricular haemorrhage in preterm infants. Arch Dis Child 1984; 59:637.

172. Cooke RWI. Early and late cranial ultrasonographic appearances and outcome in very low birthweight infants. Arch Dis Child 1987; 62:931.

173. Clancy RR, Tharp BR, Enzman D. EEG in premature infants with intraventricular hemorrhage. Neurology 1984; 34:583.

174. DeVries LS, Connell JA, Dubowitz LMS, et al. Neurological, electrophysiological and MRI abnormalities in infants with extensive cystic leukomalacia. Neuropediatrics 1987; 18:61.

175. Bada HS, Korones SB, Anderson GD, et al. Obstetric factors and relative risk of neonatal germinal layer/intraventricular hemorrhage. Am J Obstet Gyecol 1984; 148:798.

176. Szymonowicz W, Yu VYU, Wilson FE. Antecedents of periventricular haemorrhage in infants weighing 1250 g or less at birth. Arch Dis Child 1984; 59:13.

177. Weindling AM, Wilkinson AR, Cook J, et al. Perinatal events which precede periventricular haemorrhage and leukomalacia in the newborn. Br J Obstet Gyaenecol 1985; 92:1218.

178. Kitchen W, Ford GW, Doyle LW, et al. Cesarean section or

vaginal delivery at 24 to 28 weeks' gestation; comparison of survival and neonatal and two-year morbidity. Obstet Gyencol 1985; 66:149.

179. Calvert SA, Hoskins EM, Fong KW, Forsyth SC. Etiological factors associated with the development of periventricular leukomalacia. Acta Paediatr Scand 1987; 76:254.

180. Rayburn WF, Donn SM, Kolin MG, Schork MA. Obstetric care and intraventricular hemorrhage in the low birth weight infant. Obstet Gynecol 1983; 61:408.

181. Levene MI, Fawer CL, Lamont RF. Risk factors in the development of intraventricular haemorrhage in the preterm neonate. Arch Dis Child 1982; 57:410.

182. Cooke RWI. Factors associated with periventricular haemorrhage in very low birthweight infants. Arch Dis Child 1981; 56:425.

183. Bejar R, Coen RW, Merritt TA, et al. Focal necrosis of the white matter (periventricular leukomalacia): sonographic, pathologic, and electroencephalographic features. AJNR 1986; 7:1073.

184. Skullerud K, Westre B. Frequency and prognostic significance of germinal matrix hemorrhage, periventricular leukomalacia, and pontosubicular necrosis in preterm neonates. Acta Neuropathol 1986; 70:257.

185. Nakamura Y, Fujiyoshi Y, Fukuda S, et al. Cystic brain lesion in utero. Acta Pathol Jpn 1986; 36:613.

186. Pevsner PH, Garcia-Bunuel R, Leeds N, Finklestein M. Subependymal and intraventricular hemorrhage in neonates. Early diagnosis by computed tomography. Radiology 1976; 119:111.

187. van de Bor M, Verloove-Vanhorick SP, Brand R, et al. Incidence and prediction of periventricular-intraventricular hemorrhage in very preterm infants. J Perinat Med 1987; 15:333.

188. Lebed MR, Schifrin BS, Waffran F, et al. Real-time B scanning in the diagnosis of neonatal intracranial hemorrgage. Am J Obstet Gynecol 1982; 142:851.

189. Teberg AJ, Hotrakitya S, Wu PYK, Yeh SY, Hoppenbrouwers T. Factors affecting nursery survival of very low birth weight infants. J Perinat Med 1987; 15:297.

190. Amato M, Gambon R, Von Muralt G, Huber P. Neurosonographic and biochemical correlates of periventricular leukomalacia in low-birth-weight infants. Pediatr Neurosci 1987; 13:84.

191. Altman DI, Volpe JJ. Cerebral blood flow in the newborn infant: measurement and role in the pathogenesis of periventricular and intraventricular hemorrhage. Adv Pediatr 1987; 34:111.

192. Crothers B, Paine RS. The natural history of cerebral palsy. Cambridge: Harvard University Press, 1959.

19

The Scope and Limitations of Neurologic and Behavioral Assessments of the Newborn

Anneliese F. Korner, Ph.D.

The Historical Origins of Neonatal Assessments
The Scope, Diverse Purposes, and Inherent Limitations
    of Different Neonatal Assessments
  Assessing the Infant's Condition at Birth
  Assessing the Infant's Gestational Age
  Neonatal Neurologic Assessments
  Neonatal Behavioral Assessments
  Neonatal Maturity Assessments
Conclusions

This chapter begins with a historical account of the beginnings of neonatal assessments and is followed by an overview of the theoretic and empiric issues that determine the scope and limitations of neonatal assessment techniques. This overview includes a discussion of the purposes of various neonatal assessment techniques, the uses that have been made of these assessments, and the problems inherent in reliably measuring the neonate's capabilities. Also discussed is the developmental and clinical validity of neonatal assessment as well as the problems inherent in achieving predictive or prognostic validity in relating neonatal assessment to later developmental outcomes. These issues are illustrated with examples from a variety of neonatal assessment procedures. Space limitations do not permit a full description of most of the neonatal assessments that have been developed over the years, but the reader is given a fairly comprehensive list of references to most of the procedures described in the literature. More fully described are three different types of neonatal examinations—one that assesses the neurologic integrity of full-term infants,[1] another that describes the behavioral repertoire and social responsiveness of full-term infants,[2] and a third and recently developed one that focuses primarily on

assessing the differential maturity of functioning of preterm infants as they grow to term.[3] The chapter concludes with a discussion of what might reasonably be expected from neonatal assessments and what are unrealistic expectations.

THE HISTORICAL ORIGINS OF NEONATAL ASSESSMENTS

Although there is considerable evidence that interest in the neonate's capabilities dates back to antiquity, it was not until the 19th century that careful observations about the newborn's sensory endowment began to appear in scientific publications.[4-7] In the first half of the 20th century a fairly large number of systematic studies of neonates began to appear. An overview of these studies can be found in Peiper's scholarly encyclopedic volumes.[8-9] Peiper not only summarized what was known prior to 1960 about the neonate's sensory repertoire and responsiveness, but he described most of the reflexes and behavioral responses of neonates that still are being assessed today. Interest in the neonate's behavioral and neurologic repertoire began to intensify in the early 1960s. With the advent of more sophisticated and more systematic observational methods, instrumentation, experimental design, and statistical techniques, infant research has become ever more prolific since then and has brought with it an awareness that the neonate's competencies are far greater than had formerly been anticipated.

Systematic and comprehensive assessment procedures for evaluating neonates and young infants began to appear in the early 1930s and 1940s.[10-13] In 1932 Charlotte Bühler and Hildegard Hetzer,[10] two Viennese psychologists, published their first edition of *Kleinkindertests*. A little later in the 1930s, Bayley's infant scales were published.[11,12] In 1941 the first edition of *Developmental*

Preparation of this chapter was assisted by grant MH 36884 from the National Institute of Mental Health, Prevention Research Branch, Division of Clinical Research. The author's research reported in this chapter was also supported by grant MH 36884 as well as by grant RR-81 from the General Clinical Research Center in the Division of Human Resources, National Institute of Health.

239

Diagnosis by Gesell and Amatruda[13] appeared. In the 1950s four different types of assessment procedures were developed. One was designed to evaluate the infant's condition at birth[14] and another to test the neurologic maturity of the newborn;[15] a third type was designed to discriminate between normal and compromised neonates[16] and a fourth to detect specific neurologic deficits.[17-18] After 1960 the field of neonatal assessment grew steadily and continues to grow today.[1-3, 19-41]

THE SCOPE, DIVERSE PURPOSES, AND INHERENT LIMITATIONS OF DIFFERENT NEONATAL ASSESSMENTS

Assessing the Infant's Condition at Birth

To determine the infant's condition at birth, the most commonly used assessment is that developed by Apgar.[14] Even though the Apgar rating system only inferentially assesses neurologic and behavioral responses, this method of evaluating the infant's condition at birth is briefly described here because the medical conditions underlying poor Apgar scores can profoundly affect the results of early and sometimes even later neurologic and behavioral examinations.

The infant's Apgar score is the sum of five subscores ranging from 0 to 2 each, based on ratings of the infant's heart rate, respiratory effort, muscle tone, reflex irritability, and color at one minute and five minutes after birth. In some centers ratings are also made after two, 10, 15, and 20 minutes. Two very large studies with subject populations of 27,715 and 17,221 infants have shown the usefulness of Apgar scoring at one and five minutes after birth.[42, 43] In both studies low scores were closely associated with neonatal mortality in the first month of life, with the largest number of deaths occurring in the first two days.[43] Additionally, results from the Collaborative Project[43] showed that low five-minute Apgar scores were strongly associated with neurologic morbidity at one year of age. It should be emphasized that these results estimate the probability of death or morbidity in *groups* of infants rather than predicting for individual infants. Further, it should be stated that Apgar ratings are not nearly so valid for preterm infants as they are for evaluating the condition at birth of full-term infants. This is true because the majority of the Apgar signs are as strongly influenced by the infant's immaturity as they are by the infant's condition at birth. By definition, the younger the infants are gestationally, the poorer their respiratory effort and muscle tone are apt to be and the less likely they are to cry. It might be useful to develop an Apgar score for preterm infants that would take into account the infant's gestational age.

Such a system would make a meaningful distinction between the infant's condition and the confounding aspects of his or her immaturity.

Assessing the Infant's Gestational Age

The development of methods for assessing infant gestational age was a major advance for neonatology and the clinical care of preterm infants as well as for developmental research. Prior to the advent of gestational age assessment techniques, the infant's postconceptional age was judged mostly by weight. Classifying the infant's degree of immaturity by weight can be misleading, particularly in those who are small or large for gestational age.

The two most common methods for estimating infant gestational age are by assessing the neurologic maturity of functioning and by judging the infant's external appearance (e.g., skin color and opacity, breast size, amount of lanugo). Both approaches were first used in 1966, Robinson[20] taking the neurologic approach and Farr et al[21] defining external characteristics to assess gestational age. In 1970 Dubowitz et al[25] combined the two approaches by using 11 of Farr's external characteristics and 10 neurologic items, most of which were part of the Saint-Anne Dargassies[15] and Amiel-Tison[24] examinations. In their standardization study Dubowitz et al[25] included only infants whose mothers reliably knew the date of their last menstrual period and who had not been taking oral contraceptives for 12 months prior to conception. The results of this study showed that in assessing the combination of neurologic and external signs, the correlation with gestational age was 0.93, with an error of prediction of $\pm$ 2 weeks using 95 percent confidence limits. For the external signs alone the correlation was 0.91 with an error of prediction of $\pm$ 2.4 weeks, and for the neurologic signs alone the correlation was 0.89 with an error of prediction of $\pm$ 2.6 weeks.

Because the full Dubowitz assessment frequently cannot be used with very ill preterm infants and because neonatologists often find that they do not have the time to administer the full examination, a series of shortened versions of the assessment were developed.[29, 32, 33] The best known and the most widely used version of the shortened gestational age assessment is that by Ballard et al.[33] The Ballard assessment includes only 12 of the 21 Dubowitz items, equally divided into neurologic maneuvers and external signs. In developing the shortened assessment, the same babies were examined with the Ballard and the full Dubowitz examinations, resulting in a correlation of 0.97 between the two assessments.

Even though the existing gestational age assessments are of tremendous utility for making clinical decisions, the incidences of error from all estimates are of great concern to investigators who are engaged in developmental studies that rely heavily on knowing infants' accurate ages. If, for example, a study is designed to determine how the sleep or the behavioral functioning of an infant at 32 weeks gestational age differs from that of a 34-week-old preterm infant, erroneous gestational age estimates will greatly affect the clarity of the differences. Or when, in a controlled intervention study, assignment to groups is made by using gestational age in a blocked design, errors in gestational age estimates will also blur the results.

Two recent studies have underscored this problem. One report indicated that the Dubowitz examination may systematically overestimate the gestational age of preterm infants, especially if they are black, were born to hypertensive mothers, and their gestations were less than 33 weeks.[44] Another study in which the Ballard assessment was used with 1,246 preterm infants at eight different institutions confirmed this bias in that the mean neurologic estimated gestational age exceeded the mean estimated date of confinement at every one of the eight sites.[45] Estimates based on external characteristics correlated more strongly with estimates of estimated dates of confinement and were more accurate than the combined neurologic and physical signs.

It is often not realized that even when the dates of the mother's last menstrual cycle are reliably known, estimating the infant's gestational age from the maternal dates has a minimum error rate of ±1 week. Although ovulation occurs most frequently between the 12th and the 16th days of the cycle, there is considerable variation, with ovulation taking place not uncommonly between the eighth and the 20th days.[46] That there are no error-free methods of assessing gestational age is also underscored by estimates from head circumference or ultrasonography, which have variable error rates and most frequently underestimate the age of small-for-date infant.[47,48] In biologic terms these variations should not be surprising because rates of maturation and physical growth vary with older children as well. In the area of gestational age estimates, these varying maturational rates are manifested in the most startling, if not ludicrous way: For example, twins or triplets not infrequently are judged to be discrepant in gestational age by more than two or three weeks.

In our own developmental studies we have tried to come to grips with the seemingly insurmountable problem of knowing the infant's age by including in our studies only infants whose gestational age estimates are all within a two-week range. Because of the prevalence of discrepancies in gestational age estimates in excess of two weeks, we pay a heavy price in having to exclude a large number of infants from our studies. We make a further attempt to reduce the error of the gestational age estimation of infants whose estimates are all within a two-week range by averaging the estimates available.*

---

*For a further elucidation of the many complex issues involved in gestational age estimation, see the scholarly review by Casaer and Akiyama.[49]

Neonatal Neurologic Assessments

Not all assessments called neurologic examinations are neurologic in the traditional sense, namely, designed to diagnose specific neurologic syndromes or deviations. Even though some neurologic examinations have this goal,[1, 17, 30, 35, 36, 40] other assessments aim mostly at studying the development of neural functions.[24, 26, 31] Still other assessments are neurologic largely by inference, in that they are designed to discriminate statistically between neurologically suspect, abnormal, and normal infants, either through comparisons of group means in performance or through empirically derived cut-off points below which the infant's performance is considered suspect or abnormal.[16, 40, 50]

Of the neurologic assessments designed to be diagnostic of specific syndromes in full-term infants, Prechtl's is by far the most comprehensive.[1, 30] The Prechtl neurologic examination, which was standardized on a large sample of full-term infants, is both a clinical and a research instrument. It is a lengthy assessment, requiring great technical skill and a fundamental understanding of the early developmental stages of the nervous system.

The examination begins with an observation period in which the infant's behavioral states, resting posture, and spontaneous motor activity (including athetoid movements and tremors) are observed. After this observation period a comprehensive group of reflexes are tested, first while the infant is in the supine position and later in the examination while the baby is in the prone position or is held in the upright position. Testing of reflexive behavior includes the motor and vestibular systems, the eyes and skin, rooting, and sucking. Also included in the examination is a systematic check of the infant's resistance against passive movements and the range and power of active movements. Throughout the examination the infant's behavioral states, respirations, motor activity, posture, asymmetry of response, and skin color are observed.

Central to the Prechtl examination are two very important concepts:

1. The optimal behavioral state or states in which most of the test items must be administered are specified. This is important, because certain reflexes and other responses will be either present or absent, diminished or exaggerated, depending on the infant's behavioral state. Even though Prechtl recommends a specified sequence in the elicitation of responses, he suggests that if the baby is not in an appropriate state, he or she should be either aroused or pacified in order to achieve the appropriate state. If mild rocking or cuddling is not effective, the examination should be terminated and repeated when the baby is in a more adequate state.

2. In his scoring system Prechtl specifies which of the infant's responses are optimal. The sum of optimal scores can provide information regarding the overall integrity of an infant's nervous system. Further, the absence of optimal scores in certain areas of functioning

can provide differential diagnostic clues. The Prechtl examination also can be used to arrive at a diagnosis of specific clinical syndromes. For example, when frequent asymmetries are noted in the infant's motor responses, posture, and spontaneous motility, a diagnosis of hemisyndrome is made. Other syndromes involve abnormal reactivity on the part of the infant, such as consistent hyperexcitability or apathy. To arrive at an adequate diagnostic picture of the integrity of the infant's nervous system, repeated Prechtl examinations are essential.

Prechtl[51] repeatedly has stressed that to be diagnostically valid, a neurologic examination has to be comprehensive. He recommends that one clinically evaluate the infant's overt signs of abnormalities until such time that the infant can tolerate a complete examination. Even though Touwen et al[52] in Prechtl's laboratory have developed a short standardized neurologic screening test, this assessment is not designed to be a substitute for the full neurologic examination. The screening test is used primarily to select infants who require a full diagnostic neurologic evaluation. The proviso that only complete neurologic assessments are valid, however, has not been adhered to by others who have developed shortened versions of the Prechtl examination. Thus, Schulte et al[53] and Joppich and Schulte[54] developed neurologic assessments modeled after the Prechtl assessment that were applicable to sick newborns, and Aylward[35,41] developed a Prechtl type of assessment suitable for preterm infants.

Another comprehensive neurologic examination is that by Lilly and Victor Dubowitz.[36] This assessment is applicable to preterm and full-term infants. The Dubowitz neurologic assessment includes fewer tests of specific reflexes than does the Prechtl examination[1, 30] but includes many behavioral items from the Brazelton assessment.[2] Most heavily emphasized is the evaluation of the infant's movements and tone. Because the results of the Dubowitz examination are based on an item by item analysis, this assessment can be shortened by administering only those items that are compatible with the infant's medical condition. In comparing infants who had intraventricular hemorrhage with infants who did not, the authors found significant diagnostic differences in the infants with intraventricular hemorrhage who were born before 36 weeks' gestational age. More infants with intraventricular hemorrhage had low tone and motility, tight popliteal angles, and roving eye movements and were more frequently incapable of visual tracking than were infants without intraventricular hemorrhage. Dubowitz and Dubowitz[36] stressed the importance of repeated assessments. They also emphasized that frequently it is not the initial severity of the neurologic signs that is important for prognosis, but their persistence.

In considering the scope and limitations of neonatal neurologic assessment, a distinction must be made between an examination's usefulness in diagnosing abnormalities in the neonatal period (concurrent validity) and its potential for prognosticating later neurologic defects and deviant development (predictive validity). There is general agreement that it is important to perform repeated assessments during the neonatal period, not only to validate the diagnostic impressions gained but to assess whether and to what degree the infant's condition improves. Steady improvement and disappearance of abnormal responses during the neonatal period are considered by most to be a good prognostic sign.[55]

When neurologic assessments for neonates were first developed, it of course was hoped that they would be instrumental in long-range predictions of neurologic impairment or developmental deviation. In the many studies that have appeared in the literature, there is consensus that on a probabilistic basis, infants who were normal at birth will remain normal in childhood unless they sustain significant central nervous system insults after the neonatal period. It is equally clear that infants diagnosed as showing neurologic impairment during the neonatal period statistically have a significantly higher *probability* of having neurologic problems in later childhood than do individuals diagnosed as being normal neonates.[16, 18, 30, 55, 56] This implies that predictions are limited to groups of infants and cannot be made for individuals.

This fact was clearly demonstrated in a comprehensive literature review by Hadders-Algra[56] that covered dozens of studies and thousands of infants. This fact also was highlighted in Hadders-Algra's own follow-up study of the correlates of brain dysfunction in children who as neonates were given Prechtl neurologic assessments.[56] One repetitive theme that emerged from most of the studies was that adverse environmental conditions such as poor socioeconomic and familial circumstances had a much greater impact on developmental outcome than did perinatal and neonatal complications,[56] a finding also stressed in Sameroff and Chandler's earlier review.[57]

Little is known about the mechanism by which many infants who as neonates show evidence of neurologic deficits become normally functioning children. It is not that the neonatal neurologic assessments, if done repeatedly and by experienced examiners, are likely to yield unreliable or clinically invalid results. It has been postulated that the disappearance of abnormal neonatal responses may be a function of the plasticity and adaptive capacity of the developing brain, which may permit recovery from temporary central nervous system insults or compensation for permanent brain lesions.[55] At any rate, the eventual normality of a majority of children who as neonates showed clear indications of neurologic deviancy should not be taken as a contraindication to performing neonatal neurologic assessments. A large array of studies have shown that neonates judged to be abnormal are at significantly greater risk for later neurologic deficits than their normal counterparts. It therefore is imperative that these high risk infants be followed closely so that remedial intervention can be made available as needed.[51, 56, 58]

Neonatal Behavioral Assessments

Not infrequently behavioral examinations are called neurobehavioral assessments, because much of the newborn's behavior is governed by and is an expression of the extent and the limitations of his or her neurologic repertoire. Several neurobehavioral assessments have been developed over the last 30 years, both for different and for overlapping purposes.

One of the earliest and psychometrically most rigorous behavioral assessments was Rosenblith's modification of the Graham Behavior Test.[16] In the 1960s Rosenblith[19] collected normative data in a large sample of full-term neonates who participated in the Collaborative Perinatal Research Project. The Rosenblith assessment includes a general maturity scale that consists mostly of motor items, a sensory maturity scale that tests visual and auditory responsivity, and a variety of ratings of the infant's irritability and muscle tone. In using her assessment, Rosenblith reported high interobserver and test-retest reliabilities. The test was used to study individual differences at birth among newborns, to predict Bayley performance at eight months,[59] and to study the relation between special sensitivities in newborns and later abnormalities.[60, 61] Except for good prognostication of later abnormality in single cases of light sensitivity, prediction of the developmental status of the sample to eight months was modest.

The most widely used neonatal behavioral assessment is the one developed by Brazelton.[2] The original purpose of this examination was to study individual differences in full-term infants in order to document the effects of the infant's individuality on the earliest parent-infant interaction and relationship. The Brazelton assessment (NBAS) also was designed to identify the precursors to later tempermental and personality differences. The scope of purposes for which Brazelton's assessment has since been used has expanded considerably. The following are some of the domains in which the Brazelton examination has been utilized: studies of high risk infants,[62-68] studies of the effects of obstetrical medication[69-71] and maternal substance abuse,[72-75] cross-cultural comparisons of newborn behavior,[76-79] prediction of later development,[80-82] and as a form of intervention.[83-86] In the latter the Brazelton assessment has been used to demonstrate the infant's behavioral repertoire to parents, either to educate them about the capabilities of their newborn or to enhance their sensitivity to the infant's behavioral cues.*

The Brazelton assessment consists of 27 nine-point

scales that include test items and observations in the following domains: habituation to sensory stimuli during sleep, orientation to inanimate and animate auditory and visual stimuli, motor maturity, activity, tone, the lability, range, and regulation of the infant's states, as well as some indications of the infant's autonomic stability.[2, 39] Optimal states for the assessment of each test item are specified. A flexible approach to the administration of the assessment is recommended. Also included in the examination are 18 reflex items scored on a four-point scale. These items serve as a screen for gross neurologic abnormalities. A detailed neurologic evaluation is recommended when three or more abnormal scores are obtained.

Even though many of the test items overlap with those used in other assessments,[1, 16, 19, 24] several aspects of the Brazelton examination are highly original. One of these is the testing of the infant's response and orientation to the human voice and face. These items assess individual differences in the infant's earliest capacity for interacting with caregivers. Other novel and very central features of the Brazelton assessment are observations of the rapidity with which infants become excited and irritable in response to the examination and infants' ability to console themselves or to be consoled. These observations have led to the widely accepted yet somewhat controversial view that neonates are already capable of organizing themselves to master and control their reactions to external and internal stimuli.[87] Scoring of the Brazelton assessment is based on the best performance the infant can achieve on each item. Horowitz et al[88] introduced an additional scoring system that considered the infant's "modal" response to the test items. The "modal" score was designed to capture the infant's more typical behavior, characterizing how a baby is apt to respond to his or her caregiver at home.

Even though the Brazelton examination was designed for use with full-term infants, it frequently has been used with preterm infants as well. This gradually led Brazelton[39] and his colleagues[38, 88] to develop supplementary scales, applicable to preterm infants. Additionally, Als et al[38] developed an elaborate offshoot of the Brazelton examination (the APIB), which is used primarily with preterm infants.

One of the most common uses of neurobehavioral assessments has been to determine in what way the behavior of preterm infants grown to term differs from that of infants born at term.[34, 89, 90] Such studies have shown that the development of preterm infants grown to term is uneven, some functions being accelerated, others retarded, and still others undistinguishable from those of full-term babies. One problem that may have confounded the results of these studies is that the medical complications that preterm infants frequently incur seem to have a greater impact on their development than does their prematurity. Another problem that may have confounded the results of some of these studies is that

---

*For a more complete list of the different types of studies done with this assessment, see the article by Brazelton et al[87] on this subject.

just born, full-term infants were used most frequently as controls for the preterm infants. Judging from the study by Palmer et al,[91] differences between the full-term and the preterm infants may disappear or diminish greatly when the full-term infants become a few days old.

Palmer et al administered the Dubowitz neurologic examination to preterm infants at term and to one-day-old and five-day-old full-term infants. In comparing 11 test items on day 1, the groups differed significantly in nine instances. By day five the difference between the groups was no longer significant on four items, and differences had decreased in magnitude on four additional items. Behaviorally, the just born, full-term infants had a good deal more flexion and tone than when they were five days old. Considering the fact that the one-day-old full-term infants had just been delivered from a very confining environment, this difference is not surprising. Clearly, although it is less convenient to study full-term infants after they have left the hospital, evidence from this study suggests that this would be the method of choice in any preterm and full-term comparisons.

Even though the scope and purposes of neurobehavioral assessments are broad, these techniques also have definite limitations. Although, on the whole, most neurobehavioral assessments have concurrent validity and measure what they are designed to assess, there is always the potential, as there is with other neonatal assessments, that any given examination may be unreliable for any number of reasons. Sequential assessments are always preferable to single examinations, not only because repeated assessments promise to capture the infant's characteristic responses better than any single examination, but because they also highlight directions of change. As is the case with neurologic examinations, the predictive validity of neurobehavioral assessments to later development is, at best, modest.

There are a number of intrinsic and extrinsic factors that make prediction problematic. For one, little is known about how the neurobehavioral functions tested in the neonatal period are linked to functions tested later in childhood. In follow-up studies, well-standardized tests like the Bayley or the Stanford-Binet test are commonly administered with the tacit assumption that the neonatal and childhood test results should be strongly correlated. Because the behavior patterns observed and functions tested in neonates are for the most part developmentally age specific, it is unrealistic to expect that the types of tests used later in development will show direct links to the earlier assessments. Quite apart from these intrinsic measurement problems, longitudinal research has shown repeatedly that the single most powerful influence on child development is not so much the innate givens, but the socioeconomic and familial circumstances in which children are raised.[57, 92-95]

Neonatal Maturity Assessments

By far the best standardized and most widely known maturity assessments are the Bayley Scales of Infant Development[96] and the Gesell Developmental Schedules.[13] Both assessments are applicable for testing the developmental status over the entire span of infancy. Although these assessments are applicable to full-term infants who are less than one month old, these instruments measure a relatively narrow range of neonatal function and are more suitable for evaluating the maturity of older infants. Therefore, neither the Bayley nor the Gessell assessment has been widely used during the neonatal period.

Neonatal maturity assessments for preterm infants include, of course, the techniques for estimating infant gestational age, already mentioned.[21, 25-27, 33] However, these procedures are not suitable for the longitudinal study of developing functions, in that these assessments are applicable and valid only during the first few days of life. A group of French neonatal neurologists first assessed and systematically documented the maturational course of neural functions in subjects ranging from preterm infants aged 28 weeks after conception to term infants.[15, 17, 24, 31] As neurologists, these investigators of course were interested in identifying early neurologic deficits, but they did this appropriately in the context of gathering normative data relating to preterm infant functioning. Thus Saint-Anne Dargassies[15] and later Amiel-Tison[24] systematically illustrated the age differences in functioning of preterm infants in two-week increments.

Both neurologic and neurobehavioral assessments have been used to assess the relative maturity of preterm and full-term infants, [2, 35-39] even though these assessments were not structurally designed for this specific purpose. In many of these assessments the highest scores on individual scales are considered to be the most mature, even though there are many exceptions to this rule. In some assessments the most mature or optimal response is at times the lowest or the middle score of a scale,[2] or somewhere between the highest and the lowest score.[1, 36] In addition, only rarely has the developmental validity of the scores considered to be the most mature been tested statistically.

The most recent development in the area of neonatal maturity assessment is the procedure developed by Korner et al.[3] Development of a pilot version of the Neurobehavioral Maturity Assessment for Preterm Infants (NB-MAP) began in 1977.[3] Development of this procedure was prompted by the need to monitor the developmental progress of preterm infants who participated in a randomized controlled longitudinal intervention study.[97] In developing this instrument, we started from the assumption that the most relevant and most important goal of any intervention would be to facilitate the normality of the infants' developmental course so that their ultimate development and maturity would not be too different from that of full-term newborns within the normal range.[98] Unfortunately we could not use any of the pre-existing maturity assessments for preterm infants,[15, 17, 24, 31] because none of these examinations characterized preterm infants' performance in less than two-week age intervals. Because it was unrealistic to expect that experimental and control groups would differ in the maturity of functioning in excess of two weeks, it was necessary to develop a procedure that potentially could reveal more subtle differences in performance.

Because preterm infants have a finite neurobehavioral repertoire, most of the test items in the NB-MAP examination, of necessity, overlap with those used in other assessments.[3, 99, 100] Nevertheless this procedure differs from most others in a number of important ways:

1. In line with our goal of testing the maturity of the infant's functioning, only test items that had shown age changes in previous work were included in the procedure. In the further selection of the test items, our first priority was to include in the assessment only conceptually and clinically meaningful maneuvers. Additionally, a scoring system was devised in which the scores of each scale were ordered from the least to the most mature responses.

2. In developing the assessment we excluded aversive maneuvers such as the Moro and pinprick reflexes. In order not to fatigue the infants by excessive handling, approximately half the assessment time is spent in observing them. Infants become eligible for testing at 32 weeks' postconceptional age provided they are medically stable. We found empirically that we were able to carry out the complete assessment in almost all 32-week-old infants without causing undue fatigue.

3. In developing the maturity assessment, we chose to use a truly invariant sequence of item presentation designed to bring about the kind of behavioral states that are most likely to elicit the best possible responses from preterm infants. Even though we were keenly aware that the infants' states strongly influence their responses,[101] we found empirically that with young preterm infants the requirement of a predetermined state before administering each item was not feasible. The attempt to achieve the appropriate predetermined states through various rousing or soothing maneuvers would have greatly prolonged the examination, fatigued the infant, or failed altogether. For this reason we chose to build into the assessment a standard sequence of rousing, soothing, and alerting items that maximized the chance of testing the various functions in appropriate states and minimized the need to intervene with some infants more than with others. This approach prevented the examination from becoming a different procedure for each infant and guaranteed that the examination would be comparable from one infant to the next. This strategy also

provided the opportunity to study systematically the age changes in the infants' states in response to a standard sequence of identical events.[102]

4. The unique aspect of the NB-MAP procedure was that the psychometric soundness of the items was made a precondition for their inclusion in this assessment. To prevent untested and unreliable items from being included in the examination, the test-retest reliability on two consecutive days had to be a minimum of 0.6. Test items were grouped into clusters that had conceptual cohesion and face validity and that were then tested to determine whether they had statistical cohesion as well. Unreliable and noncohesive test items were eliminated from the test, as were redundant clusters. The remaining clusters then were tested for developmental validity based on whether they showed significant changes with age. With this approach, nine reliable and developmentally valid dimensions emerged: motor development and/or vigor; two items measuring resistance to passive movement (popliteal angle and scarf sign); alertness and orientation; maturity of vestibular response; and four state-related items consisting of the percentage of state ratings the infant was asleep; the percentage of state ratings the infant was crying while awake; the vigor of crying; and the infant's excitability in response to being handled. All these dimensions showed significant increases with age except for sleep, which decreased significantly as the infants grew to term.

The Neurobehavioral Maturity Assessment (NB-MAP) can be used for a number of purposes when the maturity of infant functioning is the key issue—assessing the effects of intervention studies, clinical trials, and changes in the care of preterm infants; monitoring the developmental progress in individual infants; and, potentially, making a contribution to basic knowledge regarding the nature and sequence of preterm infants' behavioral development. Additionally, the NB-MAP can be used for ancillary purposes, although these are secondary to its prime objective of measuring the maturity of functioning of preterm infants. The assessment highlights gross neurologic malfunctioning and thus can point to the need for a full neurologic work-up. The NB-MAP also can be used to study the stability of individual differences in developmentally changing preterm infants, a purpose for which this assessment has already been used in a recent study.[103]

One of the prime purposes of all maturity assessments is to provide some indication of whether the development of a given infant proceeds normally or shows significant developmental lags. Both the Bayley and the Gesell Developmental Schedules, which have been standardized on large samples of infants who mostly were older than full-term neonates, accomplish this purpose very well. It is not clear whether the developmental guidelines provided by the Saint-Anne Dargassies and Amiel-Tison assessments were derived from large samples of preterm infants. However, the fact that these assessments characterize infant performance only in two-week age intervals has certain clinical advantages: If the performance in a preterm infant *consistently* lags by more than two weeks, it is clear that the developmental progress in that infant should be closely monitored. Because the NB-MAP assessment is developmental in structure, it also can be used to generate developmental guidelines. Because normative guidelines must be based on large samples from many different populations, much further research with this instrument is needed. Even when such normative guidelines are established, it is important to be aware that these must be used judiciously in clinical contexts. Preterm infants are a very heterogeneous group whose performance is readily influenced by variability in state and health status. It therefore is important to use normative guidelines primarily to identify infants who on repeated examination show developmental lags so that appropriate follow-up and remedial intervention can be instituted.

Maturity assessments fare no better in predicting long-range developmental outcome than do neurologic and behavioral assessments. Even the Bayley assessment, a reliable and well-standardized assessment that uses the same test structure for infants aged one to 30 months, shows only modest and at times poor predictability from one age to another. Understandably, prediction is best for adjacent ages and worsens as the age span increases between assessments. Contrary to original hopes, Bayley results do not predict later IQ's of school-age children or adults, except in cases of severe retardation. It appears that it was not the intent of Saint-Anne Dargassies and Amiel-Tison to predict later intelligence from their assessments of preterm infants, nor is it our intent to do so with the NB-MAP test.

The same inherent conceptual problems exist with the neonatal maturity assessments as with the neurologic and behavioral assessments: Early capabilities in age-specific functions are not necessarily linked to later competencies. The functions tested at early ages differ from those tested later. Additionally, the socioeconomic and familial circumstances in which the children are raised strongly affect their development.[57, 92] All these limitations regarding the predictive validity of maturity assessments, however, do not negate the tremendous usefulness of these assessments, including those administered during the neonatal period, in providing a reliable and valid estimate of the infant's developmental status at the time of testing relative to that of other infants of the same age.[104, 105] These tests thus can be used profitably to identify infants demonstrating developmental delays or those who are at risk for such delays.

CONCLUSIONS

Summing up the scope and limitations of neonatal assessments, whether designed to test the infant's neurologic integrity, neurobehavioral repertoire, or developmental status, there is general concensus about the following:

1. Many neonatal assessment techniques yield reliable and valid information regarding the infant's current status, provided that repeated examinations are given by an experienced examiner who carefully follows the standard instructions for each assessment technique. There are no short-cuts to these provisos, no matter how much the busy clinician might wish otherwise. In practice, it would be desirable at least to use standard screening techniques in intensive care nurseries, so that infants who show deviation of any kind will be targeted for a more complete work-up. If the deviation is confirmed, it is imperative that close follow-up be instituted, because early remedial intervention may be indicated.

2. Although repeated careful assessments done with well-standardized procedures provide reliable and valid information about a child's neonatal functioning, the cumulative research evidence indicates that prediction from these assessments to later development is generally poor. This really is not surprising when one considers the plasticity and adaptive capacity of the developing brain and the tremendous and continuous effect of socioeconomic and familial circumstances that maintain, foster, or depress the developmental course in young children.[55, 57]

3. Although prediction in regard to later development in the population as a whole is generally poor, research findings consistently demonstrate that neonates identified as having neurologic deviations, behavioral peculiarities, or developmental lags are at a significantly greater risk for later deviant development. Although the majority of these infants outgrow their original difficulties, particularly when raised in a supportive familial environment, there is an increased risk that some will continue to show later developmental problems. This risk is based on statistical estimates from group findings. In a similar vein, neonates found to be normal at birth have a high probability of becoming normal children unless they encounter significant problems after the neonatal period. This implies that predictions are limited to groups of at-risk infants only.

4. The cumulative evidence described clearly indicates that in questions relating to malpractice, one must differentiate between the usefulness of assessments during the neonatal period and the relevance of these assessments for later development. *Repeated* and careful assessments during the neonatal period with the use of well-standardized techniques, administered by experienced examiners, are not likely to produce many false positive or false negative test results. At the same time, the evidence gathered during the neonatal period cannot be used to explain with any certainty the deviation of a child's later development. Even though early deviation places an infant at greater risk for later abnormality, this prediction is a statistical estimate derived from group data. For the most part, these predictions are not applicable to individual children.

I thank Valerie A. Thom, Nancy M. Lane, and Janet Constantinou for their helpful review of this chapter.

REFERENCES

1. Prechtl HFR, Beintema D. The neurological examination of the fulterm newborn infant. Little club clinics in developmental medicine. No. 12. London: William Heinemann, 1964.
2. Brazelton TB. Neonatal behavioral assessment scale. Clinics in developmental medicine. No. 50. S.I.M.P. Philadelphia: JB Lippincott, 1973.
3. Korner AF, Kraemer HC, Reade EP, et al. A methodological approach to developing an assessment procedure for testing the neurobehavioral maturity of preterm infants. Child Dev 1987; 58:1478.
4. Sigismund B. Kind und welt, 1856. Altenburg, 1897.
5. Kussmaul A. Über das seelenleben des neugeboreuen menschen. Leipzig, 1859.
6. Darwin C. The expression of emotions in man and animals. London: Murray, 1873.
7. Preyer W. Die Sehle des Kindes 4. Auflag. Leipzig, 1895.
8. Peiper A. Die Hirntätigkeit des Sauglings. Berlin: Springer, 1928.
9. Peiper A. Cerebral function in infancy and childhood. (Translation of the third revised German edition by B. Nagler and H. Nagler.) New York: Consultants Bureau, 1963.
10. Bühler CH, Hetzer H. Kleinkindertests. Leipzig, 1932.
11. Bayley N. The California first-year mental scale. Berkeley, California: University of California Press, 1933.
12. Bayler N. The California infant scale of motor development. Berkeley, California: University of California Press, 1936.
13. Gesell A, Amatruda CS. Developmental diagnosis: normal and abnormal child development. New York: Hoeber, 1941.
14. Apgar V. A proposal for a new method of evaluation of the newborn infant. Curr Res Anesth Analg 1953; 32:260.
15. Saint-Anne Dargassies S. Méthode d'examen neurologique du nouveau-né. Et Néonatales 1954; 3:101.
16. Graham FK, Matarazzo RG, Caldwell BM. Behavioral differences between normal and traumatized newborns. II. Standardization, reliability and validity. Psychol Monogr 1956; 70:No. 428.
17. André-Thomas Y, Chesni Y, Saint-Anne Dargassies S. In: MacKeith RC, ed. The neurological examination of the infant. London: Medical Advisory Committee of the National Spastics Society, 1960.
18. Paine RS. Neurological examination of infants and children. Pediatr Clin North Am 1960; 7:471.
19. Rosenblith JF. The modified Graham behavior test for neonates: test-retest reliability, normative data and hypotheses for future work. Biol Neonate 1961; 3:174.
20. Robinson RJ. Assessment of gestational age by neurological examination. Arch Dis Child 1966; 41:437.
21. Farr V, Mitchell RG, Neligan GA, Parkin JM. The definition of some external characteristics used in the assessment of gestational age in the newborn infant. Dev Med Child Neurol 1966; 8:507.
22. Milani-Comparetti A, Gidoni EA. Routine developmental examination in normal and retarded children. Dev Med Child Neurol 1967; 9:631.
23. Frankenberg W, Dobbs J. The Denver developmental screening test, J Pediatr 1967; 71:181.
24. Amiel-Tison C. Neurological evaluation of the maturity of newborn infants. Arch Dis Child 1968; 43:89.
25. Dubowitz LMS, Dubowitz V, Goldberg C. Clinical assessment of gestational age. J Pediatr 1970; 77:1.
26. Finnström O. Studies on maturity in newborn infants. III. Neurological examination. Neuropadiatrie 1971; 3:72.
27. Finnström O. Studies on maturity in newborn infants. II. External characteristics. Acta Paediatr Scand 1972; 61:24.
28. Parmelee AH Jr. Newborn neurological examination. Unpublished manuscript, August 1974.
29. Parkin JM, Hey EN, Clowes JS. Rapid assessment of gestational age at birth. Arch Dis Child 1976; 51:259.
30. Prechtl H. The neurological examination of the full-term new-

31. Saint-Anne Dargassies S. Neurological development in the full-term and premature neonate. New York: Elsevier–North Holland, 1977.
32. Capurro H, Konichezky S, Fonseca D, Caldeyro-Barcia R. A simplified method for diagnosis of gestational age in the newborn infant. J Pediatr 1978; 93:120.
33. Ballard JL, Novak KK, Driver M. A simplified score for assessment of fetal maturity of newly born infants. J Pediatr 1979; 95:769.
34. Kurtzberg D, Vaughan HG Jr, Daum C, et al. Neurobehavioral performance of low-birthweight infants at 40 weeks' conceptional age: comparison with normal fulterm infants. Dev Med Child Neurol 1979; 21:590.
35. Aylward GP. Neurological development in preterm infants. JSAS catalogue of selected documents in psychology 1981; 11:31 (Ms. 2245).
36. Dubowitz LMS, Dubowitz V. The neurological assessment of the preterm and fulterm newborn infant. Philadelphia: JB Lippincott, 1981.
37. Als H, Lester BM, Tronick EC, Brazelton TB. Towards a research instrument for the assessment of preterm infants' behavior (APIB). In Fitzgerald HE, Lester BM, Yogman MW, eds. Theory and research in behavioral pediatrics. Vol. I. New York: Plenum, 1982:35.
38. Als H, Lester BM, Tronick EC, Brazelton TB. Manual for the assessment of preterm infants' behavior (APIB). In: Fitzgerald HE, Lester BM, Yogman MW, eds. Theory and research in behavioral pediatrics. Vol. I. New York: Plenum, 1982:65.
39. Brazelton TB. Neonatal behavioral assessment scale. 2nd ed. Philadelphia: JB Lippincott, 1984.
40. Ellison PH, Horn JL, Browning CA. Construction of an infant neurological international battery (INFANIB) for the assessment of neurological integrity in infancy. Phys Ther 1985; 65:1326.
41. Aylward GP, Verhulst SJ, Colliver JA. Development of a brief infant neurobehavioral optimality scale: longitudinal sensitivity and specificity. Dev Neuropsychol 1985; 1:265.
42. Apgar V, James LS. Further observations on the newborn scoring system. Am J Dis Child 1962; 107:419.
43. Drage JS, Berendes H. Apgar scores and outcome of the newborn. Pediatr Clin North Am 1966; 13:635.
44. Spinnato JA, Sibai BM, Shaver DC, Anderson GD. Inaccuracy of Dubowitz gestational age in low birthweight infants. Obstet Gynecol 1984; 63:491.
45. Constantine NA, Kraemer HC, Kendell-Tackett KA, et al. Use of physical and neurological observations in assessment of gestational age in low birthweight infants. J. Pediatr 1987; 110:921.
46. Prichard JA, MacDonald PC, Gant NF, eds. Williams obstetrics, 17th ed. Norwalk, Connecticut: Appleton-Century-Crofts, 1985:43.
47. Usher R, McLean F. Intrauterine growth of live-born Caucasian infants at sea level: standards obtained from measurements in seven dimensions of infants born between 25 and 44 weeks of gestation. J Pediatr 1969; 74:901.
48. Campbell S. The prediction of fetal maturity by ultrasonic measurement of the biparietal diameter. J Obstet Gynecol 1969; 76:603.
49. Casaer P, Akiyama Y. The estimation of the post-menstrual age: a comprehensive review. Dev Med Child Neurol 1970; 12:697.
50. Howard J, Parmelee AH Jr, Kopp CD, Littman B. A neurological comparison of preterm and fulterm infants at term conceptional age. J Pediatr 1976; 88:995.
51. Prechtl HFR. Assessment methods for the newborn infant, a critical evaluation. In: Stratton P, ed. Psychobiology of the human newborn. London: John Wiley, 1982:21.
52. Touwen BCL, Bierman-Van Endenburg M, Jurgens-Van der Zee A. The neurological screening of fulterm newborn infants. Dev Med Child Neurol 1977; 19:739.
53. Schulte FJ, Michaelis R, Fillipp E. Neurologie des Neu-

born infant. 2nd ed. Clinics in developmental medicine. No. 63. S.I.M.P. Philadelphia: JB Lippincott, 1977.

geborenen. I Mitteilung. Ursache und klinische Symptomatologie von Functions-störungen des Nervensystems bei Neugeborenen. Zeit Kinderheilk 1965; 93:242.

54. Joppich G, Schulte FJ. Neurologie des Neugeborenen. New York: Springer Verlag, 1968.

55. Parmelee AH, Michaelis R. Neurological examination of the newborn. In: Hellmuth J, ed. Exceptional infant. Vol. 2. Studies in abnormalities. London: Butterworths. 1971.

56. Hadders-Algra M. Correlates of brain dysfunction in children—a follow-up study. Groningen: Drukkerij Van Denderen, 1987.

57. Sameroff A, Chandler M. Reproductive risk and the continuum of care-taking casualty. In: Horowitz FD, ed. A review of child development research. Vol. 4. Chicago: University of Chicago Press, 1975:187.

58. Brown JV. Current behavioral tools for testing neurological function in the newborn. In: Neonatal neurological assessment and outcome. Report of the 77th Ross conference on pediatrics. Columbus, Ohio: Ross Laboratories, 1980:99.

59. Rosenblith JF. Relation between neonatal behaviors and those at 8 months. Dev Psychol 1974; 10:779.

60. Anderson RB, Rosenblith JF. Light sensitivity in the neonate: a preliminary report. Biol Neonate 1964; 7:83.

61. Anderson-Huntington RB, Rosenblith JF. Reports on newborns with questionable light sensitivity. Biol Neonate 1972; 20:81.

62. Als H, Tronick E, Adamson L, Brazelton TB. The behavior of the full-term yet underweight newborn. Dev Med Child Neurol 1976; 18:590.

63. Lester BM, Zeskind PS. Brazelton scale and physical size correlates of neonatal cry features. Infant Behav Dev 1979; 4:393.

64. Sepkoski C, Garcia-Coll C, Lester BM. The cumulative effect of obstetric risk variables on newborn behavior. In: Lipsitt LT, Field TM, eds. Infant behavior and development: perinatal risk and newborn behavior. Norwood, New Jersey: ABLEX, 1982.

65. Telzrow RW, Snyder DM, Tronick E, et al. The behavior of jaundiced infants undergoing phototherapy. Dev Med Child Neurol 1980; 22:317.

66. Nelson CA, Horowitz FD. The short-term behavioral sequelae of neonatal jaundice treated with phototherapy. Infant Behav Dev 1982; 5:289.

67. Yogman MW, Cole P, Als H, Lester BM. Behavior of newborns of diabetic mothers. Infant Behav Dev 1982; 5:331.

68. Thompson RJ, Cappelman MW, Zeitschel KA. Neonatal behavior of infants of adolescent mothers. Dev Med Child Neurol 1979; 21:474.

69. Standley K, Soule AB, Copans SA, Duchowny MS. Local-regional anesthesia during childbirth: effect on newborn behavior. Science 1974; 186:634.

70. Horowitz FD, Ashton J, Culp RE, et al. The effect of obstetric medication on the behavior of Israeli newborns and some comparisons with American and Uruguayan infants. Child Dev 1977; 48:1607.

71. Kuhnert BR, Harrison MJ, Linn PL, Kuhnert PM. Effects of maternal epidural anesthesia on neonatal behavior. Anesth Analg 1984; 63:301.

72. Soule AB, Standley K, Copans SA, Davis M. Clinical uses of the Brazelton neonatal scale. Pediatrics 1974; 54:583.

73. Kaplan SL, Kron RE, Litt M, et al. Correlations between scores of the Brazelton neonatal assessment scale, measures of newborn sucking behavior, and birthweight in infants born to narcotic addicted mothers. In: Ellis NR, ed. Aberrant development in infancy: human and animal studies. Vol 8. Hillsdale, New Jersey: Erlbaum, 1975.

74. Chasnoff IJ, Hatcher R, Burns WJ. Polydrug-and methadone-addicted newborns: a continuum of impairment? Pediatrics 1982; 70:210.

75. Streissguth AP, Barr HM, Martin DC. Maternal alcohol use and neonatal habituation assessed with the Brazelton scale. Child Dev 1983; 54:1109.

76. Freedman EG, Freedman N. Behavioral differences between Chinese-American and European-American newborns. Nature 1969; 224:1127.

77. Brazelton TB, Tronick E, Lechtig A, et al. The behavior of nutritionally deprived Guatemalan infants. Dev Med Child Neurol 1977; 19:364.

78. Garcia-Coll CT, Sepkoski C, Lester BM. Cultural and biomedical correlates of neonatal behavior. Dev Psychobiol 1981; 14:147.

79. Dixon S, Keefer C, Tronick E, Brazelton TB. Perinatal circumstances and newborn outcome among the Gusii of Kenya: assessment of risk. Infant Behav Dev 1982; 5:11.

80. Sostek AM, Anders T. Relationships among the Brazelton neonatal scale, Bayley infant scales and early temperament. Child Dev 1977; 48:320.

81. Vaughn BE, Taraldson B, Crichton L, Egeland B. Relationships between neonatal behavioral organizations and infant behavior during the first year of life. Infant Behav Dev 1980; 3:47.

82. Lester BM. Data analysis and prediction. In: Brazelton TB, ed. Neonatal behavioral assessment scale. 2nd ed. Philadelphia: JB Lippincott, 1984.

83. Anderson C, Savin DB. Enhancing responsiveness in mother-infant interaction. Infant Behav Dev 1983; 6:361.

84. Liptak GS, Keller BB, Feldman AW, Chamberlain RW. Enhancing infant development in parent practitioner interaction with the Brazelton neonatal assessment scale. Pediatrics 1983; 72:71.

85. Myers BJ. Early intervention using Brazelton training with middle-class mothers and fathers of newborns. Child Dev 1982; 53:462.

86. Widmayer SM, Fields TM. Effects of Brazelton demonstration on early interactions of preterm infants and their teenage mothers. Infant Behav Dev 1980; 3:79.

87. Brazelton TB, Nugent JK, Lester BM. Neonatal behavioral assessment scale. In: Osofsky JD. Handbook of infant development. New York: John Wiley & Son, 1987:780.

88. Horowitz FD, Sullivan JW, Linn P. Stability and instability in the newborn infant: the quest for illusive threads. In: Samaroff AJ, ed. Organization and stability of newborn behavior: a commentary on the Brazelton neonatal behavioral assessment scale. Monogr Soc Res Child Dev 1978; 43:29.

89. Ferrari F, Grosoli MV, Fontane G, Cavazutti GB. Neurobehavioral comparison of low-risk preterm and full-term infants at term conceptional age. Dev Med Child Neurol 1983; 25:450.

90. Paludetto R, Mansi P, Rinaldi T, et al. Behavior of preterm newborns reaching term without any serious disorder. Early Hum Dev 1982; 6:357.

91. Palmer PG, Dubowitz LMS, Verghote M, Dubowitz V. Neurological and neurobehavioral differences between preterm infants at term and full-term newborn infants. Neuropediatrics 1982; 13:183.

92. Samaroff AJ, Seifer R, Barochas R, et al. Intelligence quotient scores of 4-year-old children: social-environmental risk factors. Pediatrics 1987; 79:343.

93. Escalona SK. Babies at double hazard: early development of infants at biologic and social risk. Pediatrics 1982; 70:670.

94. Beckwith L, Cohen SE. Home environment and cognitive competence in preterm children during the first five years. In: Gottfried A, ed. Home environment and early cognitive development. New York: Academic Press, 1984:235.

95. Broman SH, Nichols PL, Kennedy WA. Preschool IQ: prenatal and early development correlates. Hillsdale, NJ: Erlbaum, 1975.

96. Bayley N. Manual for the Bayley scales of infant development. New York: Psychological Corporation, 1969.

97. Korner AF, Schneider P, Forrest T. Effects of vestibular-proprioceptive stimulation on the neurobehavioral development of preterm infants: a pilot study. Neuropediatrics 1983; 14:170.

98. Korner AF. Preventive intervention with high-risk newborns: theoretical, conceptual and methodological perspectives. In: Osofsky JD, ed. Handbook for infant development. 2nd ed. New York: Wiley-Interscience, 1987:1066.

99. Korner AF, Thom VA, Forrest T. Neurobehavioral maturity assessment for preterm infants (NB-MAP): a manual of instructions. 1986 revision, unpublished.

100. Korner AF, Thom VA, Forrest T. Demonstration videotape. Neurobehavioral maturity assessment of preterm infants (NB-MAP), 1986 revision.

101. Korner AF. State as a variable, as obstacle, and as mediator of stimulation in infant research. Merrill-Palmer Q 1972; 18:77.

102. Korner AF, Brown BW Jr, Reade EP, et al. State behavior of preterm infants as a function of development, individual and sex differences. Infant Behav Dev 1988; 111:111.

103. Korner AF, Brown BW Jr. Dimiceli S, et al. Stable individual differences in developmentally changing preterm infants: a replicated study. Child Dev, in press.

104. Bayley N. Development of mental abilities. In: Mussen PH, ed. Carmichael's manual of child psychology. Vol. 1. New York: Wiley, 1970:1163.

105. Lewis M, McGurk H. Evaluation of infant intelligence scores true or false. Science 1972; 179:1174.

20

The Medicolegal Imperative: Placental Pathology and Epidemiology

Geoffrey Altshuler, M.B., B.S., M.D. and Allen A. Herman, M.B., Ch.B., Ph.D.

Placental Use Within the Legal Imperative
Logistics of Placental Triage
Clinical Indications for Placental Examination
Examination Techniques
The Status of Placental Pathology Texts
Rationale for a Focused Approach to the
    Clinicopathic Significance of Placental
    Abnormalities
A Lexicon of Placental Abnormalities
    Noninfectious Lesions
      Acute Meconium Staining
      Chronic Meconium Staining
        Caveats in Regard to Meconium Staining
      Lesions of Reduced Placental Perfusion
        Acute Placental Ischemia
        Chronic Placental Ischemia
        Acute Infarcts
        Chronic Infarcts
        Caveat in Regard to Placental Ischemia
      Nucleated Red Blood Cells
      Intimal Cushions
      Fetal Thrombosis
      Avascular Villi
      Chorangiosis
      Intravillous Hemorrhage
      Hydrops
      Dysmaturity
      Amnion Nodosum
    Infectious Lesions
      Membranitis
      Chorioamnionitis
      Perivillositis
      Villitis
        Villitis of Unknown Etiology
        Basal Villitis

Introduction to Epidemiologic Concepts
    Epidemiologic Methods
      The Cohort Study
      The Case Control Study
    The Importance of Pathogenic Concepts to
      Epidemiologic Methods
      Caveat in Regard to Epidemiologic Study
        of Placental Findings
      Placental Factors in Studies of Perinatal Asphyxia
    Methods of a Study
      The Population Studied
      Method of Placental Scoring
      Univariate Analysis
      The Epidemiologic Model for Logistic Regression
        Analysis
      Complementary Additions to the Logistic
        Regression Analysis
      The "Chronic" Model
      The "Acute" Model
Discussion

In high risk perinatal medicine the placenta is an important surgical pathology specimen. It is an objective diary, related to the outcome of pregnancy. Placental findings often reveal evidence of fetal disease and negative outcome that is unrelated to clinical management. A survey of the American College of Obstetricians and Gynecologists reveals that 73 percent of its Fellows have been sued at least once in their careers.[1] In this chapter we discuss the importance of the placenta in regard to the legal imperative. Attorneys and insurance companies realize that placental findings may strongly affect judgments against physicians. They now encourage obstetricians and pediatricians to have placentas examined by pathologists, according to the principles indicated in the present chapter.

PLACENTAL USE WITHIN THE LEGAL IMPERATIVE

Comprehensive gross and light microscopic placental examinations should not be performed when normal newborns are born after normal pregnancies and deliveries. This does not preclude a nurse practitioner or pathology technician from completing a placental checklist, for all deliveries; an example is illustrated in Figure 20–1. For additional archival purposes, representative tissues from all placentas can be processed inexpensively with an automatic tissue processor. The prepared paraffin blocks can be stored conveniently for many years. If they are needed for a lawsuit, even a long time thereafter, they can be processed into light microscopic slides. In many cases findings in placental examinations can prevent loss of litigation. The cost of placental archives is therefore justifiable.

LOGISTICS OF PLACENTAL TRIAGE

If placentas are not immediately archived, they should be stored promptly at 4°C. In many hospitals placentas are stored in freezers. It is difficult to document changes of meconium in frozen placentas, and when subsequent light microscopic examination is carried out, the villi are found to have severe artifacts.

ID number					_____	
Date of birth					_____	
Length of cord (cm)						
Diameter of cord (cm)						
Cord insertion	Centr.	Eccen.	Margl.	Velam.		
Number of vessels					_____	
True knot in cord				Yes	No	
Insertion of membranes						
	Marginal	Circummarginate	Circumvallate			
Color of fetal surface	Blue-gray	Green	Other			
Subchorionic fibrin						
A. Patchy	Diffuse					
B. Slight	Moderate	Severe				
Amnion nodosum				Yes	No	
Cysts				Yes	No	
Placenta proper						
A. Complete				Yes	No	
B. Succenturiate				Yes	No	
C. Bipartite				Yes	No	
Hemorrhage				Yes	No	
Trimmed weight (gm)						
Dimensions						
A. Length (largest diameter, cm)						
B. Width (smallest diameter, cm)						
C. Thickness (depth, cm)						

Figure 20–1   Gross Placental Examination Form

We disagree with Naeye's claim that refrigeration causes troublesome artifacts.[2] On the other hand, storage in formalin causes artifactual distention of blood vessels. This obscures opportunity to evaluate causes of true placental vascular dilatation, e.g., fetal heart failure, umbilical cord obstruction, and rare intrathoracic or other fetal masses that obstruct placental venous return. Those placental findings are important; they represent detrimental fetal situations that often are not clinically recognizable.

With regard to microbiologic tests, we have found that refrigeration at 4°C is an appropriate means of storage. Nonspecific contamination does not occur even when specimens are submitted for culture on the fourth postnatal day. Refrigeration enhances the chances of isolating *Listeria Monocytogenes*.

CLINICAL INDICATIONS FOR PLACENTAL EXAMINATION

The following are circumstances in which there is a great likelihood of associated placental abnormalities: recurrent reproductive failure (a maternal history of stillbirth, spontaneous abortion, or prematurity in one or more pregnancy), diabetes, dysmorphia, dysmaturity, erythroblastosis, multiple births, and meconium staining. Naeye[2] has advocated that all grossly abnormal placentas should be examined. Most of those placentas are not associated with abnormalities in the associated newborns. It thus seems to be very unreasonable to charge a parent for such an examination.

EXAMINATION TECHNIQUES

Methods of placental examination have been established by Benirschke.[3] For standard surgical pathology use, buffered formalin is recommended.[4] Formalin is convenient, and unlike Bouin's fixative, it can be used for long-term storage. An additional disadvantage of Bouin's fixative is that it obscures light microscopic identification of bacteria.[5]

Many pathologists restrict placental samples to three paraffin embedded blocks. To optimize the diagnosis of placental dysmaturity and villitis, representative tissues should include placental tissue near the umbilical cord insertion site, two sections of placenta from nonmarginal superficial placental sites, and two sections of nonmarginal placenta with the maternal floor. A segment of umbilical cord and membrane roll should also be processed. Within the aforementioned tissues there should be no more than one lateral part of the placenta. Because of nonspecific degenerative changes, appearances in that part may confuse pathologists who are unfamiliar with placentas. Samples of grossly obvious lesions should always be processed.

THE STATUS OF PLACENTAL PATHOLOGY TEXTS

Benirschke and Driscoll's tome remains the landmark against which textbooks of placental pathology must be judged.[6] Those authors have provided major information regarding placental lesions and the outcome of associated neonates.

Fox[7] has written a readable textbook, but some of his statements are incorrect and provocative. For example, on page 248: "Histological examination of the placenta of a macerated fetus is of no value whatsoever."

Perrin[8] has edited an excellent monograph of placental pathology; it is comprehensive and has a good bibliography.

Naeye and Tafari[9] have incorporated much data into a textbook of pregnancy risk factors. They have strongly asserted that chorioamnionitis is caused by infection and that it causes prematurity, morbidity, and mortality. This important concept was pioneered by Benirschke[10] and Blanc[11] many years ago.

RATIONALE FOR A FOCUSED APPROACH TO THE CLINICOPATHOLOGIC SIGNIFICANCE OF PLACENTAL ABNORMALITIES

In innumerable articles there is documentation of the relationship between abnormal placentas and negative outcomes in associated newborns; the Collaborative Perinatal Study provides the best example.[12] Causes of perinatal morbidity and mortality, however, frequently remain a mystery.[13] Our approach to the epidemiologic investigation of fetal disease is to categorize individual placental abnormalities into pathogenetic groups. Singly or in combination, these placental factors may be associated with pregnancy failure.

A LEXICON OF PLACENTAL ABNORMALITIES

Many physicians who care for the fetus and newborn are unaware that the placenta is a clinically important specimen. To simplify the pathology of the placenta, the following information is provided.

Noninfectious Lesions

Acute Meconium Staining

Discharge of fetal intestinal content initially produces a bright green, slimy change across the placenta and its membranes. At light microscopic examination one sees acute necrosis of the amniotic epithelium. When this is unaccompanied by reparative or degenerative epithelial changes and when there is no meconium within macrophages of the subamniotic connective tissue, the typical clinical history is that the meconium discharge occurred less than two hours prior to delivery.

Chronic Meconium Staining

After meconium has been present across its surface for a couple of hours, a placenta develops a brown-green color. At light microscopic examination one sees meconium-laden macrophages within the membranes, the placental subamniotic connective tissue, and the umbilical cord. The longer the period of time between meconium discharge and fetal delivery, the more brown the placenta becomes. Light microscopic examination then shows numerous, deeply located meconium-laden macrophages across the placental chorion and within the umbilical cord. The following caveats have important medicolegal implications.

Caveats in Regard to Meconium Staining.

1. Empiric knowledge is the only means by which a placental pathologist can estimate meconium discharge.

2. Intrapartum discharge of meconium generally is regarded as being of no clinical significance if the meconium is removed from the newborn's oropharynx immediately after the head is delivered. Although this is usually true, exceptions may occur. The causes that lead the fetus to discharge the meconium may have more impact on the outcome of the newborn than the meconium itself.

3. Pathologic findings in chronic meconium discharge necessitate caution in the interpretation of meconium effects. One of us (G.A.) has performed three autopsies in which there had been a history of meconium discharge that occurred more than three hours prior to delivery. The associated placentas had typical features of chronic meconium staining. The neonates had expired only a few hours after delivery. Their lungs did not have any signs of meconium aspiration. All this is understandable when one recalls that a fetus may cease breathing in circumstances of chronic fetal disease.[14]

4. Meconium discharge commonly occurs as a result of fetal distress, but it does not invariably produce perinatal asphyxia. There are many instances of acutely and chronically acquired fetal asphyxia that are unaccompanied by meconium discharge. Alternately, as we show later in this chapter, acute meconium staining is significantly associated with postnatal asphyxia.

5. Miller and colleagues[15] studied the effects of meconium on epithelium within a sterile in vitro system. The changes resembled those of delivered meconium-stained placentas. The time sequence of the in vivo changes cannot be assumed to be the same as that of the

experimental model. Many mothers who experience meconium discharge additionally have cervicitis and chorioamnionitis. Meconium by itself does not produce inflammation.[16] When infection is present, however, meconium produces severe chorioamnionitis. Temporal changes of amniotic epithelium and meconium-laden macrophages cannot then be interpreted reliably.

6. Despite the foregoing reservations, a pathologist often can determine whether there has been an episode of meconium discharge within or beyond two hours of delivery.

Lesions of Reduced Placental Perfusion

In pathophysiologic states and with decidual arteriopathy, there may be a substantial reduction in uteroplacental blood flow. A common example of the former is severe abuse of cigarettes. A common example of the latter is pregnancy-induced hypertension. Singly or in combination, four placental changes accompany the aforementioned circumstances: acute ischemia, chronic ischemia, acute infarction, and chronic infarction. We often have seen these changes associated with fetal hypoxia and acidosis.

Acute Placental Ischemia. The placental changes that result from acute deprivation of placental blood flow are often not recognizable by the naked eye. Characteristic light microscopic features of reduced placental perfusion include contracted villi and increased numbers of syncytiotrophoblastic knots (Fig. 20–2).

Chronic Placental Ischemia. Chronic reduction of uteroplacental blood flow is commonly accompanied by the proliferation of placental X cells throughout villi that are entrapped by fibrin (Fig. 20–3).

Acute Infarcts. Sometimes, when placentas are focally deeply congested in appearance, they have light microscopic features of acute infarction. Acute placental infarcts are often not grossly recognizable.

Chronic Infarcts. When placentas have grossly obvious gray-tan infarcts, the light microscopic findings resemble the changes of chronic ischemia already described.

Caveat in Regard to Placental Ischemia. Because exceptional cases occur, there can be no absolute correlation between placental ischemia and perinatal morbidity or mortality. In a situation of 15 years' clinical follow-up, an 80 percent incidence of placental ischemia and infarction has been seen (by G.A.) to be unaccompanied by psychomotor or other negative outcomes. Urinary estriol studies and placental glycoprotein immunohistochemical markers are indirect measures of placentofetal reserve;[17,18] they are not absolute determinants of fetal outcome.

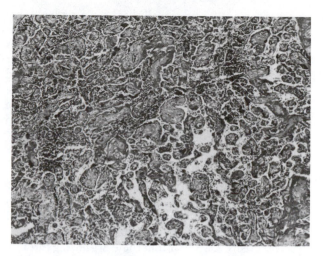

Figure 20-2   Acute placental ischemia. The villi are contracted, and there are numerous syncytiotrophoblastic knots. (Original magnification 50X.)

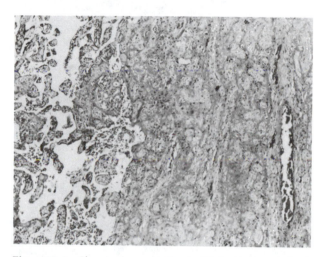

Figure 20-3   Chronic placental ischemia. Fibrinoid change is dominant across the right aspect of this illustration. The X cells in this particular picture have nuclei that look granular; they are prominent at the central part of the picture. (Original magnification 50X.)

Nucleated Red Blood Cells

Interpretation of cellular detail in light microscopic slides depends on tissue fixation. When placentas are at room temperature for many hours, their autolytic stromal cells condense and resemble nucleated red blood cells. Proper storage of placentas at 4°C prevents that artifact and makes possible accurate light microscopic determination of fetal nucleated red blood cells. The nuclei of these cells have a typical light microscopic appearance (Fig. 20–4). They are smaller than mononuclear leukocytes. The ratio of nucleated red blood cells to leukocytes in fetal placental blood vessels is always pathologic when it exceeds 1:1.5. In severe disease, erythroblasts accompany nucleated red blood cells. The cause of these cells traditionally has been described as Rh or similar disease. We therefore must now emphasize that prophylactic treatment against Rh disease has almost eradicated immunohemolytic disease and that nowadays the typical cause of placental nucleated red blood cells is idiopathic chronic fetal hypoxia. We have found an 85 percent concordance of nucleated red blood cells in fetal placental blood vessels with nucleated red cell counts in postdelivery peripheral blood specimens.

Intimal Cushions

In clinical situations of fetal hypoxia and acidosis, we frequently have seen lamination of fibrin along the endothelial surface of the umbilical cord and fetal placental veins. De Sa[19] found these organizing thrombi to be associated with emboli and thrombi in other organs (Fig. 20–5).

Fetal Thrombosis

Thrombotic lesions in fetal placental blood vessels commonly are associated with spontaneous abortion and with stillbirth.[20] All phases of thrombosis are seen, including fibrin deposition and recanalization. Classic studies of intravascular coagulation indicate the commonest causes of these lesions to be hypoxia, acidosis, and infection (Fig. 20–6).[21]

Avascular Villi

The ultimate consequence of a deficient blood supply to a fetal placental terminal villus is that it will develop avascularity. These lesions commonly are associated with organized fetal placental thrombi and with uteroplacental vasculopathy (Fig. 20–7).

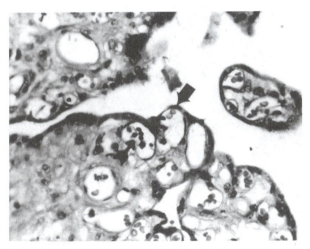

Figure 20-4 Fetal nucleated red blood cells. Note the size of these cells at the lower left arrow, in comparison with the size of the mature red blood cells at the upper right arrow. (Original magnification 300×.)

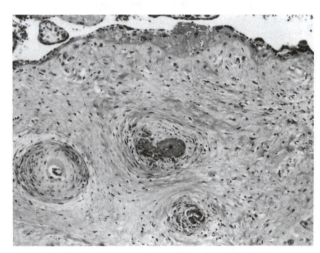

Figure 20-6 Fibrin thrombus in central blood vessel. (Original magnification 120×.)

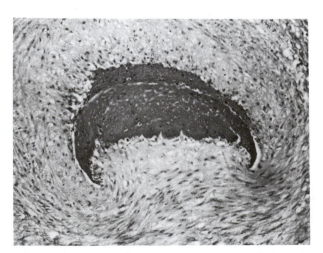

Figure 20-5 Fetal placental vascular intimal cushion. This picture shows an arc of fibrin beneath numerous tightly packed red blood cells. (Original magnification 120×.)

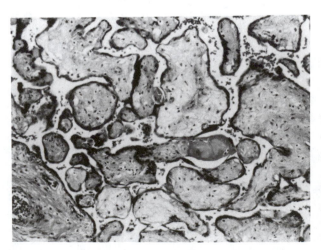

Figure 20-7 Avascular villi. Only the villus at the lower left has a blood vessel. (Original magnification 120×.)

Chorangiosis

Abnormalities of numerically increased capillaries within placental villi have been seen for many years.[22] A few years ago a convenient definition was provided.[23] There should be at least 10 different light microscopic areas in 10 different placental areas, with 10 villi that have 10 capillary lumens in each villus. The vessels may be present in more than one plane of section. Chorangiosis is different from congestion, in which the vasculature is numerically normal. The excessive vascularity of chorangiosis may be masked by edema of high output fetal cardiac failure (Fig. 20–8). Chorangiosis never occurs in normal pregnancies and deliveries. It has been reported to be present in the placentas of 5 percent of the neonates in an intensive care unit.[23] Its great importance is that more than 25 percent of those neonates either die or have congenital anomalies. Not uncommonly chorangiosis occurs in placentas that have villitis (Fig. 20–9). Because of its frequent occurrence with pre-eclampsia and diabetes, we speculate that chorangiosis involves chronic low grade hypoxia resulting from uteroplacental vasculopathy and uteroplacental insufficiency.

Intravillous Hemorrhage

In many pathology textbooks and articles, hemorrhagic lesions have been described as resulting from hypoxia. In the placental villus the cause of this includes damage to the endothelium of delicate capillaries.

Hydrops

Placental edema is accurately identifiable only when it is accompanied by water-laden stromal cells. Variable concentrations of alcohol used in tissue processing cause variable degrees of tissue shrinkage. Because of this, the degree of placental edema cannot be judged by the size of the villi. Causes of placental hydrops include fetal heart failure, immunohemolytic anemia, and chronic intrauterine infection (especially from cytomegalovirus).

Dysmaturity

Throughout gestation, placental villi become smaller, and their trophoblastic surface features syncytiotrophoblast with occasional cellular knots. Third trimester placentas that have large villi with numerous stromal cells, a lack of syncytiotrophoblast, and syncytiotrophoblastic knots are pathologic (Fig. 20–10). The cause of this abnormal development is usually not apparent. Examples of placental dysmaturity are chorangiosis, diabetes, and immunohemolytic anemia.

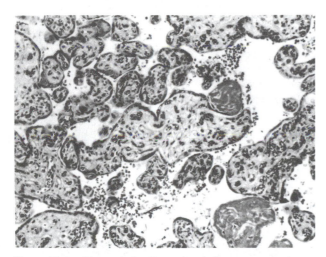

Figure 20–8 Chorangiosis. Clear colored edema or stroma is seen about the numerous capillaries in these villi. (Original magnification 120×.)

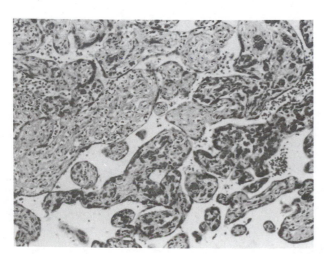

Figure 20–9 Proliferative villitis (at left) and chorangiosis (at right). (Original magnification 70×.)

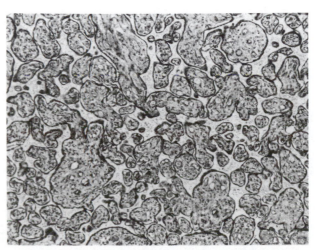

Figure 20–10 Diffuse dysmaturity of placental villi. Compare the large size of these villi and the almost total lack of syncytiotrophoblastic knots with the ischemic changes shown in Figure 20–2. (Original magnification 50×.)

Amnion Nodosum

Lesions of conglutinated squames and vernix of fetal skin have long been known as amnion nodosum. Causes have been recognized as chronic leakage of amniotic fluid and nonfunctioning fetal kidneys (absent or dysplastic kidneys). Because of resultant lung compression, the fetal lung may not develop and it becomes hypoplastic. Diffuse epithelial degeneration with foci of amniotic squamous balls often accompany amnion nodosum. On rare occasions they may occur unaccompanied by amnion nodosum. These changes have recently been described as being associated with fetal lung hypoplasia.[24]

Infectious Lesions

Membranitis

Acute and chronic inflammation of the extraplacental membranes is called membranitis. Exudative patterns are typically present with bacteria, *Mycoplasma* and *Chlamydia*. Focal necrotizing lesions are signs of cytomegalovirus and herpes simplex virus infection.

Chorioamnionitis

Emigration of fetal leukocytes from the chorionic vessels to the amniotic surface is called chorioamnionitis. This inflammation invariably is associated with membranitis and often is associated with umbilical cord vasculitis and funisitis (inflammation within the umbilical cord). When infectious antigens penetrate into the amniotic cavity, they chemotactically attract fetal leukocytes. This is the pathogenetic mechanism by which umbilical cord vasculitis and funisitis can occur with chorioamnionitis. Each of these inflammatory lesions results from infection that ascends from the cervix.

Perivillositis

Intervillositis and perivillositis are indicators of blood-borne infection. These are terms of convenience and are almost interchangeable. When the inflammation is dominant within the maternal sinusoids, the first term is more appropriate. When the inflammation is concentrated about villous tissue, the term perivillositis is preferred.

Villitis

Inflammation of the villi has the same connotation as inflammation elsewhere (Figs. 20–9, 20–11). Acute inflammation features exudative or necrotizing changes with polymorphonuclear leukocytes. The lymphocytic, plasmacytic, and lymphohistiocytic forms of villitis are characteristic of chronic infection. Several patterns of inflammation may be present within the single chronically inflamed placenta, including necrotizing villitis. A relatively monomorphous proliferation of histiocytes within villi warrants the term "granulomatous." Many organisms are known to produce granulomatous lymphadenopathy; usually, however, the specific cause is not identified. This is also true for granulomatous villitis.

Villitis of Unknown Etiology. There are characteristic or pathognomonic features associated with several infectious causes of placental villitis.[25] Villitis of unknown etiology denotes that the causative infection is neither clinically nor pathologically apparent.[26] Sander[27] has claimed that hemorrhagic endovasculitis is a unique vascular lesion. In fact, 75 percent of his initially reported cases occurred with villitis of unknown etiology.[27] It is therefore preferable to recognize hemorrhagic endovasculitis as one of several patterns of villitis of unknown etiology that can be present simultaneously with other inflammatory patterns. Moreover, with spontaneous abortions and stillbirths, hemorrhagic endovasculitis commonly appears in thrombotic lesions that lack inflammatory cells (Figs. 20–12, 20–13). Sander et al[28] have acknowledged that "intravascular coagulation may be basic to the entire process."

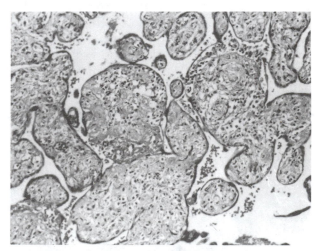

Figure 20–11   Proliferative villitis and developing fibrinoid necrosis in the villus toward the upper left. (Original magnification 120×.)

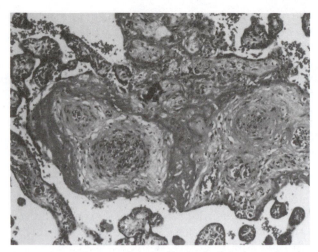

Figure 20-12 Precursor lesions of hemorrhagic endovasculopathy. Note the fine granular appearance of the damaged red blood cells in the obliterated fetal villous blood vessels. (Original magnification 120×.)

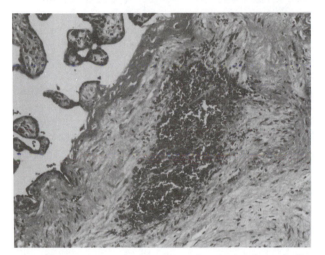

Figure 20-13 Hemorrhagic endovasculopathy in placental villus. (Original magnification 120×.)

Basal Villitis. Lymphocytic cells are often present within the decidua of the placental membranes and the placental floor. We assume that this correlates with the prevalence of infection in the lower genital tract of pregnant mothers. Basal villitis implies that there are many chronic inflammatory cells and that the inflammation has spread to involve contiguous villi.

INTRODUCTION TO EPIDEMIOLOGIC CONCEPTS

The placenta is frequently neglected in epidemiologic studies. It has a wide range of responses to pathologic processes and thus has the potential for clarifying causal pathways of perinatal risk factors. Epidemiologists now realize that findings of placental analysis augment conventional studies of exposure-disease relationships.[29] There are three commonly used, basic types of epidemiologic studies: clinical trials, cohort studies, and case control studies. Since placental factors are not easily amenable to experimental manipulation, we will not discuss clinical trials.

Epidemiologic Methods

The Cohort Study

In a cohort study the investigators identify two or more groups of pregnant women at various levels of risk of poor perinatal outcome. These cohorts are defined at a common point of entry to observation. This usually occurs at the first prenatal visit.[30] The women are followed to the end of pregnancy or to another endpoint of concern. The numbers of poor outcomes are counted. The direction of the inquiry or investigation is from cause to effect.

The Collaborative Perinatal Project is a good example of a cohort study.[12] Between 1959 and 1966, data relating to sociodemographic, prenatal, and intrapartum risk factors were collected from 53,518 pregnancies in 12 regionally different United States medical centers. A number of investigators have used these data to examine the relationship between various risk factors and poor perinatal outcome. Examples include perinatal hypoxia and cerebral palsy, coitus and chorioamnionitis, and coitus with perinatal morbidity and mortality.[31-33].

In a cohort study we measure the frequency with which poor outcomes occur at a given point in time (the incidence). The contrast in incidence between exposed and nonexposed cohorts forms the basis of the measure of association. The relative risk is the ratio of the incidence in the exposed group relative to the incidence in the unexposed group (relative risk = I_E/I_U). These considerations are illustrated in Table 20–1. Exposed (or at-risk) women who have poor pregnancy outcome are represented by "a," those with good outcome are designated "b," the nonexposed (low risk) women who have poor outcome are designated "c," and "d" designates the nonexposed women with good pregnancy outcome. The risk of a poor perinatal outcome in the exposed women is given by the incidence (a/a + b) of poor outcome in the exposed women. This risk is divided by the incidence (c/c + d) of poor outcome among unexposed women to give the relative risk. The relative risk is a measure of the association between exposure and outcome.

The incidences of poor pregnancy outcome are usually relatively small. Thus, in a perinatal cohort study a large population is required to demonstrate a given effect. This number can be reduced by a historical cohort study. This is easy to construct when pregnancy data are available. It obviates the need to follow the women in real time. Although a historical cohort study uses previously collected data, it has the same prospective or forward direction of inquiry as a classic cohort study.

TABLE 20–1   A Fourfold Table of a Cohort Study

	Poor Perinatal Outcome	
	Present	Absent
Exposed	a	b
Not exposed	c	d
	Direction of inquiry	

Confounding influences associated with risk factors and outcome commonly occur in exposed and nonexposed women.[34] Randomization of cases chosen for clinical trials theoretically removes confounders, because it ensures similarity of the study groups. In both cohort and case control studies, however, confounders can cause substantial errors in regard to data and conclusions. The concept of confounders is important; it is discussed in the next section of this chapter.

The Case Control Study

When investigators perform perinatal case control studies, they gather "cases" of babies with poor outcomes and "controls" of babies who are well. Both groups of mothers are then questioned about their exposure to specific risk factors. Their perinatal records are examined. The direction of the inquiry is backward, i.e., from effect to cause.

In a case control study the relative risk cannot be calculated precisely. That consideration pertains because the incidence of poor outcomes in the unexposed population is incompletely known. The precise incidence of the factor to be studied in the unexposed population depends on knowledge of the relative frequency of that factor in the total population from which the control group was selected. However, if poor pregnancy outcome is uncommon (less than 10 percent in the population exposed to the risk factor), and if cases and controls are selected from the same population, the odds ratio is a close estimate of the relative risk.

A schematic demonstration of the case control study is shown in Table 20–2. In that table, "a" represents poor pregnancy outcome within the exposed (at-risk) group, "b" is the exposed group free of poor outcome, "c" is the nonexposed group who have a poor outcome, and "d" is the group free of risk and poor

TABLE 20–2   A Fourfold Table of a Case Control Study

	Poor Pregnancy Outcome	
	Present	Absent
Exposed	a	b
Not exposed	c	d
	Direction of inquiry	

outcome. The odds ratio is given by ad/bc and represents the odds that a poor pregnancy outcome will occur in women exposed to a specific risk factor.

Case control studies are common because they provide a practical and easy method for studying rare diseases. The ease of computerized execution of the case control study can result in misleading findings. To reach a reliable conclusion about causality, on the basis of case control studies, requires care in the analysis and interpretation of data.

The troublesome problem of confounding is central to both cohort and case control studies. A simple illustration of this is demonstrated in Table 20–3. The exposure variable, the disease variable, and the confounder are dichotomous variables. Each is either present or absent (see Table 20–3). The relative risk, calculated according to whether the confounder is present or absent, is substantially different from the crude relative risk. Those risks, in Table 20–3, are, respectively, 1.02, 1.86, and 4.00.

When there is confounding in a data set, the Mantel-Haenszel procedure can be used to compensate for that issue. The Mantel-Haenszel procedure provides a summary relative risk, which adjusts for the effect of the confounder.[35] In Table 20–3, whereas the crude relative risk is 4.00, the Mantel-Haenszel adjusted relative risk is 1.13. At a more sophisticated level a multivariate statistical procedure can be used to adjust for confounding. Linear logistic regression analysis is an example of this.[36] Logistic regression computer packages are commercially available and can be implemented with ease.[37,38]

The Importance of Pathogenetic Concepts to Epidemiologic Methods

In epidemiologic studies of placental findings and fetal outcome, it is important to use statistical models that are based on pathogenetic principles. Univariate analysis usually shows a strong association between chorioamnionitis and complications of prematurity, because chorioamnionitis causes premature onset of labor. The reason that umbilical cord vasculitis and funi-

TABLE 20–3   An Example of Confounding in a Cohort Study

	Confounder					
	Present		Absent			
	Poor Outcome		Poor Outcome		Poor Outcome	
	Present	Absent	Present	Absent	Present	Absent
Exposed	194	706	6	94	200	800
Not exposed	21	79	29	871	50	950
	Relative risk = 1.02		Relative risk = 1.86		Relative risk = 4.00	
					Mantel-Haenszel relative risk = 1.13	

sitis similarly relate to fetal outcome is that, together with chorioamnionitis, they result from ascending intra-uterine infection.

Logistic regression analysis takes interacting or dependent considerations into account. It identifies factors that are independently significant. The number of factors that are significant depends on the manner in which the statistical model is constructed. When pathogenetically unrelated placental lesions are entered into a logistic regression analysis, a smaller number of significant findings is identified than when a smaller number of pathogenetically related factors is submitted to logistic regression study.

With analyses in which unrelated pathologic factors are processed, the computer program causes a loss of true relationships and removes important risk factors from the data set. The factors are lost because of the frequency with which they occur. For example, if two risk factors occur relatively frequently in the same data set, they often are identified with one another and are jointly removed. This consideration ultimately affects the study population at large.

Caveat in Regard to Epidemiologic Study of Placental Findings

The use of pathogenetic principles in the construction of epidemiologic investigation is the optimal means by which causality can be determined from pathologic abnormalities.

Placental Factors in Studies of Perinatal Asphyxia

Innumerable investigators have studied relationships of various obstetrical and neonatal risks to various outcomes of pregnancy. Throughout the last few years there have been an enormous number of litigations in behalf of patients who have suffered cerebral palsy and other afflictions. Epidemiologic investigations of placental lesions, their pathogenesis, and their associations have been numerically lacking. In the context of the present legal imperative, our attention focuses on perinatal asphyxia as the outcome variable of placental lesions that are indicative of hypoxic phenomena.

Methods of a Study

Population Studied

All 892 of the patients had been hospitalized in the neonatal intensive care unit of the Oklahoma Children's Memorial Hospital. They had been delivered at the adjacent Oklahoma Memorial Hospital or had been born at community or regional district hospitals. No information was processed as to the number of babies that were born at the respective hospitals, and we did not investigate other demographic data. The neonates were hospitalized between November 1983 and August 1987. Criteria for the diagnosis of perinatal asphyxia were selected by the attending clinicians and included at least two of the following: a history of cesarean section done because of late decelerations or other obstetrical signs of fetal distress, an Apgar score of 3 or less at the fifth postnatal minute, postnatal hypoglycemia (30 mg per deciliter or less), disseminated intravascular coagulation of the newborn, postnatal acidosis (pH 7.2 or less), and neonatal seizures within the first 24 hours after delivery. Neonates with these factors were selected as cases (n = 193); the remaining neonates were used as controls (n = 699).

Method of Placental Scoring

Our routine scores of gross and light microscopic placental lesions are made on a 0 through 3+ basis or are listed as present or absent. In the investigation reported here we recorded scores of less than (1+) to be absent and items of (1+) or more to be present. For some items we used a grading system of absent, grade 1, and grade 1+ (i.e., any score greater than 1).

Univariate Analysis

In the interest of space, we will not detail information relating to our statistical contingency tests. Let us just report that the initial approach was to evaluate the following 17 variables by univariate analysis: acute and chronic meconium staining, abruptio placentae, acute and chronic infarcts, acute and chronic ischemia, fetal thrombi, fetal vascular intimal cushions, chorangiosis, fetal nucleated red blood cells, placentomegaly, dysmaturity, hydrops, membranitis, chorioamnionitis, and villitis. The univariate association between placental factors and asphyxia was analyzed using odds ratios with 95 percent confidence intervals.[38] Acute and chronic meconium staining, abruptio placentae, acute and chronic infarcts, acute and chronic ischemia, fetal thrombi, fetal vascular intimal cushions, chorangiosis, fetal nucleated red blood cells, gestational age, and birth weight were significantly associated with perinatal asphyxia in the univariate analysis. Placental membranitis and chorioamnionitis were not significantly associated with perinatal asphyxia. This is noteworthy because membranitis and chorioamnionitis are now generally accepted as major causes of prematurity. That does not mean, however, that they are causes of asphyxia, morbidity, or mortality.

The Epidemiologic Model for Logistic Regression Analysis

We developed a case control study to explore the relationship between placentally mediated fetal hypoxic damage and neonatal asphyxia. Of all the pathologic changes described in our lexicon, we selected those listed in Table 20–4 to be the lesions that best represent the pathogenesis of fetal hypoxia.

Earlier in this chapter we emphasized the need to use pathogenetic concepts in the construction of statistical analyses. We then explained that, when this is not done, important risk factors can be lost because of their frequent occurrence with other factors in the same data set. Chorangiosis and dysmaturity evolve throughout a substantially longer period of time than do the other chronic lesions listed in Table 20–4. We hypothesize that most instances of fetal nucleated red blood cell production evolve very slowly. Lack of a priori proof of this does not negate the validity of the overall statistical model or hypothesis. In subgrouping the chronic factors in this fashion (Table 20–4), we are constructing a hypothesis for investigation; we are not making a conclusion.

Rationalization as to why some of the lesions of Table 20–4 are categorized as acute and others as chronic is not necessary for the purpose of this chapter. Suffice it to say that, in broad terms, the factors that cause these lesions are considered to evolve throughout a period of less than, or more than, 24 hours.

The acute and chronic factors listed in Table 20–4 were entered into multiple linear logistic regression analyses,[36] using the BMDP package program.[38] The factors were entered into the program by grouping them according to the following:

1. All seven acute factors were entered into the first set. This included acute ischemia, acute infarction, intravillous hemorrhage, intimal cushion, chronic meconium staining, acute meconium staining, and fetal thrombosis.

2. The chronic factors were put into the program according to three different sets. In the first set all the chronic factors were entered; these included chronic ischemia, chronic infarction, avascular villi, chorangiosis, dysmaturity, and nucleated red blood cells. The second group of chronic factors introduced into the BMDP

program was comprised of chronic ischemia, chronic infarction, and avascular villi. The third collection of chronic factors introduced into the program consisted of chorangiosis, dysmaturity, and nucleated red cells.

Complementary Additions to the Logistic Regression Analysis

Many studies of obstetrical risk factors include numerous items that depend on an interview or recall process. Examples include alcohol ingestion and cigarette use. The only clinical factors that we set as entry variables, against the clinically determined outcome of asphyxia, were gestational age, birth weight, largeness for gestational age, and smallness for gestational age.

Results of the Logistic Regression Analysis

Within "chronic" and "acute" models of placentally mediated processes studied in relation to perinatal asphyxia (Table 20–4), six factors were found to be significant: nucleated red blood cells, chronic ischemia, intimal cushions, intervillous fibrin, and acute and chronic meconium staining (Tables 20–5, 20–6).

The "Chronic" Model

Throughout the three different groupings of the six chronic factors (Table 20–4), despite the various ways in which we entered the data, the same two factors repeatedly were found to be significant. Nucleated red blood cells were a significant predictor of perinatal asphyxia in univariate (crude odds ratio [OR] = 3.97, 95 percent confidence interval [CI] = 2.3-6.8) and multivariate analysis (see Table 20–5). Chronic infarction, avascular villi, dysmaturity, and chorangiosis were found to be nonsignificant in multivariate analyses. However, as shown in Table 20–5, chorangiosis greater than 1+ was marginally significant in univariate analysis (OR = 2.02, 95 percent CI = 0.95-4.3) and in multivariate analysis (OR, adjusting for chronic ischemia, chronic infarction, avascular villi, dysmaturity, and nucleated red blood cells = 1.97, 95 percent CI = 0.9-4.3).

The "Acute" Model

The data of Table 20–6 indicate that, of the eight factors therein tested, four are significant (intimal cushions, intervillous fibrin, and acute and chronic

TABLE 20–4   Placental Signs of Potential Fetal Hypoxia

Acute Damage	Chronic Damage
Acute ischemia	Chronic ischemia
Acute infarction	Chronic infarction
Intravillous hemorrhage	Avascular villi
Intimal cushion	Chorangiosis
Chronic meconium	Dysmaturity
Acute meconium	Nucleated red blood cells
Fetal thrombosis	

TABLE 20-5   The Association Between Chronic Hypoxic Damage of the Placenta and Perinatal Asphyxia

Placental Abnormality	Controls	Cases	Crude OR	95% CI	Adjusted OR*	95% CI	Adjusted OR†	95% CI
Chronic ischemia								
Absent	650	166	1.00		1.00		1.00	
Present	49	27	2.16	1.3–3.6	1.91	1.1–3.2	1.76	1.02–3.1
Chronic infarction								
Absent	671	183	1.00		1.00		‡	
Present	28	10	1.31	0.6–2.8	0.81	0.4–1.8	‡	‡
Avascular villi								
Absent	678	183	1.00		1.00		‡	
Present	21	10	1.76	0.8–3.8	1.46	0.7–3.2	‡	‡
Chorangiosis								
Absent	629	171	1.00		1.00		‡	
Grade 1	50	11	0.81	0.4–1.6	0.77	0.4–1.5	‡	‡
Grade 1+	20	11	2.02	0.95–4.3	1.97	0.91–4.3	‡	‡
Dysmaturity								
Absent	634	172	1.00		1.00		‡	
Grade 1	50	15	1.11	0.6–2.0	1.04	0.6–1.9	‡	‡
Grade 1+	15	6	1.47	0.6–3.9	1.19	0.4–3.3	‡	‡
Nucleated red blood cells								
Absent	668	163	1.00		1.00		1.00	
Present	31	30	3.97	2.3–6.8	3.71	2.2–6.3	3.00	1.7–5.4

    * Analysis adjusted for chronic ischemia, chronic infarction, avascular villi, chorangiosis, dysmaturity, and nucleated red blood cells.
    † Analysis adjusted for chronic ischemia, intravascular hemorrhage, nucleated red blood cells, intimal cushion, chronic meconium, acute meconium, intervillous fibrin, gestational age, and birth weight small for gestational age and large for gestational age.
    ‡ Excluded from multivariate logistic regression analysis.

TABLE 20-6   The Association Between Acute Hypoxic Damage of the Placenta and Perinatal Asphyxia

Placental Abnormality	Controls	Cases	Crude OR	95% CI	Adjusted OR*	95% CI	Adjusted OR†	95% CI
Acute ischemia								
Absent	638	169	1.00		1.00		‡	
Present	61	24	1.49	0.9–2.5	1.49	0.9–2.5	‡	‡
Acute infarction								
Absent	663	179	1.00		1.00		‡	
Present	36	14	1.44	0.8–2.7	1.23	0.6–2.5	‡	‡
Intravillous hemorrhage								
Absent	678	182	1.00		1.00		1.00	
Present	21	11	1.95	0.9–4.1	1.96	0.9–4.1	1.47	0.7–3.3
Intimal cushion								
Absent	686	179	1.00		1.00		1.00	
Present	13	14	4.13	1.9–8.9	3.71	1.7–8.2	3.89	1.6–9.2
Chronic meconium								
Absent	627	149	1.00		1.00		1.00	
Present	72	44	2.57	1.7–3.9	2.67	1.8–4.1	4.25	2.5–7.2
Acute meconium								
Absent	686	182	1.00		1.00		1.00	
Present	13	11	3.19	1.4–7.2	3.44	1.5–8.0	6.05	2.4–15.1
Fetal thrombosis								
Absent	681	181	1.00		1.00		‡	
Present	18	11	2.29	1.1–4.9	0.98	0.4–2.4	‡	‡
Intervillous fibrin								
Absent	601	147	1.00		1.00		1.00	
Grade 1	81	40	2.02	1.3–3.1	2.39	1.5–3.7	1.89	1.2–3.0
Grade 1+	17	6	1.44	0.6–3.7	1.12	0.4–3.1	0.81	0.3–2.4

    * Analysis adjusted for acute ischemia, acute infarction, intravillous hemorrhage, intimal cushion, chronic meconium, acute meconium, fetal thrombosis, and intervillous fibrin.
    † Analysis adjusted for chronic ischemia, intravascular hemorrhage, nucleated red blood cells, intimal cushion, chronic meconium, acute meconium, intervillous fibrin, gestational age, and birth weight small for gestational age and large for gestational age.
    ‡ Excluded from multivariate logistic regression analysis.

meconium staining). Acute ischemia, acute infarction, intravillous hemorrhage, and fetal thrombosis were not significant (see Table 20-6). The crude OR (univariate analysis) of fetal thrombosis was significant (OR 2.29, CI 1.1-4.9). When adjustment for other factors was made, fetal thrombosis was revealed not to be significant (adjustment for acute ischemia, acute infarction, intravillous hemorrhage, intimal cushions, intervillous fibrin, and acute and chronic meconium staining produced results of OR = 0.98, CI = 0.4-2.4).

DISCUSSION

There are many obstetrical complications and abnormal laboratory or fetal monitoring findings that are important risk factors for cerebral palsy and other poor outcomes of pregnancy.[39-44] The nature of the present contribution precludes a need to review them. Although Naeye and his colleagues[9,45] have contributed to the use of the placenta in large population-based statistical studies, there has been a general failure to investigate placentas with comprehensive epidemiologic methods.

A limitation of laboratory tests and of fetal monitoring is that the findings in those examinations relate to a fixed point in time. Aside from possible problems of sensitivity, specificity, and interpretation, the result of a test carried out at a fixed point in time cannot firmly predict patient outcome. Some investigators have questioned the value of Apgar scores, the most traditional of all markers of perinatal status.[46,47]

A caveat from these considerations should be to conclude that no test or group of tests can perfectly predict patient outcome. In that context it behooves us to develop epidemiologic models from which the significance of placental lesions can be determined.

The theme of the present chapter has a three-tiered format. At the first level of consideration is the assertion that placental examinations and epidemiology are important. Next it is emphasized that hypotheses linking these two must be constructed according to pathogenetically meaningful principles. Finally, methods are provided to illustrate means by which the investigative questions could be reasonably resolved.

In this chapter we have described and discussed many lesions and considerations of placental pathology. Asphyxia is the most grievous cause of a poor pregnancy outcome and litigation. We therefore elected to pursue an epidemiologic investigation of placental lesions that are most representative of hypoxic phenomena. By logistic regression analysis, with several biologic models of data entry, we found that six placental lesions are significantly associated with perinatal asphyxia—fetal nucleated red blood cells, fetal vascular intimal cushions, chronic ischemia, intervillous fibrin, and acute and chronic meconium staining.

The significance of fetal nucleated red blood cells in regard to perinatal apshyxia may be the most important of all the foregoing findings. Examination of umbilical cord blood, taken at the time of delivery, can provide confirmatory documentation as to the numerical extent of the cells within the newborn's peripheral blood. In 1967 Fox[48] reported the relevance of nucleated red blood cells to fetal hypoxia. It is ironic that this observation has been lost in the literature. When Benirschke reviewed a draft of our present chapter, he brought Fox's article to our attention. For many years we and others had lost sight of that most important contribution. In the absence of immunohemolytic disease, placental fetal nucleated red blood cells must be interpreted as a major marker of fetal hypoxia.

Other findings of the present investigation are noteworthy. Chorioamnionitis, one of the commonest of all placental lesions and a major cause of prematurity, was not herein associated with asphyxia. Acute meconium staining, a common occurrence that often is considered unimportant clinically, was highly associated with asphyxic outcome.

The cases herein investigated were from a high risk population. From an a priori point of view, the following assertion is worthy of emphasis. Placental lesions that are found to be significant in a study of high risk patients would probably be highly significant in a study whose controls would include normal pregnancies and newborns. Thus, in the present investigation, lesions like chorangiosis—herein revealed to be marginally significant —would likely be proven to be substantially significant.

CONSIDERATIONS FOR FUTURE RESEARCH

With chorioamnionitis, the umbilical vein is the first vessel to participate in the inflammatory response. When fetuses are chronically exposed to meconium, damage of placental surface vessels and umbilical cord substance occurs. We have therefore recently hypothesized that infectious agents and meconium may produce perinatal asphyxia by means of placental and umbilical cord vasocontraction and fetal hypoperfusion. We have tested isotonic contraction of umbilical vein segments with 1 percent fresh meconium and with group B streptococcus (GBS) spent media, respectively. Our methods were similar to those of Altura and his colleagues.[49] The venous segments were suspended in Krebs-Henseleit media with carbogen at 37°C and pH 7.3 to 7.4. The average contraction caused by GBS media was 41 percent of serotonin effect, and the average contraction caused by meconium was 47 percent of that of serotonin. Boiling of the GBS spent media did not affect its ability to induce contraction. Boiling meconium for 1 hour, however, did eradicate meconium's ability to cause contraction. These observations require further investigation. Appropriate methods include experiments similar to those mentioned herein and experiments with animal models. Studies of humans could include Doppler evaluations of umbilical cord blood flow and investigations by epidemiologists.

The placenta is a diary of gestational life. To decipher its clues of perinatal disease, the final imperative should be to pursue the wisdom of epidemiologic discipline.

REFERENCES

1. Professional liability insurance and its effects: Report of a survey of ACOG's membership. Washington, DC: American College of Obstetricians and Gynecologists, 1985.
2. Naeye RL. Functionally important disorders of the placenta, umbilical cord, and fetal membranes. Hum Pathol 1987; 18:680.
3. Benirschke K. Examination of the placenta. Obstet Gynecol 1961; 18:309.
4. Altshuler G. The placenta, how to examine it, its normal growth and development. In: Naeye RL, Kissane JM, Kaufman N, eds. Perinatal diseases. Baltimore: Williams & Wilkins, 1981:5.
5. Altshuler G, Hyde S. Fusobacteria. An important cause of chorioamnionitis. Arch Pathol Lab Med 1985; 109:739.
6. Benirschke K, Driscoll SG, eds. The pathology of the human placenta. New York: Springer, 1967.
7. Fox H. Pathology of the placenta. Philadelphia: WB Saunders, 1978.
8. Perrin EVDK, ed. Pathology of the placenta. In: Roth LM, ed. Contemporary issues in surgical pathology. Vol 5. New York: Churchill Livingstone, 1984:141.
9. Naeye RL, Tafari N. Risk factors in pregnancy and diseases of the fetus and newborn. Baltimore: Williams & Wilkins, 1983.
10. Benirschke K. Routes and types of infection in the fetus and newborn. AMA J Dis Child 1960; 99:714.
11. Blanc WA. Amniotic infection syndrome: pathogenesis, morphology and significance in circumnatal mortality. Clin Obstet Gynecol 1959; 2:705.
12. Niswander KR, Gordon M. The women and their pregnancies. Philadelphia: WB Saunders, 1972.
13. Prenatal and perinatal factors associated with brain disorders. PB 87-172581. Bethesda, Maryland: National Institutes of Health, April 1985.
14. Kaplan M. Fetal breathing movements. An update for the pediatrician. Am J Dis Child 1983; 137:177.
15. Miller PW, Coen RW, Benirschke K. Dating the time interval from meconium passage to birth. Obstet Gynecol 1985; 66:459.
16. Lauweryns J, Bernat R, Lerut A, Detournay G. Intrauterine pneumonia. An experimental study. Biol Neonate 1973; 22:301.
17. Ostergard DR. Estriol in pregnancy. Obstet Gynecol Surv 1973; 28:215.
18. Altshuler G, DeBault LE. Preliminary report: immunoperoxidase-linked human placental lactogen as a histopathologic index of perinatal morbidity and mortality. Pediatr Pathol 1983; 1:469.
19. De Sa DJ. Intimal cushions in fetal placental veins. J Pathol 1973; 110:347.
20. Ornoy A, Crone K, Altshuler G. Pathological features of the placenta in fetal death. Arch Pathol Lab Med 1976; 100:367.
21. McKay DG. Disseminated intravascular coagulation. New York: Hoeber, 1965.
22. Benirschke K, Driscoll SG. The pathology of the human placenta. Berlin: Springer-Verlag, 1967:390.
23. Altshuler G. Chorangiosis. An important placental sign of neonatal morbidity and mortality. Arch Pathol Lab Med 1984; 108:71.
24. Altshuler G, Jordan J, Hyde S. Amniotic squamous balls: associations with oligohydramnios, amnion nodosum, Potter's syndrome and lung hypoplasia. Arch Gynecol (to be published).
25. Altshuler G. Placental infection and inflammation. In: Perrin EVDK, ed. Surgical pathology of the human placenta. New York: Churchill Livingstone, 1984.
26. Altshuler G, Russell P. The human placental villitides. A review of chronic intrauterine infection. Curr Top Pathol 1975; 60:63.
27. Sander CH. Hemorrhagic endovasculitis and hemorrhagic villitis of the placenta. Arch Pathol Lab Med 1980; 104:371.
28. Sander CH, Kinnane L, Stevens NG, Echt R. Haemorrhagic endovasculitis of the placenta: a review with clinical correlation. Placenta 1986; 7:551.
29. Goodman DR, James RC, Harbison RD. Placental toxicology. J Chem Toxicol 1982; 20:123.
30. Susser M, et al. Quantitative estimates of prenatal and perinatal risk factors for perinatal mortality, cerebral palsy, mental retardation and epilepsy. In: Freeman JM, ed. Prenatal and perinatal factors associated with brain disorders. NIH Publication 85-1149. Bethesda, Maryland: National Institutes of Health, 1985.
31. Nelson KB, Ellenberg JH. Antecedents of cerebral palsy: multivariate analysis of risk. N Engl J Med 1986; 315:81.
32. Naeye RL. Coitus and associated amniotic fluid infections. N Engl J Med 1979; 301:1198.
33. Klebanoff MA, Nugent RP, Rhoads GG. Coitus during pregnancy: is it safe? Lancet 1984; 2:914.
34. Kleinbaum DG, Kupper LL, Morgenstern H. In: Epidemiologic research. New York: Van Nostrand Rheinhold, 1982.
35. Mantel N, Haenszel W. Statistical aspects of data from retrospective studies of diseases. J Natl Cancer Inst 1958; 22:719.
36. Breslow N, Day N. Statistical methods for cancer research. Geneva: World Health Organization, 1980.
37. Harrell FE. The logistic procedure. In: SUGI supplemental library user's guide. SAS Institute, 1983:179.
38. Engelman L. Stepwise logistic regression. In: Dixon WJ, Brown MB, Engelman L, et al, eds. BMDP statistical software manual. Berkeley, California: University of California Press, 1985.
39. Nelson KB, Ellenberg JH. Obstetric complications as risk factors for cerebral palsy. JAMA 1984; 251:1843.
40. Vintzileos AM, Gaffney SE, Salinger LM, et al. The relationships among the fetal biophysical profile, umbilical cord pH, and Apgar scores. Am J Obstet Gynecol 1987; 157:627.
41. Dijxhoorn MJ, Visser GHA, Touwen BCL, Huisjes HJ. Apgar score, meconium and acidaemia at birth in small-for-gestational age infants born at term, and their relation to neonatal neurological morbidity. Br J Obstet Gynaecol 1987; 94:873.
42. Hollander DI, Wright L, Nagey DA, et al. Indicators of perinatal asphyxia. Am J Obstet Gynecol 1987; 157:839.
43. Josten BE, Johnson TRB, Nelson JP. Umbilical cord blood pH and Apgar scores as an index of neonatal health. Am J Obstet Gynecol 1987; 157:843.
44. Green SH. Is fetal blood sampling and pH estimation helpful or harmful? Arch Dis Child 1987; 62:1097.
45. Naeye RL, Peters EC. Antenatal hypoxia and low IQ values. Am J Dis Child 1987; 141:50.
46. Sykes GS, Molloy PM, Johnson PJ, et al. Do Apgar scores indicate asphyxia? Lancet 1982; 1:494.
47. The value of the Apgar score. Editorial. Lancet 1982; 2:1393.
48. Fox H. The incidence and significance of nucleated erythrocytes in the foetal vessels of the mature human placenta. J Obst Gynaecol Br Cmwlth 1967; 74:40.
49. Altura BM. Comparative contractile actions of different kinins on human umbilical arteries and veins. Eur J Pharmacol 1972; 19:171.

21 The Appropriateness of Intensive Care Applications

David K. Stevenson, M.D. and Amnon Goldworth, Ph.D.

Decision Making in Neonatal-Perinatal Medicine
Attempts to Regulate Physician Behavior
The "Baby Doe" Legacy
Moral Implications
Recommendations

A careful consideration of the "appropriateness" of intensive care is especially important in medical decision making related to neonates. Such consideration addresses the most fundamental character of a medical decision: whether the decision complies, inasmuch as compliance is possible, with the physician's professional charge to do what is best for the patient in terms of both saving life and preventing or treating injury (helping) and alleviating pain and suffering (not harming). Thus, the "appropriateness" of a decisive act supersedes all other characterizations, including standard or nonstandard (the level at which malpractice might be considered), correct or incorrect, and relevant or irrelevant (Fig. 21-1).

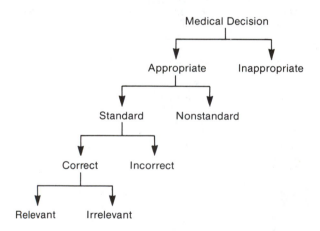

Figure 21-1 The nature of medical decision making.

This study was supported in part by a grant (RR-00081) from the General Clinical Research Centers Program of the Divisions of Research Resources, National Institutes of Health, and the Christopher Taylor Harrison Research Fund.

There is also a general concept of neonatal intensive care that involves the application of sophisticated technology (e.g., equipment, procedures, medications) to help or not harm newborn babies who are dependent on such care for their survival and avoidance of injury, pain, and suffering. However, all newborn babies are dependent and vulnerable, and all premature or sick newborns are, at least temporarily, disabled and at risk for handicaps. From a conservative (natural) perspective, any activities other than those undertaken by an infant's mother in a natural setting (professionally unassisted nuturing and caretaking practices) might be considered intensive care. Such a perspective would easily construe intravenous fluid administration or hyperalimentation as "intensive" or "heroic" undertakings, and might even consider gavage feeding in a similar light. However, what defines "intensive care" is less important than the kind of care that is appropriate for a particular individual. For example, no one would argue that maternal (or paternal) nurturing and caretaking would be inappropriate under any circumstances, but the appropriateness of any other kind of activity involving the neonate might be called into question, depending on the context in which it would be considered.

The concept of "appropriateness" not only refers to whether something is medically indicated but includes reference, in principle, to other relevant factors, such as the adequacy of facilities and staff for undertaking certain practices, the educational background, social circumstances, and financial status of the family, the social and economic resources of the community, and the ethical perspectives of the decision makers. A critical conceptual point is that "appropriateness" means more than having specific efficacy in practice, and at least suggests consideration primarily of whether having such specific efficacy might also have a possible consequence in the best interest of the patient[1] and secondarily of the family and society. As an illustration of this point, a given technology, such as a mechanical ventilator, may be construed as being a life-saving piece of equipment and "appropriate" for application to save someone's life and alleviate suffering in one context, but in another context also may be construed as an instrument of torture and "inappropriate" for application to save someone's life, because it is causing harm and contributing to suffering, despite having the same predictable effect (providing adequate oxygenation and ventilation) in each case, and supporting life for as long as it is applied in each case.

Thus, the concept of "appropriateness" is especially important in decision making in neonatal intensive care, as the issues of withholding or withdrawing of intensive care life support are considered. The complexity and difficulty of such decision making is compounded in situations in which it is believed that the child might survive with such intensive care but would be gravely impaired, although not quite to the point of being irreversibly comatose. Consideration of the "appropriateness" of intensive care reflects, in fact, the implementation of the complex professional charge of the physician. Understanding this charge is fundamental to any understanding of the decision making or appreciation of the judgments of physicians responsible for applying intensive care.

DECISION MAKING IN NEONATAL-PERINATAL MEDICINE

A medical decision is a complex phenomenon. It involves more than simply thinking logically, as one might derive a conclusion from a set of premises according to well-established and agreed upon operations of thought applied to well-described models of biologic reality. In fact, the models of medical science are imperfect and always changing. Empirical experience has a predominant role in the practice of medicine, but ethical considerations are inextricably intertwined with medical decision making. Moreover, the complex professional charge of the physician set forth in the Hippocratic tradition is the integrating force in the decision making process.

The physician's charge is twofold: to save life and to alleviate pain and suffering (Fig. 21–2). Although each charge by itself represents a challenge and an important goal, the integration of both goals into each decisive

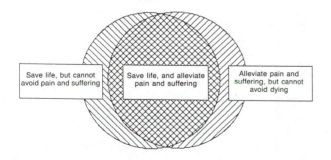

Figure 21–2 The physician's professional charge.

action represents the ultimate challenge. Thus, a physician should do good (commit acts) or avoid harm (omit acts). Committing and omitting are always companion acts in decision making by physicians and have equal importance and impact on the state of being of patients. Although the zone of overlap where saving a patient's life also alleviates pain and suffering represents the ideal, there are situations that restrict compliance in practice. That is, there are circumstances in which death cannot be avoided and only alleviation of pain or suffering is possible; conversely, life sometimes can be preserved only at the price of tremendous suffering. Moreover, the extent to which death is or is not avoidable (and within what time frame) may depend on the "amount" of suffering that the patient or decision makers are able to accept in the effort to save or prolong life. Whereas reasonable precision is commonly possible with respect to knowing about the avoidability of death, the experience of suffering remains essentially subjective; thus, judgments about its severity (especially for the neonate) are imprecise at best, and highly variable.

The decision making process that characterizes the application of intensive care must involve carefully considered commissions and omissions based on incomplete information. Furthermore, such decisions must focus on human values in addition to survival, such as the quality of survival. The experience of suffering is highly variable, any definition of suffering is subject to interpretation, and suffering is difficult to conceptualize for a neonate. However, physicians still must consider the avoidance of pain or suffering as an integral practical component of any act committed to save life.[2]

Before the advent of modern intensive care support, in particular, mechanical ventilation, the recognition of this dual charge rarely generated any conflicts. A physician might approach patient care employing a strategy of doing everything possible to save a person's life, because there was simply not too much to do. Under such circumstances the blanket application of "intensive care" could be almost uniformly "appropriate." There would be little risk of violating the tenets of preserving life and preventing pain or suffering. Avoiding suffering would often go hand in hand with avoiding dying. The therapies available were simply not potent enough to substantially modify the natural history of most life-threatening illnesses, nor were they potent enough to cause harm themselves.

The situation has become quite different with modern intensive care. An empirically determined blanket application of modern intensive care can result in prolonged pain or suffering for some individuals, as has been suggested by Fischer and Stevenson.[3] In a group of extremely premature infants, one-third might die within minutes after birth because they could not be resuscitated, and their suffering, at least in terms of duration, would be minimal. Approximately half of those surviving long enough to be admitted to the intensive care nursery eventually would die after varying lengths of time and suffering (hours to months). Of the surviving one-third of the total number of infants born alive, only 20 percent might be free of disabilities and any suffering related to their premature birth (Fig. 21–3). Thus, if saving life is the paramount objective, suffering for some individuals, including some who will not even survive, cannot be avoided in this example. As Fischer and Stevenson pointed out, this is no less in conflict with the physician's charge of preventing suffering than euthanasia is in conflict with the goal of preserving life. Although the condemnation of euthanasia is almost universal, there has been general acceptance of treatment strategies that virtually ensure suffering. A more critical consideration of the ''appropriateness'' of therapeutic strategies in particular cases is now required.[4]

ATTEMPTS TO REGULATE PHYSICIAN BEHAVIOR

There are difficulties in attempting to regulate newborn intensive care or the behavior of physicians responsible for making decisions in this setting. Because all newborn babies are dependent and vulnerable, and all premature or sick newborns are at least temporarily disabled and at risk for handicaps, it has been tempting to provide general guidelines for their care. However, the ability to predict the outcome for individual infants is extremely limited,[5,6] even for infants with certain chromosomal and genetic abnormalities. The most important limitation, however, is one often overlooked by physicians themselves, as well as by lawyers attempting to understand the decision making of the physician in the context of a particular case. This limitation relates to the misapplication of statistical data derived from analysis of samples of subject populations in attempting to predict an individual subject's survival or injuries. Prediction with respect to the individual is always uncertain, and general information about populations of infants with similar problems is, at best, a limited guide for reasonable

decision making in individual cases because statistical information describes samples or populations and not individuals. Thus, if general understanding of the circumstance is the goal, reference to such information is appropriate for assessing the reasoned opinions of the physician, but the information is inadequate, if not irrelevant, for assessing the particular decision making process of the physician taking care of a particular infant. This subtle but important distinction between what is generally true and what is specifically the case, and what is reasonable and what is correct or incorrect, sits at the center of the malpractice crisis. Perhaps the most instructive examples of this critical conceptual and practical interface between law and medicine, besides malpractice, have been the attempts to regulate physician behavior, in particular with respect to newborn intensive care. The history of such attempts has been chronicled previously (Fig. 21–4)[7-9]

THE ''BABY DOE'' LEGACY

Decisions to withhold or withdraw treatment from newborns attracted considerable attention in the 1970s because of several cases involving infants with clearly identified severe congenital defects. Public attention was focused on the process by which these decisions were made. However, one infant in particular, ''Baby Doe,'' who died in Bloomington, Indiana, in 1982 after his parents refused corrective surgery for birth defects accompanying Down syndrome, served as the impetus for notification to health care providers that Section 504 of the Rehabilitation Act of 1973, which prohibits discrimination on the basis of handicap, applied to the treatment of infants born with disabilities. The US Department of Health and Human Services published its final version of the Baby Doe rule in 1984[10] and followed this with the closely related Child Abuse Amendments of 1984 and the Child Abuse Rule of 1985, both of which attempted to define the terms of the Baby Doe regulations and exceptions to its require-

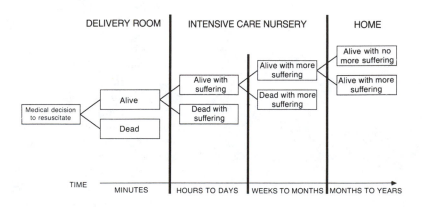

Figure 21–3   The consequences of uncertainty.

4/9/82   "Infant Doe" born with Down's syndrome and esophageal atresia with tracheoesophageal fistula; parents refuse surgery; juvenile court judge upholds parents; baby dies 5 days later

4/30/82   President Reagan instructs the Secretary of Health and Human Services (HHS) to notify health care providers of the applicability of §504 of the Rehabilitation Act of 1973 to the treatment of handicapped patients (newborns)

5/18/82   HHS notifies hospitals of the applicability of §504 and establishes investigative procedures for noncompliance

3/7/83   HHS issues an interim final rule

4/14/83   Interim final rule declared invalid

7/5/83   HHS issues a proposed rule, with 60-day comment period

10/11/83   Baby "Jane Doe" born with myelomeningocele, microencephaly, hydrocephalus, and other birth defects

10/15/83   Lawrence Washburn, a right-to-life attorney, contacts New York Supreme Court Judge Frank DeLuca

10/16/83   Washburn files a petition that, if successful, would require baby Jane Doe to be treated surgically

10/18/83   Judge Tanenbaum appoints William Weber as guardian *ad litem* for baby Jane Doe without notice to the hospital or parents

10/19/83   Hearings commence on the petition before Judge Tanenbaum

10/20/83   Judge Tanenbaum upholds Washburn's petition

10/21/83   Five justices of the New York Supreme Court, Appellate Division, reverse Judge Tanenbaum's decision

10/24/83   An appeal is filed in the New York State Court of Appeals

10/27/83   HHS advises university hospital that it is initiating legal action for noncompliance with §504

10/28/83   New York Court of Appeals upholds baby Jane Doe's parents' right to withhold surgery

11/2/83   US Justice Department files a petition in US District Court against university hospital for noncompliance with §504

11/4/83   Arguments begin in the US District Court

11/8/83   New York State Attorney General's Office files a brief in US District Court, arguing that the federal government does not have jurisdiction in this case

11/10/83   Six organizations representing the disabled file an amicus curiae brief supporting the federal government's request to inspect the medical records

11/17/83   Judge Leonard Wexler denies the federal government's request

11/18/83   Justice Department files notice of appeal

12/12/83   US Supreme Court refuses Mr. Weber's request that it hear the case of baby Jane Doe

12/23/83   Washburn initiates a class action suit on behalf of baby Jane Doe and other newborn infants similarly situated

12/30/83   Washburn files a motion to appoint a new guardian *ad litem* for baby Jane Doe

1/12/84   HHS issues final rules, effective Feb. 13, 1984, on "Nondiscrimination on the Basis of Handicap; Procedures and Guidelines Relating to Health Care for Handicapped Infants"

1/20/84   Judge Roger J. Miner refuses Washburn's request

2/2/84   US House of Representatives passes the child abuse protection bill (HR 1904)

2/23/84   Second Circuit US Court of Appeals affirms the district court's ruling in university hospital's favor that the federal government be denied access to baby Jane Doe's medical records

3/1/84   Washburn appeals the decision of Jan 20, 1984

3/8/84   Shunt surgery performed on baby Jane Doe

3/12/84   American Medical Association and American Hospital Association file suit in US District Court seeking to invalidate HHS regulations

3/28/84   Baby Jane Doe discharged from university hospital

4/19/84   Washburn withdraws his appeal to the US Court of Appeals

7/26/84   After negotiation with hospital associations, physician groups, and disability and right-to-life groups, the US Senate passes its version of the Child Abuse Protection Bill (S 1003); unlike HR 1904, S 1003 defines "withholding medically indicated treatment"

8/16/84   Justice Department announces it will not continue efforts to obtain baby Jane Doe's medical records

9/84   Both houses pass an amended bill

10/2/84   Justice Department appeals the US District Court's decision in May that invalidated the Baby Doe rules published in January

10/9/84   President Reagan signs the Child Abuse Amendments in 1984

12/10/84   Proposed rule published in the *Federal Register*; comments for consideration are to be received by Feb 8, 1985

2/7/85   Public Policy Council of the American Societies of Academy Pediatrics (the American Pediatric Society, the Association of Medical School Pediatric Department Chairman, and the Society for Pediatric Research) sends missive to National Center on Child Abuse and Neglect, US Children's Bureau "to express deep concern regarding the impact of the proposed rules, 45 CFR Part 1340, for implementation of Public Law 98-457, the Child Abuse Amendments of 1984, and the accompanying interim model guidelines for establishment of infant care review committees"

Figure 21-4   Summary of events leading up to the "Baby Doe" rule. (From Stevenson DK, Ariagno RL, Kutner JS, et al. The "Baby Doe" rule. JAMA 1986; 255:1909.)

ments. Although the Supreme Court of the United States declared the Baby Doe rule invalid, the Child Abuse Amendments of 1984 and the Child Abuse Rule have remained law.

The Child Abuse and Neglect Prevention and Treatment Program (or "Child Abuse Rule") is a final rule that implements the Child Abuse Amendments of 1984 (Public Law 98-457). The amendments supplement the Child Abuse Prevention and Treatment Act (Public Law 92-247, 42USC 5101, et seq.), signed into law in 1974. The Child Abuse Rule mandates "that, in order to qualify for basic State grants under the Act, States must have had, by October 9, 1985 (within one year of enactment), programs or procedures or both in place within the State's Child Protective Service (CPS) system for the purpose of responding to reports of medical neglect, including instances of the withholding of medically indicated treatment (including appropriate nutrition, hydration, and medication) for disabled infants with life threatening conditions." The Child Abuse Rule defines "withholding of medically indicated treatment" as "failure to respond to an infant's life threatening conditions by providing treatment (including appropriate nutrition, hydration, and medication), which, in the treating physician's reasonable medical judgment, will be most likely to be effective in ameliorating or correcting all such conditions." Furthermore, "exceptions to the requirement to provide treatment (but not the requirement to provide appropriate nutrition, hydration, and medication) may be made only in cases in which: 1) the infant is chronically and irreversibly comatose; or 2) the provision of such treatment would merely prolong dying or not be effective in ameliorating or correcting all the infant's life threatening conditions or otherwise be futile in terms of the survival of the infant; or 3) the provision of such treatment would be virtually futile in terms of the survival of the infant and the treatment itself under such circumstances would be inhumane."

Because all newborn babies are dependent and vulnerable, and all premature or sick newborns are at least temporarily disabled and at risk for handicaps, the law would seem to have general applicability by its design. A practical problem encountered relates to the absence of reference to "quality of life" considerations in the Child Abuse Rule. That is, the rule, by its omission of specific comments, suggests that parents' and doctors' perceptions of quality of life should play no part in decision making in newborn intensive care. The rule implies that the decision instead should be based on an assessment of the child's chance for survival, taking into account the risk of inhumane treatment. What at first might have seemed an innocent statement of principle initiated in a laudable spirit of respect for persons, no matter what the disabilities, becomes transformed through attempts at implementation into a potential threat to the professional integrity of the physician, the natural role of the parents, and the well-being of the patient.

For example, quality of life issues are often clearly expressed for the adult patient who has some frame of reference because a past and a known future can serve as reference. Such is not the case for the infant who has no history as a social person, and an unknown future. It is also a fact that it is difficult to include an objective evaluation of the quality of life in the decision making process for infants, because they have an almost unbelievable potential for recovery from serious injuries, which may be grossly manifest at the time the decision making is undertaken. The converse is also true. Infants who appear normal at birth may, in fact, develop serious disabilities, which become apparent only later in life. Extremely variable outcomes in terms of function can even be observed among infants with known genetic or developmental syndromes. This extraordinary degree of uncertainty (in cases in which certainty may have been assumed by the legal profession and the public) is represented by a gray area or ambiguous zone in which some mental or physical disability can be anticipated in a sick newborn, but the extent of the disability cannot be established. Thus, the assumption of the "Baby Doe" and Child Abuse Rules that many different conditions affecting individual patients can be lumped under a few general categories with predictable outcomes is misleading, if not simply wrong. Because of the dual commitment of the physician to help and not harm the infant, the physician must weigh the likelihood of survival with the degree of suffering experienced by an infant who cannot articulate his suffering or express his will, and not simply consider that "the treatment itself under such circumstances would be inhumane." Even the exceptions specified in the Child Abuse Rule may be inadequate for the treatment of many infants. The more common case, in which an infant has been given mechanical ventilation for a long period of time and it is not know precisely what the chances of survival are (although they are certainly poor) and what pain the infant is experiencing, is left unaddressed.

Thus, the Child Abuse Rule ignores the reality of medical practice with all its uncertainties in the care of critically ill infants and assumes a complete base of information, which is in fact rarely available, and assumes that treatment results are more predictable than they really are. Moreover, it assumes that with precise knowledge of the infant's condition at birth, treatment options are clear and simple conclusions to be derived from premises. This is far from true. The regulations create an illusion of acceptable and unacceptable courses of action that are not easily applied to the daily dilemmas arising in delivery rooms and intensive care nurseries. The physician often may have to make a decision about the "appropriateness" of intensive care if it is thought that the child will survive with intensive care, but will be gravely impaired but not quite to the point of being irreversibly comatose. The "appropriateness" of therapeutic options needs to be considered, including the option to withdraw life support and let the neonate die.[11] The decision making process becomes more difficult if no meaningful prediction can be made regarding whether the neonate is likely to survive, and it is likely but not certain that he or she will have grave disabilities. The legal profession should exercise great caution as it is asked to address or resolve such issues.

MORAL IMPLICATIONS

A major problem is the absence of any reference to quality of life considerations in the Child Abuse Rule. The reason for this omission was enunciated as follows:

The physician's "reasonable medical judgment" concerning medically indicated treatment must be one that would be made by a reasonably prudent physician, knowledgeable about the case and the treatment possibilities with respect to the medical conditions involved. It is not to be based on subjective "quality of life" or other abstract concepts.[12]

In a later document the Department of Health and Human Services continued to refer to "the subjective opinions about the future 'quality of life' of a retarded or disabled person."[13] This characterization of quality of life judgments appears to be supported by the diversity of positions taken by doctors, lawyers, ethicists, and theologians concerning such judgments when applied to the noncomatose or nondying infant. Consider the following sampling of viewpoints:

In its discussion of the omission or withdrawal of treatment of seriously ill neonates, the President's Commission for the Study of Ethical Problems in Medicine and Biomedical and Behavioral Research pointed out that efforts to save the lives of seriously ill newborns often leaves those who survive with inherited or iatrogenic disabilities. One then may ask whether or to what extent the expectation of such disabilities should be taken into account in deciding whether to treat or not to treat. The Commission concluded "that a very restrictive standard is appropriate: such permanent handicaps justify a decision not to provide life-sustaining treatment only when they are so severe that continued existence would not be a net benefit to the infant."[14] The Commission added that "in all surrogate decision making, the surrogate is obligated to try to evaluate benefits and burdens from the infant's own perspective."[15] The Commission's standard calls for treatment if the infant is not suffering pain or never develops any capacity for social interaction or lives only a short time. A different viewpoint is presented by Father Richard A. McCormick, as follows:

The meaning, substance, and consummation of life is found in human relationships, and the qualities of justice, respect, concern, compassion, and support that surround them.... One who must support his life with disproportionate effort focuses the time, attention, energy, and resources of himself and others not precisely on relationships. Such concentration easily becomes overconcentration and distorts one's view of and weakens one's pursuit of these very relational goods that define our growth and flourishing. The importance of relationships gets lost in the struggle for survival.

Life is not a value to be preserved in and for itself. To maintain that would commit us to a form of medical vitalism that makes no human or Judeo-Christian sense. It is a value to be preserved precisely as a condition for other values, and therefore insofar as these other values remain attainable. Since these other values cluster around and are rooted in human relationships, it seems to follow that life is a value to be preserved only insofar as it contains some potentiality for human relationships.[16]

The essential feature of McCormick's guideline for omitting or withdrawing life-sustaining treatment is that "life is a value to be preserved only insofar as it contains some potentiality for human relationships." An important difference between McCormick and the President's Commission is that in those instances in which there are no human interactions, the latter requires treatment and the former calls for its omission or cessation.

Dr. H. Tristram Engelhardt Jr., presents a third approach, which maintains that we have a duty not to treat when treatment would merely prolong suffering. Englehardt draws attention to the fact that a number of suits have been initiated that were based on the legal concept of "wrongful life" and then explains that

The concept of tort for wrongful life is transferrable in part to the painfully compromised existence of children who can only have their life prolonged for a short, painful and marginal existence. The concept suggests that allowing life to be prolonged under such circumstances would itself be an injury of the person whose painful and severely compromised existence would be made to continue.... The concept of injury for continuance of existence, the proposed analogue of the concept of tort for wrongful life, presupposed that life can be a negative value such that the medical maxim *primum non nocere* ("first do no harm") would require not sustaining life.[17]

In a fourth approach Professor Robert Weir[18] argues that neonates are potential persons and as such have claims to life that can be overridden only by "detriment-benefit judgments made for the infant's sake." He observes that there are infants for whom the harms of congenital conditions or of ineffective treatments are such that the detriment outweighs the benefit. He concludes that such harms can be viewed as conditions worse than death:

In extreme, relatively rare circumstances an extension of a seriously defective infant's life can represent a greater harm than does nontreatment resulting in death. In such cases ... to withhold the treatment in order to bring about the infant's death is to do something less harmful to the infant than would treatment resulting in an extension of the infant's life for an indeterminate period of time. Infants in these extreme circumstances can rightfully be said to be better off dead precisely because death represents a lesser harm for them than enduring an injurious, tortured existence.[19]

Weir adds a proviso that nontreatment decisions should be made within major diagnostic categories. To make such decision "across major diagnostic lines is to engage in unfair quality-of-life assessments, because any less-than-normal infant will lose out in such a comparison."[20]

Comparisons of the four positions relating to quality of life judgments just presented indicate that the President's Commission emphasizes the net benefit to the infant, McCormick emphasizes the potentiality for human relations, Englehardt focuses on the injury to the infant, and Weir combines the positions of the President's Commission and Englehardt, but insists that such judgments should be governed by diagnostic categories. Given these differences, as well as others not mentioned, the government appeared to be correct in disallowing quality-of-life judgments. But then the government should have disallowed parts of its own policy. This becomes clear when we look at what is said in opposition to quality-of-life judgments in terms of the sanctity of life approach represented by Rabbi Moshe Tendler in the following passage:

As you know, the ethical foundation of our society, of western civilization is a biblical one.... There are certain indispensable foundations for an ethical system and one of them is the sanctity of human life. This concept has a corollary; that is that human life is of infinite value. This in turn means that a piece of infinity is also infinite and a person who has but a few moments to live is of no less value than a person who has 70 years to live. And likewise, a person who is handicapped and cannot serve the needs of society is no less a man and no less entitled to the same price tag—a price tag inscribed with an infinite price. A handicapped individual is a perfect specimen when viewed in an ethical context. This value is an absolute value. It is not relative to life expectancy, to state of health, or to usefulness to society....[21]

The government asserts that an exception to treatment may be made when such treatment "would merely prolong dying or not be effective in ameliorating or correcting all the infant's life threatening conditions or otherwise be futile in terms of survival of the infant."[22] But treatment that prolongs dying prolongs life, and any life, according to the sanctity-of-life ethic, is of infinite value and is therefore worth preserving. For the sanctity-of-life advocate it is always wrong to allow human life to end regardless of its length or quality. But for the government there are circumstances as expressed in its exception to treatment in which efforts to save a life may cease.

There is a more moderate form of the sanctity-of-life approach, which maintains that we have a prima facie rather than an absolute obligation to sustain life. A prima facie obligation is one that tells us what we ought to do in the presence of other relevant considerations. Although not explicitly stated, this may come close to what the government had in mind. However, the moderate sanctity-of-life position does not avoid quality-of-life judgments, for it is these that permit us to override the prima facie obligations to treat.

An alternative position advanced by the legal theorist John A. Robertson,[23] although not taking a sanctity-of-life approach, appears to reinforce the government's stand by attacking any use of quality-of-life judgments as applied to infants who are able to survive. Robertson discusses several circumstances in which the omission or cessation of treatment seems to be called for. One involves the infant's experiencing severe physical pain; the other involves the suffering of the infant as caused by living a life devoid of social interactions. With reference to the first, he observes that the pain may not be constant or may be controlled by analgesics. Thus, unless the pain is chronic or unmanageable, one may not justifiably conclude that life is not worth living. With reference to the second, Robertson offers two alternatives. The first is to accept the premises but to question the amount of suffering experienced in the particular case. He believes that this eliminates the justification of death over life except in the most extreme instances of psychosocial deprivation. The second is to dismiss the quality-of-life approach entirely.

He observes that the absence of schooling or social interaction for defective individuals may be due to the social attitudes of healthy ones. Many of the former who are nonambulatory can be trained to do satisfying work. Nor should we assume that a nonproductive existence for those who cannot be so trained is necessarily an unhappy one. Thus, we cannot conclude for one and all that the lives of those who suffer from psychosocial deprivation are not worth living. However, there are infants who suffer from the extremes of malformation or retardation so that their ability to interact with others is minimal. In response to this consideration Robertson says:

In what sense can the proxy validly conclude that a person with different wants, needs, and interests, if able to speak, would agree that such a life were worse than death?... Compared with the situation and life prospects of a "reasonable man," the child's potential quality of life indeed appears dim. Yet a standard based on healthy, ordinary development may be entirely inappropriate to the situation. One who has never known the pleasures of mental operation, ambulation, and social interaction surely does not suffer from that loss as much as one who has. While one who has known these capacities may prefer death to a life without them, we have no assurance that the handicapped person, with no point of comparison, would agree. Life and life alone, whatever its limitations, might be of sufficient worth to him.[24]

Robertson's main point is that proxy judgments of the quality of life of defective children are not justified. Life, whatever its character, may be of worth to the defective individual. Therefore we have no moral right to omit or withdraw life-supporting treatment. This is consistent with the government's prohibition against the omission or cessation of treatment for the biologically viable infant. However, Robertson's argument can lead to a radically different conclusion. If we cannot make the appropriate quality-of-life judgment, it is also possible that life *may not* be of any worth to the defective individual. Thus, no judgment is possible as to which is the proper course of action: treatment or nontreatment. Given this outcome, we can no longer comfort ourselves with the dictum, "When in doubt, treat." Once it is recognized that to treat and save may create the conditions for a deeply deprived life that has no worth to the defective individual, we cannot hide behind the problematic view that to intervene with life-rescuing efforts is always in the patient's interest.

Are we then to be left with no other option for deciding what to do in terms of the interests of the infant but to randomize the giving or withdrawing of treatment? Is the decision to treat or not to treat to be a matter of the toss of a coin? The answer is no.

It should be noted that, notwithstanding differences among physicians, ethicists, lawyers, and theologians concerning the quality-of-life criteria under which the omission or cessation of life-saving treatment for infants is justified, there is considerable agreement that some defective infants should not receive such treatment. In this respect the government clearly stands as one against many. In addition, differences in quality-of-life judgments do not rule out the possibility of broad support for an appropriate moral policy based on quality-of-life considerations. The following declaration, which is central to such a policy, would appear to be compatible with the four quality-of-life positions described earlier: It is morally wrong to employ life-saving treatment for infants who cannot be adequately compensated for the pain and suffering they experience. Here too the government stands opposed.

However, even if we could develop a moral policy that would receive total support, we would still have disagreements about the application of policy to the specific case. In this context it is of particular interest to consider the Baby Jane Doe case, which came to public attention in 1983 during the uproar over the Baby Doe case. Baby Jane Doe was born with meningomyelocele, hydrocephalus, and microcephalus. Her parents were given the option of surgery for her spinal column and shunts to drain the excessive fluid from her head or, as a second "conservative" option, no medical treatment other than antibiotics to protect her from infection to her spinal column, as well as food and water. Doctors believed that without surgery Baby Jane Doe would live for several weeks to two years. The parents chose the second option. In commenting on this case, Professor Fred M. Frohock observed

One nagging thought about the Baby Jane Doe case is that there might not be any right answer in the dispute. No evidence was ever presented to suggest that the parents of the little girl were negligent or in any way irrational. No unusual superstitions or religious beliefs inform their views. They are Catholics who assert that religion played no part in their decision. They seemed in all respects genuinely concerned with the welfare of their child. The treatment they chose was conservative, ruling out those surgical interventions which would repair the spinal opening and drain the fluid from the brain. It is true that the parents may have decided against surgery on the expectation that the child would then die very quickly. But the parents may have been prepared to say that a short life with higher quality is better than a long life with severe disabilities.[25]

When there is no right answer, we must identify and accept those that are reasonable. Reasonable decisions are based on a grasp of the treatment options and the probabilities of their outcomes, which are guided by a coherent moral perspective. Since different individuals have different moral perspectives, there can be differences in the reasonable decisions reached concerning the same case. But, as Professor Earl E. Shelp pointed out, "These decisions warrant respect within a society that acknowledges its pluralism and protects the freedom of particular moral communities and agents to create, discover and pursue their concrete view of the good."[26] In those circumstances in which the best that we can hope for are reasonable judgments rather than consensus on the part of those who serve as surrogates for a defective infant, any rule or law, such as the government's Child Abuse Rule, which aborts such decisions, must be viewed as arbitrary and morally unwarranted.

RECOMMENDATIONS

Governmental law makers and private practice lawyers should understand that physicians' decisions are contextual phenomena, and represent more than logical conclusions derived from precisely known premises through reasoned arguments. Their judgments may be correct or incorrect, and still well reasoned in either case. Likewise, they can be poorly reasoned, and correct or incorrect in either case. It is also important to understand that the goals of the physician in decision making must reflect not only a commitment to saving life, but also to alleviating suffering, and therefore must consider the "appropriateness" of therapeutic options, not simply their possibility in a particular case. Moreover, the efficacy of an option is not sufficient for choosing it.

The possible harmful effect of attempts by the federal government to monitor physicians' decisions may be substantial, and may encourage abuse of applications of medical technology that neither increase the chance of survival nor reduce suffering. A more constructive approach would be government support for research to prevent injury and illness in mothers and infants, for social programs in medical care serving handicapped infants and their families, as well as increased support for prenatal care that has been demonstrated to reduce the risk of handicaps.

With respect to malpractice, although the public deserves the right to receive at least the standard care, some mistakes cannot be avoided because of the uncertainties of medical practice. These should not be automatically construed as malpractice without careful consideration of the context in which the practices were performed and the reasonability of the judgments made. Moreover, injury and disability among patients do not always indicate mistakes, and necessitate a decision about culpability. Other more generally applicable and just ways should be considered to improve the assistance for disabled individuals than by taxing the public and legal system through ad hoc procedures to mobilize financial support for injured individuals.

REFERENCES

1. Statement of the American Medical Association to the Select Education Subcommittee Committee on Education and Labor U.S. House of Representatives. RE:HR. 6492—Handicapped Infants Protection Act, September 1982. Conn Med 1983; 47:29.
2. Cassel EJ. The nature of suffering and the goals of medicine. N Engl J Med 1982; 306:639.
3. Fischer AF, Stevenson DK. The consequences of uncertainty. An empirical approach to medical decision making in neonatal intensive care. JAMA 1987; 258:1929.
4. Rhoden NK. Treating Baby Doe: the ethics of uncertainty. Hastings Cent Rep 1986; 16:34.
5. Kimble KJ, Ariagno RL, Stevenson DK, et al. Predicting survival among ventilator-dependent very low birth weight infants. Crit Care Med 1983; 11:182.
6. Zarfin J, Van Aerde J, Perlman M, et al. Predicting survival of infants of birth weight less than 801 grams. Crit Care Med 1986; 14:768.
7. Stevenson DK, Ariagno RL, Kutner JS, et al. The "Baby Doe" rule. JAMA 1986; 255:1909.
8. Weir RF. Sounding board: the government and selective nontreatment of handicapped infants. N Engl J Med 1983; 309:661.
9. Shapiro DL, Rosenberg P. The effect of federal regulations regarding handicapped newborns: a case report. JAMA 1984; 252:2031.
10. Federal Register 1984; 49:1622.
11. Whitelaw A. Death as an option in neonatal intensive care. Lancet 1986; 2:328.
12. Federal Register 1985; 49:48163.
13. Federal Register 1985; 50:14879.
14. President's Commission for the Study of Ethical Problems in Medicine and Biomedical and Behavioral Research. Deciding to forego life-sustaining treatment. 1983; 218.
15. President's Commission for the Study of Ethical Problems in Medicine and Biomedical and Behavioral Research. Deciding to forego life-sustaining treatment. 1983; 219.
16. McCormick RA. To save or let die: the dilemma of modern medicine. JAMA 1974; 229:174.
17. Englehardt HT Jr. Some qualities of life are not worth living. In: Brody BA, Englehardt HT Jr, eds. Bioethics readings and cases. Englewood Cliffs, New Jersey: Prentice-Hall, 1987:182.
18. Weir RF. Selective nontreatment of handicapped newborns. Oxford: Oxford University Press, 1984:195.
19. Weir RF. Selective nontreatment of handicapped newborns. Oxford: Oxford University Press, 1984:207.
20. Weir RF. Selective nontreatment of handicapped newborns. Oxford: Oxford University Press, 1984:235.
21. Tendler M. Quoted in Brody H. Ethical dilemmas in medicine. Boston: Little Brown, 1976:66.
22. Federal Register 1985; 50:14878.
23. Robertson JA. Involuntary euthanasia of defective newborns: a legal analysis. Stanford Law Rev 1975; 27:213.
24. Robertson JA. Involuntary euthanasia of defective newborns: a legal analysis. Stanford Law Rev 1975; 27:254.
25. Frohock FM. Special care: medical decision at the beginning of life. Chicago: University of Chicago Press, 1986:26.
26. Shelp EE. Born to die? Deciding the fate of critically ill newborns. New York: Free Press, 1986:204.

Note: Page numbers in italics indicate illustrations; those followed by t indicate tables.

A

Abdominal circumference, maternal, in intrauterine growth retardation, 27
ABO incompatibility, and hemorrhagic anemia, 149
Abruptio placentae, and cerebral palsy, 229
  and cocaine, 61
Acid-base determination, of cord blood, 39, 42
  of fetal scalp blood, 39
Acidosis, metabolic. See also *Metabolic imbalances.*
  and neonatal asphyxia, 4–5
  correction of, in neonatal resuscitation, 99–100
  fetal, and neurologic outcome, 4–5
Acquired immunodeficiency syndrome, neonatal, 85–86
Acyclovir, for congenital herpes simplex virus infection, 81, 82
  for varicella zoster infection, 83
Adrenal blood flow, in fetal hypoxia/asphyxia, 71–72
Afterload reduction, for cardiac output enhancement, 106–107
AIDS, neonatal, 85–86
Airway maintenance, in neonatal resuscitation, 97
Albumin, for hypovolemia, 102
Alcohol, teratogenicity of, 59–60
Alcohol withdrawal syndrome, neonatal, 59
Aminoglycosides, for necrotizing enterocolitis prophylaxis, 170
Aminopterin, teratogenicity of, 58t
Amnion nodosum, 256
Amniotic fluid, leakage of, 16–17
Analgesics. See also *Anesthesia.*
  administration of, 54
  direct effects of, 54–55
  neurobehavioral effects of, 55
Androgens, teratogenicity of, 58t
Anemia, and bleeding disorders, 152–153
  and refractory hypoxemia, 107
  causes of, 149
  Diamond-Blackfan, 149
  hemolytic, 151–152
    and hyperbilirubinemia, 150, 156–158
  hemorrhagic, 149–151, 149t, 150t
  management of, 107
  of prematurity, 151
Anesthesia, 46–55

and neonatal depression, 54–55
complications of, 47–52
general, contraindications to, 47
  endotracheal intubation in, 49
    failed, 48
  esophageal intubation in, 48
    failed endotracheal intubation in, 48
  induction drugs for, 49
  maternal cardiopulmonary collapse during, 47, 49–50
  maternal hypoxia during, 47
  preoxygenation in, 47
  pulmonary aspiration in, 48–49
general guidelines for, 46–47
neurobehavioral effects of, 55
regional, 50–55
  and uterine contractility, 52
  drug effects in, direct, 54–55
    indirect, 52–54
  effects of, on labor and delivery, 52
  fetal bradycardia in, 53–54
  fetal scalp injection in, 47, 55
  hypotension in, 50–51, 52–53
  in preeclampsia, 50
  indications for, 47
  intrathecal/intravascular injection of, and fetal bradycardia, 54
    detection of, 51–52
  local anesthetics for, test dose of, 51–52
    toxicity of, 47, 50, 51
  massive epidural block in, 51
  neonatal depression in, 54–55
  placental perfusion in, 52
  respiratory failure in, 50
  subdural block in, 51
  total spinal block in, 51
Angel dust, fetal effects of, 62–63
Anoxia, definition of, 65
Antacids, prior to general anesthesia, 48
Antibiotics, and cerebral palsy, 229
  for toxoplasmosis, 88
Anticholinergics, for general anesthesia, 49
Antiviral agents, for cytomegalovirus infection, 85
  for herpes simplex virus infection, 82
  for varicella zoster virus infection, 83
Apgar score, 3, 240
  and cerebral palsy, 6, 7t, 42, 231
  and meconium staining, 42
  and metabolic status, 5, 42
  and neonatal asphyxia, 42
  and neonatal seizures, 6
  in prematurity, 240
  limitations of, 231
Apnea, and anesthesia/analgesia, 54–55
  in preterm infant, 15
Apomorphine, prior to general anesthesia,

48
Arrhythmias. See also *Bradycardia.*
  and beta-mimetics, 18–19
Arterial blood gas levels, fetal, 66, 66–67, 66t, 67
  and neurologic outcome, 4–5
  in cord blood, 39, 42
  in scalp blood, 39
  neonatal, in hypoxemia, 99t, 107–111, 108t, 109t
  target range for, 99, 105
Arterial pressure, fetal, in hypoxia/asphyxia, 70, 72, 75
  neonatal, improvement of, 100–102
Arteries, great, transposition of, 108, 108t
Asphyxia, definition of, 65–66
  fetal, 65–76
    and gestational age, 69
    and meconium staining, 252–253
    cardiovascular response to, 69–73
    causes of, 66
    chronic, 76
    endocrine and metabolic response to, 73
    experimental models of, 68–69
    intrapartum monitoring of. See *Fetal monitoring.*
    neurologic response to, 74–76
    sequelae of, 65
  perinatal/neonatal, and cerebral palsy, 6–7, 7t
    and fetal blood gas levels, 4–5
    and gastrointestinal damage, 164–165
    and hypoxic-ischemic encephalopathy, 104–120. See also *Hypoxic-ischemic encephalopathy.*
    and meconium, 3–4
    and mental retardation, 8
    and neonatal neurologic syndrome, 5
    and neurologic impairment, 2–3, 4t, 8–9. See also *Neurologic impairment*
    and seizures, 5–6
    and subependymal-intraventricular hemorrhage, 233–234
    cardiovascular response to, 95
    correlative signs of, 3–5
    degree of, evaluation of, 3, 4t
    electroencephalography in, 180t, 181t, *182*, 182–183
    epidemiology of, 2–9
    intrapartum monitoring for. See *Fetal monitoring.*
    nuclear magnetic resonance spectroscopy in, 190–194
    nutritional support in, 164–165
    placental factors in, epidemiologic studies of, 259–262, 260t, 261t

Aspiration, meconium, 42
pulmonary, during general anesthesia, 48–49
Ataxia, in cerebral palsy, 223. See also *Cerebral palsy.*
Athetosis-choreoathetosis, in cerebral palsy, 224 See also *Cerebral palsy.*
Atropine, in neonatal resuscitation, 101

B

Baby Doe regulations, 266–269, *267*
Baby Jane Doe case, *267,* 271
Ballard assessment, of gestational age, 240–241
Basal villitis, placental, 257
Bayley Scales of Infant Development, 244–246
Bed rest, for preterm labor, 18
Behavioral assessment, neonatal, 243–244
Behavioral problems. See also *Neurologic impairment.*
and cytomegalovirus infection, 84
and rubella, 87
Behavioral response, to fetal hypoxia/asphyxia, 73–74
Beta-mimetics, fetal effects of, 19–20
for preterm labor, 18–21
side effects of, 18–20
tolerance to, 20
Betamethasone, for fetal lung maturity enhancement, 13
Bicarbonate, in neonatal resuscitation, 99–100
Bilirubin. See also *Hyperbilirubinemia.*
neurotoxicity of, 148, 156–157
production of, 156
Birth trauma, and cerebral palsy, 232
and intracranial hemorrhage, imaging of, 209
Bleeding. See *Hemorrhage.*
Bleeding disorders, and anemia, 152–153
Blood gas levels, fetal, 55, 66–67, 66t
and neurologic outcome, 4–5
in cord blood, 39, 42
in scalp blood, 39
neonatal, in hypoxemia, 99t, 107–108t
target range for, 99, 105
Blood group incompatibilities. See *ABO incompatibility; Rh incompatibility.*
Blood pressure, fetal, variation in, in hypoxia/asphyxia, 70, 72
neonatal, improvement of, 100–102
in hypovolemia, 101
Blood sampling, fetal, for asphyxia, 39, 42
in maternal immune thrombocytopenia, 38
Blood transfusion. See *Transfusion.*
Brachial plexus injury, 43–44
Bradycardia, fetal, in hypoxia/asphyxia, 72–73
in regional anesthesia, 53–54
neonatal, causes of, 100
management of, 100–101
Brain. See also under *Cerebral.*
congenital malformations of, and cerebral palsy, 228–229
electroencephalography in, 183
maturation of, electroencephalographic demonstration of, *178,* 178–180, *179*

Brain damage. See also *Encephalopathy; Neurologic impairment.*
and hyperbilirubinemia, 157
and hypoglycemia, 142–146
and polycythemia, 154, 156
and seizures, 138
electroencephalographic assessment of, 180–184, 180t, 181t, *182*
in fetal hypoxia/asphyxia, 74–76
in hypoxic-ischemic encephalopathy, 115–117, 115t *116, 117.* See also *Hypoxic-ischemic encephalopathy.*
Brain energy metabolism, 142
noninvasive assessment of, 189–194
Brainstem necrosis, in hypoxic-ischemic encephalopathy, 116, 119
Brazelton neurobehavioral assessment, 243
Breast feeding, and jaundice, 157–158
and necrotizing enterocolitis, 169, 171
Breathing movements, fetal, in hypoxia/asphyxia, 73–74
Breech presentation, 35–36, 35t, 36t
and cerebral palsy, 229
Bretylium, for bupivacaine cardiotoxic reaction, 51
Bronchopulmonary dysplasia, electroencephalographic abnormalities in, 182–183
encephalopathy in, 182–183
in preterm infant, 15
Broviac catheter, for total parenteral nutrition, 164
Brow presentation, 35
Bupivacaine, side effects of, 47, 50, 51
Busulfan, teratogenicity of, 58t
Butorphanol, intrapartum, 54

C

Calcium, in neonatal resuscitation, 102
Calcium channel blockers, for preterm labor, 24
and ritodrine, 25
Cancer chemotherapeutic agents, teratogenicity of, 58t
Carbon monoxide, fetal exposure to, with maternal smoking, 155
Cardiac arrhythmias. See also *Bradycardia.*
and beta-mimetics, 18–19
Cardiac compression, in neonatal resuscitation, 97
Cardiac disease. See *Heart disease.*
Cardiac malformations, and maternal diabetes, 102, 105–106
ductus-dependent, 111, 111t
Cardiac output, fetal, redistribution of, in hypoxia/asphyxia, 70, 73
neonatal, assessment of, 100
decreased, signs of, 100
maintenance of, 105–107
resuscitative enhancement of, 100–102
Cardiogenic shock, treatment of, 106
Cardiomyopathy, neonatal hypertrophic, and maternal diabetes, 102, 105–106
Cardiopulmonary collapse, maternal, during general anesthesia, 47, 49–50
Cardiotonic therapy, immediate, 102
supportive, 105–106
Cardiovascular collapse, in fetal hypoxia/asphyxia, 74–75
maternal, in regional anesthesia, 50–51
Cardiovascular depression. See

Depression, neonatal.
Cardiovascular system, fetal, 66–68
Cardioversion, in neonatal resuscitation, 101
Case control study, 258, 258t
Catecholamines, for cardiac output enhancement, 102, 106
Catheterization, central venous, in total parenteral nutrition, 164
in neonatal resuscitation, 98
umbilical artery, and necrotizing enterocolitis, 170
in total parenteral nutrition, 163–164
Central venous catheterization, in total parenteral nutrition, 163–164
Central venous pressure, invasive measurement of, for hypovolemia, 101
Cephalic version, external, 36, 36t
Cephalopelvic disproportion, 37, 37t
Cerclage, cervical, 12
Cerebellar necrosis, in hypoxic-ischemic encephalopathy, 116, 119
Cerebellar sclerosis, in hypoxic-ischemic encephalopathy, 116
Cerebral blood flow, autoregulation of, 115
in fetal hypoxia/asphyxia, 72, 74–76
in hypoxic-ischemic encephalopathy, 114–115
in preterm infant, 115
noninvasive measurement of, 186–189
Cerebral edema, and fetal hypoxia/asphyxia, 74, 75–76
in hypoxic-ischemic encephalopathy, 119
imaging of, 216–218, *218, 219*
Cerebral infarction, focal, in hypoxic ischemic encephalopathy, imaging of, 216
periventricular hemorrhagic, imaging of, 212, *214*
Cerebral metabolism and biochemistry, noninvasive assessment of, 189–194
Cerebral oxygenation, noninvasive measurement of, *194,* 194–195
Cerebral palsy, 221–235
and Apgar score, 6, 7t, 42, 231
and birth trauma, 232
and birth weight, 224t, 227–228
and breech presentation, 229
and congenital infections, 229
and congenital malformations, 228–229
and fetal (nonperinatal) hypoxia/asphyxia, 76
and fetal monitoring, 230–231
and gestational age, 224t, 227
and head circumference, 228
and hypoxic-ischemic encephalopathy, 226–227, 231–235
and intracranial hemorrhage, 232, 233
and intrauterine growth retardation, 224t, 227–228
and maternal age, 227
and maternal neurologic disorders, 227
and meconium staining, 230
and mental retardation, 223–224
and neonatal asphyxia, 225–226, 230–235
and neonatal neurologic status, 231–235
and neonatal seizures, 136, 137, 232
and neonatal stroke, 232

and periventricular leukomalacia, 233–235
and placental abnormalities, 229
and prematurity, 224t, 227, 232–233
and race, 227
and reproductive history, 227
and seizures, 232
and socioeconomic status, 227
and subependymal-intraventricular hemorrhage, 233–234
and suboptimal obstetric care, 226–227
and twin gestation, 230
and umbilical cord length, 229
ataxia in, 223
athetosis-choreoathetosis in, 223
brain morphology in, 224–225
clinical phenotypes of, 222–223
definition of, 222
diagnosis of, time of, 222
dystonia in, 225
epidemiology of, 6–7, 7t, 224, 225–230, 224t
familial, 225–226
hemiplegia in, 223
historical overview of, 222
pathologic findings in, 225
perinatal risk factors in, 226–227
postnatal, 225–226
prepregnancy and pregnancy risk factors in, 227–230
prevalence of, 224, 224t
quadriplegia in, 223
radiologic findings in, 225
spastic diplegia in, 223
spastic syndromes in, 223
Cerebral response, to fetal hypoxia/asphyxia, 74–76
Cerebral vascular occlusion, in hypoxic-ischemic encephalopathy, 115
Cerebrospinal fluid, in congenital syphilis, 89
Cerebrovascular accident, neonatal, and cerebral palsy, 232
Cervical cerclage, 12
Cesarean section, anesthesia for. See Anesthesia, general.
for preterm delivery, 13
with dysfunctional labor, 37, 37t
with genital herpes, 81
with macrosomia, 43
with malpresentation, 35
with maternal immune thrombocytopenia, 38–39
with shoulder dystocia, 43
Chest compression, in neonatal resuscitation, 97
Child Abuse Rule, 266–269, 267
Chlorambucil, teratogenicity of, 58t
Chlordiazepoxide, teratogenicity of, 57, 58t
Chloroprocaine, fetal tolerance of, 54
Chlorpromazine, for anesthesia induction, 50
for neonatal narcotic withdrawal, 60
Chorangiosis, 255, 255, 261t
Choreoathetosis, in cerebral palsy, 223. See also Cerebral palsy.
Chorioamnionitis, 16–17, 256
and cerebral palsy, 229
and meconium staining, 253
Chorioretinitis, and toxoplasmosis, 88
Chronic lung disease, in preterm infant, 15

Cigarette smoking, maternal, fetal effects of, 155–156
Cimetidine, prior to general anesthesia, 48
Circulation, fetal-maternal, 66, 66–68, 66t, 67
impaired. See Asphyxia; Hypoxia.
preferential, in fetal hypoxia/asphyxia, 69–73
umbilical, reduction of, fetal cardiovascular response to, 71
uterine, in fetal hypoxia/asphyxia, 70, 73
Circulatory collapse, maternal, during general anesthesia, 47, 49–50
Coagulopathies, 152–153
Cocaine, fetal/neonatal effects of, 61–62
Cohort study, 257–258, 258t
Colchicine, teratogenicity of, 58t
Colloid, for hypovolemia, 101–102
Compound presentation, 35
Compression, cardiac, in neonatal resuscitation, 97
Computed tomography, in cerebral edema, 217, 219
in cerebral palsy, 225
in focal cerebral infarction, 216
in hypoglycemic encephalopathy, 218
in hypoxic-ischemic encephalopathy, 196
with diffuse injury, 217–218, 219
in multicystic encephalomalacia, 217, 219
in periventricular leukomalacia, 209–216, 211, 213–215
in subarachnoid hemorrhage, 209
in subependymal-intraventricular hemorrhage, 197–209
single photon emission, for cerebral blood flow measurement, 187
time of injury in, 225
Confounders, epidemiologic, 258, 258t
Congenital abnormalities, and alcohol, 59–60
and cerebral palsy, 228–229
and illicit drug use, 60–63
and therapeutic drug use, 57, 58t
cardiac, and maternal diabetes, 102, 105–106
ductus-dependent, 111, 111t
Congenital infections. See Infection, congenital.
Congenital malformations, and cerebral palsy, 228–229
Consultation, for extended intensive care, 111–112
Cord. See Umbilical cord.
Cord pH values, and Apgar score, 5
Coronary blood flow, in fetal hypoxia/asphyxia, 71
Cortical infarction, in hypoxic-ischemic encephalopathy, 115–116, 115t, 116, 119
Corticosteroids, for fetal lung maturity enhancement, 13
for preterm membrane rupture, 17
teratogenicity of, 58t
Coumarin, teratogenicity of, 58t
Cricoid pressure, for endotracheal intubation, for general anesthesia, 49
Crystalloid, for hypovolemia, 101–102
Cyanosis. See Asphyxia; Hypoxia.
Cyclophosphamide, teratogenicity of, 58t

Cyst, porencephalic, post-hemorrhagic, 207
Cystic encephalomalacia, imaging of, 217–218, 218
Cysts, in multicystic encephalomalacia, 218, 219
periventricular, benign, imaging of, 213, 215, 216, 218
in periventricular leukomalacia, 211, 212, 213–215
Cytomegalovirus infection, congenital, 83–85

D

Deafness, and congenital syphilis, 89
and cytomegalovirus infection, 84, 85
and rubella, 86–87
and toxoplasmosis, 88
Decision-making, in neonatal-perinatal medicine, 264t, 265, 265–266, 266
Deep gray nuclei, necrosis of, in hypoxic-ischemic encephalopathy, 116, 116, 119
Deflection malpresentation, 35
Defibrillation, in neonatal resuscitation, 101
Delivery, analgesia and anesthesia for. See Analgesics; Anesthesia.
and malpresentation, 35, 36, 229
and maternal immune thrombocytopenia, 38–39
and maternal infections, 37–38
cesarean. See Cesarean section.
episiotomy in, 39–40
forceps, 40–41
and cerebral palsy, 232
in preterm delivery, 40
outlet, with episiotomy, 39–40
in intrauterine growth retardation, 28
in macrosomia, 42–44
preterm. See also Labor, preterm; Prematurity.
causes of, 12
episiotomy in, 40
induced, after membrane rupture, 17
management of, 12–13
outlet forceps in, 40
prevention of, 12
vaginal vs. cesarean route for, 13
route of, and subependymal-intraventricular hemorrhage, 233
traumatic
and cerebral palsy, 232
and intracranial hemorrhages, imaging of, 209
vacuum, 41
Depression, neonatal. See also Asphyxia; Hypoxia; Respiratory distress.
and analgesia/anesthesia, 54–55
and cerebral palsy, 230–231
resuscitation in. See Resuscitation.
Developmental delay. See also Intellectual impairment; Neurologic impairment.
and acquired immunodeficiency syndrome, 85
and cytomegalovirus infection, 85
and rubella, 87
Dexamethasone, for fetal lung maturity enhancement, 13
Dextrose, for neonatal hypoglycemia, 144, 145t
Diabetes mellitus, maternal, and

neonatal hypertrophic
    cardiomyopathy, 143, 146
and neonatal hypoglycemia, 143,
    146. See also *Hypoglycemia.*
    beta-mimetics in, 19
Diamond-Blackfan syndrome, 149
Diazepam, for anesthesia induction, 49
    for neonatal narcotic withdrawal, 60
    teratogenicity of, 58t
Diazoxide, for hypoglycemia, 145
Diet. See *Nutritional support.*
Diethylstilbestrol, teratogenicity of, 58t
Diphenylhydantoin, teratogenicity of, 58t
2,3-Diphospho-glycerate, and hemolytic
    anemia, 152
Disseminated intravascular coagulation,
    153
Disseminated neonatal herpes virus
    infection, 80–81
Diuretics, for pulmonary parenchymal
    disease, 110
Dobutamine, for cardiac output
    enhancement, 102, 106
Dopamine, for cardiac output
    enhancement, 102, 106
    toxicity of, 106
    with nitroprusside, 107
Drugs, analgesics. See *Analgesics.*
    and electroencephalographic
        abnormalities, 181
    and hyperbilirubinemia, 157, 158
    anesthetic. See *Anesthesia.*
    placental transfer of, 54, 57
    recreational, fetal/neonatal effects of,
        57, 59–63
    teratogenic, 57–63, 58t
    therapeutic, fetal/neonatal effects of,
        57, 58t
Dubowitz gestational age assessment,
    240–241
Dubowitz neurologic assessment, 242
Ductal patency, 110
Ductal shunting, and hypoxemia, 108,
    108t, 109t
Ductus arteriosus, patency of, persistent,
    109–110
    therapeutic maintenance of, 111
Ductus arteriosus blood flow, in fetal
    hypoxia/asphyxia, 71
Ductus venosus blood flow, in fetal
    hypoxia/asphyxia, 71
Dystonia, in cerebral palsy, 223. See also
    Cerebral palsy.

E

Eclampsia. See *Preeclampsia.*
Edema, cerebral, and fetal
    hypoxia/asphyxia, 74, 75–76
    in hypoxic-ischemic encephalopathy,
        119
    imaging of, 216–218, *218*
    placental, 224
    pulmonary, and beta-mimetics, 19
Electrical impedance plethysmography, for
    cerebral blood flow measurement, 189
Electrocardiography, in neonatal
    resuscitation, 97
Electroencephalography, 176–185
    abnormal patterns on, 180–184
        in bronchopulmonary dysplasia,
            182–183

in congenital brain malformations,
    183
in herpes encephalitis, 184
in inborn errors of metabolism, 183
in intraventricular hemorrhage, 183,
    184
in periventricular leukomalacia, 182,
    183–184
nonpathologic causes of, 181
continuous monitoring with, 184–185
delta brushes in, 178, *179*
dysmature background activity on
    significance of, 183
frontal sharp waves in, 178, *179*
in iatrogenic paralysis, 183
in neonatal encephalopathy, 118,
    119–120, 180–184, 180t, 181t, *182*
    predictive value of, 180–183, 181t
in neonatal seizures, *126–129,*
    130–134, *131–134,* 132t
    interpretation of, 138–139
interburst interval in, 184
interpretation of, 178
maturational changes on, 178–180,
    179, 180
sleep patterns on, 178, 179, *179*
suppression burst patterns in, 184
technical aspects of, 177–178
temporal theta bursts in, 178, *179*
Encephalitis, herpes,
    electroencephalography in, 184
    herpes simplex virus, 80–81
    rubella, 86
    varicella zoster, 83
Encephalomalacia, multicystic, imaging
    of, 217–218, *219*
Encephalopathy. See also *Brain damage.*
    bilirubin, 148, 156–157
    electroencephalographic assessment of,
        180–184, 180t, 181t, *182*
    human immunodeficiency virus, 85–86
    hypoxic ischemic, 113–120. See also
        Hypoxic-ischemic encephalopathy.
    postasphyxial, 5
    static, 223. See also *Cerebral palsy.*
Endocrine response, to fetal
    hypoxia/asphyxia, 73
Endotracheal intubation, in general
    anesthesia, 48, 49
    in neonatal resuscitation, 97
Enteral feeding. See *Nutritional support.*
Enterocolitis, necrotizing. See *Necrotizing
    enterocolitis.*
Ephidrine, for maternal anesthesia-
    induced hypotension, 53
Epidemiology, case control study in, 258,
    258t
    cohort study in, 257–258, 258t
    confounders in, 258, 258t
    logistic regression analysis in,
        260, 260t
    methods of, 257–258
    of placental factors in perinatal
        asphyxia, 259–262, 260t, 261t
    pathogenetic concepts and, 258–259
    univariate analysis in, 258, 259
Epidural anesthesia. See *Anesthesia,
    regional.*
Epidural hematoma, imaging of, 209
Epilepsy. See *Seizures.*
    maternal, and cerebral palsy, 227
Epinephrine, and uterine blood flow,
    53–54

and uterine contractility, 52
    for test dose, in regional anesthesia, 52
    in neonatal resuscitation, 100–101
Episiotomy, 39–40
Erb's palsy, 43–44
Erythroblastosis fetalis, and neonatal
    hypoglycemia, 144
Erythrocytes, first postnatal day, normal
    values for, 149t
    packed. See also *Transfusion.*
        for anemia, 107
        for hypovolemia, 102
    placental nucleated, 253–254, *254*
        and perinatal asphyxia, 259–262,
            261t
Erythropoiesis, failure of, causes of, 149
Erythropoietin, fetal production of, 156
Esophageal intubation, in general
    anesthesia, 48
Ethics, and treatment decisions, 264–272.
    See also *Intensive care.*
Etomidate, for anesthesia induction, 49,
    50
External cephalic version, of breech
    presentation, 36, 36t
Extracorporeal membrane oxygenation,
    and intracranial hemorrhage, 209,
    210

F

Face presentation, 35
Facial abnormalities, in fetal alcohol
    syndrome, 59
Feeding. See *Nutritional support.*
Fenoprofen, for preterm labor, 23
Fentanyl, for anesthesia induction, 49
Fetal alcohol effect, 59
Fetal alcohol syndrome, 59–60
    and mental retardation, 8
Fetal assessment, in intrauterine growth
    retardation, 26–28
Fetal membranes, preterm rupture of,
    12–13, 16–17. See also *Prematurity.*
Fetal monitoring, intrapartum, 39, 42
    and cerebral palsy, 230–231
    and hypoxia/asphyxia, 70, 72, 73
    and maternal immune
        thrombocytopenia, 38–39
    and meconium staining, 41
    and neonatal seizures, 6
    cord blood sampling in, 39, 42
    effectiveness of, 230–231
    in preterm delivery, 13
    scalp blood sampling in, 39
Fluid therapy, for cardiac output
    enhancement, 101–102
Forceps delivery, 40–41
    and cerebral palsy, 232
    in preterm delivery, 40
    outlet, with episiotomy, 39–40
Fresh frozen plasma. See also
    Transfusion.
    for disseminated intravascular
        coagulation, 153
    for hypovolemia, 101, 102
Furosemide, for pulmonary parenchymal
    disease, 110

G

Gastrointestinal tract, development of,
    161t
    incomplete, complications of, 162t

hypoxic ischemic damage to, 164–165
    and necrotizing enterocolitis 169–170
Gavage feeding, 160–161. See also
    Nutritional support.
General anesthesia. See *Anesthesia,
    general.*
Genital herpes, 38, 79–82
Gentamicin, for necrotizing enterocolitis
    prophylaxis, 170
Gesell Development Schedules, 244–246
Gestational age, assessment of, 240–241
    electroencephalographic, 178–180,
        180, 181
Glial fatty metamorphosis, in hypoxic-
    ischemic encephalopathy, 116
Glial scar, in periventricular leukomalacia,
    imaging of, 212–216, *217*
Glucagon, for hypoglycemia, 145
Glucocorticoids, for fetal lung maturity
    enhancement, 13
Glucose, and brain damage, in fetal
    hypoxia/asphyxia, 75
    and brain energy metabolism, 142
    in resuscitation, 97, 98–99
    measurement of, in hypoglycemia, 144
    neonatal, normal values for, 142
    screening for, 144
Group B streptococcal infection,
    maternal, 38
Growth retardation, intrauterine, 25–28
    and cerebral palsy, 227–228
    and chronic fetal hypoxia/asphyxia,
        76
    and maternal smoking, 155
    and preeclampsia, 155
    placental, and cerebral palsy, 229

H

Head circumference, and cerebral palsy,
    228
Hearing loss, and cytomegalovirus
    infection, 84, 85
    and rubella, 86–87
    and toxoplasmosis, 88
    in congenital syphilis, 89
Heart, congenital malformations of, and
    maternal diabetes, 102, 105–106
    ductus-dependent, 111, 111t
    fetal, 67, 68
Heart disease, congenital, and rubella, 86
    therapeutic maintenance of ductal
        patency for, 111, 111t
    maternal, anesthesia in, 49
Heart rate, fetal, monitoring of. See *Fetal
    monitoring.*
    neonatal, pharmacologic enhancement
        of, 100–101
Hematocrit, neonatal, in hyperviscosity
    syndrome, 153–154
    in polycythemia, 153–154, *154*
    target level for, 107
Hematologic disorders, 148–158
Hematologic values, normal neonatal,
    148, 149t
Hematoma, epidural, imaging of, 209
    subdural, 209
Hemiplegia, in cerebral palsy, 223. See
    also *Cerebral palsy.*
Hemodynamics, fetal-maternal, *66,*
    66–68, 66t, *67*
    abnormal. See *Asphyxia, Hypoxia.*

Hemoglobin, cord blood, normal values
    for, 149t
    fetal, 66
    neonatal, 107
Hemolysis. See also *Rh incompatibility.*
    and anemia, 151–152
    and hyperbilirubinemia, 150, 156–158
    neonatal, causes of, 151t
Hemophilia, 152–153
Hemorheologic disorders, neonatal, and
    maternal smoking, 155–156
    and preeclampsia, 155–156
Hemorrhage, fetal-to-maternal, 149, 150
    intracranial, and extracorporeal
        membrane oxygenation, 209, *210*
        imaging of, 198–209
    intraparenchymal, 198, *205, 206, 210*
    intraventricular. See *Intraventricular
        hemorrhage.*
    intravillous placental, 255, 261t
    maternal, management of, 49–50
    neonatal, acute vs. chronic, 150, 150t
        causes of, 149–151, 149t
        clinical features, of, 150t
        closed space, 150–151
        treatment of, 150, 150t
        types of, 149t
    periventricular, in hypoxic-ischemic
        encephalopathy, 117, 120
    subarachnoid, computerized
        tomography of, 209
        in hypoxic-ischemic encephalopathy,
            117
    subependymal-intraventricular. See
        *Subependymal-intraventricular
        hemorrhage.*
Hemorrhagic disorders, and anemia,
    152–153
Hepatic blood flow, in fetal
    hypoxia/asphyxia, 71
Hepatic rupture, 157
Herpes encephalitis,
    electroencephalography in, 184
Herpes simplex virus infection, 38, 79–82
Herpes zoster virus infection maternal, 82
High forceps delivery. See *Forceps
    delivery.*
Hormonal response, to fetal
    hypoxia/asphyxia, 73
Human immunodeficiency virus infection,
    85–86
Hyaline membrane disease, hypoxemia in,
    108t, 109–110
Hydration, for preterm labor, 18
Hydrocephalus, in hypoxic-ischemic
    encephalopathy, 117
    post-hemorrhagic, imaging of, *200,
        201,* 207
Hydrocortisone, for hypoglycemia, 145,
    145t
Hydrops, placental, 255
Hyperbilirubinemia, 148, 156–158
    and breast feeding, 157–158
    in preterm infant, 14–15
Hyperglycemia, and beta-mimetics, 19
Hyperinsulinemia, neonatal, 143
Hyperoxia test, 107–108, 108t
Hyperoxia-hyperventilation test, 108–109,
    108t
Hypertension, maternal. See
    Preeclampsia.
    pulmonary, and hypoxemia, 108t,
        109t, 110–111

Hypertrophic cardiomyopathy, neonatal,
    and maternal diabetes, 102, 105–106
Hyperventilation, assisted, 105
Hyperviscosity syndrome, 153–154
    and maternal smoking, 155–156
    and preeclampsia, 155–156
    as epiphenomenon, 156
Hypoglycemia, 98–99
    and birth weight, 143
    and erythroblastosis fetalis, 144
    and inborn errors of metabolism, 144
    and hypoxic-ischemic encephalopathy,
        114
    and pituitary disorders, 144
    brain damage in, mechanism of,
        142–143
    clinical features of, 143–144
    definition of, 142
    drug-induced, 143–144
    etiology of, 143–144, 143t
    imaging in, 218
    outcome of, 145–146, 145t
    treatment of, 144–145, 145t
Hypokalemia, and beta-mimetics, 19
Hypopituitarism, and neonatal
    hypoglycemia, 144
Hypotension, in regional anesthesia,
    50–51, 52–53
Hypothermia, in preterm infant, 14
Hypovolemia, maternal, 49–50
    neonatal, correction of, 101–102, 152
Hypoxemia. See also *Asphyxia; Hypoxia.*
    evaluation of. See also *Blood gas levels.*
        medicolegal aspects of, 104–105,
            111–112
    fetal, intrapartum, monitoring for, 39,
        42
    neonatal, physiologic classification of,
        99t
    refractory, evaluation and
        management of, 107–111, 108t
Hypoxia. See also *Asphyxia; Hypoxemia.*
    definition of, 65
    fetal, 65–76
        and gestational age, 69
        and maternal smoking, 155
        and preeclampsia, 155
        cardiovascular response to, 69–73
        causes of, 66
        chronic, 76
        endocrine and metabolic response to,
            73
        neurologic response to, 74–76
        sequelae of, 65. See also *Neurologic
            impairment.*
    maternal, and general anesthesia, 47
        fetal cardiovascular response to,
            69–70, 71
    neonatal, and ischemic encephalopathy,
        104–120. See also *Hypoxic
        ischemic encephalopathy.*
        and necrotizing enterocolitis,
            169–170
        resuscitation in, 94–102. See also
            Resuscitation, neonatal.
    physiologic classification of, 99, 99t
    sequelae of. See *Brain damage;
        Neurologic impairment.*
Hypoxic-ischemic encephalopathy,
    113–120
    and cerebral palsy, 231–235
    and neurologic impairment, 119–120,
        136

and periventricular leukomalacia,
   imaging of, 209–216, *211,*
   213–215, 217
and seizures, 119–120, 136
and subependymal intraventricular
   hemorrhage, imaging of, 197–207,
   199–208
cerebral edema in, 216–217, *218*
clinical features of, 117–120
clinicopathologic syndromes in,
   119–120
diffuse, imaging of, 216–218, *218, 219*
electroencephalography in, 118,
   119–120, 180t, 181t, *182,* 182–183
focal infarction in, imaging of, 217
imaging in, 114, *115,* 186–187, *187,*
   190–194, 196–219
management of, 118–119
   future prospects for, 120, *120*
multicystic encephalomalacia in,
   217–219, *219*
neuropathology of, 115–117, 115t, *116,*
   117
nuclear magnetic resonance spectroscopy
   in, 190–194
pathophysiology of, 113–115
positron emission tomography in,
   186–187, *188*
prognosis in, 120
risk factors for, 233–234

I

IgA, secretory, 169
Immune thrombocytopenia, maternal,
   and delivery, 38–39
Immunization, rubella, 87
   varicella zoster, 83
Inborn errors of metabolism,
   electroencephalography in, 183
Indomethacin, for persistent patent
   ductus arteriosus, 110
   for preterm labor, 23–24
   with ritodrine, 25
Induction drugs, for general anesthesia,
   49, 50
Infarction, cerebral, focal, in hypoxic-
   ischemic encephalopathy, imaging
   of, 216
      periventricular hemorrhagic, imaging
      of, 212, *214*
   placental, 253, 261t
      and cerebral palsy, 229
Infection, bacterial, and necrotizing
   enterocolitis, 170
   congenital, and anemia, 149
      and cerebral palsy, 229
   cytomegalovirus, 83–85
   herpes simplex virus, 79–82
   human immunodeficiency virus,
      85–86
   rubella virus, 86–87
   Toxoplasmosis gondii, 87–88
   Treponema pallidum, 88–89
   varicella zoster virus, 82–83
   intrauterine, and preterm membrane
      rupture, 16–17
   and labor and delivery, 37–38
   placental, *256,* 256–257, *257*
Inotropic drugs, for cardiac output
   maintenance, 105–106
   for cardiac output enhancement, 102
   in resuscitation, 102

Intellectual impairment. See also *Mental
   retardation; Neurologic impairment.*
   and cytomegalovirus infection, 84, 85
   and rubella, 86–87
Intensive care, and quality of life
   considerations, 269–271
   appropriateness of, 264–272
   Baby Doe regulations and, 266–269,
      267
   decision-making in, 264t, *265,*
      265–266, *266*
   extended, 104–112
      consultation and referral for,
         111–112
      medicolegal aspects of, 104–105,
         111–112
   immediate. See *Resuscitation, neonatal.*
   moral implications of, 269–271
   regulation of physician behavior in,
      266, *267*
Intervillositis, placental, 256
Intracranial hemorrhage. See *Hemorrhage.*
Intralipid, and hyperbilirubinemia, 158
Intraparenchymal hemorrhage, imaging
   of, 198, *205, 206, 209, 210*
Intrauterine growth retardation. See
   Growth retardation, intrauterine.
Intraventricular hemorrhage, and
   extracorporeal membrane
   oxygenation, 207–209, *210*
   and maternal immune
      thrombocytopenia, 38–39
   electroencephalography in, 183, 184
   grading of, 197
   imaging of, 197–209, *199–208, 210*
   in hypoxic-ischemic encephalopathy,
      117, 120
   in preterm infant, 14
   neonatal, with maternal immune
      thrombocytopenia, 38–39
   sequelae of, *199–201,* 207
Intubation, endotracheal, in general
   anesthesia, 48, 49
   in neonatal resuscitation, 97
   esophageal, in general anesthesia, 48
Iodides, teratogenicity of, 58t
Ischemia, cerebral. See also *Hypoxic-
   ischemic encephalopathy.*
   gut, and necrotizing enterocolitis
      169–170
   myocardial, and beta-mimetics, 19
   placental, 253, *253,* 261t
Isoproterenol, in neonatal resuscitation,
   100–101

J

Jaundice. See *Hyperbilirubinemia.*

K

Kernicterus, 156–157. See also
   Hyperbilirubinemia.
   and cerebral palsy, 223. See also
      Cerebral palsy.
   in preterm infant, 14–15
Ketamine, for anesthesia induction, 49
Ketone bodies, and brain energy
   metabolism, 142
Kleihauer-Behtke method, 149, 150

L

Labor, abnormal, 36–37, 37t
   and malpresentation, 35, 36

anesthesia for. See *Anesthesia.*
   normal, 36, *36, 37*
   pain in, management of. See
      Analgesics, Anesthesia.
   fetal effects of, 55
   preterm, 17–25. See also *Delivery,
      preterm; Prematurity.*
   and preterm membrane rupture, 16
   bed rest for, 18
   causes of, 12, 17
   definition of, 17
   hydration for, 18
   prevention of, 12
   sedation for, 18
   tocolytics for, 18–25. See also
      Tocolytics.
Laceration, perineal, and episiotomy, 40
Lactate, and brain damage, in fetal
   hypoxia/asphyxia, 74–75
Lactic acid, fetal, and neurologic
   outcome, 4–5
Large for gestational age. See
   Macrosomia.
Laryngoscopy, fiberoptic, prior to general
   anesthesia, 49
Learning disabilities. See *Intellectual
   impairment.*
Leukomalacia, periventricular. See
   Periventricular leukomalacia.
Lidocaine, fetal tolerance of, 54
   for general anesthesia, in
      hypertension/toxemia, 49
   for tests dose, in regional anesthesia, 52
Liver, blood flow in, in fetal
   hypoxia/asphyxia, 71
   rupture of, 151
Local anesthesia. See *Anesthesia, local.*
Logistic regression analysis, 259, 260, 260t
Low birth weight. See also *Growth
   retardation, intrauterine;
   Prematurity.*
   and hypoglycemia, 143
   and maternal smoking, 155
   and preeclampsia
   definition of, 11
   incidence of, 11–12
   neurologic outcome with, 12
Low forceps delivery, 40, 41
   definition of, 40
   in preterm delivery, 40
Lung. See also under *Pulmonary,
   Respiratory.*
Lung maturity, fetal, enhancement of,
   glucocorticoids for, 13

M

Macrosomia, 42–43
   and hypoglycemia, 143
   and shoulder dystocia and brachial
      plexus injury, 43–44
Magnesium sulfate, for preterm labor,
   21–23
   with ritodrine, 24
Magnetic resonance imaging, in hypoxic-
   ischemic encephalopathy, 196
   in periventricular leukomalacia,
      212–216, *217*
Magnetic resonance spectroscopy,
   189–194
Malpractice, 271–272
   and multifactorial nature of neurologic
      impairment, 8, 75
Malpresentation, 34–36, 35t, 36t

and cerebral palsy, 229
Mantel-Haenszel procedure, 258, 258t
Maturity assessment, neonatal, 244–246
Mechanical ventilation. See *Ventilation.*
Meconium aspiration, 42
Meconium staining, 3–4, 252–253
  and cerebral palsy, 230
  and perinatal asphyxia, 259–262, 260t,
    261t
  management of, 41–42
Membranes, preterm rupture of, 12–13,
  16–17. See also *Prematurity.*
Membranitis, placental, 256
Meningoencephalitis. See *Encephalitis.*
Meningovascular syphilis, chronic, 89
Mental retardation. See also *Intellectual
  impairment, Neurologic impairment.*
  and cerebral palsy, 223–254
  and congenital cytomegalovirus
    infection, 84–85
  and fetal alcohol syndrome, 8, 59
  and neonatal seizures, 136, 137
  and toxoplasmosis, 88
  epidemiology of, 8
  multifactorial natures of, 223–224
Mentum posterior presentation, persistent,
  35
Meperidine, intrapartum, 54
Mepivacaine, fetal tolerance of, 54
Meprobamate, teratogenicity of, 58t
Mercaptopurine, teratogenicity of, 58t
Metabolic acidosis, and neonatal asphyxia,
  4–5
  correction of, in neonatal resuscitation,
    99–100
  fetal, and neurologic outcome, 4–5
Metabolic imbalances, and beta-mimetics,
  19
  in hypoxic-ischemic encephalopathy,
    113–114, *114*
Metabolic response, to fetal
  hypoxia/asphyxia, 73
Metabolism, brain energy, 142
  cerebral, noninvasive assessment of,
    189–194
  inborn errors of,
    electroencephalography in, 183
Methylaminopterin, teratogenicity of, 58t
Metoclopramide, prior to general
  anesthesia, 48
Metocuride iodide, for paralysis
  induction, for supportive ventilation,
    105
Microcephaly, and congenital
  cytomegalovirus infection, 84–85
Midforceps delivery, 40–41
  and cerebral palsy, 233
Milk, breast. See *Breast feeding.*
Monitoring. See *Fetal monitoring.*
Moral aspects, of treatment decisions,
  264–272.
  See also *Intensive care.*
Morphine, therapeutic, for neonatal
  narcotic withdrawal, 60
Motor disabilities, and acquired
  immunodeficiency syndrome, 85
  and rubella, 87
Motor disorders, and toxoplasmosis, 88
Movement, fetal, in hypoxia/asphyxia,
  73–74
Mucocutaneous herpes simplex virus
  infection, 80–81

Muller-Hillis maneuver, 37
Multicystic encephalomalacia, imaging of,
  217–218, *219*
Muscular dystrophy, magnetic resonance
  spectroscopy in, 190
Myocardial dysfunction, treatment of,
  resuscitative, 102
  supportive, 105–107
Myocardial ischemia, and beta-mimetics,
  19

N

Naloxone, intrapartum, 54
Naprosyn, for preterm labor, 23
Narcotics, fetal addiction to, 60–61
  therapeutic, for neonatal narcotic
    withdrawal, 60
Nasogastric feeding, 160–161. See also
  Nutritional support.
Near infrared oxygen sufficiency scope,
  194, 194–195
Necrotizing enterocolitis, 165–171
  clinical features of, 165–166, 165t
  diagnosis of, 166
  epidemiology of, 165
  in preterm infant, 15
  management of, 166
  nutritional support in 166–167
  pathogenesis of, 166, *166, 167*
    and enteral feeding, 167–169
    and infectious agents, 170
    and vitamin E, 170
    immunologic factors in, 169
    ischemic-hypoxic factors in, 169–170
  prevention of, 170–171
  radiologic features of, 166
  risk factors for, *166*
  staging of, 166–167, 168t
Neonatal assessment, 239–247
  and cerebral palsy, 231–235
  behavioral, 243–244
  historical origins of, 239–240
  maturity, 244–246
  neurologic, 241–243
  of condition at birth, 231–235, 240.
    See also *Apgar score*
  of gestational age, 240–241
    electroencephalographic, 178–180,
      180, 181
  predictive value of, 246
  scope and limitations of, 246
Neonatal depression. See also *Asphyxia;
  Hypoxia; Respiratory distress.*
  and analgesia/anesthesia, 54–55
  and cerebral palsy, 230–231
  assessment of. See *Neonatal assessment.*
  resuscitation in. See *Resuscitation.*
Neonatal neurologic syndrome, 5
Neurobehavioral assessment, neonatal,
  243–244
Neurobehavioral Maturity Assessment for
  Preterm Infants, 244–246
Neuroimaging. See also specific methods
  of.
  in hypoxic-ischemic encephalopathy,
    196–219
  of cerebral edema, 216–217, *219*
  of focal cerebral infarction, 216
  of hypoglycemic encephalopathy, 218
  of hypoxic-ischemic encephalopathy,
    186–187, *188,* 190–194, 196–219

with diffuse injury, 217–218, *218,
  219*
of intracranial hemorrhages, 197–209,
  199–208, 210, 211
of multicystic encephalomalacia,
  217–218, *219*
of periventricular leukomalacia,
  209–216, *211, 213–215, 217*
Neurologic impairment. See also specific
  types of.
  and acquired immunodeficiency
    syndrome, 85–86
  and bronchopulmonary dysplasia,
    182–183
  and congenital infections, 79–89
  and cytomegalovirus infection, 84–85
  and fetal blood gas levels, 4–5
  and fetal hypoxia/asphyxia, 74–76
  and herpes simplex virus infection,
    80–81
  and hypoglycemia, 145–146
  and hypoxic-ischemic encephalopathy,
    119–120, 136
  and low birth weight, 12
  and maternal substance abuse, 57–63
  and meconium staining, 4
  and neonatal neurologic syndrome, 5
  and neonatal seizures, 5–6, 7t, 136–138
  and perinatal asphyxia, 2–3, 6–9, 7t
  and rubella, 86–87
  and syphilis, 89
  and toxoplasmosis, 87–88
  and varicella zoster infection, 82–83
  multifactorial nature of, 8–9, 75
  neonatal assessment of, 241–243
  prediction of, 246
    electroencephalographic, 180–184,
      180t, 181t, *182*
  treatment of, ethical-legal
    considerations in, 264–272. See
    also *Intensive care.*
Neuromuscular blockade, for supportive
  ventilation, 105
  electroencephalographic monitoring in,
    183
Neurosyphilis, 88–89
Neurotransmitters, in hypoxic-ischemic
  encephalopathy, 114
Nicardipine, for preterm labor, 24
Nifedipine, for preterm labor, 24
NIROS-SCOPE, *193,* 193–194
Nitrogen mustard, teratogenicity of, 58t
Nitroprusside, for anesthesia induction,
  50
  for cardiac output enhancement,
    189–194
  for hyaline membrane disease, 110
  for neonatal pulmonary hypertension,
    111
Nuclear magnetic resonance spectroscopy,
  189–194
  phosphorus, in hypoxic-ischemic
    encephalopathy, 114 *114*
  proton, 120, *120*
Nutritional support, 160–171
  enteral, 160–162
  in asphyxia, 164–165
  in management of necrotizing
    enterocolitis, 165–171, 167
  in pathogenesis of necrotizing
    enterocolitis, 167–169, 170–171
  parenteral, 162–164

O

Obstetrical anesthesia, 46–55. See also
    Anesthesia.
Obstetrical care, suboptimal, and cerebral
    palsy, 226–227
    and malpractice, 271–272
Obstetrical shock, 49–50
Ocular disorders, and cytomegalovirus
    infection, 83–85
    and rubella, 86–87
    and toxoplasmosis, 88
Oligohydramnios, in intrauterine growth
    retardation, 27
    in premature membrane rupture, 16–17
Opiates, fetal addiction to, 60–61
    intrapartum, 54
    therapeutic, for neonatal narcotic
        withdrawal, 60
Oral contraceptives, teratogenicity of, 58t
Outlet forceps delivery, 40, 41
Oxygen, arterial. See also *Blood gas
    levels.*
    target range for, 99, 105
    supplemental, in neonatal resuscitation,
        97
        prior to general anesthesia, 47
    toxicity of, 15, 99, 210, 211
Oxygen tension. See *PO₂.*
Oxygenation, and cyanosis, 152
    cerebral, noninvasive measurement of,
        194, 194–195
    extracorporeal membrane, and
        intracranial hemorrhage, 210, 211
    inadequate. See *Asphyxia, Hypoxemia,
        Hypoxia.*
    of fetal tissues, 66, 66–68, 66t, 67
Oxytocin, for dysfunctional labor, 37–37t

P

PaCO₂, target range for, 105
Pain, labor, fetal effects of, 55
    management of. See *Analgesics,
        Anesthesia.*
Pallor, neonatal, differential diagnosis of,
    152t
Pancuronium bromide, for paralysis
    induction, for supportive ventilation,
    105
Panhypopituitarism, and neonatal
    hypoglycemia, 144
PaO₂, in hypoxemia, 99t, 107–111, 108t,
    109t
    target range for, 99, 105
Paracervical block. See also *Anesthesia,
    regional.*
    and fetal bradycardia, 53
Paralysis, and brachial plexus injury,
    43–44
    induced, electroencephalographic
        monitoring in, 183
    for supportive ventilation, 105
Paregoric, for neonatal narcotic
    withdrawal, 60
Parenteral feeding. See *Nutritional
    support.*
Patent ductus arteriosus, in preterm
    infant, 14
    persistent, 110
PCP, fetal effects of, 62–63
Pentazocine, intrapartum, 54
Perinatal telencephalic
    leukoencephalopathy, 116–117

Perineal laceration, and episiotomy, 40
Periventricular cysts, benign, imaging of,
    213–215, 216, *218*
    in periventricular leukomalacia, *211,*
        212, *213–215*
Periventricular hemorrhage, in hypoxic-
    ischemic encephalopathy, 117, 120
Periventricular hemorrhagic infarction,
    imaging of, 212, *214*
Periventricular leukomalacia, and cerebral
    palsy, 233
    and stroke, 232
    electroencephalography in, *182,
        183–184*
    imaging of, 209–216, *211, 213–215,
        217*
    in hypoxic-ischemic encephalopathy,
        117, *117*
    risk factors for, 233–234
Perivillositis, placental, 256
Persistent mentum posterior presentation,
    35
Persistent patent ductus arteriosus, 110
pH determination, of cord blood, 39, 42
    of fetal scalp blood, 39
Phencyclidine, fetal effects of, 62–63
Phenobarbital, for neonatal narcotic
    withdrawal, 60
Phentolamine mesylate, for dopamine
    tissue necrosis, 106
Phosphate compounds, in hypoxic-
    ischemic encephalopathy, 114, *114*
Phosphocreatine-phosphorus ratio, in
    neonatal asphyxia, 190–191
Phosphorus nuclear magnetic resonance
    spectroscopy, in hypoxic-ischemic
    encephalopathy, 114, *114*
Phototherapy, for neonatal jaundice, 157
Physician behavior, regulation of, 266,
    267
Pituitary dysfunction, and neonatal
    hypoglycemia, 144
Placenta, abnormalities of, and cerebral
    palsy, 229
    and perinatal asphyxia, epidemiologic
        study of, 259–262, 260t, 261t
    pathogenetic classification of,
        252–257
    abruption of, and cerebral palsy, 229
    and cocaine, 61
    avascular villi in, 254, *254,* 261t
    disorders of, and fetal
        hypoxia/asphyxia, 66
    drug passage across, 54, 57
    dysmaturity of, 255, *255,* 261t
    edema of, 255
    examination of, clinical indications for,
        251
        routine, checklist for, 251, *251*
        techniques of, 251
    fetal nucleated red cells in, and
        perinatal asphyxia, 259–262, 261t
    infarction of, 253, 261t
    infectious lesions of, 256–257, 261t
    intimal cushions in, 254, *254,* 261t
    intravillous hemorrhage in, 255, 261t
    ischemia of, 253, *253,* 261t
    meconium staining of. See *Meconium
        staining.*
    noninfectious lesions of, 252–256
        and perinatal asphyxia, 259–262,
            260t, 261t
    nucleated red cells in, 253–254, *254,*

        261t
    samples of, storage of, 251
    tissue selection for, 251
    textbooks on 252
    thrombotic lesions in, 254, *254,* 261t
    villitis in, 255, *255*
Placenta previa, and cerebral palsy, 229
Placental perfusion, in regional
    anesthesia, 52–54
Plasma, fresh frozen. See also
    Transfusion.
    for disseminated intravascular
        coagulation, 153
    for hypovolemia, 101, 102
Platelet transfusion, for
    thrombocytopenia, 153
Plethysmography, electrical impedance,
    for cerebral blood flow measurement,
    189
    venous occlusion, 187–189
Pneumonia, bacterial, hypoxemia in,
    108t, 109–110
PO₂, and cyanosis, 152
    fetal-maternal levels of, *66,* 66–67, 66t,
        67
    in fetal hypoxia/asphyxia, 75
Polycythemia, 153–154, *154*
    and hyperbilirubinemia, 150, 156–158
    as epiphenomenon, 156
    diagnosis of, 156
    transfusion for, 154, 156
Pontosubicular necrosis, in hypoxic-
    ischemic encephalopathy, 116
Porencephaly, post-hemorrhagic, 207
Positive pressure ventilation. See
    Ventilation.
Positron emission tomography, for
    cerebral blood flow measurement,
    186–187, *188*
    in cerebral metabolism and
        biochemistry evaluation, 194
Postasphyxial encephalopathy, 5. See also
    *Hypoxic-ischemic encephalopathy,
    Neurologic impairment.*
Prechtl neurologic examination, 241–242
Preeclampsia, anesthesia in, 49–50
    fetal effects of, 155–156
Pregnancy. See also *Delivery; Labor.*
    optimality of, and cerebral palsy, 227
    risk factors in, for cerebral palsy,
        227–230
Preload, enhancement of, 101–102
Prematurity. See also *Labor, preterm.*
    and cerebral palsy, 224t, 227, 232–233
    and malpresentation, 34, 35
    and necrotizing enterocolitis, 165. See
        also *Necrotizing enterocolitis.*
    and periventricular leukomalacia, 233
    and preterm membrane rupture, 16
    and subependymal-intraventricular
        hemorrhage, 233
    anemia of, 151
    Apgar score in, 240
    complications of, 13–16
    electroencephalography in, continuous
        monitoring, 184–185
    exchange transfusion in, 151
    gastrointestinal tract underdevelopment
        in, complications of, 162t
    neonatal aspects of, 13–16
    neonatal assessment in, 240–246. See
        also *Neonatal assessment.*
    neurobehavioral assessment in, 243–244

nutritional support in. See *Nutritional support.*
obstetrical aspects of, 12–13
Preoxygenation, in general anesthesia, 47
Presentation, 34–36, 35t, 36t
breech, and cerebral palsy, 229
Pressor response, paradoxical, 95
Preterm delivery. See *Delivery, preterm.*
Preterm rupture of membranes, 12–13, 16–17. See also *Prematurity.*
Procarbazine, teratogenicity of, 58t
Prolapse, umbilical cord, in malpresentation, 34–35
Prostaglandin E₁, for maintenance of ductus arteriosus patency, 111
Prostaglandin synthetase inhibitors, for preterm labor, 23–24
Pulmonary arterial disease, and hypoxemia, 108t, 109t, 110–111
Pulmonary aspiration, during general anesthesia, 48–49
Pulmonary blood flow, in fetal hypoxia/asphyxia, 71
Pulmonary disease, chronic, in preterm infant, 15
Pulmonary edema, and beta-mimetics, 19
Pulmonary hypertension, and hypoxemia, 108t, 109t, 110–111
Pulmonary hypoplasia, and preterm membrane rupture, 16
Pulmonary parenchymal disease, and hypoxemia, 108t, 109t, 110
Pulmonary surfactant, and respiratory distress syndrome, 13–14

Q

Quadriplegia, in cerebral palsy, 223. See also *Cerebral palsy.*
Quality of life, and treatment decisions, 269–272. See also *Intensive care.*

R

Radioiodine, teratogenicity of, 58t
Ranitidine, prior to general anesthesia, 48
Red cells. See *Erythrocytes.*
Referral, for extended intensive care, 111–112
Regional anesthesia. See *Anesthesia, regional.*
Rehabilitation Act of 1973, 266, 267
Respiration, neonatal, maladaptive, pathophysiology of, 95
Respiratory depression. See *Neonatal depression.*
Respiratory distress, and anemia, 152, 153
and hypovolemia, 152, 153
and subependymal-intraventricular hemorrhage, 234
pathophysiology of, 95
resuscitation in, 94–102. See also *Resuscitation, neonatal.*
Respiratory distress syndrome, 13–14
chronic complications of, 15
prevention of, 13
Respiratory failure, in regional anesthesia, 50
Respiratory movements, fetal, in hypoxia/asphyxia, 73–74
Resuscitation, maternal, during general anesthesia, 47
neonatal, 94–102
ABC's of, 97t

anemia correction in, 152
anticipating need for, 95–96
bicarbonate in, 99–100
cardiac compression in, 97
cardiac output enhancement in, 100–102
cardiotonic therapy in, 102
drug therapy in, 97–102
for enhancement of cardiac output, 100–102
for restoration of metabolic homeostasis, 98–100
routes of administration for, 97–98
equipment for, 96, 96t
extended management after, 104–112
glucose in, 97, 98–99
guidelines for, 97
heart rate enhancement in, 100–101
hierarchy of interventions in, 97
hypocalcemia correction in, 102
hypovolemia correction in, 101–102
in meconium staining, 42
initiation of, 96–97
intubation in, 97
medicolegal aspects of, 102
objective of, 94–95
oxygen in, 97, 99
preparation for, 96, 96t
ventilatory assistance in, 97
Retardation. See *Growth retardation, intrauterine; Mental retardation.*
Retinopathy, in preterm infant, 15
Rh incompatibility, and neonatal hypoglycemia, 144
Ritodrine, 20–21
for preterm labor, in combination therapy, 24–25
Rosenblith neurobehavioral assessment, 243
Rubella, 86–87

S

Scalp blood sampling, fetal, for fetal asphyxia, 39
with maternal immune thrombocytopenia, 38
Scalp injection, inadvertent anesthetic, 47, 55
Scalp stimulation, fetal, for fetal asphyxia, 39
Secretory IgA, 169
Sedatives, for preterm labor, 18
teratogenicity of, 58t
Seizures, maternal, and cerebral palsy, 225
in regional anesthesia, 47, 50, 51
local anesthetic-induced, 50, 51
neonatal, 123–139
and brain damage, 138
and cerebral palsy, 233
and epilepsy, 123
and hypoglycemia, 145–146
and hypoxic-ischemic encephalopathy, 119–120, 136
and morbidity and death, 136–138
and neurologic outcome, 5–6, 7t, 136–138
case studies of, 136–137
clinical classification of, 123–125, 124t
clinical vs. electrographic, 134–135, 135t

diagnosis of, pitfalls in, 136–137, 138
electroencephalographic diagnosis of, 130–134, *131–134,* 132t
pitfalls in, 138–139
electroencephalographic monitoring of, long-term, 135, *136*
electrographic, 125–130, *126–134*
vs. clinical, 134–135
etiology of, 6, 135–136
and prognosis, 137
in hypoxic-ischemic encephalopathy, 118, 119
in iatrogenic paralysis, 183
incidence of, 135
multifocal onset, 129
nonepileptic, 134–135
occult, 135
overdiagnosis of, 124–125, 136–137, 138
prognosis in, 5–6, 7t, 137–138
severity of, measures of, 137–138
significance of, 135–138
sites of origin of, 129, 130t
spatial distribution of, 128–129, *129*
temporal profile of, 129–130, *130*
unifocal onset, 129
visual diagnosis of, 134–135, 135t
Shock, cardiogenic, treatment of, 106
obstetrical, 49–50
Shoulder dystocia, 43–44
Single photon emission computed tomography, for cerebral blood flow measurement, 187
Sleep patterns, electroencephalographic, 178, 179, *179*
Small for gestational age, 25, 25t
Smoking, maternal, fetal effects of, 155–156
Sodium citrate, prior to general anesthesia, 48
Spastic syndromes, in cerebral palsy, 223. See also *Cerebral palsy.*
Spectroscopy, nuclear magnetic resonance, 189–194
Spinal anesthesia. See *Anesthesia, regional.*
Spleen, rupture of, 151
Static encephalopathy, 223. See also *Cerebral palsy.*
Status marmoratus, in hypoxic-ischemic encephalopathy, 116
Steroids, for fetal lung maturity enhancement, 13
for preterm membrane rupture, 17
teratogenicity of, 58t
Streptococcal infection, group B, maternal, 38
Stroke, neonatal, and cerebral palsy, 232
Subarachnoid hemorrhage, in hypoxic-ischemic encephalopathy, 117
Subdural block, 51
Subdural hematoma, imaging of, 209
Subdural hemorrhage, imaging of, 209
Subependymal-intraventricular hemorrhage, 197
and cerebral palsy, 233
and extracorporeal membrane oxygenation, 207–209, *210*
and periventricular leukomalacia, *211,* 212
grading of, 197
imaging of, 198–207, *200–208, 210*

risk factors for, 233–234
sequelae of, *200, 201, 207*
Substance abuse, fetal/neonatal effects of, 57–63
Suctioning, for meconium staining, 41
Subdural hematoma, imaging of, 209
Subdural hemorrhage, imaging of, 209
Surfactant, pulmonary, and respiratory distress syndrome, 13–14
Syphilis, congenital, 88–89

T

Tachypnea, neonatal, and anemia, 152
Testosterone, teratogenicity of, 58t
Thalidomide, 57, 58t
Thermal regulation, in preterm infant, 14
Thioamides, teratogenicity of, 58t
Thiopental, for anesthesia induction, 49, 50
Thrombocytopenia, 153
immune, maternal, and delivery, 38–39
Thrombophlebitis, and umbilical artery catheterization, 164
Thrombosis, fetal, placental findings in, 254, *254,* 261t
Tissue perfusion, fetal, *66,* 66–68, 66t, *67*
Tocolytics, 18–25
and neonatal hypoglycemia, 143–144
beta-mimetic, 18–25
combination, 24–25
efficacy of, evaluation of, 17–18
fetal effects of, 19–20
for preterm membrane rupture, 16, 17
side effects of, 18–20
tolerance to, 20
types of, 20–25
Tolazoline, for neonatal pulmonary hypertension, 111
Tomography, computed. See *Computed tomography.*
Total intrauterine volume, in intrauterine growth retardation, 27
Total parenteral nutrition. See *Nutritional support.*
Toxemia. See *Preeclampsia.*
anesthesia in, 49–50
Toxoplasmosis, 87–88
Transfusion, fetus-to-fetus, 150
in anemia, 107, 151
in disseminated intravascular coagulation, 153
in erythroblastosis fetalis, and neonatal hypoglycemia, 144
in hemolytic anemia, 151, 152
in hyperbilirubinemia, 157–158
in hyperviscosity syndrome, 154, 156
in hypovolemia, 101, 102
in neonatal hemorrhage, 150, 150t
in polycythemia, 154, 156
in thrombocytopenia, 153
resuscitative, 101
Transposition of great arteries, 108, 108t
Transpyloric feeding, 161–162. See also *Enteral feeding.*

Treatment, withholding of, 264–272. See also *Intensive care.*
Trimethadione, teratogenicity of, 58t
Trimethylene melamine, teratogenicity of, 58t
Twins, cerebral palsy in, 230

U

Ulegyria, in hypoxic-ischemic encephalopathy, 115–116, *116*
Ultrasonography, in cerebral edema, 216–217, *218*
in focal cerebral infarction, 216
in hypoxic ischemic encephalopathy, with diffuse injury, 217–218, *218*
in intraparenchymal hemorrhage, 209, *210*
in intrauterine growth retardation, 26, 26t, *27*
in multicystic encephalomalacia, 218, *218*
in periventricular leukomalacia, 209–212, *211, 213–215, 217*
in subependymal-intraventricular hemorrhage, 198, *199–202, 204–206*
Umbilical artery catheterization, for total parenteral nutrition, 163–164
and necrotizing enterocolitis, 170
in neonatal resuscitation, 98
Umbilical artery Doppler studies, in intrauterine growth retardation, 27
Umbilical artery velocimetry, in intrauterine growth retardation, 27
Umbilical cord, abnormalities of, and blood loss, 150
blood flow in, reduction of, fetal cardiovascular response to, 71
variation in, in fetal hypoxia/asphyxia, 71
blood sampling from, in fetal asphyxia, 39, 42
in maternal immune thrombocytopenia, 38
compression of, fetal cardiovascular response to, 71
disorders of, and fetal hypoxia/asphyxia, 66
length of, and neurologic outcome, 229
prolapse of, in malpresentation, 34–35
rupture of, 150
Umbilical cord blood, normal hemoglobin values for, 149t
pH values for, and Apgar score, 5
PO$_2$ content of, *66,* 66–67, 66t
sampling of, intrapartum, 39, 42
Univariate analysis, 258, 259
Urethan, teratogenicity of, 58t
Urine output, and cardiac output, 100
Uterine artery spasm, and regional anesthesia, 53–54
Uterine blood flow, and epinephrine, 53–54
reduction of, fetal cardiovascular response to, 70, 73

Uterine contractility, and epinephrine, 52
Uterine contractions, monitoring of, for preterm labor, 12
Uterine hypertonus, and regional anesthesia, 53–54
Uteroplacental perfusion, impaired. See *Asphyxia, Hypoxia.*
normal, *66,* 66–68, 66t

V

Vaccination. See *Immunization.*
Vacuum extraction, 41
Vaginal delivery. See *Delivery.*
Varicella zoster immune globulin, 83
Varicella zoster virus infection, congenital, 82–83
Vasodilators, for cardiac output enhancement, 106–107
for hyaline membrane disease, 110
for neonatal pulmonary hypertension, 111
Venous occlusion plethysmography, for cerebral blood flow measurement, 187–189
Ventilation, for pulmonary parenchymal disease, 109–110
resuscitative, 97
supportive, 105
Ventricular enlargement, in multicystic encephalomalacia, 218, *219*
post-hemorrhagic, imaging of, *200, 201,* 207
Verapamil, for preterm labor, 24
and ritodrine, 25
Version, external cephalic, of breech presentation, 36, 36t
Vertex presentation, abnormal, 35
Very low birth weight, 11. See also *Growth retardation, intrauterine; Prematurity.*
Video encephalographic monitoring, 184–185
Villitis, placental, *256,* 256–257,
Vinblastine, teratogenicity of, 58t
Vision loss, and rubella, 86–87
and toxoplasmosis, 88
Vitamin E, and necrotizing enterocolitis, 170
Vitamin K, prophylactic, 152–153
Volume expansion, for cardiac output enhancement, 101–102
Vomiting, induction of, prior to general anesthesia, 48–49

W

Watershed infarction, in hypoxic-ischemic encephalopathy, 115–116, 119
periventricular leukomalacia as, 210
White matter lesions, in hypoxic-ischemic encephalopathy, 116–117, *117,* 119–120
Wilms' tumor, 321–322
Withdrawal, alcohol, 59
cocaine, 61
narcotic, 60